T0318649

ISCHEMIC AND TRAUMATIC BRAIN AND SPINAL CORD INJURIES

ISCHEMIC AND TRAUMATIC BRAIN AND SPINAL CORD INJURIES

Mechanisms and Potential Therapies

AKHLAQ A. FAROOQUI

Department of Molecular and Cellular Biochemistry, The Ohio State University, Columbus, Ohio, United States

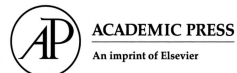

ACADEMIC PRESS

An imprint of Elsevier

Academic Press is an imprint of Elsevier
125 London Wall, London EC2Y 5AS, United Kingdom
525 B Street, Suite 1800, San Diego, CA 92101-4495, United States
50 Hampshire Street, 5th Floor, Cambridge, MA 02139, United States
The Boulevard, Langford Lane, Kidlington, Oxford OX5 1GB, United Kingdom

Library of Congress Cataloging-in-Publication Data
A catalog record for this book is available from the Library of Congress

British Library Cataloguing-in-Publication Data
A catalogue record for this book is available from the British Library

ISBN: 978-0-12-813596-9

For Information on all Academic Press publications
visit our website at https://www.elsevier.com/books-and-journals

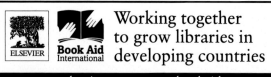

Working together
to grow libraries in
developing countries

www.elsevier.com • www.bookaid.org

Publisher: Nikki Levy
Acquisition Editor: Melanie Tucker
Editorial Project Manager: Timothy Bennett
Production Project Manager: Anusha Sambamoorthy
Cover Designer: Matthew Limbert

Typeset by MPS Limited, Chennai, India

Dedication

This monograph is dedicated to my beloved father "late Sharafyab Ahmed Sahab," uncle late Mohammed Ateeq Sahab. Their guidance and influence continue to inspire and support me.

Akhlaq A. Farooqui

Contents

2. Molecular Aspects of Ischemic Injury

3. Potential Neuroprotective Strategies for Ischemic Injuries

4. Molecular Aspects of Spinal Cord Injury

5. Potential Neuroprotective Strategies for Experimental Spinal Cord Injury

10. Summary, Perspective, and Direction for Future Research on Neurotraumatic Diseases

About the Author

Dr Akhlaq A. Farooqui is a leader in the field of signal transduction, brain phospholipases A_2, bioactive ether lipid metabolism, polyunsaturated fatty acid metabolism, glycerophospholipid-, sphingolipid-, and cholesterol-derived lipid mediators, glutamate-induced neurotoxicity and modulation of signal transduction by phytochemicals. He has discovered the stimulation of plasmalogen-selective phospholipase A_2 (PlsEtn-PLA$_2$) and diacyl- and monoacylglycerol lipases in brains from patients with Alzheimer disease. Stimulation of PlsEtn-PLA$_2$ produces plasmalogen deficiency and increases levels of eicosanoids that may be related to the loss of synapses in brains of patients with Alzheimer disease. He has published cutting-edge research on the generation and identification of glycerophospholipid-, sphingolipid-, and cholesterol-derived lipid mediators in kainic acid-mediated neurotoxicity by lipidomics. He has authored 12 monographs: *Glycerophospholipids in Brain: Phospholipase A_2 in Neurological Disorders* (2007); *Neurochemical Aspects of Excitotoxicity* (2008); *Metabolism and Functions of Bioactive Ether Lipids in Brain* (2008); *Hot Topics in Neural Membrane Lipidology* (2009); *Beneficial Effects of Fish Oil in Human Brain* (2009); *Neurochemical Aspects of Neurotraumatic and Neurodegenerative Diseases* (2010); *Lipid Mediators and their Metabolism in the Brain* (2011); *Phytochemicals, Signal Transduction, and Neurological Disorders* (2012); *Metabolic Syndrome: An Important Risk Factor for Stroke, Alzheimer Disease, and Depression* (2013); *Inflammation and Oxidative Stress in Neurological Disorders* (2014); *High Calorie Diet and the Human Brain* (2015); and *Therapeutic Potentials of Curcumin for Alzheimer Disease* (2016). All monographs are published by Springer, New York, and Springer International Publishing Switzerland. He has also published a monograph on *Neurochemical Aspects of Alzheimer's Disease*, which is published by Elsevier, New York.

In addition, he has edited 11 books: *Biogenic Amines: Pharmacological, Neurochemical and Molecular Aspects in the CNS* (2010); *Molecular Aspects of Neurodegeneration and Neuroprotection*, Bentham Science Publishers Ltd (2011); *Phytochemicals and Human Health: Molecular and pharmacological Aspects* (2011); *Beneficial Effects of Propolis on Human Health in Chronic Diseases* (2012) Vol 1; *Beneficial Effects of Propolis on Human Health in Chronic Diseases* (2012) Vol 2. These books were published by Nova Science Publishers, Hauppauge, New York. *Molecular Aspects of*

Oxidative Stress on Cell Signaling in Vertebrates and Invertebrates (2012); *Metabolic Syndrome and Neurological Disorders* (2013); *Diet and Exercise in Cognitive Function and Neurological Diseases* (2015); *Neuroprotective Effects of Phytochemicals in Neurological Disorders* (2017) were published by Wiley-Blackwell, John Wiley and Sons, Inc., Hoboken, New Jersey. *Trace Amines and Neurological Disorders: Potential Mechanisms and Risk Factors* (2016) and *Role of the Mediterranean Diet in the Brain and Neurodegenerative Diseases* (2018) were published by Elsevier, New York.

— **2018**

Preface

Neurotraumatic diseases are critical public health problem. Common neurotraumatic diseases include strokes, spinal cord injury (SCI), traumatic brain injury (TBI), concussion, and chronic traumatic encephalitis (CTE). Stroke is a metabolic trauma caused by severe reduction or blockade in cerebral blood flow due to the formation of a clot leading not only to the deficiency of oxygen and reduction in glucose metabolism, but also decrease in ATP production and accumulation of toxic products. In contrast, TBI and SCI are caused by physical trauma to the brain or spinal cord, due to falls, motorcycle and car accidents, gunshots, military action, and contact sport such as American football, boxing, wrestling, rugby, hockey, lacrosse, soccer, and skiing. Despite the differences in the origin of the pathology, stroke, SCI, and TBI share several similarities regarding their pathophysiological processes. Thus, stroke, SCI, and TBI are accompanied by overstimulation of glutamate receptor, a massive influx of Ca^{2+}, prolonged decrease in ATP, stimulation of Ca^{2+}-dependent enzyme, induction of mitochondrial dysfunction, increase in oxidative and nitrosative stress, hyperexcitability, and onset of acute neuroinflammation due to the activation of microglia and astrocytes around injury site. In addition, stroke, SCI, and TBI are accompanied by induction of apoptotic cell death. These processes result in neurodegeneration and irreversible loss of neurologic function not only through the breakdown of cellular and subcellular integrity, but also through alterations in redox and free-radical generation. Estimates of stroke, SCI, TBI, concussion, and CTE occurrence indicate that these injuries cause enormous losses to individuals, families, and communities. They result in a large number of deaths and impairments leading to permanent disabilities. Research has also shown that neurotraumatic diseases usually require long-term care and therefore incurs economic cost to health systems. For this reason, many countries need to develop surveillance systems and conduct epidemiologic studies to measure the impact of neurotraumatic diseases among their people to guide the development of more effective preventive methods. A number of methods have already proven effective, such as changes in lifestyle, use of motorcycle helmets, head supports in vehicles or on sports equipment.

In the light of above information, I have decided to provide readers with a comprehensive and cutting-edge description of pathogenesis and potential treatment strategies for neurotraumatic diseases. This monograph has 10 chapters. Chapter 1, Classification and Molecular Aspects of Neurotraumatic Diseases: Similarities and Differences With Neurodegenerative and Neuropsychiatric Diseases, describes classification, similarities, and difference among neurotraumatic, neurodegenerative, and neuropsychiatric diseases. Chapter 2, Molecular Aspects of Ischemic Injury, describes information on molecular aspects of ischemic injury. Chapter 3, Potential Neuroprotective Strategies for Ischemic Injuries, describes information on potential neuroprotective strategies for ischemic injuries. Chapter 4, Molecular Aspects of Spinal Cord Injury, describes the cutting-edge information on molecular aspects of SCI. Chapter 5, Potential Neuroprotective Strategies for Experimental Spinal Cord Injury, describes information on the potential neuroprotective strategies for experimental SCI. Chapter 6, Neurochemical Aspects of Traumatic Brain Injury, describes information on neurochemical aspects of TBI. Chapter 7, Potential Neuroprotective Strategies for Traumatic Brain Injury, describes information on potential neuroprotective strategies for TBI. Chapter 8, Molecular Aspects of Concussion and Chronic Traumatic Encephalopathy, is devoted to cutting-edge information on molecular aspects of concussion and chronic traumatic encephalopathy. Chapter 9, Potential Neuroprotective Strategies for Concussion and Chronic Traumatic Encephalopathy, summarizes studies on potential neuroprotective strategies for concussion and chronic traumatic encephalopathy. Chapter 10, Summary, Perspective, and Direction for Future Research on Neurotraumatic Diseases, provides readers with a perspective that will be important for future research work on neurotraumatic diseases. My presentation and demonstrated ability to present complicated information on signal transduction processes in neurotraumatic diseases makes this book particularly accessible to neuroscience graduate students, teachers, and fellow researchers. It can be used as supplement text for a range of neuroscience courses. Clinicians, neuroscientists, neurologists, and pharmacologists will find this book useful for understanding molecular aspects of neurotraumatic diseases and its treatment. To the best of my knowledge no one has written a monograph on pathogenesis, biomarkers, potential treatment strategies for neurotraumatic diseases. This monograph is the first to provide a comprehensive description of signal transduction processes associated with the pathogenesis and potential treatment of neurotraumatic diseases.

The choices of topics presented in this monograph are personal. They are not only based on my interest in the pathogenesis and treatment of neurotraumatic diseases, but also in areas where major progress has been made. The key objective of this monograph is to critically evaluate the information on the pathogenesis and potential treatment strategies for neurotraumatic diseases. Each chapter of this monograph contains an extensive list of references, which are arranged alphabetically to works that are cited in the text. I have tried to ensure uniformity and mode of presentation as well as a logical progression of subjects from one topic to another and have provided an extensive bibliography. For the sake of simplicity and uniformity a large number of figures with chemical structures of drugs used for the treatment of neurotraumatic diseases along with line diagrams of colored signal transduction pathways are also included. I hope that my attempt to integrate and consolidate the knowledge on pathogenesis and potential treatment strategies for neurotraumatic diseases in the brain will initiate more studies on molecular mechanisms and treatment of neurotraumatic diseases in human brain. This knowledge can be useful for the optimal health of young, boomer, and preboomer American generations.

Akhlaq A. Farooqui
Columbus, OH, United States

Acknowledgments

I thank my wife, Tahira, for critical reading of this monograph, offering valuable advice, useful discussion, and evaluation of subject matter. Without her help and participation, this monograph neither could nor would have been completed. I would also like to express my gratitude to Melanie Tucker and Timothy Bennett of Elsevier/Academic Press for their quick responses to my queries and professional manuscript handling.

Akhlaq A. Farooqui

List of Abbreviations

PtdCho	Phosphatidylcholine
PtdEtn	Phosphatidylethanolamine
PtdIns	Phosphatidylinositol
PtdIns4P	Phosphatidylinositol 4-phosphate
PtdIns(4,5)P_2	Phosphatidylinositol 4,5-bisphosphate
Ins-1,4,5-P_3	Inositol-1,4,5-trisphosphate
ARA	Arachidonic acid
DHA	Docosahexaenoic acid
EPA	Eicosapentaenoic acid
PLA$_2$	Phospholipase A$_2$
COX	Cyclooxygenase
LOX	Lipoxygenase
EPOX	Epoxygenase
APP	Amyloid precursor protein
AD	Alzheimer disease
Aβ	β-Amyloid
NFTs	Neurofibrillary tangles
CSF	Cerebrospinal fluid
GSK-3	Glycogen synthase-3
ROS	Reactive oxygen species
RNS	Reactive nitrogen species
AGE	Advanced glycation end products
APP	Amyloid precursor protein
IL	Interleukin
TNF-α	Tumor necrosis factor-alpha
NO	Nitric oxide
BBB	Blood−brain barrier
PET	Positron emission tomography
SPECT	Single-photon emission computed tomography
SCI	Spinal cord injury
TBI	Traumatic brain injury
CTE	Chronic traumatic encephalopathy
MMP-9	Matrix metalloproteinase-9
MAP kinase	Mitogen-activated protein kinase
BDNF	Brain-derived neurotrophic factor
ICAM-1	Intercellular adhesion molecule-1

Classification and Molecular Aspects of Neurotraumatic Diseases: Similarities and Differences With Neurodegenerative and Neuropsychiatric Diseases

INTRODUCTION

Brain is a highly complex organ, which is responsible for a variety of tasks including receiving and processing sensory information and the control of highly complex behaviors that allow for survival. Brain has a very high metabolic rate. It accounts for 2% of body weight, but it receives about 15% of the cardiac output and consumes approximately 25% of glucose and 20% of all inhaled oxygen at rest (Attwell et al., 2010). This enormous metabolic demand of glucose and oxygen is due to the fact that neurons are highly differentiated cells requiring large amounts of adenosine triphosphate (ATP) in order to maintain ionic gradients across cell membranes and maintain physiological neurotransmission. Neurodegeneration is a complex multifactorial process that causes neuronal death in the brain and spinal cord resulting in brain and spinal cord damage and dysfunction. Neurodegeneration is a progressive process associated with the loss of selective populations of vulnerable neurons. Neurodegeneration is regulated by many factors, including genetic abnormalities, immune system problems, and metabolic or mechanical insults to the brain and/or spinal cord tissues (Farooqui, 2010; Deleidi et al., 2015). Neurodegeneration is accompanied by oxidative stress, axonal transport deficits, protein oligomerization, aggregation, calcium deregulation, mitochondrial dysfunction, abnormal neuron–glial interactions, neuroinflammation, DNA damage, and aberrant RNA processing (Farooqui, 2010).

Diseases associated with brain, spinal cord, and nerves damage and dysfunction are called neurological disorders. The neurological consequences of neurodegeneration in patients can have devastating effects on mental and physical functioning. Several hundred neurological disorders have been described in the literature. These disorders may cause structural, neurochemical, and electrophysiological abnormalities in the brain, spinal cord, and nerves causing paralysis, muscle weakness, poor coordination, seizures, confusion, and pain (Farooqui, 2010; Kempuraj et al., 2016). Several hundreds of distinct neurological and psychiatric diseases have been reported to occur in human population. These diseases can be classified into three major groups: neurotraumatic diseases, neurodegenerative diseases, and neuropsychiatric diseases. Common neurotraumatic diseases include strokes, traumatic brain injury (TBI), spinal cord injury (SCI), chronic traumatic encephalitis (CTE), and epilepsy. Common neurodegenerative diseases are Alzheimer's disease (AD), Parkinson's disease (PD), and Huntington's disease (HD) (Farooqui, 2010). In AD, neurons of the hippocampus and entorhinal cortex are the first to degenerate, whereas in PD, dopaminergic neurons in the substantia nigra degenerate. HD is characterized by neuronal death in the basal ganglia and cortex. Amyotrophic lateral sclerosis (ALS) is accompanied by mutations in superoxide dismutase 1 (SOD1) in motor neurons. These diseases represent a primary health problem especially in the aging population (Hamer and Chida, 2009). For example, AD ranks as the sixth leading cause of death in the United States. PD, the second most prevalent neurodegenerative disease, affects 1%–2% of the population above 65 years (Bekris et al., 2010; Alzheimer's Association, 2011). Reactive oxygen species (ROS) are chemically reactive molecules, which are closely associated with the pathogenesis of neurotraumatic and neurodegenerative diseases. ROS are naturally metabolites, which are generated within the biological system. They not only play important roles in cellular activities such as inflammation, cell survival, and stressor responses, but are also associated with cardiovascular diseases, muscle dysfunction, onset of allergies, and induction of various types of cancers (Zuo et al., 2015). Owing to their reactivity, high-concentration generation of ROS in the brain can lead to oxidative stress-mediated neural cell death (Farooqui, 2010; Dias et al., 2013; Zuo et al., 2015). A common characteristic of virtually all neurodegenerative diseases is that the consequences are often devastating, with severe mental and physical effects. This is due in large part to the loss or dysfunction of neurons—a highly specialized cell type that is typically postmitotic—lost cells are not replaced. Thus, once a neuron is lost, it typically gone forever, along with its associated function. Due to aging of global population, prevalence of AD, PD, HD, and ALS is expected to increase, imposing a social and economic burden on society (Hebert et al., 2003; Kowal et al., 2013). Examples of neuropsychiatric disorders are depression, schizophrenia, some forms of bipolar affective disorders, autism, mood disorders, attention-deficit disorder, dementia, tardive dyskinesia, and chronic fatigue syndrome. Neuropsychiatric diseases involve abnormalities in cerebral cortex and limbic system (thalamus, hypothalamus, hippocampus, and amygdala). Neuropsychiatric diseases not only involve alterations in serotonergic, dopaminergic, noradrenergic, cholinergic, glutamatergic, and γ-aminobutyric acid (GABA)-ergic signaling within the visceromotor network, but are also associated with alterations in synaptogenic growth factors (brain-derived neurotrophic factor [BDNF]), fibroblast growth factor, and insulin-like growth factors (Farooqui, 2010; Williams and Umemori, 2014).

In strokes, TBI, and SCI, neurodegeneration occurs rapidly (in a matter of hours to days) because of sudden lack of oxygen, rapid decrease in ATP, disturbance in transmembrane potential, sudden collapse of ion gradients, and rapid interplay among excitotoxicity, oxidative stress, and neuroinflammation at very early stage (Farooqui, 2010). In addition, in strokes, TBI, and SCI, acute neuroinflammation develops rapidly due to the accumulation of eicosanoids and the release of proinflammatory cytokines (Farooqui, 2010). In contrast, in AD, PD, HD, and ALS, oxygen, nutrients, and reduced levels of ATP continue to be available to the neurons, and ionic homeostasis is maintained to a limited extent resulting in a neurodegenerative process, which takes many years to develop (Farooqui et al., 2010). Furthermore, in AD, PD, HD, and ALS due to abnormalities in immune system, chronic inflammation remains undetected and lingers for years, causing continued insult to the brain tissue and ultimately reaches the threshold of detection many years after the onset of the neurodegeneration (Farooqui et al., 2007; Farooqui, 2010). Currently, there are no therapeutic agents that can induce neuronal regeneration or repair damage in the affected area in the brain damaged by neurotraumatic, neurodegenerative, and neuropsychiatric diseases. Therefore, drugs to treat these pathological conditions effectively are not available (Farooqui, 2010; Allgaier and Allgaier, 2014; Gao et al., 2016).

NEURODEGENERATION IN ISCHEMIC INJURY

To function normally, brain needs an uninterrupted supply of glucose and oxygen through cerebral blood flow (CBF). Glucose and oxygen are needed for the synthesis of ATP, which is required not only for maintaining the appropriate ionic gradients across neural membranes (low intracellular Na^+, high K^+, and very low cytosolic Ca^{2+}), but also for creating optimal cellular redox potentials. Stroke is a metabolic insult caused by severe reduction or blockade in CBF, leading not only to a deficiency of oxygen and reduction in glucose metabolism, but also to a decrease in ATP production and accumulation of toxic products (Farooqui, 2010). Two major types of strokes have been described in humans: ischemic and hemorrhagic. Ischemic strokes are brought about by critical decrease in blood flow to various brain regions causing neurodegeneration. Hemorrhagic strokes are caused by a break in the wall of the artery resulting in spillage of blood inside the brain or around the brain. Ischemic stroke is subclassified into thrombotic or embolic strokes. A thrombotic stroke or infarction occurs when a clot forms in an artery supplying the brain, whereas an embolic stroke is the result of a clot formed elsewhere in the body and subsequently transported through the bloodstream to the brain. The onset of stroke is often subtle and accompanied by the breakdown of the blood—brain barrier (BBB), overstimulation of glutamate receptors by extracellular glutamate leading to neuronal excitotoxicity (Table 1.1). This process results in calcium influx and mitochondrial dysfunction resulting in the deficiency in energy (ATP) supply as well as generation of high levels of oxidants which are the key contributors to neurodegeneration through necrotic and apoptotic cell death. Excessive glutamate receptor stimulation may also produce increase in nitric oxide production which can be detrimental to neural cells, as nitric oxide interacts with superoxide to form the

TABLE 1.1   Molecular Changes in Brains of Stroke Patients

Neurochemical Changes	Reference
Release of glutamate and overstimulation of glutamate receptors	Farooqui (2010); Shen et al (2010)
Increase in Ca^{2+}-influx and stimulation of Ca^{2+}-dependent enzymes	Farooqui (2010)
Onset of mitochondrial dysfunction	Farooqui (2010); Baxter et al. (2014)
Induction of oxidative stress and increase in lipid peroxidation	Love (1999); Farooqui (2010)
Increased expression of proinflammatory cytokines and chemokines	Farooqui (2010); Kawabori and Yenari (2015)
Induction of apoptotic cell death	Farooqui (2010); Kimura-Ohba and Yang (2016)

toxic molecule peroxynitrite (Farooqui, 2010). High-level oxidant production elicits neuronal apoptosis through the actions of proapoptotic Bcl-2 family members resulting in mitochondrial permeability transition pore opening. In addition to apoptotic responses to severe stress, high levels of oxidants can induce endoplasmic reticulum stress pathways which may further contribute to induction of apoptosis. At the injury site, vascular cells (endothelial cells, vascular smooth muscle cells, adventitial fibroblasts, and neurons) promote the generation of ROS primarily via cell membrane-bound nicotinamide adenine dinucleotide phosphate oxidase (Sun et al., 2007). Other sources of ROS include uncontrolled arachidonic acid cascade and production of ROS by mitochondria during respiration. Stroke-mediated injury also triggers a robust inflammatory reaction characterized by the activation of endogenous microglia, leading to increase in expression of cytokines and chemokines (Allan et al., 2005; Farooqui and Horrocks, 2007). Stroke also results in increased cerebrovascular permeability and leakage. These processes support secondary ischemic brain injury (Brouns and De Deyn, 2009). The common stroke-mediated deficits include motor impairment (including limb spasticity), sensory impairment, language impairment (aphasia and/or dysarthria), dysphagia, cognitive impairment, visual impairment, and poststroke depression (O'Keefe et al., 2014). Because stroke-mediated brain injury disrupts functional connections in periinfarct *and* remotely connected regions, it is important to investigate brain-wide network dynamics during poststroke recovery. I propose that a better understanding of molecular mechanisms associated with neural circuit rewiring in the brain will be an important step toward developing future therapeutic strategies for recovery from stroke-mediated brain injury.

RISK FACTORS FOR STROKE

Two types of risk factors control the onset of stroke: Modifiable risk factors and nonmodifiable risk factors. Modifiable risk factors include hypertension, diabetes, heart disease, hypercholesterolemia (atherosclerosis), atrial fibrillation (most common sustained cardiac arrhythmia), high alcohol consumption, *cigarette smoke*, and oral contraceptive (Fig. 1.1), whereas nonmodifiable risk factors are age, family history of cerebrovascular diseases, gender, and race (Allen and Bayraktutan, 2008). Among modifiable risk factors, atherosclerosis is viewed as simply the deposition and accumulation of lipids and cellular debris within the wall of medium to large arteries, resulting in plaque formation and disturbance of blood flow. In atherosclerosis, alterations in endothelial

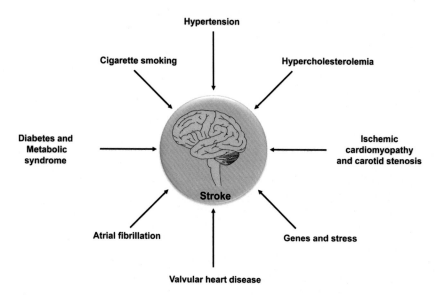

FIGURE 1.1   Factors modulating stroke.

function contribute to the formation and destabilization of plaques (Libby, 2002). According to American Stroke Association, hypertension contributes to 30%–40% stroke risk, cigarette smoking 12%–18%, and diabetes 5%–27%. Some of the above risk factors can be mitigated. Other less-well documented risk factors include geographic location, socioeconomic status, and alcoholism. It is becoming increasingly evident that chronic kidney disease (CKD) and end-stage kidney disease are important risk factors for stroke (Sanchez-Perales et al., 2010; Masson et al., 2015). Meta-analysis has indicated a strong direct relationship between albuminuria and stroke risk. Any degree of albuminuria increases stroke risk by 68%, and for every 25 mg/mmol increase in albuminuria, stroke risk increases by 10% (Masson et al., 2015). Interestingly, the effect of glomerular filtration rate and albuminuria appear to be additive with no evidence of interaction (Masson et al., 2015). These findings are consistent through categories of CKD and albuminuria, gender and patient risk groups (diabetes, hypertension, and smoking), and types of stroke. Patients on dialysis have the highest stroke risk at 2–7 times higher than non-CKD patients, with a 3–5 times higher mortality (US Renal System, 2009; Ovbiagele, 2011; Wang et al., 2014a,b). It is predicted that about two-thirds of patients on dialysis above 75 years may die within a year of a stroke (US Renal System, 2009). Modifiable risk factors are known to have profound effects on the structure and function of blood vessels as well as on their interface with circulating blood. Many of the established risk factors such as lifestyle alter vascular structure by promoting atherosclerosis and stiffening of arteries as well as by inducing narrowing, thickening, and tortuosity of arterioles and capillaries (Allen and Bayraktutan, 2008; Iadecola and Davisson, 2008). In brain, above-mentioned morphological alterations are often associated with reductions in resting CBF and marked alterations in CBF regulation. Mild hyperhomocysteinemia can also increase the risk for clinical manifestations of stroke, probably due to the pleiotropic biochemical properties of homocysteine (Hcy) and its impact on venous and arterial atherosclerotic modifications (Steele et al., 2013; Petras et al., 2014; Williams et al., 2014). Hcy acts by suppressing NO production by endothelial cells and platelets and increasing the production of ROS by the release of arachidonic acid from the platelets. Hcy inhibits not only glutathione peroxidase through the proliferation of endothelial cells (Petras et al., 2014), but also methyl-transferases, to suppress DNA repair and promote apoptotic cell death (Petras et al., 2014; Williams et al., 2014). Thus, converging evidence suggests that aging, hypertension, diabetes, and hypercholesterolemia impair vital adaptive mechanisms that promote adequate brain perfusion (Arrick et al., 2007; Kitayama et al., 2007; Iadecola and Davisson, 2008). In addition, it is also proposed that appropriate distribution of oxygen, glucose, and other nutrients by the cerebral vasculature is critical for optical cognitive performance. Thus, the cerebral microvasculature is a key site of vascular resistance and a preferential target for small-vessel disease. While deleterious effects of vascular risk factors on microvascular function are known, the contribution of this dysfunction to cognitive deficits is less clear.

BIOMARKERS FOR STROKE

As stated above, brain damage after ischemic injury develops rapidly from a complex signaling cascade involving excitotoxicity, oxidative stress, and neuroinflammation. Early excitotoxicity contributes to fast necrotic cell death, which leads to the core of the infarction. The ischemic penumbra that surrounds the infarct core suffers milder insults. In this area, both mild excitotoxic and inflammatory mechanisms contribute to delayed cell death involving biochemical characteristics of apoptosis (Farooqui, 2010). These processes produce several metabolites (biomarkers), which is measured in blood, cerebrospinal fluid (CSF), or tissue to determine the onset of stroke. Early diagnosis of stroke is difficult because the presence of BBB slows the release of brain tissue proteins into blood after stroke, delaying the release of glial and neuronal proteins. The permeability of the BBB during the first 48 hours after onset of stroke is influenced by the extracellular enzymic activation. Stroke-mediated damage to the brain may occur during reperfusion (Farooqui, 2010), and many potential blood markers of cerebral ischemia and inflammation, which contribute to pathogenesis of stroke, are found in other conditions that mimic stroke, such as severe myocardial infarction and brain infection. This suggests that the early diagnosis of stroke is difficult because there are no reliable and specific, very sensitive, accessible, standardized, cost-effective biomarkers are available (García-Berrocoso et al., 2010; Liu et al., 2017). In addition, it is unlikely that a single biomarker will reflect the complete picture of stroke, which is a multifaceted complex metabolic injury (Farooqui, 2010). Combining biomarkers from multiple cellular pathways may be a better way of diagnosing stroke. Thus, few biomarkers of stroke have been described for processes closely associated with pathophysiology of stroke. These processes include onset of inflammation, endothelial dysfunction, and blood coagulation/thrombosis (Jickling and Sharp, 2011; Kim et al., 2013). Many proteins [brain natriuretic peptide, D-dimer (a product of fibrin degradation), C-reactive protein, low-density lipoprotein, troponins, neuron-specific enolase (NSE), fibrinogen, fibronectin, UCH-L1, S100β, von Willebrand factor (vWF), ICAM, VCAM, interleukin-6 (IL-6), and tumor necrosis factor-α (TNF-α)], neurotransmitters, glutamate, and lipid mediators (metabolites of arachidonic acid metabolism) are altered in blood and CSF of stroke patients. Among the above-mentioned biomarkers, D-dimer, fibrinogen, fibronectin, vWF factor, and thrombomodulin are biomarkers of endothelial dysfunction (Fig. 1.2). In addition, myelin basic protein, which is one of the main components of myelin sheath, can be detected in the CSF and blood within first hours after the onset of stroke. Furthermore, PARK-7 and malondialdehyde are biomarkers of oxidative stress. Matrix metalloproteinase-9 has been widely investigated for its role in the disruption of the BBB and extracellular matrix following stroke (Kernagis and Laskowitz, 2012; Turner and Sharp, 2016). An important development in evaluating the risk of ischemic stroke is the use of lipoprotein-associated phospholipase A$_2$ (Lp-PLA$_2$), a circulating enzyme involved in inflammation that is an independent predictor of future stroke among healthy individuals (Oei et al., 2005). In fact, the Food and Drug Administration (FDA) has approved recently the blood measurement of Lp-PLA$_2$ to predict the risk of cardiovascular and cerebrovascular events, supporting the view that early ischemic stroke detection may permit physicians to prescribe lifestyle changes in order to reduce some risk factors or establish preventive treatments.

Another important CSF and blood biomarker for stroke can be the presence of microRNA (mRNA), which are composed of a group of endogenous and noncoding small RNAs which control expression of

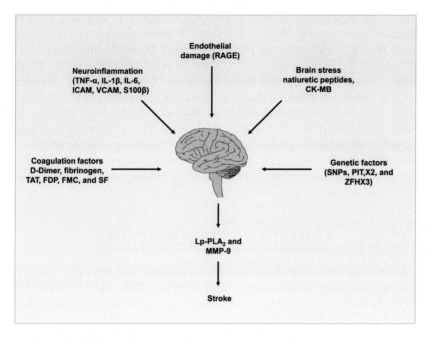

FIGURE 1.2 Biomarkers for stroke. *BNP*, brain natriuretic peptide; *CK-MB*, creatine kinase isoform MB; *FDP*, fibrin/fibrinogen degradation products; *FMC*, fibrin monomer complex; *SF*, soluble fibrin; *sRAGE*, soluble advanced glycation end products receptor; *TAT*, thrombin–antithrombin complex; *TNF-α*, tumor necrosis factor alpha; *IL-1β*, interleukin-1β; *IL-6*, interleukin-6; *vWF*, von Willebrand factor; *MMP-9*, matrix metalloproteinase; *Lp-PLA2*, lipoprotein-associated phospholipase A_2.

complementary target mRNAs. Significant changes have been reported to occur in the gene expressions in minutes to hours after the onset of stroke. In animal models of stroke, it is shown that circulating miR-125b-2[*], miR-27a[*], miR-422a, miR-488, and miR-627 are markedly increased and these miRNAs can be used as biomarkers for stroke (Sepramaniam et al., 2014). miR-290 elevated at 24 hours after reperfusion (Jeyaseelan et al., 2008). Similarly, miR-10a, miR-182, miR-200b, and miR-298 are increased in both blood and brain 24 hours after ischemia/reperfusion (Liu et al., 2010). Similarly, increased hsa-miR-106b-5P and hsa-miR-4306 and decreased hsa-miR-320e and hsa-miR-320d in plasma may be novel biomarkers for the early detection of acute stroke in humans (Wang et al., 2014a,b). Other studies have indicated that miR-30a, miR-126, and let-7b may be useful biomarkers for ischemic stroke in humans (Long et al., 2013). The successful translation of this information in clinical practice has proved difficult. This may be due to the heterogeneity of ischemic stroke. Based on the above information, the rapid diagnosis of stroke remains a major challenge for patient management and therapeutic intervention. Converging evidence suggests that currently there is no single biomarker approved to identify stroke etiology. However, at present, in most hospitals, the diagnosis of ischemic stroke is made solely on clinical grounds after diagnosing hemorrhagic lesions by computed tomography (CT) and magnetic resonance imaging (MRI). Once such a diagnosis is made, patients benefit from thrombolytic therapy administered within 4.5 hours of stroke onset (Jickling and Sharp, 2011; Kim et al., 2013; Stanca et al., 2015). This is tempting to suggest that the availability of specific biomarkers for rapid diagnosis of stroke will be highly beneficial not only for diagnosis and determining eligibility for intravenous thrombosis, but also for assessing the response to the treatment.

ANIMAL MODELS FOR STROKE

Animal models of stroke are an indispensable tool not only for investigating mechanisms of ischemic cerebral injury, but also for developing novel antiischemic regimens (Braeuningers and Kleinschnitz, 2009; Herson and Traystman, 2014). Several animal models have been developed in small animals (mice, rats, and rabbits) to study the pathogenesis and treatment of stroke. These models include permanent middle cerebral artery occlusion (MCAo) model, thromboembolic clot model, endothelin model, and embolic stroke model (Fluri et al., 2015). Among these animal models, two rodent animal stroke models are commonly used in laboratory research: one is transient or permanent MCAo model and the other is thromboembolic clot model (Fluri et al., 2015). In the MCAo model, a nylon monofilament is advanced through the internal carotid artery to occlude the MCA. In this model, the decrease in blood flow in the brain is measured by Doppler flowmetry with a probe placed over the MCA territory. Restoration of blood flow (reperfusion) can be achieved by withdrawing the occluding suture. Permanent MCAo (no reperfusion) is achieved usually by electrocoagulation or photochemically induced thrombosis of the MCA. Other animal models induce a global or forebrain ischemia by four-vessel occlusion in rat or bilateral common carotid artery occlusion in gerbil, which lacks the circle of Willis and thus has no collateral blood flow. Global models mimic the complete loss of blood flow to the brain that occurs during cardiac arrest. The MCAo model is used to study pathophysiological processes or neuroprotective agents in stroke, whereas the thromboembolic clot model is more convenient for investigating the thrombolytic agents and pathophysiological processes after thrombolysis (Fluri et al., 2015). Each model has its strengths and weaknesses. In general, majority of stroke animal models do not sufficiently resemble the clinical reality of cerebral ischemia (Endres et al., 2008). Thus, ischemic injury in the rodent animal model under experimental conditions is not homologous to pathological stroke in human subject because there are substantial anatomical differences between the rodent and human brains, particularly that the rodent brain has a higher gray-to-white matter ratio compared to the human brain. In addition, in animal model studies, occlusion of blood vessel is performed by artificial methods, whereas in stroke patient's in vivo occlusion occurs through the clot formation. Animal model studies ignore the effect of clot-derived substances (thrombin, a trypsin-like allosteric serine protease) that may be flushed into the ischemic region by residual flow, possibly confounding the ischemic insult (Feuerstein et al., 2008). Thrombin activates astrocytes and microglial cells and promotes neuroinflammation not only by modulating p38 mitogen-activated protein kinase, c-Jun N-terminal kinase, PAR-1, PAR-3, and PAR-4 (Suo et al., 2002, 2003), but also by releasing cyclooxygenase-2, inducible nitric oxide synthase, TNF-α, interleukin-$1\alpha/\beta$ (IL-$1\alpha/\beta$), IL-6, IL-12, and boosts CD40 expression and all potent proinflammatory factors (Suo et al., 2002). Another major problem associated with studies on animal stroke models is that studies are mostly conducted in young animals without any comorbidity. These models differ from human stroke, which particularly affects elderly people who have various cerebrovascular risk factors. Furthermore, in ischemic stroke patients, occlusion occurs in large or small vessels and may be secondary to in situ thrombosis, artery-to-artery embolism, or cardiac embolism. This type of injury may affect very different areas of the human brain (Ford, 2008). The consequences of small-vessel occlusion may differ from that of large-vessel occlusion with respect to the effect of neuroprotection, and good animal models of small-vessel occlusion have not been developed (Ford, 2008). Furthermore, the rate of induction of other pathophysiological processes such as neuroinflammation, cortical spreading depolarizations, and stem-cell-mediated regeneration in human subjects can be different from rodent stroke models (Endres et al., 2008). These observations indicate that unlike the standard animal model of permanent or temporary MCAo, clinical stroke injury in patients is a very heterogeneous process in which drug distribution and levels of biomarkers indicating recovery in various regions of brain should be monitored with sensitive neuroimaging techniques (Ford, 2008; Green, 2008; Walberer and Rueger, 2015). It is proposed that noninvasive in vivo imaging studies should be performed using MRI and positron emission tomography (PET). These neuroimaging tools (SPECT and PET) allow the monitoring key pathophysiological processes associated with stroke over time. The use of SPECT and PET not only provide information on CBF (Walberer et al., 2012) and brain edema (Walberer et al., 2008), but also about neuroinflammation (Walberer et al., 2014), and stem-cell-mediated regeneration (Rueger et al., 2010, 2012). PET is essential in the transfer of the concept of the penumbra to clinical stroke and thereby may have a great impact on developing treatment strategies. Converging evidence suggests that mimicking all aspects of human stroke in one animal model is not possible because ischemic stroke is itself a very heterogeneous neurological disorder. Animal model studies have demonstrated a relatively short window of opportunity (30−90 minutes) for the effective treatment of stroke. This short window of opportunity has not worked in human clinical studies (Ginsberg, 2008; Hill et al., 2013).

NEURODEGENERATION IN SCI

SCI is caused by physical trauma to the spine from falls, motorcycle and car accidents, gunshots, and contact sport (American football, wrestling, rugby, hockey, lacrosse, soccer, and skiing). Traumatic SCI has a two-phase pathology characterized by primary and secondary injuries (Oyinbo, 2011). Primary injury can be attributed to the physical compression of the spinal cord, stretching of the nervous tissue, or disruption of local blood supply. Primary injury not only results in the deformation of spinal cord and narrowing of the spinal cord canal, but also produces dramatic changes in spinal cord volume. Mechanical damage to the spinal cord in the primary injury may also impact blood vessels, immediately inducing intraspinal hemorrhage or reducing blood supply. Pathologically, primary injury occurs rapidly in a limited area of spinal cord producing direct damage of neurons, glial, or endothelial cells rupturing cell membranes, releasing neuronal intracellular contents (Sekhon and Fehlings, 2001), and producing hemorrhage, edema, and ischemia (Sun et al., 2016). In contrast, the secondary injury develops over the hours and days after SCI, producing behavioral and functional impairments due to increase in excitatory amino acids and ROS. These neurochemical changes promote the activation of microglial cells, astrocytes, and oligodendrocytes. Activation of microglial cells and astrocytes induces expression of proinflammatory cytokines (TNF-α, IL-1, and IL-6) and chemokines [monocyte chemotactic protein 1, C−C motif chemokine ligand 20 (CCL20)] causing neuroinflammation, whereas involvement of oligodendrocytes is related to the demyelination. In addition, secondary injury also produces alterations in local ionic concentrations, loss of regulation of local and systemic blood pressure, reduced spinal cord blood flow, breakdown of the BBB, penetration of serum proteins into the spinal cord, apoptosis, activation of calpain proteases, accumulation of neurotransmitter, increase in production of free radicals/lipid peroxidation, and imbalance of activated metalloproteinases. Furthermore, secondary injury is also accompanied by macrophages and polymorphonuclear leukocyte infiltration, and activation of macrophages and vascular endothelial cells generate oxygen free radicals and other cytotoxic by-products (Bramlett and Dietrich, 2004). Furthermore, the release of excess of glutamate and failure of reuptake by astrocytes result in excitotoxicity around adjacent neurons (Li and Stys, 2000). Over time, astrocytes proliferate and surround the perilesional zone, creating an irregular mesh-like barrier of interwoven cell processes (Yuan and He, 2013). At the injury site, reactive oligodendrocyte precursor cells rapidly divide and accumulate and along with fibroblast deposition promote the formation of glial scar. This process is accompanied by increased expression and deposition of chondroitin sulfate proteoglycans (CSPGs), neural/glial antigen 2 (NG2), and tenascin at the injury site (Ahuja et al., 2016). CSPGs and myelin glycoproteins act via the Rho-ROCK (rho-associated protein kinase) pathway to inhibit neurite outgrowth by signaling growth cone collapse through effector kinases (Forgione and Fehlings, 2014). These neurochemical mechanisms severely restrict endogenous neural circuit regeneration and oligodendrocyte remyelination at a cellular level in the injured spinal cord (Ahuja et al., 2016). SCI often results in severe motor dysfunction, such as complete paralysis. These patients typically cannot only walk, but they also lose bowel, bladder, and sexual functions.

RISK FACTORS FOR SCI

Although an SCI is usually the result of an accident and can happen to anyone, certain factors may predispose you to a higher risk of sustaining an SCI, including gender, age, risky behavior, and osteoporosis (Coelho and Beraldo, 2009). Thus, SCIs affect a disproportionate amount of men. In fact, males account for 80% and females account for only about 20% of SCIs in the United States. More SCIs occur in 16−30 years old humans due to participation in contact sports and car or motorcycle accidents. SCIs due to fall are common in males above 65 years than in younger ones. Humans with bone and joint disorders such as arthritis or osteoporosis are at risk of SCIs (Barss et al. 2008; Coelho and Beraldo, 2009).

BIOMARKERS FOR SCI

Several biomarkers can be used for the diagnosis of SCI. These biomarkers include neurofilaments, cleaved-Tau, microtubule-associated protein 2 (MAP2), myelin basic protein, NSE, S100β, and glial fibrillary acidic protein (GFAP; Van Middendorp et al., 2011; Yokobori et al.,

2015). Changes in the above biomarkers also occur in TBI and CTE, so these biomarkers are not specific for SCI. Investigators are now started to study miRNA in SCI (Nieto-Diaz et al., 2014; Martirosyan et al., 2016). Microarray data from rodent contusion models of SCI have indicated that SCI produces alterations in the global mRNA expression patterns (Nieto-Diaz et al., 2014). Variations in mRNA abundance largely result from alterations in the expression of the cells at the damaged spinal cord. However, mRNA expression levels after SCI are also influenced by the infiltration of immune cells to the injury site as well as the death and migration of specific neural cells after injury (Nieto-Diaz et al., 2014). Bioinformatic analysis of microarray data has been used to identify specific variations in mRNA expression underlying transcriptional changes in target genes, which contribute to key neurochemical events in the SCI. Direct evidences on the role of mRNAs in SCI are scarcer, although recent studies have identified that several mRNAs (miR-21, miR-486, miR-20) involved in key mechanisms of the SCI such as cell death and astrogliosis (Nieto-Diaz et al., 2014). These miRNAs are produced in the nucleus by RNA polymerase II and processed by a variety of proteins before entering the cytoplasm as pre-miRNA. In the cytoplasm, the enzyme called dicer 1 ribonuclease type III, or DICER1contributes to the processing of the pre-miRNA duplex into a single-stranded miRNA sequence". This single-stranded miRNA sequence incorporate itself into an RNA silencing complex, which interacts with an mRNA sequence to perform downregulation either through its degradation or by inhibiting translation in the targeted mRNA. Studies on mRNA expression patterns at different time points following rat SCI using microarray have indicated that the induction of a specific mRNA expression pattern follows moderate contusive SCI at 7 days after SCI. miRNA downregulation is paralleled by mRNA upregulation, strongly supporting the view that miRNAs regulate transcriptional changes following SCI. Bioinformatic analyses have indicated that changes in mRNA expression affect key processes in SCI physiopathology, including inflammation and apoptosis. mRNA expression not only changes the invasion of immune cells at the injury site, but also produces changes in miRNAs, which are specific for spinal cord cells. It is proposed that miRNAs can be used as biomarkers for SCI (Yunta et al., 2012). Conventional MRI can also be used to assess macroscopic changes in the injured spinal cord, as it does not adequately address axonal injury in the white matter.

ANIMAL MODELS FOR SCI

As stated earlier, animal models of neurotraumatic diseases are needed for studying (a) molecular mechanisms of diseases;

(b) elucidating genotype–phenotype relationships; (c) validation of diagnostic biomarkers and therapeutic targets; and (d) development and testing of new drugs prior to launching costly clinical trials. Animal models of SCI have been developed in rats, mice, dogs, rabbits, and guinea pigs. Rodents are used most commonly in preliminary studies, as they are relatively inexpensive, readily available, and have demonstrated similar functional, electrophysiological, and morphological outcomes to humans following SCI (Metz et al., 2000; Kundi et al., 2013). Nonhuman primate SCI models have also been developed using marmosets, macaques, and squirrel monkeys (Iwanami et al., 2005). Several models have been developed using several injury procedures including (a) weight drop SCI model, (b) photochemical SCI model, (c) Ischemia-reperfusion SCI model, (d) excitotoxic SCI model, and (e) inflammatory SCI model (Kundi et al., 2013; Zhang et al., 2014). These models vary in terms of the animal utilization, site of injury infliction, and injury mechanism. Based on the mechanism of injury, SCI models can be classified as contusion, compression, distraction, dislocation, transection, or chemical. Contusion models, in which a transient force is applied to displace and damage the spinal cord, include weight drop, electromagnetic, and air pressure devices (Gruner, 1992; Strokes, 1992; Scheff et al., 2003; Kundi et al., 2013). Most of the animal models of SCI have been developed to simulate the biomechanics and neuropathology of human injury. Among these models, the weight drop model in rats remains the most widely used method of producing SCI experimentally. This technique offers the advantage of being clinically relevant, because most human injuries involve tissue damage due to rapid movement of the vertebral column with the impact of bone against the spinal cord. Rat SCI models also allow us to understand how neuronal circuitry changes following SCI and how recovery can be promoted by enhancing spontaneous regenerative mechanisms and by counteracting intrinsic inhibitory factors. Rat SCI model studies have also revealed possible routes to rescuing circuitry and cells in the acute stage of injury. However, due to the complexity of human SCI, no one model can encompass all aspects of SCI (Kundi et al., 2013; Kjell and Olson, 2016). Above SCI models have been developed to produce a consistent, easily reproducible, and graded injury that mediates SCI pathology in humans as closely as possible.

Studies on rat models of SCI provide an important mammalian model for SCI in the laboratory. Rat model of SCI have not only provided information on inflammation, scarring, and myelination at cellular and molecular levels, but also gave opportunity to evaluate treatment strategies for SCI in the laboratory (Kjell and Olson, 2016). Rat models of SCI have also facilitated the development of robust tests for assessing the recovery of locomotor and sensory functions. Rat models have also allowed us to understand how neuronal circuitry changes following SCI and how recovery can be promoted by enhancing spontaneous regenerative mechanisms and by counteracting intrinsic inhibitory factors (Kjell and Olson, 2016). Rat SCI models have also revealed information on replacement therapies for SCI, including grafts and bridges, stem primarily from rat studies.

NEURODEGENERATION IN TBI

TBI is caused by the damage to the brain from an external mechanical force. Like SCI, TBI is also caused by an impact to the head due to motorcycle and car accidents, contact sports, fall (particularly in seniors), and gunshots. TBI consists of two broadly defined components: a primary injury, attributable to the mechanical insult that occurs at the time of trauma to neurons, axons, glia, blood vessels, and integrity of the BBB as a result of shearing, tearing, or stretching; and a secondary injury, attributable to the series of systemic and local neurochemical and pathophysiological changes involving peripheral immune cells and activation of resident neural cells, triggering the release of molecular mediators such as cytokines, growth factors, and adhesion molecules, and activation of a complex network of pathways. Secondary injury develops over a period of hours to days and months following the primary injury (Raghupathi, 2004; Stoica and Faden, 2010). Among various neurochemical processes, oxidative stress, excitotoxicity, increase in intracellular calcium, activation of calcium-dependent enzymes (calpain, phospholipase A_2, nitric oxide synthase, caspases), neuronal apoptosis, and lipid degradation play a central role in secondary brain injury-mediated neurodegeneration in TBI (Vosler et al., 2009; Petronilho et al., 2010). Other neurochemical and neurophysiological changes following TBI involve the initiation of an acute inflammatory responses, including infiltration of peripheral blood cells, mitochondrial dysfunction, and activation of resident immunocompetent cells, as well as the release of numerous immune mediators such as interleukins and chemotactic factors (Stahel et al., 2000). Neurochemical and neurophysiological changes in the secondary injury contribute to the development of many of the neurologic deficits observed after TBI. In addition, TBI is also accompanied by the increase in intracranial pressure, which may account for local hypoxia and ischemia as well as secondary hemorrhage and herniation, leading to initiation and execution of multiple neuronal cell death mechanisms (Andriessen et al., 2010). The delayed onset of these changes suggests that there is a window for therapeutic intervention (pharmacologic or other) to prevent progressive tissue damage and improve functional recovery after TBI (Loane et al., 2015). TBIs are classified as mild and severe TBIs, based on neurochemical and clinical findings (Kraus, 1993). Mild TBI is the most common head injury, accounting for approximately 70%—90% of all traumatic brain injuries (Nordstrom et al., 2013). Mild TBI is defined as a head trauma resulting in a brief loss of consciousness and/or alteration of mental state. Mild TBI is usually benign, but occasionally causes persistent and sometimes progressive symptoms with no gross pathology, such as hemorrhage or abnormalities that are observed on a conventional CT scan of the brain (McCrory et al., 2009). Most symptoms of mild TBI (concussion) are resolved spontaneously over a fairly short period of time. No effect is observed on memory. In contrast, severe TBI may result in long consciousness with impaired thinking or memory, movement, sensation (e.g., vision or hearing), or emotional functioning (e.g., personality changes, depression). These issues not only affect individuals, but can also have lasting effects on families and communities.

RISK FACTORS FOR TBI

Many cases of TBI are caused by motorcycle and car accidents and contact sports among young adults (15 and 24 years). Among seniors (75 years and older), fall is an important risk factor for TBI (Rutland-Brown et al., 2006). Men are nearly three times as likely to die as women. Several studies have indicated that genetic factors play an important role in the interindividual variability in TBI and in predicting functional and cognitive outcomes following brain injury (McAllister, 2010; Waters et al., 2013; Weaver et al., 2014). These variations are caused by changes in the DNA sequence within a given gene and are referred to as genetic polymorphisms.

Although symptoms of TBI can be resolved within a year after injury, 70%—90% of patients endure prolonged and often permanent neurocognitive dysfunctions. It is now becoming increasingly evident that TBI can lead to early onset of dementia (Barnes et al, 2014; Gardner et al., 2014) as well as PD and other degenerative conditions (Gardner and Yaffe, 2015; Gardner et al., 2015). In particular, TBI is a strong environmental risk factor in the development of AD. Recent gene expression studies have indicated that the upregulation of key pathways leading to AD and PD provoked by mild, moderate, or severe forms of TBI (Tweedie et al., 2013; Greig et al, 2014). TBI is also a leading cause of acquired epilepsy (Campbell et al., 2014). In veterans, 57% of seizures can be linked to TBI (Salinsky et al., 2015). Immediately following injury, the brain undergoes distinct electrophysiological changes, which can be detected with electroencephalography (Schmitt and Dichter, 2015). Seizures not only account for heightened morbidity and mortality in the early stages following TBI, but also remain the leading cause of death several years following TBI (Rao and Parko, 2015). Collective evidence suggests that TBI is an important risk factor for several neurological diseases.

BIOMARKERS FOR TBI

Putative biomarkers for severe TBI include levels of total Tau protein, NSE, S100β (a Ca-binding protein), GFAP, ubiquitin C-terminal hydrolase-L1 (UCH-L1), MAP2, IL-6, and IL-10. Among these, some biomarkers are derived from neuronal origin, whereas others are of glial origin. These biomarkers are elevated in CSF of TBI patients. Delayed elevations in levels of some of these biomarkers are also observed in the blood after following TBI (Zetterberg et al., 2013; Adrian et al., 2016). The diagnosis of TBI can be made after neurological examination by neuroimaging cranial CT scanning and MRI. However, CT scanning has low sensitivity toward diffuse brain damage and confers exposure to radiation. In contrast, MRI can provide information on the extent of diffuse TBI. However, widespread application of MRI is restricted due not only to cost, but also to limited availability in many hospitals. CT, MRI, and counseling are often used to diagnose postconcussive syndrome, posttraumatic epilepsy, or CTE (Bogoslovsky et al., 2016). Despite the above-mentioned biomarkers and procedures, FDA has not approved a specific biomarker for clinical use in TBI in adults and children.

ANIMAL MODELS FOR TBI

The development of animal models of TBI is vital to study the pathophysiology of TBI. Animal models of TBI not only share the ultimate goals of reproducing reproducible patterns of brain damage observed in humans, but also allow testing of potential therapeutic agents for neuroprotection. Animal models have been developed using several techniques. These models include: (a) controlled cortical impact (CCI) TBI model (Shear et al., 2004; Wolff et al., 2008), fluid percussion (FP) injury TBI model (Thompson et al., 2005), (c) weight drop TBI model (Zohar et al., 2003; Schwulst et al., 2013), (d) impact acceleration TBI model (Marmarou et al., 1994), blast TBI model (Bauman et al., 2009), (e) repetitive TBI model (Longhi et al., 2009; Shitaka et al., 2011), (f) mild TBI

(Shultz et al., 2011; DeWitt et al., 2013; Prins et al., 2013). Among these models, FP injury TBI model, CCI model, and weight drop injury model are the most commonly used to generate injuries with characteristics of mild or severe TBI (Namjoshi et al., 2013). FP injury is generated by rapid injection of saline through a craniotomy into the epidural space, which causes the brain to move within the skull. CCI injury is produced by the rapid compression of brain tissue by an air-driven piston through a craniotomy. Neurodegeneration occurs within the compressed brain tissue, inducing a contusion core, which usually develops within days after injury. Finally, the weight drop model involves the release of a weight from a known height directly onto the closed skull to produce general movement of the brain. Each animal model has individual advantages and disadvantages, and although originally developed in rats, they have subsequently been effectively used in mice either with or without modifications. Clearly, mice are smaller, often less expensive, easier to handle, and provide a wide opportunity for genetic manipulations to understand mechanisms, using knockout and knockin technology. In contrast, rats have larger brains, and more readily allow time-dependent plasma as well as CSF sampling. It is important to note that rodent models of TBI require the use of anesthetic agents that clearly limit immediate postinjury behavioral evaluations in relation to orientation, memory, and level of consciousness. Based on animal model studies, it can be mentioned that there are similarities as well as differences in cellular and molecular events in human and rodent TBI. It should be kept in mind that there are substantial anatomical differences between the rodent and human brains, particularly that the rodent brain has a higher gray-to-white matter ratio compared to the human brain. Furthermore, notable differences exist between rodent and human brains in terms of brain geometry, craniospinal angle, and gyral complexity (Morales et al., 2005). In addition, natural circumstances that exist in human TBI during contact sports or fall or motorcycle and car accidents or boxing cannot be reproduced in the laboratory settings. Most models mimic either focal or diffuse brain injury, whereas the clinical reality suggests that each patient has an individual form of TBI characterized by various combinations of focal and diffuse patterns of tissue damage. This is additionally complicated by the occurrence of secondary insults such as hypotension, hypoxia, ischemia, extracranial injuries, modalities of traumatic events, age, gender, and heterogeneity of medical treatments and preexisting conditions. Although no single animal TBI model perfectly mimics the symptoms of human TBI (Marklund and Hillered 2011), cross-validation across animal models has indicated that neuroinflammation is a consistent feature of TBI and its early mitigation has benefits. Collective evidence suggests that an ideal animal model of TBI does not exist.

NEURODEGENERATION IN NEURODEGENERATIVE DISEASES

Neurodegenerative diseases are a heterogeneous group of multifactorial debilitating neurological disorders, which are characterized by the progressive loss of neurons leading to central nervous system dysfunction. The molecular mechanisms contributing to the pathogenesis of neurodegenerative diseases is not fully understood. However, it is speculated that neurodegeneration in specific population of neurons in neurodegenerative diseases is caused not only by the accumulation of misfolded proteins, their dysfunctional trafficking, and induction of mitochondrial dysfunction, but also due to the onset of excitotoxicity, oxidative stress, and neuroinflammation (Farooqui, 2010). Among the above-mentioned processes, the accumulation of misfolded proteins may be a major event in the pathogenesis of neurodegenerative diseases. In addition, interplay between environmental and genetic factors along with synaptic failure, altered metal homeostasis, and failure of axonal and dendritic transport may also contribute to neurodegeneration in neurodegenerative diseases (Farooqui, 2010). Now it is well established that AD, PD, HD, and ALS have different clinical and pathological features, such as the accumulation of β-amyloid ($A\beta$) in nucleus basalis, hippocampus, and entorhinal cortex in AD, α-synuclein (α-syn) deposition in substantia nigra in PD, accumulation of mutated huntingtin (Htt) in neurons of the basal ganglia in HD, and changes in activity of mutated Cu/Zn-SOD1 in motor neurons in ALS. However, the molecular mechanisms associated with the pathogenesis of above neurodegenerative diseases such as mitochondrial dysfunction, excitotoxicity, oxidative stress, and neuroinflammation appear to overlap considerably (Farooqui, 2010; Xie et al., 2014) (Fig. 1.3). Common characteristic features of the above-mentioned neurodegenerative diseases are accumulation of specific misfolded protein and increase in the rate of cross-talk among excitotoxicity, oxidative stress, and neuroinflammation. These processes along with the activation of microglial cells and astrocytes may lead to devastating consequences with severe mental and physical effects related to the neurodegeneration, onset of cognitive dysfunction, dementia, and alterations in high-order brain functions, which are related to the entorhinal cortex, hippocampus, limbic system, and neocortical areas.

RISK FACTORS FOR NEURODEGENERATIVE DISEASES

Important risk factors for neurodegenerative diseases include aging, positive family history (genes), long-term consumption of western diet

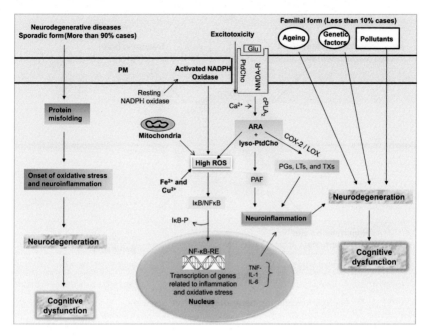

FIGURE 1.3 Factors modulating neurodegeneration and cognitive dysfunction. *PM*, plasma membrane; *Glu*, glutamate; *NMDAR*, N-methyl-ᴅ-aspartate receptor; *PtdCho*, phosphatidylcholine; *lyso-PtdCho*, lysophosphatidylcholine; *cPLA₂*, cytosolic phospholipase A₂; *PAF*, platelet activating factor; *ARA*, arachidonic acid; *COX-2*, cyclooxygenase-2; *LOX*, lipoxygenase; *PGs*, prostaglandin; *LTs*, leukotrienes; *TXs*, thromboxanes; *ROS*, reactive oxygen species; *NF- κB*, nuclear factor-κB; *NF-κB-RE*, nuclear factor-κB response element; *TNF-α*, tumor necrosis factor-α; *IL-1β*, interleukin-1β; *IL-6*, interleukin-6.

(high-calorie diet), sedentary lifestyle (lack of exercise), and environmental and genetic factors (Fig. 1.4). Among various neurodegenerative diseases, apolipoprotein E4 (APOE4) genotype is a powerful risk factor for developing AD. In addition, mutations in three genes that are inherited in an autosomal dominant fashion have also been linked to rare familial, early-onset forms of AD. These genes include those encoding APP, presenilin 1 (PS1), and presenilin 2 (PS2) (Farooqui, 2017). Similarly, mutations in at least four genes have been linked to PD, including α-syn (*PARK1*), parkin (*PARK2*), DJ-1 (*PARK7*), and PTEN (phosphatase and tensin homolog deleted on chromosome 10)-induced kinase 1 (*PINK1*, also known as *PARK6*) (Polymeropoulos et al., 1997; Kitada et al., 1998; Bonifati et al., 2003; Valente et al., 2004). At the genetic level, HD is characterized by an expanded CAG repeat encoding a polyglutamine (polyQ) tract in exon 1 of the HD gene. This gene encodes for huntingtin. Normal HD alleles have 37 or fewer glutamines in this polymorphic tract; more than 37 of these residues may contribute

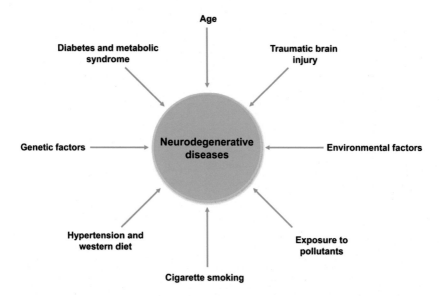

FIGURE 1.4   Factors modulating neurodegenerative diseases.

to the onset of HD (Rubinsztein et al., 1996). The length of the CAG tract is directly correlated with disease onset, with longer expansions leading to earlier onset of HD. Transgenic mouse model (SOD1^{G93A}) of SOD1−ALS has been developed, expressing approximately 20−24 copies of the human coding sequence with the G93A mutation, under control of the human *SOD1* promoter (Gurney et al., 1994). Since the development of this model, over 20 other SOD1 models have been created, and SOD1 transgenic rodents have been used as the primary rodent models of ALS. Other potential risk factors for the onset of neurodegenerative diseases are hypertension, diabetes, smoking, TBI, depression, socioeconomic status, ethnicity, smoking, and education (Fig. 1.4). Neurotoxic metals such as lead, mercury, aluminum, cadmium and arsenic, as well as some pesticides (Monnet-Tschudi et al., 2006) and metal-based nanoparticles have been involved in AD due to their ability to increase beta-amyloid (Aβ) peptide and the phosphorylation of Tau protein (P-Tau), causing deposition of senile/ amyloid plaques and induction of neurofibrillary tangles (NFTs), which are characteristics of AD (Farooqui, 2010, 2017). The exposure to lead, manganese, solvents, and some pesticides (rotenone) (Monnet-Tschudi et al., 2006) has been related to hallmarks of PD such as mitochondrial dysfunction, alterations in metal homeostasis, and aggregation of proteins such as α-syn, which is a key constituent of Lewy bodies (LB), a crucial factor in PD pathogenesis (Chin-Chan et al., 2015). Common

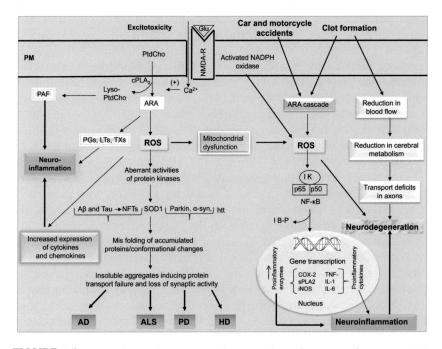

FIGURE 1.5 Molecular mechanisms contributing to the pathogenesis of neurotraumatic and neurodegenerative diseases. *Glu*, glutamate; *NMDAR*, N-methyl-D-aspartate receptor; *PtdCho*, phosphatidylcholine; *lyso-PtdCho*, lysophosphatidylcholine; *cPLA₂*, cytosolic phospholipase A_2; *PAF*, platelet activating factor; *ARA*, arachidonic acid; *COX-2*, cyclooxygenase-2; *PGs*, prostaglandin; *LTs*, leukotrienes; *TXs*, thromboxanes; *ROS*, reactive oxygen species; *Aβ*, beta-amyloid; *TNF-α*, tumor necrosis factor-α; *IL-1β*, interleukin-1β; *IL-6*, interleukin-6; *NTFs*, neurofibrillary tangles; *α-syn*, α-synuclein; *SOD1*, superoxide oxide dismutase 1; *htt*, mutated hungtingtin; *AD*, Alzheimer's disease; *PD*, Parkinson's disease; *ALS*, amyotrophic lateral sclerosis; *HD*, Huntington disease.

mechanisms of environmental pollutants to increase Aβ, P-Tau, α-syn, and neuronal death have been reported, including the oxidative stress mainly involved in the increase of Aβ and α-syn, along with the reduced activity/protein levels of Aβ degrading enzyme (IDE)s such as neprilysin or insulin IDE (Fig. 1.5).

BIOMARKERS FOR NEURODEGENERATIVE DISEASES

A probable diagnosis of neurodegenerative diseases can be made with a confidence of >85%−90%, based on clinical criteria, including medical history, physical examination, laboratory tests, neuroimaging (PET and MRI), and neuropsychological evaluation. Exact diagnosis (100%) of a neurodegenerative disease can be made only after the death of the patient at the autopsy. As stated above, AD, PD, HD, and ALS are accompanied by the accumulation of Aβ in AD, α-syn in PD, mutated huntingtin (Ht) in HD, and mutated Cu/Zn-SOD1 in ALS. Levels of these peptides and protein in CSF and blood have been used as biomarkers for AD, PD, HD, and ALS. Enzyme-linked immunosorbent assay for Aβ, α-syn, Htt, and SOD1 has been developed and used in many clinical laboratories (Fjorback et al., 2007; Xia et al., 2009; Massai et al., 2013; Keskin et al., 2016). It is also reported that mRNAs can be used to identify the neurodegenerative disease. Some mRNAs are differentially associated with AD, PD, HD, and ALS by modulating the expression of important genes involved in Aβ, α-syn, Htt, SOD1 production, and neuroinflammation (Goodall et al., 2013; Van den Hove et al., 2014). The main problems in developing ideal biomarkers for neurodegenerative diseases have been the slow understanding of pathogenesis of neurodegenerative diseases, unavailability of histopathological and biochemical diagnosis during patient lifetime, and lack of information on progression and treatment of neurodegenerative diseases. Furthermore, it is important have a complete understanding of how biomarkers for neurodegenerative diseases change over time throughout disease progression. To determine and evaluate whether a treatment is working, it is of utmost importance to choose biomarkers that are most relevant and specific to a specific neurodegenerative disease (Farooqui, 2017).

ANIMAL MODELS FOR NEURODEGENERATIVE DISEASES

Animal models of AD are needed not only to understand the molecular mechanisms underlying the pathogenesis of neurodegenerative diseases, but also to study the contribution of genetic and environmental risk factors involved in the pathogenesis of a neurodegenerative diseases. In addition, animal models are also used for developing diagnostic tests and investigating the therapeutic effects of drugs on neuropathology and cognitive function in neurodegenerative diseases. In addition, animal models are also needed to establish the pharmacodynamics and pharmacokinetic parameters and toxicity analysis of new drugs for the treatment of neurodegenerative. The use of mice (*Mus musculus*) for the development of animal models offer several advantages over invertebrate and higher models. Mice are closely related to humans than invertebrate models such as yeast, worms, or flies (Saraceno et al., 2013). Whole genome of a mouse has been mapped. The proportion of mouse genes with a single identifiable ortholog in the human genome is approximately 80%. This makes the mouse an ideal model for investigating environmental and genetic manipulations, which are not feasible in higher primates and humans (Saraceno et al., 2013). Transgenic mice have proved useful in reproducing lesions seen in a neurodegenerative disease such as the senile plaques and NFTs in AD (Langui et al., 2007). Symptoms of PD can be induced in mice by injecting a neurotoxin called 1-methyl-4-phenyl-1,2,3,6-tetrahydropyridine (Meredith and Rademacher, 2011). Injections of N-methyl-D-aspartate receptor (NMDAR) agonists (kainic acid, quinolinic, and nitropropionic acid) into the striatum of rodents or nonhuman primate produces the patterns of neuronal damage in HD (Coyle and Schwarcz, 1976; Beal et al., 1991, 1993). Transgenic mice have proved useful in reproducing symptoms of ALS (McGoldrick et al., 2013).

NEURODEGENERATION IN NEUROPSYCHIATRIC DISEASES

Neuropsychiatric diseases are multisystem and multifactorial mental disorders caused by abnormalities in cerebral cortex and limbic system (thalamus, hypothalamus, hippocampus, and amygdala). Neuropsychiatric diseases include schizophrenia, some forms of bipolar affective disorders, autism, mood disorders, depression, attention-deficit disorder, dementia, tardive dyskinesia, atypical spells, irritability, and organic mental disorder (Miyoshi and Morimura, 2010; Lyketsos, 2006). Many neuropsychiatric disorders, including autism spectrum disorder, attention-deficit/hyperactivity disorder, mental retardation, and schizophrenia can be triggered by alterations to neural development. The molecular mechanisms of neuropsychiatric diseases are not fully understood. However, it is becoming increasingly evident that changes in neurotransmitters (dopamine, serotonin, GABA, and glutamate), neuropeptides (vasopressin), cytokines (IL-6 and TNF-α), neuron–microglia interactions, and gene environmental interactions along with decrease in BDNF, low magnesium, and overactivity of hypothalamic–pituitary–adrenal (HPA) axis may contribute to the pathogenesis of major depression (Varghese and Brown, 2001; Sen et al., 2008; Dowlati et al. 2010; Wohleb, 2016; Wohleb and Delpech, 2016) (Fig. 1.6). In addition to the above processes, neuropsychiatric diseases are also accompanied by excessive shortening of telomeres. The length of telomeres is negatively correlated with the longitude of nonmedicated depression and the level of IL-6. IL-6 is considered to be a biomarker of neuroinflammation. Exact mechanisms associated with telomerase shortening remain unknown. However, it is hypothesized that oxidative stress and neuroinflammation affect the structure of replication fork in the vicinity of telomeres contributing to the onset of depression (Simon et al., 2006; Wolkowitz et al., 2011).

ISCHEMIC AND TRAUMATIC BRAIN AND SPINAL CORD INJURIES

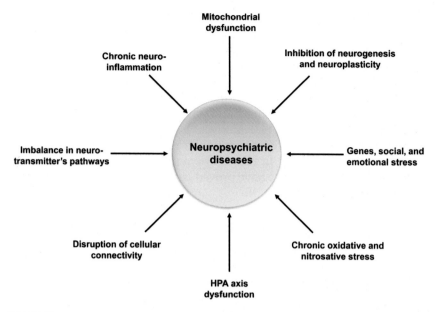

FIGURE 1.6   Processes modulating neuropsychiatric diseases.

Critically short telomeres can also cause neural cells to undergo senescence, apoptosis, and genomic instability, which correlate with poorer health and predicts mortality.

Although the above-mentioned neuropsychiatric disorders share common patterns of symptoms and treatments, there are no validated and specific biomarkers that define the underlying molecular mechanisms in the central brain. An important characteristic of neuropsychiatric disorders is the abnormality in signal transduction processes associated with cognitive function, learning and memory, as well as communication. At the molecular level, these processes are not only regulated by overexpression or underexpression of genes, but also by changes in levels of neurotransmitters and proinflammatory arachidonic acid metabolites (Miyoshi and Morimura, 2010). There is a growing body of evidence supporting the view that neuropsychiatric disorders are the consequences of dysregulation of complex intracellular signaling cascades and neuronal networks, rather than the consequences of deficits or excesses of individual neurotransmitters (Quinones and Kaddurah-Daouk, 2009). At the cellular level, many neuropsychiatric diseases involve an increase in the concentration of intracellular Ca^{2+} within the inhibitory neurons that is driven by an increase in the entry through the NMDARs and through activation of the phosphoinositide signaling pathway that generates inositol trisphosphate ($InsP_3$) that releases Ca^{2+} from the internal stores. Furthermore, neuropsychiatric disorders are also linked with gray matter atrophy caused by decrease in neuronal and glial cell size, increase in cellular packing density, disruption in neuronal connectivity, abnormalities in neurocircuits in specific brain area particularly in the dorsolateral prefrontal cortex, and distortions in neuronal orientation (Arnold and Trojanowski, 1996; Blitzer et al., 2005). Both macro- and microcircuitry changes in limbic system can contribute to the onset of neuropsychiatric condition (Benes, 2000). Among neuropsychiatric diseases, depression is linked with multiple biochemical abnormalities, such as vascular pathological changes, autonomic functional changes, psychomotor changes, hypercoagulability, abnormality in the adrenal system, and HPA axis hyperactivity leading to low self-esteem (Evans et al., 2005). These abnormalities may produce profound effects on memory and behavior in persons both with and without cognitive impairment. In addition, these changes not only contribute to the increased risk for MCI and dementia, but are also linked with accelerated cognitive decline in the old age (Wilson et al., 2007). All these changes can profoundly affect mood, sleep, learning, and memory (Lucassen et al., 2010). Depression also occurs in neurotraumatic (stroke, SCI, and TBI) and neurodegenerative diseases (AD and PD). Here, symptoms of depression are due to age-related changes in signal transduction processes that contribute to neurotransmission and neuroplasticity in the brain (Blitzer et al., 2005; Arciniegas and Kaufer, 2006). This suggests that there is an overlap in molecular mechanisms that contribute to alterations in neurotransmission and neuroplasticity in neuropsychiatric, neurodegenerative, and neuropsychiatric diseases.

RISK FACTORS FOR NEUROPSYCHIATRIC DISEASES

Epidemiologic studies have indicated that maternal obesity and metabolic complications increase the risk of attention-deficit hyperactivity disorder, autism spectrum disorders, anxiety, depression, schizophrenia, eating disorders (food addiction, anorexia nervosa, and bulimia nervosa), and impairments in cognition in offspring (Rivera et al., 2015). It is proposed that stress exposure affects the neurobiology of mental health disorders through dysregulation of neuroimmune systems. It is shown that repeated stress exposure causes microglia activation and recruitment of peripheral monocytes to the brain contributing to the development of anxiety- and depressive-like behavior. Furthermore, stress-associated immune changes contribute to physiological processes that support neuroplasticity. Thus, stress-mediated perturbations in neuroimmune function along with mild oxidative stress, chronic neuroinflammation, and mitochondrial dysfunction can lead to impaired neuronal responses and synaptic plasticity deficits that underlie behavioral symptoms of neuropsychiatric disorders (Wohleb and Delpech, 2016).

BIOMARKERS FOR NEUROPSYCHIATRIC DISEASES

As stated above, an important goal of biomarker research is to improve the accuracy of diagnosis of neuropsychiatric diseases for improving the outcome for the patient. At present, there is no highly specific, sensitive, and reproducible biomarker(s) for neuropsychiatric diseases because these diseases are not only multifactorial disorders in their etiology, but also have heterogeneous onset and expression. So, it is unlikely that any one specific biomarker will greatly impact diagnosis and treatment of neurodegenerative diseases (Boksa, 2013). Based on omics technology, it is proposed that it may be possible to identify proteins in body fluids such as CSF, serum, or blood. However, the diagnosis of neuropsychiatric disorders is clinically performed by focusing on observable symptoms and behaviors along with neuroimaging and neurophysiological findings rather than on underlying psychodynamic processes (Patel, 2014). Understanding the descriptive symptoms for mental disorders is vital to properly diagnose each neuropsychiatric disease. Risk factors in neuropsychiatric diseases include not only neurotransmitter and cytokines changes, but also disruption of cellular connectivity, decrease in neurogenesis, alterations in microcircuitry, along with decrease in neuroplasticity. It has been hypothesized that there are early and common molecular changes in the brain that may serve as sensitive indicators of brain molecular stress and that can be predictive of neuropathological changes that increase the risk for neuropsychiatric diseases (Quinones and Kaddurah-Daouk, 2009).

ANIMAL MODELS FOR NEUROPSYCHIATRIC DISEASES

Animal modeling of human neuropsychiatric disorders is an extremely challenging topic due to the subjective nature of key symptoms, lack of biomarkers, objective diagnostic tests, and slow understanding of their pathophysiology (Nestler and Hyman, 2010). In addition, it is difficult to establish psychiatric diagnoses of hallucinations, delusions, sadness, guilt in animals compared to humans. However, when there are reasonable correlations in animals, including abnormal social behavior, motivation, working memory, emotion, and executive function, the information and conclusion can be only approximate (Nestler and Hyman, 2010). In spite of the above challenges, valid animal models for schizophrenia (Arguello et al., 2010), depression (Cryan et al., 2002; Nestler et al., 2002), bipolar disorders (Einat and Manji, 2006; Malkesman et al., 2009), and autism (Moy and Nadler, 2008) have been developed and used for research in many laboratories.

FACTORS CONTRIBUTING TO INCREASED FREQUENCY OF NEUROTRAUMATIC, NEURODEGENERATIVE, AND NEUROPSYCHIATRIC DISEASES

The prevalence of neurotraumatic, neurodegenerative, and neuropsychiatric diseases has increased considerably in the 21st century and is still increasing with a significant rate. Although traumatic injuries to brain and spinal cord result in SCI and TBI due to car, motorcycle accidents, contact sports, and military action, reasons for the increase in occurrence and commencement of stroke and neurodegenerative, neuropsychiatric diseases remain elusive. Several factors may facilitate the onset of stroke, neurodegenerative, and neuropsychiatric diseases in human population (Farooqui et al., 2007; Farooqui, 2009). These factors include age, healthy diet, environmental factors, and, to certain extent, genetic factors (Farooqui, 2009; Farooqui and Farooqui, 2009). Thus, long-term consumption of western diet, which is enriched in processed food, high in carbohydrates and salt, low in fiber, and has preservatives (toxins) may not only affect: (a) glycemic load, (b) fatty acid alterations, (c) macronutrient alterations, and (d) micronutrient density, but also produce changes in acid−base balance, sodium−potassium ratio, and decrease levels of antioxidants and micronutrients (Cordain et al., 2005). Western diet is enriched in ω-6 fatty acids, which, on the one hand, through enzymic oxidation produce high levels of proinflammatory eicosanoids (prostaglandins, leukotrienes, and thromboxanes) and, on the other hand, through nonenzymic oxidation can excessively produce high levels of oxidative stress (ROS). High levels of ROS have been reported to stimulate transcription factor NF-κB, which upon translocation to the nucleus promotes expression of proinflammatory cytokines and chemokines (Fig. 1.5). In addition, long-term consumption of western diet also produces oxidative stress through the production of AGEs. These metabolites play an important role in neurodegenerative process. Furthermore, long-term consumption of western diet also produces hyperglycemia. Sustained high levels of glucose are known to induce type 2 diabetes and metabolic syndrome. These pathological conditions are risk factors for stroke, AD, PD, and depression (Farooqui et al., 2012; Farooqui, 2013).

Under physiological conditions, astrocytes regulate the concentrations of ions, glutamate, and water, store glycogen, and offer metabolic support to neurons, in addition to regulating synaptogenesis, forming the BBB and defending against oxidative damage (Ransohoff and Brown, 2012; Wake et al., 2012). In contrast, in neurotraumatic and neurodegenerative diseases, brain damage disturbs astrocyte-driven ion and glutamate homeostasis resulting in the substantial release of glutamate, K^+ ions, and ROS. These processes contribute to neurotoxicity

(Heneka et al., 2010) through downregulation of glutamate transporters in astrocytes, leading to the onset of glutamate-induced excitotoxicity (Allaman et al., 2011). Brain injury (neurodegeneration) in neurotraumatic and neurodegenerative diseases not only puts lots of stress on the regulatory function of astrocytes, microglia, and oligodendrocytes, but also promotes the release of ATP and onset of many damage-associated molecular patterns, thus activating microglial cells, neurons, mast cells, and astrocytes to produce cytokines, chemokines, and complement (Amor et al., 2014; Skaper et al., 2014). It should be noted that very early activation of astrocytes in stroke, TBI, and neurodegenerative diseases (AD, PD, and ALS) are necessary for reactive astrogliosis (Sofroniew, 2014), whereas activation of microglia under these conditions leads to phagocytosis of dead or dying cells and debris and expression of cytokines and neurotoxic substances that can exacerbate cell damage (Bonifati and Kishore, 2007).

CONCLUSION

Neurodegeneration is a complex multifactorial process that causes neuronal death in brain and spinal cord, resulting in brain and spinal cord damage and dysfunction. Neurodegeneration is accompanied by oxidative stress, axonal transport deficits, protein oligomerization, aggregation, calcium deregulation, mitochondrial dysfunction, abnormal neuron–glial interactions, neuroinflammation, DNA damage, and aberrant RNA processing. Neurodegeneration occurs in neurotraumatic, neurodegenerative, and neuropsychiatric diseases. These diseases are accompanied by structural, neurochemical, and electrophysiological abnormalities in the brain, spinal cord, and nerves causing paralysis, muscle weakness, poor coordination, seizures, confusion, and pain. Common neurotraumatic diseases include strokes, TBI, SCI, and CTE. In ischemic and traumatic brain and spinal cord injuries, neurons degenerate rapidly (in minutes to hours) because of the sudden lack of oxygen, a quick drop in ATP, and alteration in ion homeostasis. Common neurodegenerative diseases are AD, PD, HD, and ALS (Farooqui, 2010). Neurodegenerative diseases involve accumulation of misfolded proteins and onset of neurodegeneration in specific population of neurons. In neurodegenerative diseases, some oxygen, nutrients, and ATP are available to the neurons, ion homeostasis is maintained to a limited extent, and neurodegeneration takes a longer time period (years) to die. Neuropsychiatric disorders are depression, schizophrenia, some forms of bipolar affective disorders, autism, mood disorders, attention-deficit disorder, dementia, tardive dyskinesia, and chronic fatigue syndrome. Neuropsychiatric diseases involve the abnormalities in signal transduction processes in cerebral cortex and limbic system (thalamus, hypothalamus, hippocampus, and amygdala). Growing evidence indicates that there is a considerable overlap in risk factors, molecular mechanisms (excitotoxicity, oxidative stress, and neuroinflammation) of neurodegeneration in neurotraumatic, neurodegenerative diseases, and neuropsychiatric disorders. However, there are remarkable differences in molecular, clinical, and neurophysiological aspects of neurotraumatic, neurodegenerative diseases, and neuropsychiatric disorders.

References

Adrian, H., Mårten, K., Salla, N., Lasse, V., 2016. Biomarkers of traumatic brain injury: temporal changes in body fluids. eNeuro 3, pii: ENEURO.0294-16.2016.

Ahuja, C.S., Martin, A.R., Fehlings, M., 2016. Recent advances in managing a spinal cord injury secondary to trauma. F1000Res 5, pii: F1000.

Allaman, I., Belanger, M., Magistretti, P.J., 2011. Astrocyte—neuron metabolic relationships: for better and for worse. Trends Neurosci. 34, 76—87.

Allan, S.M., Tyrrell, P.J., Rothwell, N.J., 2005. Interleukin-1 and neuronal injury. Nat. Rev. Immunol. 5, 629—640.

Allen, C.L., Bayraktutan, U., 2008. Risk factors for ischaemic stroke. Int. J. Stroke 3, 105—116.

Allgaier, M., Allgaier, C., 2014. An update on drug treatment options of Alzheimer's disease. Front. Biosci. (Landmark Ed). 19, 1345—1354.

Alzheimer's Association, 2011. Alzheimer's disease facts and figures. Alzheimer's Dementia 2011 (7), 208—244.

Amor, S., Peferoen, L.A.N., Vogel, D.Y.S., et al., 2014. Inflammation in neurodegenerative diseases—an update. Immunology 142, 151—166.

Andriessen, T.M., Jacobs, B., Vos, P.E., 2010. Clinical characteristics and pathophysiological mechanisms of focal and diffuse traumatic brain injury. J. Cell. Mol. Med. 14, 2381—2392.

Arciniegas, D.B., Kaufer, D.I., 2006. Joint Advisory Committee on Subspecialty Certification of the American Neuropsychiatric Association; Society for Behavioral and Cognitive Neurology. Core curriculum for training in behavioral neurology and neuropsychiatry. J. Neuropsychiatry Clin. Neurosci. 18, 6—13.

Arguello, P.A., Markx, S., Gogos, J.A., Kraiorgou, M., 2010. Development of animal models for schizophrenia. Dis. Model. Mech. 3, 22—26.

Arnold, S.E., Trojanowski, J.Q., 1996. Recent advances in defining the neuropathology of schizophrenia. Acta Neuropathol. (Berl). 92, 217—231.

Arrick, D.M., Sharpe, G.M., Sun, H., Mayhan, W.G., 2007. nNOS-dependent reactivity of cerebral arterioles in Type 1 diabetes. Brain Res. 1184, 365—371.

Attwell, D., Buchan, A.M., Charpak, S., Lauritzen, M., Macvicar, B.A., Newman, E.A., 2010. Glial and neuronal control of brain blood flow. Nature 468, 232—243.

Barnes, D.E., Kaup, A., Kirby, K.A., Byers, A.L., Diaz-Arrastia, R., et al., 2014. Traumatic brain injury and risk of dementia in older veterans. Neurology 83, 312—319.

Barss, P., Djerrari, H., Leduc, B.E., Lepage, Y., Dionne, C.E., 2008. Risk factors and prevention for spinal cord injury from diving in swimming pools and natural sites in Quebec, Canada: A 44-year study. Accid. Anal. Prev. 40, 787—797.

Bauman, R.A., Ling, G., Tong, L., Januszkiewicz, A., Agoston, D., et al., 2009. An introductory characterization of a combat-casualty-care relevant swine model of closed head injury resulting from exposure to explosive blast. J. Neurotrauma 26, 841−860.

Baxter, P., Chen, Y., Xu, Y., Swanson, R.A., 2014. Mitochondrial dysfunction induced by nuclear poly(ADP-ribose) polymerase-1: a treatable cause of cell death in stroke. Transl. Stroke Res 5, 136−144.

Beal, M.F., Ferrante, R.J., Swartz, K.J., Kowall, N.W., 1991. Chronic quinolinic acid lesions in rats closely resemble Huntington's disease. J. Neurosci. 11, 1649−1659.

Beal, M.F., Brouillet, E., Jenkins, B.G., Ferrante, R.J., Kowall, N.W., et al., 1993. Neurochemical and histologic characterization of striatal excitotoxic lesions produced by the mitochondrial toxin 3-nitropropionic acid. J. Neurosci. 13, 4181−4192.

Bekris, L.M., Mata, I.F., Zabetian, C.P., 2010. The genetics of Parkinson disease. J. Geriatr. Psychiatry Neurol. 23, 228−242.

Benes, F.M., 2000. Emerging principles of altered neural circuitry in schizophrenia. Brain Res. Brain Res. Rev. 31, 251−269.

Blitzer, R.D., Iyengar, R., Landau, E.M., 2005. Postsynaptic signaling networks: cellular cogwheels underlying long-term plasticity. Biol. Psychiatry 57, 113−119.

Bogoslovsky, T., Gill, J., Jeromin, A., Davis, C., Diaz-Arrastia, R., 2016. Fluid biomarkers of traumatic brain injury and intended context of use. Diagnostics (Basel) 6, pii: E37.

Boksa, P., 2013. A way forward for research on biomarkers for psychiatric disorders. J. Psychiatry Neurosci. 38, 75−77.

Bonifati, D.M., Kishore, U., 2007. Role of complement in neurodegeneration and neuroinflammation. Mol. Immunol. 44, 999−1010.

Bonifati, V., Rizzu, P., van Baren, M.J., Schaap, O., Breedveld, G.J., et al., 2003. Mutations in the *DJ-1* gene associated with autosomal recessive early-onset parkinsonism. Science 299, 256−259.

Braeuninger, S., Kleinschnitz, C., 2009. Rodent models of focal cerebral ischemia: procedural pitfalls and translational problems. Exp. Transl. Stroke Med. 1, 8.

Bramlett, H.M., Dietrich, W.D., 2004. Pathophysiology of cerebral ischemia and brain trauma: similarities and differences. J. Cereb. Blood Flow Metab. 24, 133−150.

Brouns, R., De Deyn, P.P., 2009. The complexity of neurobiological processes in acute ischemic stroke. Clin. Neurol. Neurosurg. 111, 483−495.

Campbell, J.N., Gandhi, A., Singh, B., Churn, S.B., 2014. Traumatic brain injury causes a tacrolimus-sensitive increase in non-convulsive seizures in a rat model of post-traumatic epilepsy. Int. J. Neurol. Brain Disord. 1, 1−11.

Chin-Chan, M., Navarro-Yepes, J., Quintanilla-Vega, B., 2015. Environmental pollutants as risk factors for neurodegenerative disorders: Alzheimer and Parkinson diseases. Front. Cell. Neurosci. 9, 124.

Coelho, C.V.C., Beraldo, P.S.S., 2009. Risk factors of heterotopic ossification in traumatic spinal cord injury. Arq. Neuropsiquiatr. 67, 382−387.

Cordain, L., Eaton, S.B., Sebastian, A., Mann, N., Lindeberg, S., et al., 2005. Origins and evolution of the Western diet: health implications for the 21st century. J. Am. J. Clin. Nutr. 81, 341−354.

Coyle, J.T., Schwarcz, R., 1976. Lesion of striatal neurones with kainic acid provides a model for Huntington's chorea. Nature 263, 244−246.

Cryan, J.F., Markou, A., Lucki, I., 2002. Assessing antidepressant activity in rodents: recent developments and future needs. Trends Pharmacol. Sci. 23, 238−245.

Deleidi, M., Jäggle, M., Rubino, G., 2015. Immune aging, dysmetabolism, and inflammation in neurological diseases. Front. Neurosci. 9, 172.

DeWitt, D.S., Perez-Polo, R., Hulsebosch, C.E., Dash, P.K., Robertson, C.S., 2013. Challenges in the development of rodent models of mild traumatic brain injury. J. Neurotrauma 30, 688−701.

Dias, V., Junn, E., Mouradian, M.M., 2013. The role of oxidative stress in Parkinson's disease. J. Parkinson's Dis. 3, 461−491.

Dowlati, Y., Herrmann, N., Swardfager, W., Liu, H., Sham, L., et al., 2010. A meta-analysis of cytokines in major depression. Biol. Psychiatry 67, 446−457.

Einat, H., Manji, H.K., 2006. Cellular plasticity cascades: genes-to-behavior pathways in animal models of bipolar disorder. Biol. Psychiatry 59, 1160−1171.

Endres, M., Engelhardt, B., Koistinaho, J., et al., 2008. Improving outcome after stroke: overcoming the translational roadblock. Cerebrovasc. Dis. 25, 268−278.

Evans, D.L., Charney, D.S., Lewis, L., Golden, R.N., Gorman, J.M., et al., 2005. Mood disorders in the medically ill: scientific review and recommendations. Biol. Psychiatry 58, 175−189.

Farooqui, A.A., 2009. Beneficial Effects of Fish Oil on Human Brain. Springer, New York.

Farooqui, A.A., 2010. Neurochemical Aspects of Neurotraumatic and Neurodegenerative Diseases. Springer, New York.

Farooqui, A.A., 2013. Metabolic Syndrome: An Important Risk Factor For Stroke, Alzheimer Disease, and Depression. Springer, New York.

Farooqui, A.A., 2017. Neurochemical Aspects of Alzheimer Disease: Risk Factors, Pathogenesis, Biomarkers, and Potential Treatment Strategies. Academic Press, San Diego.

Farooqui, T., Farooqui, A.A., 2009. Aging: an important factor for the pathogenesis of neurodegenerative diseases. Mech. Ageing Dev. 130, 203−215.

Farooqui, A.A., Horrock, L.A., 2007. Glycerophospholipids in Brain. Springer, New York.

Farooqui, A.A., Ong, W.Y., Horrocks, L.A., Chen, P., Farooqui, T., 2007. Comparison of biochemical effects of statins and fish oil in brain: the battle of the titans. Brain Res. Rev. 56, 443−471.

Farooqui, A.A., Ong, W.Y., 2010. Lipid mediators in the nucleus: Their potential contribution to Alzheimer's disease. Biochim Biophys Acta. 1801, 906−916.

Farooqui, A.A., Farooqui, T., Panza, F., Frisardi, V., 2012. Metabolic syndrome as a risk factor for neurological disorders. Cell. Mol. Life Sci. 69, 741−762.

Feuerstein, G.Z., Zaleska, M.M., Krams, M., Wang, X., Day, M., et al., 2008. Missing steps in the STAIR case: a translational medicine perspective on the development of NXY-059 for treatment of acute ischemic stroke. J. Cereb. Blood Flow Metab. 28, 217−219.

Fjorback, A.W., Varming, K., Jensen, P.H., 2007. Determination of alpha-synuclein concentration in human plasma using ELISA. Scand. J. Clin. Lab. Invest. 67, 431−435.

Fluri, F., Schuhmann, M.K., Kleinschnitz, C., 2015. Animal models of ischemic stroke and their application in clinical research. Drug Des. Dev. Ther. 9, 3445−3454.

Ford, G.A., 2008. Clinical pharmacological issues in the development of acute stroke therapies. Br J Pharmacol 153 (Suppl 1), S112−S119.

Forgione, N., Fehlings, M.G., 2014. Rho-ROCK inhibition in the treatment of spinal cord injury. World Neurosurg 82, e535−e539.

Gao, L.B., Yu, X.F., Chen, Q., Zhou, D., 2016. Alzheimer's disease therapeutics: current and future therapies. Minerva Med. 107, 108−113.

García-Berrocoso, T., Fernández-Cadenas, I., Delgado, P., Rosell, A., Montaner, J., 2010. Blood biomarkers in cardioembolic stroke. Curr. Cardiol. Rev. 6, 194−201.

Gardner, R.C., Yaffe, K., 2015. Epidemiology of mild traumatic brain injury and neurodegenerative disease. Mol. Cell. Neurosci. 66, 75−80.

Gardner, R.C., Burke, J.F., Nettiksimmons, J., Kaup, A., Barnes, D.E., et al., 2014. Dementia risk after traumatic brain injury vs nonbrain trauma: the role of age and severity. JAMA Neurol. 71, 1490−1497.

Gardner, R.C., Burke, J.F., Nettiksimmons, J., Goldman, S., Tanner, C.M., et al., 2015. Traumatic brain injury in later life increases risk for Parkinson disease. Ann. Neurol. 77, 987−995.

Ginsberg, M.D., 2008. Neuroprotection for ischemic stroke: past, present and future. Neuropharmacology 55, 363–389.

Goodall, E.F., Heath, P.R., Bandmann, O., Kirby, J., Shaw, P.J., 2013. Neuronal dark matter: the emerging role of microRNAs in neurodegeneration. Front. Cell. Neurosci. 7, 178.

Green, A.R., 2008. Pharmacological approaches to acute ischaemic stroke: reperfusion certainly, neuroprotection possibly. Br J Pharmacol 153 (Suppl. 1), S325–S338.

Greig, N.H., Tweedie, D., Rachmany, L., Li, Y., Rubovitch, V., et al., 2014. Incretin mimetics as pharmacologic tools to elucidate and as a new drug strategy to treat traumatic brain injury. Alzheimers Dement. 10 (1 Suppl.), S62–S67.

Gruner, J.A., 1992. A monitored contusion model of spinal cord injury in the rat. J. Neurotrauma 9, 123–128.

Gurney, M.E., Pu, H., Chiu, A.Y., Dal Canto, M.C., Polchow, C.Y., et al., 1994. Motor neuron degeneration in mice that express a human Cu,Zn superoxide dismutase mutation. Science 264, 1772–1775.

Hamer, M., Chida, Y., 2009. Physical activity and risk of neurodegenerative disease: a systematic review of prospective evidence. Psychol. Med. 39, 3–11.

Hebert, L.E., Scherr, P.A., Bienias, J.L., Bennett, D.A., Evans, D.A., 2003. Alzheimer disease in the US population—prevalence estimates using the 2000 census. Arch. Neurol. Chicago 60, 1119–1122.

Heneka, M.T., Rodriguez, J.J., Verkhratsky, A., 2010. Neuroglia in neurodegeneration. Brain Res. Rev. 63, 189–211.

Herson, P.S., Traystman, R.J., 2014. Animal models of stroke: translational potential at present and in 2050. Future Neurol. 9, 541–551.

Hill, M.D., Martin, R.H., Mikulis, D., Wong, J.H., Silver, F.L., et al., 2013. Safety and efficacy of NA-1 in patients with iatrogenic stroke after endovascular aneurysm repair (ENACT): a phase 2, randomised, double-blind, placebo-controlled trial. Lancet Neurol. 11, 942–950.

Iadecola, C., Davisson, R.L., 2008. Hypertension and cerebrovascular dysfunction. Cell Metab. 7, 476–484.

Iwanami, A., Yamane, J., Katoh, H., Nakamura, M., Momoshima, S., Ishii, H., et al., 2005. Establishment of graded spinal cord injury model in a nonhuman primate: the common marmoset. J. Neurosci. Res. 80, 172–181.

Jeyaseelan, K., Lim, K.Y., Armugam, A., 2008. MicroRNA expression in the blood and brain of rats subjected to transient focal ischemia by middle cerebral artery occlusion. Stroke 39, 959–966.

Jickling, G.C., Sharp, F.R., 2011. Blood biomarkers of ischemic stroke. Neurotherapeutics 8, 349–360.

Kawabori, M., Yenari, M.A., 2015. Inflammatory responses in brain ischemia. Curr. Med. Chem. 22, 1258–1277.

Kempuraj, D., Thangavel, R., Natteru, P.A., Selvakumar, G.P., Saeed, D., et al., 2016. Neuroinflammation induces neurodegeneration. J. Neurol. Neurosurg. Spine 1, pii: 1003.

Kernagis, D.N., Laskowitz, D.T., 2012. Evolving role of biomarkers in acute cerebrovascular disease. Ann. Neurol. 71, 289–303.

Keskin, I., Forsgren, E., Lange, D.J., Weber, M., Birve, A., et al., 2016. Effects of cellular pathway disturbances on misfolded superoxide dismutase-1 in fibroblasts derived from ALS patients. PLoS ONE 11, e0150133.

Kim, S.J., Moon, G.J., Bang, O.Y., 2013. Biomarkers for stroke. J. Stroke 15, 27–37.

Kimura-Ohba, S., Yang, Y., 2016. Oxidative DNA damage mediated by intranuclear MMP activity is associated with neuronal apoptosis in ischemic stroke. Oxid. Med. Cell Longev 2016, 6927328.

Kitada, T., Sakawa, S., Hattori, N., Matsumine, H., Yamamura, Y., et al., 1998. Mutations in the parkin gene cause autosomal recessive juvenile parkinsonism. Nature 392, 605–608.

Kitayama, J., Faraci, F.M., Lentz, S.R., Heistad, D.D., 2007. Cerebral vascular dysfunction during hypercholesterolemia. Stroke 38, 2136–2141.

Kjell, J., Olson, L., 2016. Rat models of spinal cord injury: from pathology to potential therapies. Dis. Model. Mech. 9, 1125–1137.

Kowal, S.L., Dall, T.M., Chakrabarti, R., Storm, M.V., Jain, A., 2013. The current and projected economic burden of Parkinson's disease in the United States. Mov. Disord. 28, 311–318.

Kraus, J.F., 1993. Epidemiology of head injury. In: Cooper, P.R. (Ed.), Head Injury, 3rd edn Williams & Wilkins, Baltimore, pp. 1–25.

Kundi, S., Bicknell, R., Ahmed, Z., 2013. Spinal cord injury: current mammalian models. Am. J. Neurosci. 4, 1–12.

Langui, D., Lachapelle, F., Duyckaerts, C., 2007. Animal models of neurodegenerative diseases. Med. Sci. (Paris). 23, 180–186.

Li, S., Stys, P.K., 2000. Mechanisms of ionotropic glutamate receptor-mediated excitotoxicity in isolated spinal cord white matter. J. Neurosci. 20, 1190–1198.

Libby, P., 2002. Inflammation in atherosclerosis. Nature 420, 868–874.

Liu, D.-Z., Tian, Y., Ander, B.P., Xu, H., Stamova, B.S., et al., 2010. Brain and blood microRNA expression profiling of ischemic stroke, intracerebral hemorrhage, and kainate seizures. J. Cereb. Blood Flow Metab. 30, 92–101.

Liu, P., Li, R., Antonov, A.A., Wang, L., Li, W., Hua, Y., et al., 2017. Discovery of metabolite biomarkers for acute ischemic stroke progression. J. Proteome Res. 16, 773–779. Available from: https://doi.org/10.1021/acs.jproteome.6b00779 [Epub ahead of print].

Loane, D.J., Stoica, B.A., Faden, A.I., 2015. Neuroprotection for traumatic brain injury. Handb. Clin. Neurol. 127, 343–366.

Long, G., Wang, F., Li, H., et al., 2013. Circulating miR-30a, miR-126 and let-7b as biomarker for ischemic stroke in humans. BMC Neurol. 13, 178.

Longhi, L., Perego, C., Ortolano, F., Zanier, E.R., Bianchi, P., et al., 2009. C1-inhibitor attenuates neurobehavioral deficits and reduces contusion volume after controlled cortical impact brain injury in mice. Crit. Care Med 37, 659–665.

Love, S., 1999. Oxidative stress in brain ischemia. Brain Pathol 9, 119–131.

Lucassen, P.J., Meerlo, P., Naylor, A.S., van Dam, A.M., Dayer, A.G., et al., 2010. Regulation of adult neurogenesis by stress, sleep disruption, exercise and inflammation: implications for depression and antidepressant action. Eur. Neuropsychopharmacol. 20, 1–17.

Lyketsos, C., 2006. Lessons from neuropsychiatry. J. Neuropsychiatry Clin. Neurosci. 18, 445–449.

Malkesman, O., Austin, D.R., Chen, G., Manji, H.K., 2009. Reverse translational strategies for developing animal models of bipolar disorder. Dis. Mod. Mech. 2, 238–245.

Marklund, N., Hillered, L., 2011. Animal modeling of traumatic brain injury in preclinical drug development: where do we go from here? Br. J. Pharmacol. 164, 1207–1229.

Marmarou, A., Foda, M.A., van den Brink, W., Campbell, J., Kita, H., et al., 1994. A new model of diffuse brain injury in rats. Part I: Pathophysiology and biomechanics. J. Neurosurg. 80, 291–300.

Martirosyan, N.L., Carotenuto, A., Patel, A.A., Kalani, M.Y., Yagmurlu, K., et al., 2016. The role of microRNA markers in the diagnosis, treatment, and outcome prediction of spinal cord injury. Front. Surg 3, 56.

Massai, L., Petricca, L., Magnoni, L., Rovetini, L., Haider, S., et al., 2013. Development of an ELISA assay for the quantification of soluble huntingtin in human blood cells. BMC Biochem. 14, 34.

Masson, P., Webster, A.C., Hong, M., Turner, R., Lindley, R.I., et al., 2015. Chronic kidney disease and the risk of stroke: a systematic review and meta-analysis. Nephrol. Dial. Transplant 30, 1162–1169.

McAllister, T.W., 2010. Genetic factors modulating outcome after neurotrauma. PM R 2 (12 Suppl. 2), S241–S252.

McCrory, P., Meeuwisse, W., Johnston, K., Dvorak, J., Aubry, M., Molloy, M., et al., 2009. Consensus statement on concussion in sport—the 3rd International Conference on Concussion in Sport held in Zurich, November 2008. Phys. Sportsmed. 37, 141–159.

McGoldrick, P., Joyce, P.I., Fisher, E.M.C., Greensmith, L., 2013. Rodent models of amyotrophic lateral sclerosis. Biochim. Biophys. Acta 1832, 1421–1436.

Meredith, G.E., Rademacher, D.J., 2011. MPTP mouse models of Parkinson's disease: an update. J. Parkinsons Dis. 1, 19–33.

Metz, G., Curt, A., van de Meent, H., Klusman, I., Schaw, M.E., Dietz, V., 2000. Validation of the weight-drop contusion model in rats: a comparative study of human spinal cord injury. J. Neurotrauma 17, 1–17.

Miyoshi, K., Morimura, Y., 2010. In: Miyosi, K., Morimura, Y., Maeda, K. (Eds.), Clinical Manifestations of Neuropsychiatric Disorders in Neuropsychiatric Disorders. Springer, New York, pp. 3–15.

Monnet-Tschudi, F., Zurich, M.G., Boschat, C., Corbaz, A., Honegger, P., 2006. Involvement of environmental mercury and lead in the etiology of neurodegenerative disease. Rev. Environ. Health. 21, 105–117.

Morales, D.M., Marklund, N., Lebold, D., Thompson, H.J., Pitkanen, A., et al., 2005. Experimental models of traumatic brain injury: do we really need to build a better mousetrap? Neuroscience 136, 971–989.

Moy, S.S., Nadler, J.J., 2008. Advances in behavioral genetics: mouse models of autism. Mol. Psychiatry 13, 4–26.

Namjoshi, D.R., Good, C., Cheng, W.H., Panenka, W., Richards, D., et al., 2013. Towards clinical management of traumatic brain injury: a review of models and mechanisms from a biomechanical perspective. Dis. Model. Mech. 6, 1325–1338.

Nestler, E.J., Hyman, S.E., 2010. Animal models of neuropsychiatric disorders. Nat. Neurosci 13, 1161–1169.

Nestler, E.J., Gould, E., Manji, H., Buncan, M., Duman, R.S., et al., 2002. Preclinical models: status of basic research in depression. Biol. Psychiatry 52, 503–528.

Nieto-Diaz, M., Esteban, F.J., Reigada, D., Muñoz-Galdeano, T., Yunta, M., et al., 2014. MicroRNA dysregulation in spinal cord injury: causes, consequences and therapeutics. Front. Cell. Neurosci. 8, 53.

Nordstrom, A., Edin, B.B., Lindstrom, S., Nordstrom, P., 2013. Cognitive function and other risk factors for mild traumatic brain injury in young men: nationwide cohort study. BMJ 346, f723.

Oei, H.H., van der Meer, I.M., Hofman, A., Koudstaal, P.J., Stijnen, T., et al., 2005. Lipoprotein-associated phospholipase A_2 activity is associated with risk of coronary heart disease and ischemic stroke: the Rotterdam study. Circulation 111, 570–575.

O'Keefe, L.M., Doran, S., Mwilambu-Tshilobo, Conti, L.H., Venna, V.R., et al., 2014. Social isolation after stroke leads to depressive-like behavior and decreased BDNF levels in mice. Behav. Brain Res 260, 162–170.

Ovbiagele, B., 2011. Chronic kidney disease and risk of death during hospitalization for stroke. J. Neurol. Sci. 301, 46–50.

Oyinbo, C.A., 2011. Secondary injury mechanisms in traumatic spinal cord injury: a nugget of this multiply cascade. Acta Neurobiol. Exp. (Wars) 71, 281–299.

Patel, S., 2014. Role of proteomics in biomarker discovery: prognosis and diagnosis of neuropsychiatric disorders. Adv. Protein Chem. Struct. Biol. 94, 39–75.

Petras, M., Tatarkova, Z., Kovalska, M., Mokra, D., Dobrota, D., et al., 2014. Hyperhomocysteinemia as a risk factor for the neuronal system disorders. J. Physiol. Pharmacol. 65, 15–23.

Petronilho, F., Feier, G., de Souza, B., Guglielmi, C., Constantino, L.S., et al., 2010. Oxidative stress in brain according to traumatic brain injury intensity. J. Surg. Res. 164, 316–320.

Polymeropoulos, M.H., et al., 1997. Mutation in the alpha-synuclein gene identified in families with Parkinson's disease. Science 276, 2045–2047.

Prins, M.L., Alexander, D., Giza, C.C., Hovda, D.A., 2013. Repeated mild traumatic brain injury: mechanisms of cerebral vulnerability. J. Neurotrauma 30, 30–38.

Quinones, M.P., Kaddurah-Daouk, R., 2009. Metabolomics tools for identifying biomarkers for neuropsychiatric diseases. Neurobiol. Dis. 35, 165–176.

Raghupathi, R., 2004. Cell death mechanisms following traumatic brain injury. Brain Pathol. 14, 215–222.

Ransohoff, R.M., Brown, M.A., 2012. Innate immunity in the central nervous system. J. Clin. Invest. 122, 1164–1171.

Rao, V.R., Parko, K.L., 2015. Clinical approach to posttraumatic epilepsy. Semin. Neurol. 35, 57–63.

Rivera, H.M., Christiansen, K.J., Sullivan, E.L., 2015. The role of maternal obesity in the risk of neuropsychiatric disorders. Front. Neurosci. 9, 194.

Rubinsztein, D.C., Leggo, J., Coles, R., Almqvist, E., Biancalana, V., et al., 1996. Phenotypic characterization of individuals with 30–40 CAG repeats in the Huntington disease (HD) gene reveals HD cases with 36 repeats and apparently normal elderly individuals with 36–39 repeats. Am. J. Hum. Genet. 59, 16–22.

Rueger, M.A., Backes, H., Walberer, M., Neumaier, B., Ullrich, R., et al., 2010. Noninvasive imaging of endogenous neural stem cell mobilization in vivo using positron emission tomography. J. Neurosci. 30, 6454–6460.

Rueger, M.A., Muesken, S., Walberer, M., Jantzen, S.U., Schnakenburg, K., et al., 2012. Effects of minocycline on endogenous neural stem cells after experimental stroke. Neuroscience 215, 174–183.

Rutland-Brown, W., Langlois, J.A., Thomas, K.E., Xi, Y.L., 2006. Incidence of traumatic brain injury in the United States, 2003. J. Head Trauma Rehabil. 21, 544–548.

Salinsky, M., Storzbach, D., Goy, E., Evrard, C., 2015. Traumatic brain injury and psychogenic seizures in veterans. J. Head Trauma Rehabil. 30, E65–E70.

Sanchez-Perales, C., Vazquez, E., Garcia-Cortes, M.J., Borrego, J., Polaina, M., et al., 2010. Ischaemic stroke in incident dialysis patients. Nephrol. Dial. Transplant 25, 3343–3348.

Saraceno, C., Musardo, S., Marcello, E., Pelucchi, S., Di Luca, M., 2013. Modeling Alzheimer's disease: from past to future. Front. Pharmacol. 4, 77.

Scheff, S.W., Rabchevsky, A.G., Fugaccia, I., Main, J.A., Lumpp Jr., J.E., 2003. Experimental modeling of spinal cord injury: characterization of a force-defined injury device. J. Neurotrauma 20, 179–193.

Schmitt, S., Dichter, M.A., 2015. Electrophysiologic recordings in traumatic brain injury. Handb. Clin. Neurol. 127, 319–339.

Schwulst, S.J., Trahanas, D.M., Saber, R., Perlman, H., 2013. Traumatic brain injury-induced alterations in peripheral immunity. J. Trauma Acute Care Surg. 75, 780–788.

Sekhon, L.H., Fehlings, M.G., 2001. Epidemiology, demographics, and pathophysiology of acute spinal cord injury. Spine 26 (24 Suppl.), S2–S12.

Sen, S., Duman, R., Sanacora, G., 2008. Serum brain-derived neurotrophic factor, depression, and antidepressant medications: meta-analyses and implications. Biol. Psychiatry 64, 527–532.

Sepramaniam, S., Tan, J.-R., Tan, K.-S., DeSilva, D.A., Tavintharan, S., et al., 2014. Circulating microRNAs as biomarkers of acute stroke. Int. J. Mol. Sci. 15, 1418–1432.

Shear, D.A., Tate, M.C., Archer, D.R., Hoffman, S.W., Hulce, V.D., Laplaca, M.C., et al., 2004. Neural progenitor cell transplants promote long-term functional recovery after traumatic brain injury. Brain Res. 1026, 11–22.

Shen, H., Yuan, Y., Ding, F., Hu, N., Liu, J., Gu, X., 2010. Achyranthes bidentata polypeptides confer neuroprotection through inhibition of reactive oxygen species production, Bax expression, and mitochondrial dysfunction induced by overstimulation of N-methyl-D-aspartate receptors. J. Neurosci. Res. 88, 669–676.

Shitaka, Y., Tran, H.T., Bennett, R.E., Sanchez, L., Levy, M.A., et al., 2011. Repetitive closed-skull traumatic brain injury in mice causes persistent multifocal axonal injury and microglial reactivity. J. Neuropathol. Exp. Neurol. 70, 551–567.

Shultz, S.R., MacFabe, D.F., Foley, K.A., Taylor, R., Cain, D.P., 2011. A single mild fluid percussion injury induces short-term behavioral and neuropathological changes in the Long-Evans rat: support for an animal model of concussion. Behav. Brain Res. 224, 326–335.

Simon, N.M., Smoller, J.W., McNamara, K.L., Maser, R.S., Zalta, A.K., et al., 2006. Telomere shortening and mood disorders: preliminary support for a chronic stress model of accelerated aging. Biol. Psychiatry 60, 432–435.

Skaper, S.D., Facci, L., Giusti, P., 2014. Mast cells glia and neuroinflammation: partners in crime? Immunology 141, 314–327.

Sofroniew, M.V., 2014. Multiple roles for astrocytes as effectors of cytokines and inflammatory mediators. Neuroscientist 20, 160–172.

Stahel, P.F., Shohami, E., Younis, F.M., Kariya, K., Otto, V.I., et al., 2000. Experimental closed head injury: analysis of neurological outcome, blood–brain barrier dysfunction, intracranial neutrophil infiltration, and neuronal cell death in mice deficient in genes for pro-inflammatory cytokines. J. Cerebral Blood Flow Metab. 20, 369–380.

Stanca, D.M., Mărginean, I.C., Soriţău, O., Mureşanu, D.F., 2015. Plasmatic markers for early diagnostic and treatment decisions in ischemic stroke. J. Med. Life 8, 21–25.

Steele, M.L., Fuller, S., Maczurek, A.E., Kersaitis, C., Ooi, L., et al., 2013. Chronic inflammation alters production and release of glutathione and related thiols in human U373 astroglial cells. Cell. Mol. Neurobiol. 33, 19–30.

Stoica, B.A., Faden, A.I., 2010. Cell death mechanisms and modulation in traumatic brain injury. Neurotherapeutics 7, 3–12.

Strokes, B.T., 1992. Experimental spinal cord injury: a dynamic and verifiable injury device. J. Neurotrauma 9, 129–134.

Sun, G.Y., Horrocks, L.A., Farooqui, A.A., 2007. The role of NADPH oxidase and phospholipases A2 in mediating oxidative and inflammatory responses in neurodegenerative diseases. J. Neurochem. 103, 1–16.

Sun, X., Jones, Z.B., Chen, X.M., Zhou, L., So, K.F., Ren, Y., 2016. Multiple organ dysfunction and systemic inflammation after spinal cord injury: a complex relationship. J. Neuroinflammation 13, 260.

Suo, Z., Wu, M., Ameenuddin, S., Anderson, H.E., Zoloty, J.E., et al., 2002. Participation of protease-activated receptor-1 in thrombin-induced microglial activation. J. Neurochem. 80, 655–666.

Suo, Z., Wu, M., Citron, B.A., Gao, C., Festoff, B.W., 2003. Persistent protease-activated receptor 4 signaling mediates thrombin-induced microglial activation. J. Biol. Chem. 278, 31177–31183.

Turner, R.J., Sharp, F.R., 2016. Implications of MMP9 for blood–brain barrier disruption and hemorrhagic transformation following ischemic stroke. Front. Cell. Neurosci. 10, 56.

Thompson, H.J., Lifshitz, J., Marklund, N., Grady, M.S., Graham, D.I., et al., 2005. Lateral fluid percussion brain injury: a 15-year review and evaluation. J. Neurotrauma 22, 42–75.

Tweedie, D., Rachmany, L., Rubovitch, V., Lehrmann, E., Zhang, Y., et al., 2013. Exendin-4, a glucagon-like peptide-1 receptor agonist prevents mTBI-induced changes in hippocampus gene expression and memory deficits in mice. Exp. Neurol. 239, 170–182.

US Renal Data System, 2009. USRDS 2009 Annual Data Report: Atlas of End-Stage Renal Disease in the United States. Bethseda, MD: National Institutes of Health. National Institute of Diabetes and Digestive and Kidney Diseases.

Valente, E.M., Abou-Sleiman, P.M., Caputo, V., Muqit, M.M., Harvey, K., et al., 2004. Hereditary early-onset Parkinson's disease caused by mutations in *PINK1*. Science 304, 1158–1160.

Van den Hove, D.L., Kompotis, K., Lardenoije, R., Kenis, G., Mill, J., Steinbusch, H.W., et al., 2014. Epigenetically regulated microRNAs in Alzheimer's disease. Neurobiol. Aging 35, 731–745.

van Middendorp, J.J., Goss, B., Urquhart, S., Atresh, S., Williams, R.P., et al., 2011. Diagnosis and prognosis of traumatic spinal cord injury. Global Spine J. 1, 1–8.

Varghese, F.P., Brown, E.S., 2001. The hypothalamic–pituitary–adrenal axis in major depressive disorder: a brief primer for primary care physicians. Prim. Care Companion J. Clin. Psychiatry 3, 151–155.

Vosler, P.S., Sun, D., Wang, S., Gao, Y., Kintner, D.B., et al., 2009. Calcium dysregulation induces apoptosis-inducing factor release: cross-talk between PARP-1- and calpain-signaling pathways. Exp. Neurol. 218, 213–220.

Wake, H., Moorhouse, A.J., Nabekura, J., 2012. Functions of microglia in the central nervous system—beyond the immune response. Neuron Glia Biol. 7, 47–53.

Walberer, M., Rueger, M.A., 2015. The macrosphere model—an embolic stroke model for studying the pathophysiology of focal cerebral ischemia in a translational approach. Ann. Transl. Med. 3, 123.

Walberer, M., Ritschel, N., Nedelmann, M., Volk, K., Mueller, C., et al., 2008. Aggravation of infarct formation by brain swelling in a large territorial stroke: a target for neuroprotection? J. Neurosurg. 109, 287–293.

Walberer, M., Backes, H., Rueger, M.A., Neumaier, B., Endepols, H., et al., 2012. Potential of early [(18)F]-2-fluoro-2-deoxy-D-glucose positron emission tomography for identifying hypoperfusion and predicting fate of tissue in a rat embolic stroke model. Stroke 43, 193–198.

Walberer, M., Jantzen, S.U., Backes, H., Rueger, M.A., Keuters, M.H., et al., 2014. In-vivo detection of inflammation and neurodegeneration in the chronic phase after permanent embolic stroke in rats. Brain Res. 1581, 80–88.

Wang, W.H., Guan, S., Zhang, L.Y., Lei, S., Zeng, Y.J., 2014a. Circulating microRNAs as novel potential biomarkers for early diagnosis of acute stroke in humans. J. Stroke Cerebrovasc. Dis. 23, 2607–2613.

Wang, H.H., Hung, S.Y., Sung, J.M., Hung, K.Y., Wang, J.D., et al., 2014b. Risk of stroke in long-term dialysis patients compared with the general population. Am. J. Kidney Dis. 63, 604–611.

Waters, R.J., Murray, G.D., Teasdale, G.M., Stewart, J., Day, I., et al., 2013. Cytokine gene polymorphisms and outcome after traumatic brain injury. J. Neurotrauma 30, 1710–1716.

Weaver, S.M., Portelli, J.N., Chau, A., Cristofori, I., Moretti, L., et al., 2014. Genetic polymorphisms and traumatic brain injury: the contribution of individual differences to recovery. Brain Imaging Behav. 8, 420–434.

Williams, A.J., Umemori, H., 2014. The best-laid plans go of awry: synaptogenic growth factor signaling in neuropsychiatric disease. Front. Synaptic Neurosci. 6, 4.

Williams, S.R., Yang, Q., Chen, F., Liu, X., Keene, K.L., et al., 2014. Genomics and Randomized Trials Network; Framingham Heart Study. Genome-wide meta-analysis of homocysteine and methionine metabolism identifies five one carbon metabolism loci and a novel association of ALDH1L1 with ischemic stroke. PLoS Genet. 10, e1004214.

Wilson, R.S., Arnold, S.E., Schneider, J.A., Li, Y., Bennett, D.A., 2007. Chronic distress, age-related neuropathology, and late-life dementia. Psychosom. Med. 69, 47−53.

Wohleb, E.S., 2016. Neuron−microglia interactions in mental health disorders: "For Better, and For Worse". Front. Immunol. 7, 544.

Wohleb, E.S., Delpech, J.C., 2016. Dynamic cross-talk between microglia and peripheral monocytes underlies stress-induced neuroinflammation and behavioral consequences. Prog. Neuropsychopharmacol. Biol. Psychiatry 79, 40−48. pii: S0278-5846(16)30059-8.

Wolff, M., Gibb, S.J., Cassel, J.-C., Dalrymple-Alford, J.C., 2008. Anterior but not intralaminar thalamic nuclei support allocentric spatial memory. Neurobiol. Learn. Mem. 90, 71−80.

Wolkowitz, O.M., Mellon, S.H., Epel, E.S., Lin, J., Dhabhar, F.S., et al., 2011. Leukocyte telomere length in major depression: correlations with chronicity, inflammation and oxidative stress—preliminary findings. PLoS ONE 6, e17837.

Xia, W., Yang, T., Shankar, G., Smith, I.M., Shen, Y., Walsh, D.M., et al., 2009. A specific enzyme-linked immunosorbent assay for measuring beta-amyloid protein oligomers in human plasma and brain tissue of patients with Alzheimer disease. Arch. Neurol. 66, 190−199.

Xie, A., Gao, J., Xu, L., Meng, D., 2014. Shared mechanisms of neurodegeneration in Alzheimer's disease and Parkinson's disease. Biomed. Res. Int. 648740.

Yokobori, S., Zhang, Z., Moghieb, A., Mondello, S., Gajavelli, S., et al., 2015. Acute diagnostic biomarkers for spinal cord injury: review of the literature and preliminary research report. World Neurosurg. 83, 867−878.

Yuan, Y.M., He, C., 2013. The glial scar in spinal cord injury and repair. Neurosci. Bull. 29, 421−435.

Yunta, M., Nieto-Díaz, M., Esteban, F.J., Caballero-López, M., et al., 2012. MicroRNA dysregulation in spinal cord following traumatic injury. PLoS ONE 7, e34534.

Zetterberg, H., Smith, D.H., Blennow, K., 2013. Biomarkers of mild traumatic brain injury in cerebrospinal fluid and blood. Nat. Rev. Neurol. 9, 201−210.

Zhang, N., Fang, M., Chen, H., Gou, F., Ding, M., 2014. Evaluation of spinal cord injury animal models. Neural Regen. Res. 9, 2008−2012.

Zohar, O., Schreiber, S., Getslev, V., Schwartz, J., Mullins, P., et al., 2003. Closed-head minimal traumatic brain injury produces long-term cognitive deficits in mice. Neuroscience 118, 949−955.

Zuo, L., Zhou, T., Pannell, B.K., Ziegler, A.C., Best, T.M., 2015. Biological and physiological role of reactive oxygen species—the good, the bad and the ugly. Acta Physiol 214, 329−348.

Molecular Aspects of Ischemic Injury

INTRODUCTION

Stroke is a complex vascular and neurological disorder, which leads to death and disability worldwide (Feigin et al., 2014). About 15 million people worldwide (Feigin et al., 2014) and 800,000 people in the United States suffer stroke each year (Mozaffarian et al., 2015). On average, in the United States every 40 seconds someone has a stroke and every 4 minutes someone dies from a stroke (Mozaffarian et al., 2015) suggesting that stroke is one of the major cause of death and adult disability in the United States. As stated in Chapter 1, Classification and Molecular Aspects of Neurotraumatic Diseases: Similarities and Differences With Neurodegenerative and Neuropsychiatric Diseases, stroke is a metabolic trauma caused by severe reduction or blockade in cerebral blood flow (CBF) due to the formation of a clot. This blockade not only decreases delivery of oxygen and glucose to the brain tissue, but also results in the breakdown of blood—brain barrier (BBB) and build-up of potentially toxic products in brain (Farooqui, 2010). In the Western world, most stroke (80%) are caused by the formation of blood clot in an artery (ischemic strokes) resulting in the interruption of blood flow and supply of nutrients (glucose and oxygen) to the brain, whereas in Asian countries majorities of strokes are caused by bursting (rupturing) of an artery (hemorrhagic stroke). Approximately 12% of strokes are hemorrhagic, whereas the remaining 88% are ischemic in nature. The cessation of cerebral blood circulation induces an immediate suppression of cerebral electrical activity with periinfarct depolarization leading to repeated episodes of metabolic stress (Farooqui, 2010). Males and females respond differently to stroke-mediated brain injury. Depending on age, the incidence, prevalence, mortality rate, and disability outcome of stroke-mediated neural injury differ between the sexes (Dotson and

Offner, 2017). Females generally have strokes at older ages than males and, therefore, have a worse stroke outcome. There are also major differences in how the sexes respond to stroke at the cellular level. Immune response is a critical factor in determining the progress of neurodegeneration after stroke and is fundamentally different for males and females (Dotson and Offner, 2017). Stroke-mediated injury (infarct) damages different neuronal population in the thalamus, hippocampus, and striate visual cortex (Savitz et al., 2003, 2004). Depending on areas of the brain which are affected, there are two types of ischemia: (1) global ischemia and (2) focal ischemia. Repression of blood supply to the entire brain causes global ischemia, while occlusion of certain cerebral blood vessels causes focal ischemia. An ischemic attack produces two distinguishable areas: the infarcted core, which is the region supplied by the occluded vessel; and the penumbra, which is the area between the lethally damaged core and normally perfused territory, which receives some collateral blood flow from unaffected vessels (Astrup et al., 1981; Hossmann, 1994). Neural cells within the ischemic core are often irreversibly damaged even if blood flow is reestablished. The ischemic penumbra, however, can be defined by a moderate reduction in CBF where collateral blood vessels provide neural cells with limited metabolic nutrients to temporarily maintain homeostasis during the initial stages of ischemia, but it is nonfunctional (Heiss et al., 2004). Mechanisms of neurodegeneration in ischemic core and penumbra are different (Smith, 2004). Necrosis and apoptosis, two major modes of cell death, are implicated in ischemia. Necrosis is predominant in core tissue, whereas both necrosis and apoptosis are dominant in the penumbra (Smith, 2004).

It should be noted that stroke-mediated injury in the left hemisphere has been reported to disturb language and comprehension, which reduce the ability to communicate (Pirmoradi et al., 2016). In contrast, stroke on the right hemisphere affects the intuitive thinking, reasoning, solving problems as well as the perception, judgment and the visual—spatial functions could be impaired (Sun et al., 2014; Harris et al., 2015; Tiozzo et al., 2015; Save-Pédebos et al., 2016). Different brain regions are more sensitive to stroke-mediated neuronal injury than others. The white matter is more resilient to ischemic injury than gray matter (Mattson et al., 2001). In addition, certain populations of neurons are selectively more vulnerable to ischemic injury than other neurons. For example, in the hippocampus, CA1 pyramidal neurons are highly susceptible to ischemic injury, whereas dentate granule neurons are more resistant (Mattson et al., 2001).

Stroke-mediated brain injury also exerts a potent suppressive effect on lymphoid organs, which promotes intercurrent infections, a major determinant of stroke morbidity and mortality (Meisel et al., 2005;

Urra et al., 2009). Therefore the immune system is closely related to critical events determining the fate of the ischemic brain and the survival of stroke patients. Thus the molecular events caused by cerebral ischemia not only activate components of innate immunity, but also promote inflammatory signaling that contributes to brain damage. Inflammatory signaling contributes to early molecular events triggered by the arterial occlusion and culminating in the invasion of the brain by blood-borne leukocytes. Regardless of molecular mechanism of stroke, brain tissue is highly susceptible to oxidative stress. Brain consumes large amount of oxygen and glucose to perform its functions and meet its energy demands. In addition, it contains high concentrations of polyunsaturated fatty acids, which are vulnerable to lipid peroxidation. Moreover, brain has lower antioxidant capacity as compared to other organs in the body. Neurons are particularly vulnerable to oxidative damage in stroke-affected brain tissue due to lower levels of endogenous antioxidant, glutathione, as compared to resident glial cells (Cooper and Kristal, 1997). The main symptoms of cerebral ischemia are sudden loss of consciousness, blindness, and coordination defects, including speaking problems. The size and location of infarct is an important determinant of the long-term functional deficits resulting from ischemic stroke. The initial response to stroke is the decrease in ATP along with depolarization resulting in Na^+ influx into axons. Prolonged decrease in ATP and release of glutamate produces the overstimulation of glutamate receptors resulting in a massive influx of Ca^{2+} through the plasma membrane. This facilitates neural cell death through the stimulation of Ca^{2+}-dependent enzymes. These processes result in the stimulation of proteolysis, lipolysis, and mitochondrial dysfunction (Farooqui and Horrocks, 1994, 2007) (Fig. 2.1). Multiple mechanisms contribute to mitochondrial dysfunction during and after ischemia. Mitochondrial electron transport constitutively results in production of reactive oxygen species (ROS), including superoxide radicals and hydrogen peroxide, under normal physiological conditions along with activation of nitric oxide synthase (NOS) activity leading to oxidative and nitrosative stress causing neurodegeneration and irreversible loss of neurologic function not only through the breakdown of cellular and subcellular integrity, but also through alterations in redox, and free-radical generation (Farooqui, 2010). These processes involve the activation of Ca^{2+} dependent enzymes (phospholipases A_2, C, and D (PLA$_2$, PLC, and PLD), calcium/calmodulin-dependent kinases (CaMKs), mitogen-activated protein kinases (MAPKs) such as extracellular signal-regulated kinase (ERK), p38, and c-Jun N-terminal kinase (JNK), NOSs, calpains, calcineurin, and endonucleases). Stimulation of these enzymes brings them in contact with appropriate substrates and modulates cell survival/degeneration mechanisms (Farooqui and Horrocks, 2007). Some of these

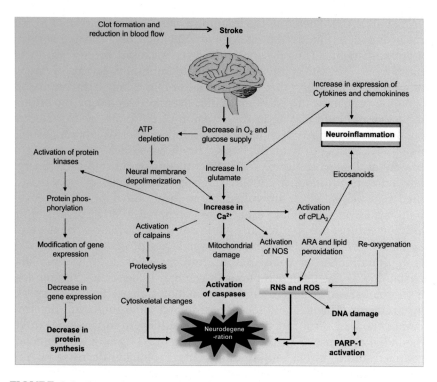

FIGURE 2.1   Neurochemical processes contributing to stroke-mediated injury in the brain.

enzymes generate proinflammatory and proapoptotic lipid metabolites, while others produce antiinflammatory and antiapoptotic products. Under normal conditions, NF-κB resides in the cytoplasm as an inactive complex bound by inhibitor proteins, Iκ-Bα and Iκ-Bβ. In response to ischemic injury, Iκ-B is either phosphorylated by Iκ-B kinase or activated by ROS. Both these processes promote the translocation of NF-κB to the nucleus, where it binds to NF-κB response element (NF-κB-RE). This binding promotes the expression of proinflammatory cytokines and chemokines. Cytokines and chemokines serve as chemical messengers. Generation of proinflammatory cytokines and chemokines facilitates neuroinflammation after the stroke-mediated neuronal injury (Fig. 2.2) (Farooqui et al., 2007; Marchesi et al., 2008). ROS can directly promote inflammation through the induction of inducible nitric oxide synthase (iNOS). This enzyme produces large amounts of nitric oxide (NO), which alter vascular structure and function through nitration and nitrosylation of critical proteins (Gunnett et al., 2005; Lima et al., 2010). Superoxide reacts with NO to produce peroxynitrite (ONOO⁻), a potent

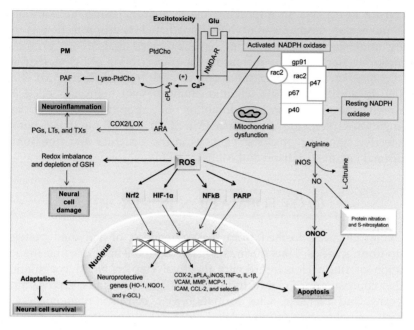

FIGURE 2.2 Sources of ROS generation in the brain and activation of transcription factors that contribute to neurodegeneration in stroke. *ARA*, arachidonic acid; *COX-2*, cyclooxygenase-2; *cPLA₂*, cytosolic phospholipase A₂; *γ-GCL*, γ-glutamylcystein ligase; *Glu*, glutamate; *HIF-1α*, hypoxia-inducible factor-1α; *HO-1*, heme oxygenase 1; *IL-1β*, interleukin-1β; *iNOS*, inducible nitric oxide synthase; *LOX*, lipoxygenase; *lyso-PtdCho*, lysophosphatidylcholine; *MMP*, matrix metalloproteinase; *NADH* quinine oxidoreductase; *NF-κB*, nuclear factor-kappaB; *NMDA-R*, N-Methyl-D-aspartic acid receptor; *NO*, nitric oxide; *Nrf2*, nuclear factor erythroid 2–related factor 2; *ONOO⁻*, peroxynitrite; *PAF*, platelet activating factor; *PARP*, poly (ADP-ribose) polymerase; *PM*, plasma membrane; *PtdCho*, phosphatidylcholine; *SPLA₂*, secretory phospholipase A₂; *TNF-α*, tumor necrosis factor-α; *VCAM*, vascular cell adhesion molecule.

nitrating agent, which causes nitration and alters vasomotor reactivity by inactivating critical endothelial and smooth muscle enzymes, and by activating the DNA repair enzyme poly-ADP-ribose polymerase leading to ATP depletion and vascular ion channel dysfunction (Pacher et al., 2007). Another potential mechanism NO-mediated damage is modification of protein groups by NO. NO covalently attaches itself to cysteine residues forming S-nitroso-thiol derivatives. This posttranslational modification significantly impacts cell survival by altering the function of critical regulatory proteins such as caspases and metalloproteases (Gu et al., 2002), and the glycolytic enzyme GAPDH (Nakamura and Lipton, 2009). These observations strongly suggest that oxidative stress, neuroinflammation, and vascular inflammation are major pathways that exert deleterious effects on the brain and blood vessels.

NF-κB also plays an important role in neuronal survival. Although, the molecular mechanism of NF-κB-mediated neuroprotection is not fully understood, recent studies have indicated that NF-κB promotes neuroprotection either by increasing the transcription of Bcl-xL (Sarnico et al., 2009) or by inducing antiapoptotic gene transcription (Pizzi et al., 2009). In addition, NF-κB activation may prevent neuronal cell death through the induction of inhibitor of apoptosis proteins and manganese-superoxide dismutase (Mn-SOD). NF-κB-mediated neuroprotective signaling produces changes in the structure and function of neuronal circuits (Mattson and Meffert, 2006).

CLOT FORMATION IN STROKE

Blood clots are formed from the aggregation of activated platelets onto fibrin meshes. Thus fibrin is a major component of clot and the formation of fibrin clots represents the final step in blood coagulation. Other components of clot include proteins, phospholipids, glycosaminoglycans, and platelets. Clot formation is a complex phenomenon in which a combination of interrelated biochemical and hemodynamic factors result in several cascade reactions causing platelet activation, deposition, aggregation, and stabilization (Lu et al., 2015; Liang et al., 2015; Wu et al., 2017). The complexity is accentuated by several feed-forward and feedback mechanisms promoting and inhibiting coagulation reactions. Therefore a comprehensive description of thrombus formation requires a model which can account for interrelated reactions involving platelet activation and aggregation, transport of platelets and chemical species in flow, and the interaction between the formed thrombus and the flow field (Sorensen et al., 1999; Fogelson et al., 2012; Kuharsky and Fogelson, 2001). Clot formation is modulated by genetic and environmental factors. These factors modulate fibrin structure in relation to thrombosis. Fibrin clots are composed of compact, highly branched networks with thin fibers. These clots are resistant to lysis. Alterations in fibrin structure have been reported in patients with several diseases including patients with acute or prior myocardial infarction, ischemic stroke, and venous thromboembolism (Lu et al., 2015). Relatives of patients with myocardial infarction or venous thromboembolism display similar fibrin abnormalities. Low-dose aspirin, statins, lowering of homocysteine, better diabetes control, smoking cessation, and suppression of inflammatory response increase clot permeability and susceptibility to lysis. Growing evidence indicates that abnormal fibrin properties represent a novel risk factor for arterial and venous thrombotic events, particularly of unknown etiology in young and middle-aged patients (Lu et al., 2015).

SOURCES OF ROS FORMATION IN STROKE-MEDIATED INJURY

Mitochondria are not only the powerhouse of the cell, but also a major source of cellular ROS (Boveris and Chance, 1973). They contain a number of enzymes that convert molecular oxygen to either superoxide or hydrogen peroxide. Under normal conditions, superoxides are scavenged either by copper/zinc-SOD (Cu/ZN-SOD or SOD-1), or by manganese-superoxide dismutase (Mn-SOD or SOD-2), which are localized in between the inner and outer mitochondrial membranes and mitochondrial matrix, respectively. These SODs dismutate superoxide to less reactive hydrogen peroxide, which can be further metabolized to water and oxygen by the catalytic activity of catalase and glutathione peroxidase. Mitochondrial uncoupling proteins also support the reduction in the production of ROS by causing mitochondrial depolarization, which reduces the potential driving electron transfer and by allowing protons to reenter the matrix, thereby bypassing ATP synthase (Kim-Han and Dugan, 2005; Hermes et al., 2016). The inner mitochondrial membrane contains the respiratory chain, which is the most important source of the intracellular ROS generation. It is estimated that 95% of ROS generated in normal (i.e., nonischemic) cells are derived from electron leak from the respiratory chain enzyme complexes (Turrens, 1997). The proton motive force is the potential energy driving proton movement into the mitochondrial matrix for ATP formation. It represents an electrochemical gradient that consists of a mitochondrial membrane potential and a proton gradient, which represent sources for mitochondrial ROS generation via electron transfer to oxygen. Other sources of ROS production in the brain include NADPH oxidases (NOX), and cyclooxygenases/lipoxygenases (COX/LOX). NADPH oxidase is present in the cytoplasm in a resting form in neurons and inflammatory cells (McCann et al., 2008). In stroke, the increase in cytosolic Ca^{2+} activates NOX, through protein kinase C (PKC) and NO derived from neuronal NOS (Girouard et al., 2009). Resting NADPH oxidase is located in the cytoplasm. Activation of this enzyme results in its translocation to plasma membrane, where it promotes ROS production (Sun et al., 2007). Another source of ROS is COX/LOX activity. These enzymes contribute to ROS production after the onset of uncontrolled ARA cascade (Farooqui, 2010). ARA is also metabolized to 4-hydroxynonenal (4-HNE). This metabolite impairs the activities of Na^+, K^+-ATPase, glucose 6-phosphate dehydrogenase, and several kinases, including JNK and p38 mitogen-activated protein kinase (p38MAPK) (Mark et al., 1997; Camandola et al., 2000). The impairment of Na^+, K^+-ATPase depolarizes neuronal membranes leading to the opening of NMDA receptor channels and influx of additional Ca^{2+} into neurons. Lysophosphatidylcholine is the other product of PLA_2 catalyzed reaction. This metabolite is converted to platelet activating factor (PAF) through acetylation. This lipid mediator contributes to neuroinflammation (Fig. 2.2). Furthermore, Ca^{2+} overload also depolarizes mitochondrial membranes (Girouard et al., 2009) producing large amounts of superoxide. Converging evidence suggests that in stroke, mitochondria not only generate ROS in the initial stage, but also contribute to ROS production during reperfusion stage. In addition, mitochondria contribute to apoptotic cell death in penumbra through the release of cytochrome c from mitochondrial membranes. Endoplasmic reticulum (ER) also contributes to stroke-mediated injury. ER not only mediates proteins processing, but also modulates intracellular calcium homeostasis and neural cell death signal activation. ER dysfunction occurs at an early stage after ischemic injury and may be the initial step in apoptotic cascades in neurons (Hayashi and Abe, 2004; Roussel et al., 2013). Other sources of ROS are invading neutrophils, activated microglia/macrophages, and cerebral blood vessels (Miller et al., 2006). It is also shown that neurons themselves generate large amounts of superoxide following transient stroke, an effect that may contribute to the progression of injury over time (Miller et al., 2006).

Many studies have demonstrated that ischemic injury causes changes in the nucleus through the involvement of DNA methylation process and DNA methyltransferases (DNMT) inhibitors can alleviate ischemia or oxidative stress-induced neural injury. In vivo, the global DNA methylation was significantly increased in infarcted tissue in model of cerebral ischemia (Endres et al., 2000, 2001). Converging evidence suggests that the role of DNA methylation in cerebral ischemia is multifaceted process, with genome-wide and gene-specific effects that control the vulnerability of the brain to ischemic injury. As stated earlier, following middle cerebral artery occlusion (MCAO) in mice, DNA methylation levels are increased in ischemic brain tissue and may be responsible for promoting cell death (Endres et al., 2000, 2001). Thus the treatment with broad-spectrum DNMT inhibitor 5-aza-2'-deoxycytidine (5-aza-dC) and zebularine (Endres et al., 2000), as well as reduced levels of DNMT1 in postmitotic neurons in transgenic mice (Endres et al., 2001), can alleviate cerebral ischemic injury. Furthermore, transgenic mice with reduced levels of neuronal DNMT1 exhibit significantly smaller infarcts following MCAO, compared with control animals. In contrast, mice without neuronal DNMT1 are not protected from cerebral ischemia. These observations support the view that the dynamic modulation of DNMT expression and the status of DNA methylation represent important mechanisms for preventing cell death in cerebral ischemia. Except for DNMTs, the expression of methyl-CpG-binding-domain (MBD)-family proteins is altered orderly within the hippocampus: MBD3 expression is significantly reduced to 3 hours after ischemia, while MBD2 expression is increased by 6 hours after ischemia, and MBD1 and MeCP2 levels are both elevated by 24 hours after ischemia (Jung et al., 2002). It is well known that histones wrap around DNA to form the nucleosome, and a variety of histone-modifying enzymes change the DNA conformation, leading to repositioning of nucleosomes, activating or preventing transcription (Kouzarides, 2007; Wang et al., 2012a). The modifications are largely reversible and allow dynamic gene expression changes in response to the cellular environment producing neuroprotective effects. Studies on pretreatment with the HDAC inhibitor, trichostatin A (TSA) have demonstrated that TSA protects against oxygen/glucose deprivation (OGD) in primary cortical neurons by enhancing histone acetylation in the promoter region of gelsolin, a pivotal mediator of actin-filament assembly—disassembly, in dose- and time-dependent manners (Meisel et al., 2006). The transcription factors Sp1 and Nrf2 contribute to the antioxidant-responsive function of HDACi. TSA through the acetylation of Sp1 transcription factor induces the expression of Catalase, Mn-SOD and p21 waf1/cip1, a cyclin-dependent kinase inhibitor. This process mitigates the glutamate-mediated oxidative neurodegeneration in vitro and 3-nitroproprionic acid-mediated neuronal death in vivo (Ryu et al., 2014). Nrf2 mediates neuroprotection in stroke through the inhibition of HDAC. Thus process involves Nrf2-mediated expression of the Keap1 and translocation of Nrf2 into the nucleus, where it promotes the expression of heme oxygenase 1 (HO-1), glutamate-cysteine ligase catalytic subunit (GCLC), and NAD(P)H:quinone oxidoreductase 1 (NQO1) in neuronal cultures and brain tissue (Wang et al., 2012a). Stroke also produces nitric oxide-mediated DNA fragmentation in neurons that would die later, but whether this is the cause or merely the result of the ischemic insult remains uncertain (Hayashi and Abe, 2004). Ischemic stroke also exerts a potent suppressive effect on lymphoid organs, which promotes intercurrent infections, a major cause of stroke-mediated morbidity and mortality (Meisel et al., 2005; Urra et al., 2009; Farooqui, 2010). Therefore, the immune system plays important roles not only in damaging neurons through neuroinflammatory processes, but also promoting brain repair through the release of growth factors in stroke patient. Thus the molecular events caused by cerebral ischemia not only activate components of innate immunity, but also promote inflammatory signaling that contributes to brain damage.

NEUROCHEMICAL CHANGES IN ISCHEMIC/REPERFUSION INJURY

Following ischemic injury, reperfusion is essential for neural cell survival. Reestablishing the blood supply to ischemic brain not only provides oxygen and glucose, but also delivers other blood-borne formed elements (platelets and leukocytes), which become activated and establish adhesive interactions with the cerebral arterial walls and neural cells (Fig. 2.3). Upon transmigration into the brain, these activated leukocytes (neutrophils, monocytes, and lymphocyte) along with astrocytes and microglial cells release their cytotoxic arsenal of ROS to exacerbate brain damage. ROS damage neural cells via a number of mechanisms including peroxidation of cell membrane and organelle lipids, oxidizing DNA, activation of matrix metalloproteinases (MMPs), calpains, and promoting opening of the mitochondrial permeability transition pore. The molecular mechanism of brain damage involves changes at both cellular and molecular levels. The activity of iNOS is incurred by cerebral ischemia. Subsequently, this leads to the production of nitric oxide, which after interaction with superoxide ($O_2^{\bullet-}$) or free iron generates peroxynitrite ($ONOO^-$), peroxyl radicals ($LOO^\bullet$), and hydroxyl radicals ($^\bullet OH$). Each of the above-mentioned free radical is capable of producing even more cellular damage than superoxide or hydrogen peroxide. Both NO and superoxide not only facilitate lipid peroxidation, DNA damage and protein modification promoting

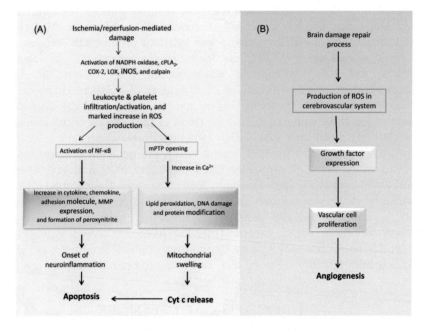

FIGURE 2.3 Neurochemical processes associated with reperfusion (A) and neural cell survival (B). *COX-2*, cyclooxygenase; *iNOS*, inducible nitric oxide synthase; *LOX*, lipoxygenase; *MMP*, matrix metalloproteinase; *mPTP*, membrane permeability transition pore; *NF-κB*, nuclear factor-kappaB; *PLA₂*, phospholipase A₂.

necrosis, but also upregulate p53 protein inducing apoptosis. As stated earlier, oxygen-derived ROS also act to enhance the inflammatory response to reperfusion via formation of oxidant-dependent proinflammatory mediators and upregulation of cytokine/chemokine and adhesion molecule expression (Fig. 2.3). Thus, while following ischemic injury, there is cellular demand for replenishment of oxygen which is met by reestablishing the blood supply, the reintroduction of molecular oxygen to the tissues results in ROS formation that is detrimental to the reperfused brain tissue. In addition, generation of ROS during reperfusion also promotes brain repair and neural cell survival (Fig. 2.3) through the involvement of growth factors. These growth factors (nerve growth factor (NGF) and brain-derived neurotrophic factor (BDNF)) not only promote angiogenesis in cerebral arteries and neurogenesis in the brain, but also induce neural cell proliferation and differentiation and activation of MMPs. These enzymes are not only involved in diverse homeostatic, but also in pathological processes. In contrast, angiogenesis is the key step for recovery of brain tissue after stroke. In penumbral regions, increase in microvessel density has been observed in human patients (Krupinski et al., 1993). In at least one study, the number of new vessels appeared to be related to longer survival times in young ischemic stroke patients, supporting the view that active angiogenesis may be beneficial (Krupinski et al., 1994). In contrast, older patients who tend to do worse after stroke (Granger et al., 1992) seem to have reduced new vessel formation (Szpak et al., 1999) indicating that angiogenesis may improve cerebral perfusion and function as part of a network repair. The molecular mechanisms associated with abovementioned processes are not fully understood. However, it is proposed that NGF and BDNF promote cellular survival via their primary receptors TrkA and TrkB, respectively. But in contrast to these neuroprotective effects, both factors can also be neurotoxic via overactivation of the p75NTR receptor (Blochl and Blochl, 2007).

Reperfusion also produces neurochemical changes in the nucleus. Reperfusion reduces phosphorylation at Ser 394 of HDAC2, and weakens the HDAC2-FOXO3a reciprocity in mouse brain tissue. Moreover, H_2O_2, which is generated during reperfusion decreases the HDAC2-FOXO3a interaction in cerebellar granule neurons, leading to the increase in histone H4K16 acetylation in the promoter region of p21. This results in upregulation of its expression. It is shown that epigenetic regulation of FOXO3a-mediated gene expression during oxidative stress produces neuronal cell death, which can be for developing treatment for the stroke (Peng et al., 2015). In addition, H_2O_2 treatment promotes the translocation of HDAC4 from the cytoplasm into the nucleus in cultured cortical neurons, where it interacted physically with peroxisome proliferator-activated receptor-γ and represses its transcriptional activity and inhibited its prosurvival activity, thus regulating neuronal death (Yang et al., 2011).

BBB is barrier, which is composed of highly specialized cerebrovascular endothelial cells, seals brain tissue from the circulating blood. It prevents blood, bacteria, or toxins entering the brain. Another essential role of the BBB is to establish a stable ionic microenvironment that ensures appropriate firing of neurons and action potential propagation. Following ischemic injury, the BBB integrity is compromised for days to even weeks and leading to permeability of previously excluded blood-borne molecules and inflammatory cells (Strbian et al., 2008; Engelhardt and Sorokin, 2009). Ischemic brain injury is accompanied by a cascade of microvascular events contributing to the accumulation of fibrin, transmigration of leukocytes (neutrophil granulocytes, macrophages, and T-cells), generation of degrading enzymes, basal laminae breakdown with loss of astrocyte and endothelial cell contacts leading to vasogenic edema and potential hemorrhagic transformation (Strbian et al., 2008; Engelhardt and Sorokin, 2009). Induction of edema not only contributes to impedance in adequate perfusion to the affected tissue bed, but also results in local compression of microcirculation producing further perfusion deficits, a rise in intracranial pressure, and dislocation of parts of the brain (Durukan and Tatlisumak, 2007; Bektas et al., 2010). In response to cerebral vascular compromise after stroke, the brain tissue makes attempts to regenerate and restore of the BBB through vascular remodeling. Sprouting of new endothelial cells from preexisting vessels is a process referred to as angiogenesis, a process, which is controlled by growth factors (vascular endothelial growth factor, platelet-derived endothelial cell growth factor, fibroblast growth factors, and epidermal growth factor), MMPs, cytokines, and integrins (Risau, 1997; Plate, 1999). Converging evidence indicates that following ischemia/reperfusion in penumbra, neural cells are injured not only by the toxic effects of oxidative and nitrosative stress on the neurovascular unit, but also by the inhibition of astrocytic repair (Farooqui, 2010; Burrows et al., 2015).

MOLECULAR ASPECTS OF NEUROINFLAMMATION IN STROKE

Neuroinflammation is a complex host defense mechanism that isolates the damaged brain tissue from uninjured area, destroys injured cells, and repairs the extracellular matrix (ECM; Amantea et al., 2015). However, uncontrolled neuroinflammation plays a major role in the pathogenesis of various neurological disorders including stroke and neurodegenerative diseases. Two types of neuroinflammation (acute and chronic) have been reported to occur in human brain. Acute neuroinflammation, which develops rapidly after stroke, is beneficial to damage repair in the nervous system, whereas chronic neuroinflammation, which develops slowly, aggravates the pathological events occurring in the brain (Farooqui, 2014). Induction of neuroinflammation is supported by microglial cells and astrocytes to reestablish homeostasis in the brain after injury-mediated disequilibrium of normal physiology. Microglia are key modulators of the immune response and neuroinflammation in the brain. They are considered the resident immune cell of the brain. Under normal conditions, microglia are primarily involved in activity-dependent synaptic pruning and repair (Farooqui, 2014). After stroke, microglial cells undergo rapid morphologic transformation from a ramified resting state, which is characterized by many branching processes, to an active, motile amoeboid state, where they become virtually indistinguishable from circulating macrophages (Saijo and Glass, 2011; Farooqui, 2014). Active microglia can then phagocytose not only foreign organisms, but also injured brain cells (Lai and Todd, 2006; Farooqui, 2014). As stated earlier, microglial cells release soluble mediators, including cytokines, prostaglandins, oxygen and nitrogen species, proteases, and nitric oxide, which reciprocally influence and modulate neuronal function such as neuroplasticity and cognitive function. Low levels of IL-1β are required for long-term potentiation (LTP), while basal levels of TNFα are necessary for proper homeostatic trafficking of AMPA and GABA$_A$ receptors for synaptic scaling (Stellwagen and Malenka, 2006; Denes et al., 2007; Wang et al., 2007; Farooqui et al., 2007; Delpech et al., 2015). Based on these studies, it is suggested that microglia-mediated cytokine and prostaglandin synthesis can modulate neuronal responses during physiological and pathological conditions. Further studies indicate that microglia-derived cytokines can indirectly affect neurons through gliotransmission mediated by astrocytes (Santello and Volterra, 2012). In addition, ATP released by microglia has been shown to induce glutamate release by astrocytes thereby acutely exciting proximal neurons (Pascual et al., 2012). These indirect signaling pathways may be further augmented during inflammatory conditions. Other studies have shown that microglia can support adaptive synaptic plasticity through the release of neurotrophic factors, such as BDNFs (Parkhurst et al., 2013), supporting the view that microglial cell activation can be beneficial for producing BDNF and clearing away dead tissue and debris after ischemia. Converging evidence suggests that following stroke, microglial cells produce chemoattractants (cytokines and chemokines), reactive oxygen and nitrogen species, proteases, and nitric oxide (Denes et al., 2007; Wang et al., 2007; Farooqui et al., 2007), with the subsequent infiltration of blood-derived cells (leukocytes)

(Jin et al., 2010; Iadecola and Anrather, 2011; Kim et al., 2016) (Table 2.1). The infiltration of leukocytes involves three major steps (rolling, adhesion, and transendothelial migration). These steps facilitate the access of leukocytes to the brain through the endothelial wall. Activated leukocytes, especially neutrophils, result in further damage of ischemic lesions through reperfusion or secondary injury mechanisms (Guha and Mackman, 2001). The interaction between leukocytes and the vascular endothelium is mediated by three main groups of cell adhesion molecules (CAMs): selectins (P-selectin, E-selectin, and L-selectin), the immunoglobulin superfamily (intercellular adhesion molecules, e.g., ICAM-1, 2 and vascular cell adhesion molecule-1 or VCAM-1) and integrins (CD11a−c) (DeGraba, 1998; Emsley and Tyrrell, 2002). Several studies have indicated that inhibition of leukocyte adhesion by targeting various adhesion molecules may prevent leukocytes from entering ischemic brain and resulting in reduction in the extent of neurologic injury (Clark et al., 1997).

Activation of microglia following ischemia/reperfusion injury also contributes to the resolution of inflammation, by releasing IL-10 and tumor growth factor (TGF)-β, and to the late reparative processes by

TABLE 2.1   Effects of Stroke on Activities of Microglial Cells and Astrocytes

Cell Types	Detrimental Effects	Beneficial Effects
Astrocytes	Expression of TNF-α, IL-1 and MMPs. Development of edema, inhibition of axon regeneration and disruption of BBB	Extracellular glutamate uptake, synthesis and release of neurotrophic factors, rebuilding of BBB, and neurovascular unit
Microglial cells	M-1 phenotype: production of proinflammatory cytokines, including TNF-α and IL-1β, production of ROS and RNS, and proteases, such as MMPs	M-2 phenotype: resolution of inflammation (IL-10 and TGF-β release, production of arginase and phagocytic activity). Late reparative processes by producing growth factors (IGF-1, brain-derived neurotrophic factor and glial cell line-derived neurotrophic factor)
Neutrophils	Microvessel obstruction, ROS production and release of MMPs that contribute to BBB damage and exacerbate inflammation	N2 phenotype: promote resolution of inflammation
Dendritic cells	Upregulation of MHCII and costimulatory molecules that prompt activation of lymphocytes	

BBB, blood−brain barrier; IGF-1, insulin/insulin-like growth factor-1; IL-10, interleukin-10; MHCII, MHC class II molecules; MMP, matrix metalloproteinase; RNS, reactive nitrogen species; ROS, reactive oxygen species; TGF-β, tumor growth factor-β.

phagocytic activity and growth factors production. Indeed, after ischemia, microglia/macrophages differentiate toward several phenotypes: the M1 proinflammatory phenotype is classically activated via toll-like receptors (TLRs) or interferon-γ, whereas M2 phenotypes are alternatively activated by regulatory mediators, such as ILs 4, 10, 13, or TGF-β. Thus immune cells exert a dualistic role on the evolution of ischemic brain damage, since the classic phenotypes promote injury, whereas alternatively activated M2 macrophages or N2 neutrophils prompt tissue remodeling and repair. After stroke, microglia are rapidly activated by ATP, which is released by damaged neurons and other glial cells (Table 2.1). This ATP interacts with P2X7 receptors to prompt production and the release of proinflammatory cytokines and chemokines (Denes et al., 2007). Stimulation of microglia also relies on TLR4 stimulation, fractalkine receptor (CX3CR1) modulation, and/or reduced CD200 receptor stimulation evoked by ischemia-induced disturbance of neuron-microglia cross-talk (Dénes et al., 2008; Dentesano et al., 2012). Moreover, the increased release of specific neurotransmitters, such as glutamate and γ-aminobutyric acid, may elicit an inflammatory or a neuroprotective phenotype in microglia by signaling through NOX (Mead et al., 2012).

In the brain astrocytes play several important roles, such as regulating the external environment of neurons, participating in the physical structuring of the brain, providing metabolites to neurons, maintaining ionic balance, modulating neurotransmission (Clarke and Barres, 2013; Ouyang et al., 2014), and maintaining the BBB integrity. During stroke, astrocytes have the potential to either protect neurons via abovementioned mechanisms, or exacerbate injury not only by secreting glutamate and proinflammatory molecules, but also by promoting edema formation (Pekny and Nilsson, 2005; Nagai et al., 2007). In addition, normal astrocytes protect neurons against oxidative stress and excitotoxicity (Khakh and Sofroniew, 2015). Astrocytes are also capable of directly transferring the healthy mitochondria to neurons, and that suppression of this transfer worsens injury following cerebral ischemia. Astrocyte "activation" and glial scar formation postinjury have traditionally been considered detrimental to stroke recovery, but reactive astrocytes have been demonstrated to have the capacity to promote neuroplasticity via secretion of neurotrophic factors (BDNF and TDF), cholesterol, and thrombospondins (Liu and Chopp, 2015). It is also reported that astrocytes within the hippocampus CA1 are more sensitive to ischemic injury, and with a higher degree of mitochondrial dysfunction compared to dentate gyrus astrocytes, and that disruption of mitochondrial homeostasis in local astrocytes following cerebral ischemia contributes to CA1 neuronal cell death (Ouyang et al., 2007, 2013a,b). Collective evidence supports a potential role of mitochondria in neuronal-astrocyte communication, and position astrocytes as central for maintenance of neuronal metabolism and bioenergetics in response to cell stress and recovery from stroke (Turrens, 1997).

After the ischemic injury, perivascular astrocytes release cytokines and activate metalloproteases (MMPs), a zinc-endopeptidases. These processes contribute to BBB disruption and vasogenic edema, whereas at later stages, they provide neuroprotection through the uptake of extracellular glutamate, BBB regeneration, and neurotrophic factors release (Amantea et al., 2010; Rossi et al., 2007; del Zoppo, 2009). The release of MMP also disrupts ECM among neural cells. Ischemic injury-mediated activation of astrocytes in the brain increases the expression of glial fibrillary acidic protein leading to reactive gliosis, which is characterized by specific neurochemical, structural, and functional changes (Pekny and Nilsson, 2005) such as the increased production of intermediate filament proteins (also known as nanofilament proteins) and remodeling of the intermediate filament system of astrocytes. Activation of astrocytes following ischemic injury contributes to the expression of many genes and characteristic morphological changes involved in stroke-mediated injury. Activation of astrocytes following stroke also participate in neuroinflammation by expressing major histocompatibility complex (MHC) and costimulatory molecules, developing Th2 (antiinflammatory) immune responses and suppressing interleukin-12 (IL-12) expression (Dong and Benveniste, 2001; Takada et al., 2005; Farooqui, 2010). Astrocytes are also capable of secreting inflammatory factors such as cytokines, chemokines, and iNOS (Dong and Benveniste, 2001; Hewett et al., 1996; Farooqui, 2010).

Converging evidence thus suggests that activated microglia, astrocytes, and leukocytes, neutrophils, macrophages, dendritic cells, and T lymphocytes interact with each other via intricate signaling pathways supporting and intensifying neuroinflammation. Although, earlier studies indicate that neurons play a passive role in neuroinflammation, recent studies indicate that neurons contribute to neuroinflammation by providing many of their products (i.e., neuropeptides and transmitters), as well as the neuronal membrane proteins CD22, CD47, CD200, CX3CL1 (fractalkine), ICAM-5, neural cell adhesion molecule, semaphorins and C-type lectins. All these neuronal factors regulate neuroinflammation (Tian et al., 2009). In addition, neurons express low levels of MHC molecules and actively promote T-cell apoptosis via the Fas−Fas ligand pathway (CD95−CD95L). Two types of neuroinflammation, (1) acute inflammation and (2) chronic inflammation, have been reported to occur in human brain. Acute neuroinflammation develops rapidly, whereas chronic inflammation develops slowly. Chronic neuroinflammation differs from acute inflammation in that it is below the threshold of pain perception. As a result, the immune system continues to attack at the cellular level. Chronic inflammation lingers for years causing continued insult to the brain tissue reaching the threshold of detection (Wood, 1998). Acute inflammation occurs in the stroke, whereas chronic neuroinflammation occurs in neurodegenerative diseases and initiating pathogenesis of chronic disease. Systemic inflammatory status prior to and at the time of stroke is a key determinant of acute outcome and long-term prognosis (McColl et al., 2009). Inhibiting neuroinflammatory responses after stroke can slow or retard brain injury and, therefore, improve neurological outcome (Yilmaz and Granger, 2008). Conversely, it is also reported that suppressing neuroinflammation can be detrimental and long-term functional recovery can be worse when neuroinflammation after stroke is inhibited (Jin et al., 2013; Patel et al., 2013). Taken together, neuroinflammatory responses after ischemic insult can be beneficial or detrimental, probably depending on the stage of stroke and environments; nevertheless, more research is needed to elucidate the role of neuroinflammation during stroke.

At the molecular level, neuroinflammation is supported by inflammatory lipid mediators such as proinflammatory eicosanoids (prostaglandins (PGs), leukotrienes (LTs), thromboxanes (TXs)), PAF (Fig. 2.4), and neurotoxic mediators such as cytokines (tumor necrosis factor-alpha

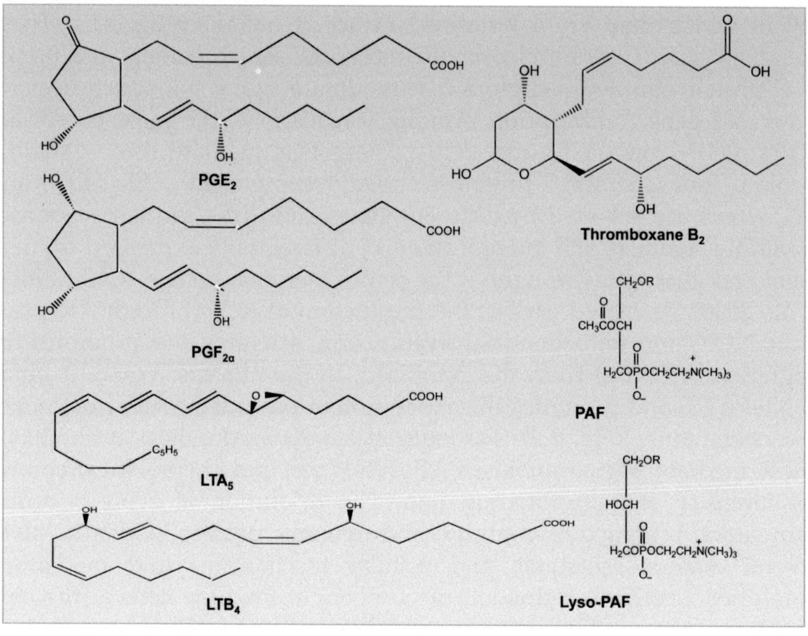

FIGURE 2.4   Chemical structures of arachidonic acid-derived eicosanoids.

TABLE 2.2   NF-κB-Mediated Stimulation of Cytokines, Chemokines, and Adhesion Molecules Following Ischemic Injury

Target	Effect	Reference
TNF-1α	Upregulation	Al-Bahrani et al. (2007)
IL-1, IL-8, IL-6	Upregulation	Al-Bahrani et al. (2007); Tuttolomondo et al. (2008)
MCP-1	Upregulation	Terao et al. (2009)
Macrophage inflammatory protein-1α (MIP-1α)	Upregulation	Terao et al. (2009)
Adhesion molecules	Upregulation	Wen et al. (2006)

(TNF-α), interleukin-1beta (IL-1β), IL-6, IL-8, IL-33, chemokine (C—C motif) ligand 2 (CCL2), CCL5, MMPs, soluble intracellular adhesion molecule-1 (sICAM-1) and E-selectin), which are upregulated due to the activation of NF-κB (Table 2.2) (Al-Bahrani et al., 2007; Tuttolomondo et al., 2008; Terao et al., 2009; Wen et al., 2006; Farooqui et al., 2007; Kamouchi et al., 2011). PGs, LTs, and TXs are generated by the stimulation of $cPLA_2$, COX-2, and 5-LOX on neural membrane phospholipids (Phillis et al., 2006; Farooqui and Horrocks, 2007). Because of their amphiphilic nature, eicosanoids can cross cell membranes and leave the cell in which they are synthesized to act on neighboring cells. These metabolites act through eicosanoid receptors, which belong to a family of G-protein-coupled receptors that modulate signal transduction pathways and gene transcription. Among various PGs, the most potent are PGD_2, PGE_2, and PGF_2 and PGE_2. These PGs mediate their signaling through four distinct G-protein-coupled receptors, EP_1, EP_2, EP_3, and EP_4, which are encoded by different genes and differ in their responses to various agonists and antagonists and differentially expressed on neuronal and glial cells throughout the central nervous system (CNS; Phillis et al., 2006). As stated earlier, the production of ROS through ARA cascade, NOX, and mitochondrial dysfunction, activates and promotes the migration of NF-κB from the cytoplasm to the nucleus, where it binds to NF-κB-RE and promotes the expression of proinflammatory cytokines and chemokines (Fig. 2.2) (Farooqui et al., 2007; Marchesi et al., 2008). These mediators (eicosanoids, PAF, cytokines, and chemokines) control the intensity of neuroinflammation. The resolution of acute neuroinflammation is an active, complex, and dynamic process, which involves several distinct metabolic and cellular mechanisms and mediators. Resolution results in reduction of numbers of immune cells at the core of ischemic site, and clearance of apoptotic cells and debris by increased phagocytic activity (Rossi et al., 2006; Serhan, 2010; Farooqui, 2011). At the molecular level, the resolution of acute inflammation is orchestrated by lipid mediators called lipoxins, resolvins, neuroprotectins, and

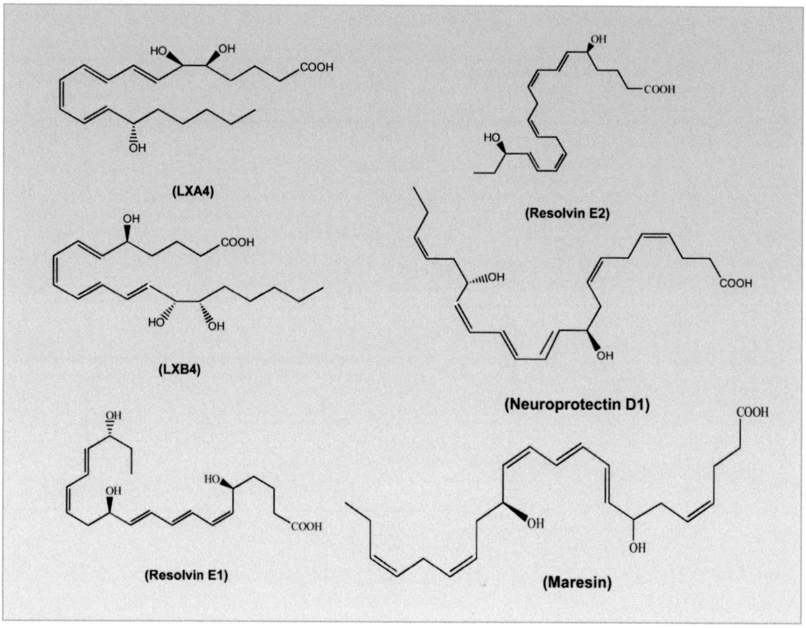

FIGURE 2.5   Chemical structures of lipoxins, resolvins, neuroprotectins, and maresins.

maresins (Serhan, 2009, 2010; Farooqui, 2011) (Fig. 2.5). Lipoxins are derived from ARA, whereas resolvin 1 and 2 are generated by eicosapentaenoic acid (EPA) and D series resolvins (Rvs), neuroprotectins (NPDs), and maresins (MaR) are derived from docosahexaenoic acid (DHA). Among DHA-derived lipid mediators, NPD1 has been reported to play endogenous neuroprotective role by inhibiting apoptotic DNA damage, upregulating antiapoptotic proteins Bcl-2 and Bcl-xL, and downregulating proapoptotic Bax and Bad expression. NPD1 also inhibits oxidative stress-induced caspase-3 activation and IL-1β-stimulated COX-2 expression along with expression of cytokines and chemokines (Fig. 2.6) (Bazan, 2005; Marcheselli et al., 2003; Serhan et al., 2008). In addition, this lipid mediator also inhibits the release of proinflammatory PGs, LTs, and TXs. Lipoxins, resolvins, and protectins decrease vascular permeability and retard PMN recruitment, while promoting recruitment of monocytes, neutrophils, and stimulating efferocytosis (Serhan et al., 2008).

STROKE-MEDIATED DAMAGE TO NEURAL CELLULAR COMPONENTS

It is well known that neural membranes are composed of glycerophospholipids (phosphatidylcholine (PtdCho), phosphatidylethanolamine

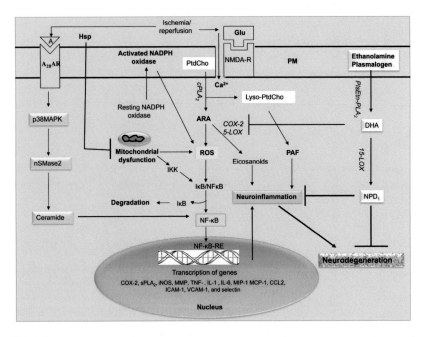

FIGURE 2.6 Effect of neuroprotection D1 (NPD1) on neuroinflammation and neurode-generation via apoptosis. *A*, Adenosine; $A_{2B}AR$, A2B adenosine receptor; *ARA*, arachidonic acid; *CCL2*, chemokine (C–C motif) ligand 2; *COX-2*, cyclooxygenase-2; *cPLA$_2$*, cytosolic phospholipase A$_2$; *DHA*, docosahexaenoic acid; *Glu*, glutamate; *ICAMs*, intercellular adhesion molecules; *IKK*, IκB kinase; *IL-1β*, interleukin-1beta; *IL-6*, interleukin-6; *iNOS*, inducible nitric oxide synthase; *5-LOX*, 5-lipoxygenase; *15-LOX*, 15-lipoxygenase; *lyso-PtdCho*, lysophosphatidylcholine; *MCP-1*, monocyte chemoattractant protein-1; *MIP1*, macrophage inflammatory protein-1; *NF-κB*, nuclear factor-κB; *NMDA-R*, N-methyl-D-aspartate receptor; *nSMase*, neutral sphingomyelinase; *PAF*, platelet activating factor; *PlsEtn*, plasmalogen; *PlsEtn-PLA$_2$*, plasmalogen-selective phospholipase A$_2$; *PtdCho*, phosphatidylcholine; *ROS*, reactive oxygen species; *TNF-α*, tumor necrosis factor-alpha; *VCAM-1*, vascular cell adhesion protein-1.

(PtdEtn), phosphatidylserine (PtdSer), and phosphatidylinositol (PtdIns)), sphingolipids (ceramide and gangliosides), and cholesterol. Phospholipid bilayer not only serves as a permeability barrier between extracellular and intracellular compartments, but also act as storage depots for generation of lipid mediators (Farooqui and Horrocks, 2007). Sphingolipids are composed by a long-chain sphingoid base backbone (e.g., sphingosine), an amide-linked long-chain fatty acid and one of various polar head groups, that defines the various classes of sphingolipid subtypes, such as a hydroxyl group in ceramide, phosphorylcholine in sphingomyelin (SM), and carbohydrates in glycosphingolipids (GLSs). Like phospholipids, sphingolipids and cholesterol are also reservoir for lipid mediators (Farooqui, 2011). Interactions between phospholipids and sphingolipids are involved in maintaining lipid asymmetry, a dynamic process, which is necessary in maintaining normal neural membrane functions such as neuroplasticity and vesicular transport (Farooqui and Horrocks, 2007). Cholesterol has a dual role: regulation of protein–sphingolipid interactions through a fine tuning of sphingolipid conformation (indirect effect), and facilitation of pore (or channel) formation through direct effect (Farooqui and Horrocks, 2007). As stated earlier, following stroke, brain tissue responds to oxygen deprivation with the initiation of rapid changes in bioenergetic metabolism to ensure ion and metabolic homeostasis. At the same time, influx of Ca^{2+} stimulates $cPLA_2$ and accelerates the cleavage of membrane phospholipids leading to changes in neural membrane composition and increase in free fatty acid concentration. The breakdown of phospholipid generates specific messengers that participate in signaling cascades that can either promote neuronal protection or cause injury (Farooqui and Horrocks, 2007). The net impact of signaling events affects the final outcome of the stroke. In addition, massive influx of Ca^{2+} initiates a cascade of events including the induction of mitochondrial dysfunction, ROS production, and activation of other Ca^{2+}-dependent enzymes including NOSs, protein kinases, COX-2, and 5-LOX (Phillis et al., 2006). Lysophospholipids, the degradation product of phospholipids is converted to PAF through acetylation. This lipid mediator not only contributes to neuroinflammation, but also modulates a variety of neural cell functions such as upregulation of MAPKs and ERKs, JNK, and p38 kinases in primary hippocampal neurons in vitro (Farooqui, 2010). While perfusion is a life-saving intervention, it can exacerbate brain damage. Although compromised energy metabolism is restored shortly after reperfusion, alterations in membrane phospholipid composition may lead to the accumulation of ARA-derived nonenzymic lipid mediators (4-hydroxynonenal, acrolein, malondialdehyde, isoprostanes, isofurans, and isoketals), which not only produce neurotoxic effects, but may cause oxidative stress supporting the view that plasma and mitochondrial membranes are the first responders as well as contributors of reperfusion-induced neuronal injury (Farooqui and Horrocks, 2007; Farooqui, 2010). In contrast, nonenzymic oxidation of DHA produces 4-hydroxy-2E-hexenal (4-HHE) (Farooqui, 2010). Increase in levels of nonenzymic mediators of ARA and DHA metabolism, calcium overload, neuroinflammation, and apoptosis are closely associated with neuronal injuries after ischemia (Farooqui, 2010). During cerebral ischemia–reperfusion injury, ceramide accumulation in astrocytes activates neutral sphingomyelinase 2 (nSMase2) by the A2B adenosine receptor $(A_{2B}AR)$/p38MAPK pathway. This accumulation of ceramide in astrocytes can also contribute to the upregulation of expression proinflammatory cytokines (Fig. 2.6).

Stroke-mediated decrease in ATP markedly reduces protein synthesis at the translational step. However, reperfusion restores the protein synthesis in all neurons except in vulnerable neurons, such as those in CA1 region of hippocampus. Events associated with stroke/reperfusion disaggregate polyribosomes, where proteins are synthesized into monosomes after reperfusion (Abe et al., 1995). It is also reported that stroke-mediated increase in Ca^{2+} influx activates many protein degrading enzymes including calpain, calcineurin, and caspases, which mediate the progressive proteolysis of structural proteins including spectrin, tubulin, eIF2, and eIF4 (DeGracia and Montie, 2004; DeGracia, 2004). In selectively vulnerable neurons, calpain-mediated proteolytic degradation of eIF4G and cytoskeletal proteins alter translation initiation mechanisms that substantially reduce total protein synthesis and impose major alterations in message selection, downregulate survival signal transduction, and caspase activation (DeGracia and Montie, 2004; DeGracia, 2004). Class IIa HDAC4 is a large protein with an extended N-terminal regulatory domain and a C-terminal tail. HDAC4 is highly expressed in the brain (Darcy et al., 2010), and neuronal activity depends and modulated by the nucleocytoplasmic shuttling of HDAC4 (Chawla et al., 2003). Stroke-mediated brain damage upregulates the level of phosphorylated HDAC4 and this upregulation is required for postischemia angiogenesis (Liu et al., 2017). The inhibition of HDAC4 phosphorylation can result in a significant decrease in the angiogenic responses from the ischemic brain tissues. Based on this information, it is suggested that the phosphorylation of HDAC4 is essential for angiogenesis after cerebral ischemia. Phosphorylation of HDAC4 is also increased in endothelial cells hypoxia model and suppression of HDAC4 phosphorylation inhibits the tube formation and migration of endothelial cells in vitro. In addition, the inhibition of angiogenesis and blockade of HDAC4 phosphorylation suppresses the expression of genes downstream of HIF-VEGF signaling in vitro and in vivo. These results support the view that phosphorylated HDAC4 may serve as an important regulator in stroke-induced angiogenesis. The protective mechanism of phosphorylated HDAC4 is associated with HIF-VEGF signaling, implicating a novel therapeutic target in stroke (Liu et al., 2017).

Two mechanisms contribute to nucleic acid's damage in cerebral ischemia/reperfusion injury. The first mechanism is mediated by nonspecific nucleases (Liu et al., 1997; Enari et al., 1998). This type of nucleic acid damage is irreversible and is caused by DNA fragmentation (Chen et al., 1997). DNA fragmentation is mediated either by proteases (Liu et al., 1997) or by neuronal NOS (Huang et al., 2000) and becomes apparent at least a few hours to a few days after cerebral ischemia, depending on the duration of ischemia. The second type of damage is oxidative DNA damage. This type of nucleic acid damage occurs early after ischemia (within the first 30 minutes of reperfusion) (Huang et al., 2000; Lin et al., 2000). In addition to DNA strand breaks (Huang et al., 2000; Chen et al., 1997), this type of DNA damage consists of base modifications (Liu et al., 1997; Cui et al., 1999) and DNA lacking a base (Huang et al., 2000). This type of damage not only involves ROS, NO, but also $^{\bullet}$OH (Epe et al., 1996). This type of DNA lesions is generally reversible by DNA repair mechanisms with the exception of those in RNA (Epe et al., 1996). On the other hand, oxidative DNA lesions in the mitochondrial DNA (mtDNA) of the human brain accumulate with age. It is not clear how the brain repairs oxidative DNA lesions in both the mitochondria and nuclei, although evidence suggests DNA repair processes exist in general population. Converging evidence suggests that the etiology of ischemia/reperfusion injury is multifactorial process, which may involve brain damage through the involvement of abnormal cross among phospholipids, sphingolipids, and cholesterol-derived lipid mediators. Under normal conditions, homeostasis among enzymes of phospholipid, sphingolipid, cholesterol metabolism is based not only on optimal levels of lipid mediators and organization of signaling network, but also on the complexity and interconnectedness of their metabolism. However, under ischemia/reperfusion, marked elevations in levels of lipid mediators disturb the signaling networks, and resulting in loss of communication among lipids, proteins, and nucleic acid metabolism. This process not only threatens the integrity of neural cell metabolic homeostasis, but may also promote neural cell death through apoptosis (Farooqui and Horrocks, 2007). In addition, ischemia/reperfusion injury may disturb the integrity of various subcellular fractions, which is needed for modulating regular cellular functions such as cell proliferation, differentiation, communication, and controlled adaptive responses through interactions among lipid mediators (Farooqui, 2011).

ISCHEMIA/REPERFUSION-MEDIATED ALTERATIONS IN ENZYME ACTIVITIES

Ischemia/reperfusion injury evokes a large number of neurochemical and immunological processes, which have been identified and characterized in animal experiments (Taoufik and Probert, 2008). Neurochemical alterations include rapid changes in neurotransmitters (glutamate and GABA), activation of Ca^{2+}-dependent enzymes, increased expression of immediate early, apoptotic, and neuroprotective, changes in activity of transcription factors, adhesion molecules along with neurotrophic mediators. These neurochemical changes are accompanied on the microscopical level by the growing of axons and formation of new synapses in the perilesional vicinity and in remote locations in functionally related areas in the affected and contralesional "nonaffected" hemisphere (Frost et al., 2003; Dancause et al., 2005). In particular, they occur when animals recover in an enriched environment or are subjected to dedicated training (Biernaskie and Corbett, 2001). As mentioned earlier, ischemic/reperfusion injury activates many enzymes including $cPLA_2$, PLC, NOS, protein kinases, calpains, calcinurin, and endonucleases (Farooqui, 2010). Many of these enzymes are activated by Ca^{2+}, which enters neurons through NMDA receptor and voltage-dependent Ca^{2+} channels at the plasma membrane level and mobilization of Ca^{2+} from intracellular stores through PLC-mediated generation of PtdIns-3 is indispensable for neural injury. Immunocytochemical studies indicate that both reactive astrocytes and microglia contain elevated levels of $cPLA_2$ following ischemia/reperfusion injury (Clemens et al., 1996). Following focal cerebral ischemia/reperfusion injury, $cPLA_2$ is activated through phosphorylation of p38MAPK (Nito et al., 2008). It is suggested that the p38MAPK/$cPLA_2$ pathway plays a key role in inducing oxidative stress, promoting BBB disruption with initiating secondary vasogenic edema following ischemia–reperfusion injury (Nito et al., 2008). In addition, stroke-mediated injury also upregulates the Rho/ROCK pathway. Increase in Rho and ROCK expression has been observed in neurons and astrocytes of the ischemic hemisphere of rodents and human within hours of stroke (Brabeck et al., 2003) leading to an increase in ROCK activity (Yano et al., 2008). In astrocytes, increase in ROCK activity not only contributes to reactive astrogliosis and glial scar formation, but also induces changes in actin dynamics, which is responsible for the morphological changes associated with reactive astrogliosis (Amano et al., 2010). These changes are controlled by Arp2/3 signaling, which lies upstream of the Rho/ROCK pathway. Astrocytic cultures that adopt a reactive morphology following Arp2/3 inhibition have been shown to have a higher proportion of active GTP-bound Rho than inactive GDP-bound Rho. These morphological changes are reversed upon ROCK inhibition (Murk et al., 2013). Thus it would appear that the Rho/ROCK pathway is essential for reactive astrogliosis.

ISCHEMIA/REPERFUSION-MEDIATED ALTERATIONS IN GENES

Cerebral ischemia/reperfusion injury is one of the strongest stimulus for gene induction in the brain (Millán and Arenillas, 2006). Many genes including inflammatory responses, neuronal apoptosis, immediate early genes (IEGs), antiapoptotic genes, Hsp genes, genes encoding growth

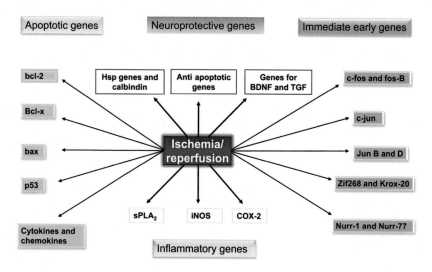

FIGURE 2.7   Effect of cerebral ischemia on gene expression.

BDNF, and transforming growth factor (TGF), and genes for proinflammatory cytokines, chemokines have been found to be induced by brain ischemia/reperfusion injury (Fig. 2.7). Some of the above-mentioned genes (cytokines, chemokines, iNOS, COX-2, and sPLA$_2$) promote neuroinflammation and neurodegeneration, while others induce neuroprotection and recovery (BDNF, TGF, and antiapoptotic genes). Ischemia also modulates proapoptotic proteins (Bax, Bad, and Bcl-XS). These proapoptotic proteins can heterodimerize with tBID and antiapoptotic proteins, Bcl-2 or Bcl-XL, via their BH3 domains (Sugawara et al., 2004; Webster et al., 2006).

IEGs represent the first wave of gene expression following ischemic injury. Examples are *c-fos, fosB c-jun, jun-B, jun-D, zif268, Krox20,* and *Nurr77*. IEGs are induced in cerebral cortex and hippocampal regions of the ischemic brain (Fig. 2.7). BDNF, Neuritin, and activity-regulated cytoskeleton-associated protein (Arc) belong to a subgroup of IEGs, which have been implicated in synaptic plasticity, a process that refers to morphologically observable changes of synapses. IEGs act as transcription factors and may represent third or fourth messengers in an intracellular cascade of stimulus transcription coupling, which converts neuronal excitation into a complex program of cellular responses that finally results in the regulation of target gene expression (Gass et al., 1993). The development of microarray procedures has allowed the profiling of gene expression following ischemic insult (Yakubov et al., 2004; Büttner et al., 2009). Oligonucleotide microarrays' studies in complete global ischemia model have indicated the presence of 576 transcripts, which are significantly altered in response to ischemic injury. Four hundred nineteen transcripts are upregulated and 157 are downregulated. Reperfusion-induced transcript changes occur in a time-dependent manner. Thus 1 hour of reperfusion alters 39 transcripts, while 6 hours of reperfusion produces changes in 174 transcripts, and 24 hours of reperfusion causes changes in 462 transcripts. Quantitative real-time reverse transcription PCR studies of 18 selected genes show excellent agreement with the microarray results. Analyses of gene ontology patterns and the most strongly regulated transcripts show that the immediate response to ischemia/reperfusion is mediated by the induction of specific transcription factors and stress genes. Delayed gene expression response is characterized by inflammation and immune-related genes. These results support the view that the response of brain tissue to ischemia is an active, specific, and coordinated process (Büttner et al., 2009). Converging evidence suggests that ischemia/reperfusion injury is accompanied by induction and suppression of many genes, which produce remarkable functional changes in the injured brain. In the late phase of ischemia/reperfusion, promote the induction of Hsps and apoptosis-related genes. These genes are associated with neuronal survival (Yagita et al., 2008) and are expressed mainly in the glial cell mitochondria in this phase of ischemia/reperfusion (Yagita et al., 2008). Hsp75 binds translocase of the inner membrane to form an ATP-dependent motor that imports mitochondrial proteins into the matrix (Voos et al., 1999). Hsp75 also associates with other mitochondrial proteins including Hsp60, voltage-dependent anion-selective channel, and nicotinamide adenine dinucleotide dehydrogenase, thus making it an important part of the mitochondrial machinery (Schwarzer et al., 2002). Focal ischemia increases the induction of Hsp (Massa et al., 1995). Increase in Hsp75 levels is associated with protection against apoptotic death (Taurin et al., 2002). Preclinical and clinical studies demonstrate that stroke promotes neurogenesis in the adult brain (Kee et al., 2001; Macas et al., 2006), and in an experimental stroke model, blockage of newly generated neuroblasts exacerbates spontaneous neuronal survival and recovery (Wang et al., 2012a,b).

ISCHEMIA/REPERFUSION-MEDIATED CHANGES IN CYTOKINES, CHEMOKINES, AND ADHESION MOLECULES

Cytokines are small secreted proteins released by cells, which have a specific effect on the interactions and communications between cells. Examples of cytokines are tumor necrosis factor (TNF-α), IL-1, IL-8, and

IL-6. Similarly, chemokines are small chemotaxic molecules that possess the ability to induce chemotaxis in nearby responsive cells. Examples of chemokines are monocyte chemoattractant protein-1 (MCP-1), macrophage inflammatory proteins-1α (MIP-1α) and cytokine-induced neutrophil chemoattractant. In addition, chemokines are characterized by the presence of conserved cysteine residues in their N-terminal sequences. Based on the spacing of their first two cysteine residues, they are classified into four distinct subgroups, C chemokines (i.e., one N-terminal cysteine), CC chemokines (i.e., two adjacent N-terminal cysteines), CXC chemokines (i.e., one amino acid between the two N-terminal cysteines), and finally CX3C chemokines (i.e., three amino acids between the two N-terminal cysteines) (Fernandez and Lolis, 2002). Ischemia/reperfusion injury increases the expression of proinflammatory cytokines as well as chemokine in different regions of rat brain as well as in cell culture experiments (Al-Bahrani et al., 2007; Tuttolomondo et al., 2008; Minami and Satoh, 2003). Lower levels of proinflammatory cytokines and higher expression of antiinflammatory cytokines are associated with lower infarct size and a better clinical outcome (Lakhan et al., 2009). On the other hand, number of proinflammatory cytokines contribute to neuroprotection and poststroke plasticity that promotes neural cell restorative processes and brain tissue remodeling (Russo et al., 2011; Liguz-Lecznar and Kossut, 2013). Original elevation of cytokine expression during acute inflammation starts as early as several hours and is associated with recruitment of different types of cells into the ischemic area, including neutrophils, lymphocytes, monocytes, and activation of resident microglia, astrocytes, and endothelial cells (Perera et al., 2006). Activation of microglia and astrocytes leading to additional release of proinflammatory factors can last for up to several weeks after stroke (Liguz-Lecznar and Kossut, 2013). Thus both neural as well as nonneural cells contribute to the production of cytokine and chemokine. These inflammatory mediators are also involved in cellular intercommunication through autocrine, paracrine, or endocrine mechanisms leading to leukocyte recruitment in the injured tissue (Mehta et al., 2007). In addition, cytokine also contributes to interconnection between brain and the immune system through hormonal cascades and cell-to-cell interactions. In contrast, chemokines (specifically CC and CXC) promote the recruitment of neutrophils and monocytes inducing phagocytic activity (Kochanek and Hallenbeck, 1992). Stroke not only stimulates the generation and release of cytokines and chemokines, but also increases the number of cytokine and chemokine receptors in the brain. It is shown that mRNA expression for TNF-α, IL-1β, IL-6, MCP-1, and MIP-1α is induced in the rat brain after focal cerebral ischemia. Cytokine and chemokine signaling is associated with the postischemic inflammatory response. The intercommunication actions of cytokines and chemokines involve a complex network linked to feedback loops and cascades. These inflammatory mediators produce their effects by interacting with specific membrane-associated receptors that are composed of a membrane-spanning region (an extracellular ligand-binding region) and an intracellular region that is activated by binding of cytokines and chemokines and hence conveying a signal from cytoplasm to the nucleus (Rothwell and Relton, 1993). Overlapping signaling pathways for the actions of these inflammatory mediators involves ROS, TLR activation, and the nuclear factor NF-κB system in ischemic injury. The balance between pro- and antiinflammatory cytokines and chemokines not only determines the prowess of the immunological response, but also influences the fate of the injured neurons following ischemic insult. In addition to cytokines and chemokines, microglia also express adhesion molecules including selectin, immunoglobulin superfamily, integrins and MMPs, which intensify and support neuroinflammation (Farooqui et al., 2007). In addition to proinflammatory cytokines, chemokines, and adhesion molecules, ischemia/reperfusion injury also results in altered expression of antiinflammatory cytokines.

CAMs are transmembrane proteins located on the cell surface. They interact with other cells or with the ECM in the process called cell adhesion. In addition to cytokines, CAMs (vascular cell adhesion molecule type 1, intercellular adhesion molecule type 1), endothelial leukocyte adhesion molecule-1 (ELAM-1), CD11/CD18 integrins, P-selectin, and metalloproteinases are also induced and participate in the early and delayed phases of ischemic damage (Koistinaho and Hökfelt, 1997). Proinflammatory cytokines and adhesion cell molecules play important roles in early neurological deterioration and infarct volume. Following ischemia/reperfusion injury, the vasculature endothelium promotes inflammation through upregulation of adhesion molecules such as ICAM, VCAM-1; ELAM, E-selectin, and P-selectin. The accumulation and infiltration of leukocytes in the brain is a complex process involving interactions between several CAMs and chemokines (Frijns and Kappell, 2002; Simundic et al., 2004). Interactions between leukocytes and endothelial surface result in adherence of leukocytes to the endothelial cells causing diapedesis (Fig. 2.8). At the molecular level, this process involves interactions of endothelial cell E- and P-selectins with the L-selectin, which is found on the surface of leukocytes (Frijns and Kappell, 2002). Blocking the activity of P-selectin by treatment with its monoclonal antibodies (ARP 2−4, RMP-1) after the onset of the ischemic injury does not reduce the infarct volume significantly (Suzuki et al., 1999) indicating that the involvement of P-selectin in the inflammatory response after ischemic injury starts early. Firm adhesion and activation of leukocytes is mediated by binding of the CD11/CD18 complex to CAMs, such as ICAM-1, VCAM-1, platelet-endothelial cell adhesion

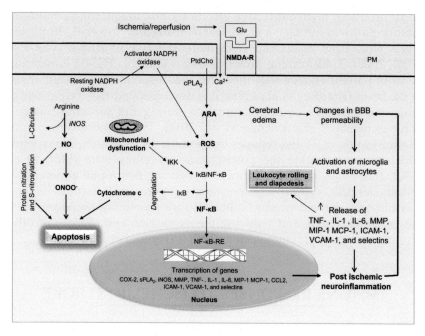

FIGURE 2.8 Effect of cerebral ischemia on BBB permeability, diapedesis, and neuroinflammation. *ARA*, arachidonic acid; *CCL2*, chemokine (C—C motif) ligand 2; *COX-2*, cyclooxygenase-2; *cPLA₂*, cytosolic phospholipase A₂; *Glu*, glutamate; *ICAMs*, intercellular adhesion molecules; *IKK*, IκB kinase; *IL-1β*, interleukin-1beta; *IL-6*, interleukin-6; *iNOS*, inducible nitric oxide synthase; *lyso-PtdCho*, lysophosphatidylcholine; *MCP-1*, monocyte chemoattractant protein-1; *MIP1*, macrophage inflammatory protein-1; *NF-κB*, nuclear factor-κB; *NMDA-R*, N-methyl-D-aspartate receptor; *NO*, nitric oxide; *ONOO⁻*, peroxynitrite; *PM*, plasma membrane; *PtdCho*, phosphatidylcholine; *ROS*, reactive oxygen species; *TNF-α*, tumor necrosis factor-alpha; *VCAM-1*, vascular cell adhesion protein-1.

molecule-1 (PECAM-1), and the mucosal addressin (Frijns and Kappell, 2002; Kalinowska and Losy, 2006). Increase in circulating CAMs is closely associated with aging, which can exacerbate leukocyte infiltration (Richter et al. 2003). IL-6 and TNF-α also modulate the expression of CAMs on the endothelial cells and promote the infiltration of ischemic penumbra by leukocytes at the site of neuroinflammation (Frijns and Kappell, 2002).

Antiinflammatory cytokines include interleukin-10 (IL-10) and transforming growth factor-β (TGF-β). IL-10 produces antiinflammatory effects not only by inhibiting the expression of interleukin-1β (IL-1β), TNF-α, and interleukin-8 (IL-8), but also by lowering cytokine receptor activation in animal studies (Zhang and An, 2007; Ooboshi et al., 2005). In in vitro ischemia/reperfusion models, IL-10 protects murine cortical and cerebellar neurons from excitotoxic damage and OGD by activating survival pathways supporting the view that

IL-10 produces neuroprotective effects by downregulating proinflammatory pathways (Sharma et al., 2011). Clinically, lower IL-10 plasma levels have been associated with increased risk of stroke (Van Exel et al., 2002). Transforming growth factor-β (TGF-β): TGF-β1 is regarded as an important endogenous mediator that responds to ischemic injury in the brain (Knuckey et al., 1996). It is demonstrated that TGF-β acts by inhibiting excessive neuroinflammation during the subacute phase of brain ischemia (Cekanaviciute et al., 2014). Furthermore, intracarotid administration of TGF-β reduces the number of circulating neutrophils, which may ameliorate the postischemic no-reflow state (Mori et al., 1992). TGF-β may also act not only by reducing neutrophil adherence to endothelial cells, suppressing the release of potentially harmful oxygen- and nitrogen-derived products, but also by promoting angiogenesis in the penumbral area, and reducing the expression and efficacy of other proinflammatory cytokines such as TNF-α (Pantoni et al., 1998).

IMMUNE RESPONSES TO ISCHEMIC STROKE

The BBB protects the brain from exposure to anything harmful in the blood, which includes protection from the peripheral immune system under normal healthy conditions. Under normal conditions in healthy human brain, endogenous macrophages and microglia perform the role of immune cells. Occasionally, a T cell may enter the brain but due to the decreased expression of MHC molecules in the CNS, the T cell leaves the brain within 24—48 hours (Miller, 1999). This makes the brain an immunoprivileged organ, which is beneficial in protecting the brain from systemic inflammation. Both the innate and the adaptive immune systems contribute to inflammatory response following ischemic brain injury. Damaged neurons of the brain, in combination with glial cells which become activated after a stroke, express chemotaxic molecules, which signal to the peripheral immune system that there is an injury to the brain. Various cytokines cause upregulation of vascular adhesion molecules in endothelial cells and on immune cells. This creates a leaky BBB which allows entry of immune cells into the brain (de Vries et al., 2012). In addition, ischemic stroke also influences immune cells in the circulation, possibly through increased activation of the sympathetic nervous system and the hypothalamic-pituitary-adrenal axis (Prass et al., 2003; Haddad et al., 2002). This may lead to a reduction in circulating immune cell counts and increase the risk of infectious complications (Prass et al., 2003). Furthermore, acute immune activation may occur in response to stroke-mediated damage to components of the neurovascular unit activating the innate and adaptive arms of the immune response (Famakin, 2014). The initial immune activation is rapid, occurs via the innate immune response and leads to neuroinflammation. During stroke-mediated injury, self-epitopes, which are protected by the systemic immune system through different mechanisms may become open to adaptive immunity. This process may in turn modulate the immune system to respond to self-antigens in the brain, thus leading to autoimmunity. Therefore stroke-induced immunosuppression may help in preventing postinjury autoimmunity against CNS antigens (Kamel and Iadecola, 2012). It is also reported that the inflammatory mediators produced during the innate immune response in turn lead to recruitment of inflammatory cells and the production of more inflammatory mediators that result in activation of the adaptive immune response. Under conditions, neuroinflammation may also promote tissue repair as well as induce immunosuppression following acute stroke leading to poststroke immune-depression. Due to their ability to simultaneously modulate the fate of different genes, miRNAs are particularly well suited to act as key regulators during immune cell differentiation and activation, and their dysfunction can contribute to pathological conditions associated with neuroinflammation. Alterations in expression of several miRNAs have been reported to occur in ischemic injury, hence indicating the use of these small molecules as disease markers, immunoregulators, and new therapeutic targets (Guedes et al., 2013). To have more information on this topic, more studies should be performed to better elucidate the timing of inflammatory and antiinflammatory responses in the brain. Ischemic stroke without systemic inflammation may mediate active depression of peripheral immunity in the brain. In the absence of systemic inflammation but in the presence of local inflammatory cytokines after brain injury, an antiinflammatory response may be triggered. This response may be detrimental because it shuts down defense mechanisms, rendering the body susceptible to infection. Under these conditions, the response can in fact be considered maladaptive or inefficient (Becker, 2012).

STROKE AND ONSET OF COGNITIVE DYSFUNCTION

Cognitive dysfunction is defined as the loss of intellectual functions such as thinking, remembering, and reasoning that interfere with daily activities. Patients with cognitive dysfunction lose ability to learn, recall, concentrate, and problem solving. Cognitive function is regulated not only by neurochemical and intricate synaptic changes, but also by neuronal and glial interactions (Morrison and Baxter, 2012). Risk factors for stroke include age, ischemic heart disease, smoking, diabetes, genetic and environmental factors along with lifestyle. Cognitive dysfunction is one of the primary disability of aging process. It predisposes individuals for neurological and psychiatric disorders eventually affecting the quality of life. The intensity of cognitive decline is markedly increased not only in patients with diabetes, metabolic syndrome, atrial fibrillation, smoking, stroke, and neurodegenerative diseases, but also in patients of neuropsychiatric diseases (Schuh et al., 2011; Farooqui, 2010). Cognitive decline during aging is multifactorial process, which is controlled by several factors such as genes for oxidative stress, neuroinflammation, immune response, mitochondrial functions, growth factors, neuronal survival, and calcium homeostasis (Lu et al., 2004; Loerch et al., 2008). In general, genes that are stress responsive and related to inflammation and DNA repair are upregulated, while genes associated with neuronal growth and survival and mitochondrial functions are downregulated with advancing age in several organisms (Yankner et al., 2008). Gene expression changes during brain aging also exhibit regional differences and sexual dimorphism (Berchtold et al., 2008). The forebrain regions including superior frontal gyrus, entire cortex and hippocampal CA1 are more susceptible to aging and exhibit a large number of gene alterations (Zeier et al., 2011). Although some progress has been made on molecular aspects of cognitive dysfunction in ageing, significant work is still needed to understand molecular mechanism of cognitive dysfunction. Cytokines (TNF-α, IL-6, IL-1, and IL-10) have been reported to play an important role not only in neuroinflammation, but also in hippocampal-dependent learning and memory (McAfoose and Baune, 2009; Brombacher et al., 2017; Jeon et al., 2016). As stated earlier, during ischemic conditions, microglial cells interact with neurons, possibly via P2 $\times$ 7 receptors (Denes et al., 2007), to induce a neuroinflammatory response, which is characterized by an upregulation of cytokines. This process may alter the normal balance and physiological function of cytokines in synaptic plasticity and learning and memory. Alternatively, reduction in CBF may decrease neurogenesis due to reduction in BDNF during aging as well as following cerebral ischemia (Fig. 2.9). Because neurogenesis in the dentate gyrus declines dramatically with ageing and pathological situation, this may represent another possible cause of age-related impairment in hippocampal-dependent memory and cognitive decline. It is proposed that the decrease in synaptic plasticity and LTP may promote synaptic dysfunction, which ultimately may be responsible for cognitive dysfunction (Fig. 2.9).

The most common cognitive dysfunctions after stroke are aphasia (language impairment) and hemispatial neglect (failure to attend or respond to stimuli on the side contralateral to the stroke). Stroke may also cause hypoperfusion resulting into impairments in working memory, attention, learning, calculation, visual perception, or executive

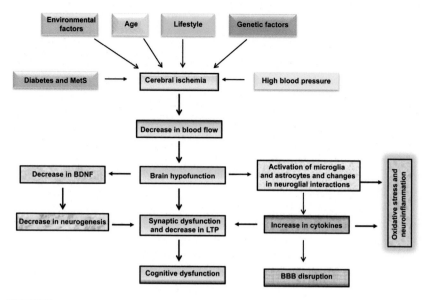

FIGURE 2.9   Contribution of cytokines in cognitive dysfunction. *BBB*, blood–brain barrier; *BDNF*, brain-derived neurotrophic factor; *LTP*, long-term potentiation.

function (i.e., decision making, organization, and problem solving). Stroke patients may also have ideomotor apraxia, an impairment in skilled movements in the absence of motor weakness or incoordination. Aphasia occurs in anywhere from 15% to one-third of patients with stroke (Inatomi et al., 2008; Engelter et al., 2006), depending on the population studied, the way language is tested, and when it is tested, and also typically occurs after left hemisphere stroke. Similar frequencies of occurrence have been reported for hemispatial neglect, with rates above 40% among patients with right hemisphere stroke (Ringman et al., 2004).

ISCHEMIC INJURY AND ITS RELATIONSHIP WITH ALZHEIMER'S DISEASE

Alzheimer's disease (AD) is a complex neurodegenerative disease, which is characterized by the accumulation of extracellular β-amyloid (Aβ) plaques (senile plaques) and intracellular neurofibrillary tangles composed of Tau amyloid fibrils (Hardy, 2009; Selkoe and Hardy, 2016; Farooqui, 2017) leading to the loss of synapses and degeneration of neurons in multiple brain regions (cortical and subcortical areas and hippocampus). It is becoming increasingly evident that early-onset AD (age onset <65 years) is primary defined by inheritable genetic risk factors: PSEN1, PSEN2, and amyloid precursor protein (APP). In contrast, late-onset AD may be controlled by modifiable risk factors, such as diet, sedentary lifestyle, sleep disturbance, smoking, heart disease, head injury, depression, alcohol consumption, and type II diabetes (Farooqui, 2017). The major single gene associated with increased late-onset AD risk is APOE. This gene is also a risk factor for cardiovascular diseases (Gungor et al., 2012). The pathogenic mechanisms underlying these two conditions seem to be connected through cerebral hypoperfusion, BBB compromise, inflammatory cell infiltration, and hemorrhagic susceptibility (Beach et al., 2007; Yarchoan et al., 2012; Farooqui, 2017). Chief among these factors are those that are associated with hypertension.

Although, ischemic stroke and AD are distinct disease entities, still they share numerous mechanisms such as neuroinflammation, immune exhaustion, and neurovascular unit compromise. In addition, cerebral ischemia and AD induce the enhancement of APP metabolism, induction of presenilins, apolipoproteins genes, and increased expression of secretases β and γ. These parameters play key roles in the generation and oligomerization of β-amyloid peptide (Aβ) (Pluta et al., 2012, 2013a). The onset of cerebral ischemia and AD is accompanied by the stimulation of β- and γ-secretases (Pluta et al., 2013b) and accumulation of Aβ. Changes in PKC activity is another important mechanistic link, which is shared by acute and chronic changes ischemia and AD (Lucke-Wold et al., 2015). In the brain, PKC isoforms play important roles in memory formation, BBB maintenance, and injury repair. Onset of brain disease states promotes functional modifications of PKC isoforms. Some mutated isoforms of PKC can contribute to neurodegeneration and cognitive decline, while other isoforms induce neuroprotection (Lucke-Wold et al., 2015). Thus cerebral ischemia alters translocation of PKC β, δ, and ζ contribute to BBB disruption and reperfusion injury. In contrast translocation of PKCε at a proper place in the membrane results in neuroprotection. Often, however, preexisting pathological conditions (diabetes, obesity, and hypertension) can lead to disrupted translocation of PKC isoforms inducing worse outcome following ischemic infarction. Similarly, PKCε also play a protective role against memory decline in AD, but toxic Aβ contributes to epigenetic downregulation of PKC isoforms (PKC β, δ, and ζ) with time. Shared pathways between the cerebral ischemia and AD such as iron-mediated toxicity and immune suppression highlight important targets in injury development and progression. Although, more studies are needed to increase our understanding about PKC activity in the brain, modulating PKC activity/translocation may enhance neuroprotective strategies for treating neurodegenerative diseases such as AD (Lucke-Wold et al., 2015). It is also reported that the complex relationship between ischemic stroke and AD is modulated and promoted by atherosclerosis and inflammatory cascade, which are characteristic features of both pathological conditions. These processes increase the risk of immune exhaustion (Brod, 2000). Furthermore, the Aβ generated by ischemic injury and one that accumulates in the pathogenesis of AD have similar characteristics in terms of induction of oxidative stress (Walsh et al., 2001). Aβ acts as a free-radical inducer. At the molecular level, interactions of Aβ with lipid bilayer result in abstraction of allylic hydrogen atom from the unsaturated acyl chains of phospholipid molecules within the lipid bilayer initiating the process of lipid peroxidation (Lauderback et al., 2001), which generates highly reactive products, such as 4-hydroxy-2-nonenal, acrolein, malondialdehyde, isoprostanes, isoketals, and isofurans, from arachidonic acid through enzymic and nonenzymic pathways (Farooqui, 2011). These metabolites can further react with proteins and enzymes, effectively amplifying the effects of Aβ to induce more free-radical formation or ROS production (Butterfield et al., 2006; Farooqui, 2011; Pocernich and Butterfield, 2012). Aβ has been reported to potently inhibit LTP, enhance long-term depression, and reduce dendritic spine density in normal rodent hippocampus. Soluble Aβ from ischemic and AD brains also disrupt the memory of a learned behavior in normal rats. These various effects can be specifically attributed to Aβ dimers. Based on this information, it is suggested that soluble Aβ oligomers extracted from AD brains potently impair synapse structure and function and that dimers are the smallest synaptotoxic species (Shankar et al., 2008). Another similarity between cerebral ischemia and AD is marked increase in BBB permeability. The normal BBB integrity is essential in protecting neural cells from systemic toxins and maintaining the necessary level of nutrients and ions for neuronal function. This BBB integrity is controlled by structural BBB components, such as tight junction proteins, integrins, annexins, and agrin and endothelial cells, astrocytes, and pericytes. BBB permeability in disrupted capillaries can also facilitate blood-to-brain delivery of circulating Aβ, exacerbating significantly increased in aged animals (Blau et al., 2012). A compromised BBB can result in neuronal cells to become vulnerable to exposure to circulating potentially proinflammatory toxic macromolecules. This suggestion is supported by observations where capillary leakage of several plasma proteins such as prothrombin, immunoglobulin G (IgG), albumin, and lipoproteins have been detected in ischemic and AD brains (Takechi et al., 2010; Zipser et al., 2007). Moreover, inflammatory processes that potentially contribute to cerebral amyloid load (Takechi et al., 2010; Zipser et al., 2007; Pallebage-Gamarallage et al., 2015), generation of inflammatory mediators, free radicals, vascular endothelial growth factor, activation of MMPs, production of various microRNAs, etc., compared to normal aged subjects. These observations support the view that alterations in BBB and activation of microglial cell- and astrocyte-mediated changes may be important risk factors for cerebral ischemia and AD. These factors also control and modulate neuron-glia crosstalk and neuronal function (Liu et al., 2012) and BBB-mediated persistence abnormalities in neuron-glia crosstalk may result in loss of cellular homeostasis leading to neurodegeneration in cerebral ischemia and AD (Raj et al., 2014). These findings support the hypothesis that brain ischemia may contribute to the etiology of sporadic AD. Potential contribution and impact of ischemia-induced activated genes on the development of sporadic AD remain to be established at both genetic and functional levels. The identification of the genes involved in sporadic AD induced by ischemia will enable to further define the events leading to AD-related abnormalities.

CONCLUSION

Stroke is a leading cause of disability and death in adults. Acute cerebral ischemia (stroke) accounts for 80% of all strokes and is due to brain arterial occlusion resulting from a clot, while >20% of patients suffer from intracranial hemorrhage. The pathogenesis of ischemic stroke is very complex. Ischemic stroke triggers a complex and highly interconnected cascade of cellular and molecular events. Stroke-mediated injury not only involves bioenergetic failure (decrease in ATP), loss of neural cell homeostasis, excitotoxicity, activation of neuronal and glial cells, and activation of PLA_2, PLC and PLD, CaMKs, MAPKs, NOS, calpains, calcinurin, and endonucleases, but also disruption of the BBB with infiltration of leukocytes. These enzymes are closely associated with neuronal cell death. Rapid neuronal cell death (necrosis) occurs in the infarct core. In contrast, apoptotic cell death occurs in the ischemic penumbra. At the cellular level, activation of microglial cells and astrocytes in stroke leads to marked elevation in production of ROS (including hydroxyl radical, superoxide anion radical, and hydrogen peroxide) and increased expression of proinflammatory cytokines and chemokines.

During ischemia/reperfusion injury, peroxynitrite and hydroxyl radical also contribute to mitochondrial dysfunction and apoptotic cell death. This provides additional mechanisms for oxidative damage. Coordination of all subcellular organelles is necessary for neuronal death cascade. However, mitochondria and nucleus play a major role in delayed neurodegeneration.

In addition, ischemic stroke is also accompanied by increased risk of the poststroke infections and onset of AD. These may be major determinants of morbidity and mortality.

References

Abe, K., Aoki, M., Kawagoe, J., Yoshida, T., Hattori, A., et al., 1995. Ischemic delayed neuronal death. A mitochondrial hypothesis. Stroke 26, 1478–1489.

Al-Bahrani, A., Taha, S., Shaath, H., Bakhiet, M., 2007. TNF-alpha and IL-8 in acute stroke and the modulation of these cytokines by antiplatelet agents. Curr. Neurovasc. Res. 4, 31–37.

Amano, M., Nakayama, M., Kaibuchi, K., 2010. Rho-kinase/ROCK: a key regulator of the cytoskeleton and cell polarity. Cytoskeleton 67, 545–554.

Amantea, D., Bagetta, G., Tassorelli, C., Mercuri, N.B., Corasaniti, M.T., 2010. Identification of distinct cellular pools of interleukin-1β during the evolution of the neuroinflammatory response induced by transient middle cerebral artery occlusion in the brain of rat. Brain Res. 1313, 259–269.

Amantea, D., Micieli, G., Tassorelli, C., Cuartero, M.I., Ballesteros, I., et al., 2015. Rational modulation of the innate immune system for neuroprotection in ischemic stroke. Front. Neurosci. 9, 147.

Astrup, J., Siesjö, B.K., Symon, L., 1981. Thresholds in cerebral ischemia—the ischemic penumbra. Stroke 12, 723–725.

Bazan, N.G., 2005. Neuroprotectin D1 (NPD1): a DHA-derived mediator that protects brain and retina against cell injury-induced oxidative stress. Brain Pathol. 15, 159–166.

Beach, T.G., Wilson, J.R., Sue, L.I., Newell, A., Poston, M., et al., 2007. Circle of Willis atherosclerosis: association with Alzheimer's disease, neuritic plaques and neurofibrillary tangles. Acta Neuropathol. 113, 13–21.

Becker, K., 2012. Autoimmune responses to brain following stroke. Transl. Stroke Res. 3, 310–317.

Bektas, H., Wu, T.-C., Kasam, M., Harun, N., Sitton, C.W., Grotta, J.C., et al., 2010. Increased blood-brain barrier permeability on perfusion CT might predict malignant middle cerebral artery infarction. Stroke 41, 2539–2544.

Berchtold, N.C., Cribbs, D.H., Coleman, P.D., Rogers, J., Head, E., et al., 2008. Gene expression changes in the course of normal brain aging are sexually dimorphic. Proc. Natl. Acad. Sci. USA. 105, 15605–15610.

Biernaskie, J., Corbett, D., 2001. Enriched rehabilitative training promotes improved forelimb motor function and enhanced dendritic growth after focal ischemic injury. J. Neurosci. 21, 5272–5280.

Blau, C.W., Cowley, T.R., O'sullivan, J., Grehan, B., Browne, T.C., Kelly, L., et al., 2012. The age-related deficit in LTP is associated with changes in perfusion and blood-brain barrier permeability. Neurobiol. Aging 33, 1005.e23–1005.e35.

Blochl, A., Blochl, R., 2007. A cell-biological model of p75NTR signaling. J. Neurochem. 102, 289–305.

Boveris, A., Chance, B., 1973. The mitochondrial generation of hydrogen peroxide. General properties and effect of hyperbaric oxygen. Biochem. J. 134, 707–716.

Brabeck, C., Mittelbronn, M., Bekure, K., Meyermann, R., Schluesener, H.J., et al., 2003. Effect of focal cerebral infarctions on lesional RhoA and RhoB expression. Arch. Neurol. 60, 1245–1249.

Brod, S.A., 2000. Unregulated inflammation shortens human functional longevity. Inflamm. Res. 49, 561–570.

Brombacher, T.M., Nono, J.K., De Gouveia, K.S., Makena, N., Darby, M., et al., 2017. IL-13-mediated regulation of learning and memory. J. Immunol. pii: 1601546.

Burrows, F.E., Bray, N., Denes, A., Allan, S.M., Schiessl, I., 2015. Delayed reperfusion deficits after experimental stroke account for increased pathophysiology. J. Cereb. Blood Flow Metab. 35, 277–284.

Butterfield, D.A., Poon, H.F., St Clair, D., Keller, J.N., Pierce, W.M., et al., 2006. Redox proteomics identification of oxidatively modified hippocampal proteins in mild cognitive impairment: insights into the development of Alzheimer's disease. Neurobiol. Dis. 22, 223–232.

Büttner, F., Cordes, C., Gerlach, F., Heimann, A., Alessandri, B., Luxemburger, U., et al., 2009. Genomic response of the rat brain to global ischemia and reperfusion. Brain Res. 1252, 1–14.

Camandola, S., Poli, G., Mattson, M.P., 2000. The lipid peroxidation product 4-hydroxy-2,3-nonenal increases AP-1-binding activity through caspase activation in neurons. J. Neurochem. 74, 159–168.

Cekanaviciute, E., Dietrich, H.K., Axtell, R.C., Williams, A.M., Egusquiza, R., et al., 2014. Astrocytic TGF-β signaling limits inflammation and reduces neuronal damage during central nervous system *Toxoplasma* infection. J. Immunol. 193, 139–149.

Chawla, S., Vanhoutte, P., Arnold, F.J.L., Huang, C.L.-H., Bading, H., 2003. Neuronal activity-dependent nucleocytoplasmic shuttling of HDAC4 and HDAC5. J. Neurochem. 85, 151–159.

Chen, J., Jin, K., Chen, M., Pei, W., Kawaguchi, K., et al., 1997. Early detection of DNA strand breaks in the brain after transient focal ischemia: implications for the role of DNA damage in apoptosis and neuronal cell death. J. Neurochem. 69, 232–245.

Clark, W.M., Lessov, N., Lauten, J.D., Hazel, K., 1997. Doxycycline treatment reduces ischemic brain damage in transient middle cerebral artery occlusion in the rat. J. Mol. Neurosci. 9, 103–108.

Clarke, L.E., Barres, B.A., 2013. Emerging roles of astrocytes in neural circuit development. Nat. Rev. Neurosci. 14, 311–321.

Clemens, J.A., Stephenson, D.T., Smalstig, E.B., Roberts, E.F., Johnstone, E.M., et al., 1996. Reactive glia express cytosolic phospholipase A_2 after transient global forebrain ischemia in the rat. Stroke 27, 527–535.

Cooper, A.J., Kristal, B.S., 1997. Multiple roles of glutathione in the central nervous system. Biol. Chem. 378, 793–802.

Cui, J., Holmes, E.H., Liu, P.K., 1999. Oxidative damage to the c-fos gene and reduction of its transcription after focal cerebral ischemia. J. Neurochem. 73, 1164–1174.

Dancause, N., Barbay, S., Frost, S.B., Plautz, E.J., Chen, D., et al., 2005. Extensive cortical rewiring after brain injury. J. Neurosci. 25, 10167–10179.

Darcy, M.J., Calvin, K., Cavnar, K., Ouimet, C.C., 2010. Regional and subcellular distribution of HDAC4 in mouse brain. J. Comp. Neurol. 518, 722–740.

DeGraba, T.J., 1998. The role of inflammation after acute stroke: utility of pursuing anti-adhesion molecule therapy. Neurology 51, S62–S68.

DeGracia, D.J., 2004. Acute and persistent protein synthesis inhibition following cerebral reperfusion. J. Neurosci. Res. 77, 771–776.

DeGracia, D.J., Montie, H.L., 2004. Cerebral ischemia and the unfolded protein response. J. Neurochem. 91, 1–8.

Delpech, J.C., Madore, C., Nadjar, A., Joffre, C., Wohleb, E.S., Laye, S., 2015. Microglia in neuronal plasticity: influence of stress. Neuropharmacology 96, 19–28.

del Zoppo, G.J., 2009. Inflammation and the neurovascular unit in the setting of focal cerebral ischemia. Neuroscience 158, 972–982.

Denes, A., Vidyasagar, R., Feng, J., et al., 2007. Proliferating resident microglia after focal cerebral ischaemia in mice. J. Cereb. Blood Flow Metab. 27, 1941–1953.

Dénes, A., Ferenczi, S., Halász, J., Környei, Z., Kovács, K.J., 2008. Role of CX3CR1 (fractalkine receptor) in brain damage and inflammation induced by focal cerebral ischemia in mouse. J. Cereb. Blood Flow Metab. 28, 1707–1721.

Dentesano, G., Straccia, M., Ejarque-Ortiz, A., Tusell, J.M., Serratosa, J., et al., 2012. Inhibition of CD200R1 expression by C/EBP beta in reactive microglial cells. J. Neuroinflamm. 9, 165.

de Vries, H.E., Kooij, G., Frenkel, D., Georgopoulos, S., Monsonego, A., et al., 2012. Inflammatory events at blood—brain barrier in neuroinflammatory and neurodegenerative disorders: implications for clinical disease. Epilepsia 53 (Suppl. 6), 45—52.

Dong, Y., Benveniste, E.N., 2001. Immune function of astrocytes. Glia 36, 180—190.

Dotson, A.L., Offner, H., 2017. Sex differences in the immune response to experimental stroke: implications for translational research. J. Neurosci. Res. 95, 437—446.

Durukan, A., Tatlisumak, T., 2007. Acute ischemic stroke: overview of major experimental rodent models, pathophysiology, and therapy of focal cerebral ischemia. Pharmacol. Biochem. Behav. 87, 179—197.

Emsley, H.C., Tyrrell, P.J., 2002. Inflammation and infection in clinical stroke. J. Cereb. Blood Flow Metab. 22, 1399—1419.

Enari, M., Sakahira, H., Yokoyama, H., Okawa, K., Iwamatsu, A., et al., 1998. A caspase-activated DNase that degrades DNA during apoptosis, and its inhibitor ICAD. Nature (London) 391, 43—50.

Endres, M., Meisel, A., Biniszkiewicz, D., Namura, S., Prass, K., Ruscher, K., et al., 2000. DNA methyltransferase contributes to delayed ischemic brain injury. J. Neurosci. 20, 3175—3181.

Endres, M., Fan, G., Meisel, A., Dirnagl, U., Jaenisch, R., 2001. Effects of cerebral ischemia in mice lacking DNA methyltransferase 1 in post-mitotic neurons. Neuroreport 12, 3763—3766.

Engelhardt, B., Sorokin, L., 2009. The blood-brain and the blood-cerebrospinal fluid barriers: function and dysfunction. Semin. Immunopathol. 31, 497—511.

Engelter, S.T., Gostynski, M., Papa, S., et al., 2006. Epidemiology of aphasia attributable to first ischemic stroke: incidence, severity, fluency, etiology, and thrombolysis. Stroke 37, 1379—1384.

Epe, B., Ballmaier, D., Roussyn, I., Briviba, K., Sies, H., 1996. DNA damage by peroxynitrite characterized with DNA repair enzymes. Nucleic Acids Res. 24, 4105—4110.

Famakin, B.M., 2014. The immune response to acute focal cerebral ischemia and associated post-stroke immunodepression: a focused review. Aging Dis. 5, 307—326.

Farooqui, A.A., 2010. Neurochemical Aspects of Neurotraumatic and Neurodegenerative Diseases. Springer, New York, NY.

Farooqui, A.A., 2011. Lipid Mediators and Their Metabolism in the Brain. Springer, New York, NY.

Farooqui, A.A., 2014. Inflammation and Oxidative Stress in Neurological Disorders. Springer International Publishing, Switzerland.

Farooqui, A.A., 2017. Neurochemical Aspects of Alzheimer's Disease: Risk Factors, Pathogenesis, Biomarkers, and Potential Treatment Strategies. Academic Press, Elsevier, London, San Diego, CA.

Farooqui, A.A., Horrocks, L.A., 1994. Excitotoxicity and neurological disorders: involvement of membrane phospholipids. Int. Rev. Neurobiol. 36, 267—323.

Farooqui, A.A., Horrocks, L.A., 2007. Glycerophospholipids in Brain. Springer, New York, NY.

Farooqui, A.A., Horrocks, L.A., Farooqui, T., 2007. Modulation of inflammation in brain: a matter of fat. J. Neurochem. 101, 577—599.

Feigin, V.L., Forouzanfar, M.H., Krishnamurthi, R., Mensah, G.A., Connor, M., et al., 2014. Global and regional burden of stroke during 1990-2010: findings from the Global Burden of Disease Study 2010. Lancet 383, 245—254.

Fernandez, E.J., Lolis, E., 2002. Structure, function, and inhibition of chemokines. Annu. Rev. Pharmacol. Toxicol. 42, 469—499.

Fogelson, A.L., Hussain, Y.H., Leiderman, K., 2012. Blood clot formation under flow: the importance of factor XI depends strongly on platelet count. Biophys. J. 102, 10—18.

Frijns, C.J.M., Kappell, L.J., 2002. Inflammatory cell adhesion molecules in ischemic cerebrovascular disease. Stroke 33, 2115–2122.

Frost, S.B., Barbay, S., Friel, K.M., Plautz, E.J., Nudo, R.J., 2003. Reorganization of remote cortical regions after ischemic brain injury: a potential substrate for stroke recovery. J. Neurophysiol. 89, 3205–3214.

Gass, P., Sprangir, M., Kiessling, M., 1993. Induction of early response genes after focal ischemia. Cerebrovasc. Dis. 3, 74–79.

Girouard, H., Wang, G., Gallo, E.F., Anrather, J., Zhou, P., et al., 2009. NMDA receptor activation increases free radical production through nitric oxide and NOX2. J. Neurosci. 29, 2545–2552.

Granger, C.V., Hamilton, B.B., Fiedler, R.C., 1992. Discharge outcome after stroke rehabilitation. Stroke 23, 978–982.

Gu, Z., Kaul, M., Yan, B., Kridel, S.J., Cui, J., et al., 2002. S-nitrosylation of matrix metalloproteinases: signaling pathway to neuronal cell death. Science 297, 1186–1190.

Guedes, J., Cardoso, A.L., Pedroso de Lima, M.C., 2013. Involvement of microRNA in microglia-mediated immune response. Clin. Dev. Immunol. 2013, 186872.

Guha, M., Mackman, N., 2001. LPS induction of gene expression in human monocytes. Cell Signal. 13, 85–94.

Gungor, Z., Anuurad, E., Enkhmaa, B., Zhang, W., Kim, K., Berglund, L., 2012. Apo E4 and lipoprotein-associated phospholipase A2 synergistically increase cardiovascular risk. Atherosclerosis 223, 230–234.

Gunnett, C.A., Lund, D.D., McDowell, A.K., Faraci, F.M., Heistad, D.D., 2005. Mechanisms of inducible nitric oxide synthase-mediated vascular dysfunction. Arterioscler. Thromb. Vasc. Biol. 25, 1617–1622.

Haddad, J.J., Saade, N.E., Safieh-Garabedian, B., 2002. Cytokines and neuro-immune-endocrine interactions: a role for the hypothalamic-pituitary-adrenal revolving axis. J. Neuroimmunol. 133, 1–19.

Hardy, J., 2009. The amyloid hypothesis for Alzheimer's disease: a critical reappraisal. J. Neurochem. 110, 1129–1134.

Harris, I.M., Wong, C., Andrews, S., 2015. Visual field asymmetries in object individuation. Conscious. Cogn. 37, 194–206.

Hayashi, T., Abe, K., 2004. Ischemic neuronal cell death and organellae damage. Neurol. Res. 26, 827–834.

Heiss, W.D., Sobesky, J., Hesselmann, V., 2004. Identifying thresholds for penumbra and irreversible tissue damage. Stroke 35, 2671–2674.

Hermes, G., Nagy, D., Waterson, M., Zsarnovszky, A., Varela, L., et al., 2016. Role of mitochondrial uncoupling protein-2 (UCP2) in higher brain functions, neuronal plasticity and network oscillation. Mol. Metab. 5, 415–421.

Hewett, S.J., Muir, J.K., Lobner, D., Symons, A., Choi, D.W., 1996. Potentiation of oxygen-glucose deprivation-induced neuronal death after induction of iNOS. Stroke 27, 1586–1591.

Hossmann, K.A., 1994. Viability thresholds and the penumbra of focal ischemia. Ann. Neurol. 36, 557–565.

Huang, D., Shenoy, A., Cui, J.K., Huang, W., Liu, P.K., 2000. In situ detection of AP sites and DNA strand breaks with 3′-phosphate ends in ischemic mouse brain. FASEB J. 14, 407–417.

Iadecola, C., Anrather, J., 2011. The immunology of stroke: from mechanisms to translation. Nat. Med. 17, 796–808.

Inatomi, Y., Yonehara, T., Omiya, S., Hashimoto, Y., Hirano, T., Uchino, M., 2008. Aphasia during the acute phase in ischemic stroke. Cerebrovasc. Dis. 25, 316–323.

Jeon, S.G., Kim, K.A., Chung, H., Choi, J., Song, E.J., et al., 2016. Impaired memory in OT-II transgenic mice is associated with decreased adult hippocampal neurogenesis possibly induced by alteration in Th2 cytokine levels. Mol. Cells 39, 603–610.

Jin, R., Yang, G., Li, G., 2010. Inflammatory mechanisms in ischemic stroke: role of inflammatory cells. J. Leukoc. Biol. 87, 779–789.

Jin, R., Liu, L., Zhang, S., Nanda, A., Li, G., 2013. Role of inflammation and its mediators in acute ischemic stroke. J. Cardiovasc. Transl. Res. 6, 834–851.

Jung, B.P., Zhang, G., Ho, W., Francis, J., Eubanks, J.H., 2002. Transient forebrain ischemia alters the mRNA expression of methyl DNA-binding factors in the adult rat hippocampus. Neuroscience 115, 515–524.

Kalinowska, A., Losy, J., 2006. PECAM-1, a key player in neuroinflammation. Eur. J. Neurol. 13, 1284–1290.

Kamel, H., Iadecola, C., 2012. Brain-immune interactions and ischemic stroke: clinical implications. Arch. Neurol. 69, 576–581.

Kamouchi, M., Ago, T., Kitazono, T., 2011. Brain pericytes: emerging concepts and functional roles in brain homeostasis. Cell. Mol. Neurobiol. 31, 175–193.

Kee, N.J., Preston, E., Wojtowicz, J.M., 2001. Enhanced neurogenesis after transient global ischemia in the dentate gyrus of the rat. Exp. Brain Res. 136, 313–320.

Khakh, B.S., Sofroniew, M.V., 2015. Diversity of astrocyte functions and phenotypes in neural circuits. Nat. Neurosci. 18, 942–952.

Kim, J.Y., Park, J., Chang, J.Y., Kim, S.H., Lee, J.E., 2016. Inflammation after stroke: the role of leukocytes and glial cells. Exp. Neurobiol. 25, 241–251.

Kim-Han, J.S., Dugan, L.L., 2005. Mitochondrial uncoupling proteins in the central nervous system. Antioxid. Redox Signal. 7, 1173–1181.

Knuckey, N.W., Finch, P., Palm, D.E., Primiano, M.J., Johanson, C.E., et al., 1996. Differential neuronal and astrocytic expression of transforming growth factor beta isoforms in rat hippocampus following transient forebrain ischemia. Brain Res. Mol. Brain Res. 40, 1–14.

Kochanek, P.M., Hallenbeck, J.M., 1992. Polymorphonuclear leukocytes and monocytes/macrophages in the pathogenesis of cerebral ischemia and stroke. Stroke 23, 1367–1379.

Koistinaho, J., Hökfelt, T., 1997. Altered gene expression in brain ischemia. Neuroreport 8, i–viii.

Kouzarides, T., 2007. Chromatin modifications and their function. Cell 128, 693–705.

Krupinski, J., Kaluza, J., Kumar, P., Kumar, S., Wang, J.M., 1993. Some remarks on the growth-rate and angiogenesis of microvessels in ischemic stroke. Morphometric and immunocytochemical studies. Patol Pol. 44, 203–209.

Krupinski, J., Kaluza, J., Kumar, P., Kumar, S., Wang, J.M., 1994. Role of angiogenesis in patients with cerebral ischemic stroke. Stroke 25, 1794–1798.

Kuharsky, A.L., Fogelson, A.L., 2001. Surface-mediated control of blood coagulation: the role of binding site densities and platelet deposition. Biophys. J. 80, 1050–1074.

Lai, A.Y., Todd, K.G., 2006. Microglia in cerebral ischemia: molecular actions and interactions. Can. J. Physiol. Pharmacol. 84, 49–59.

Lakhan, S.E., Kirchgessner, A., Hofer, M., 2009. Inflammatory mechanisms in ischemic stroke: therapeutic approaches. J. Transl. Med. 7, 97.

Lauderback, C.M., Hackett, J.M., Huang, F.F., Keller, J.N., Szweda, L.I., et al., 2001. The glial glutamate transporter, GLT-1, is oxidatively modified by 4-hydroxy-2-nonenal in the Alzheimer's disease brain: the role of Aβ(1–42). J. Neurochem. 78, 413–416.

Liang, M.-L., Da, X.W., He, A.D., Yao, G.Q., Xie, W., et al., 2015. Pentamethylquercetin (PMQ) reduces thrombus formation by inhibiting platelet function. Sci. Rep. 5, 11142.

Liguz-Lecznar, M., Kossut, M., 2013. Influence of inflammation on poststroke plasticity. Neural Plast. 2013, 258582.

Lima, B., Forrester, M.T., Hess, D.T., Stamler, J.S., 2010. S-nitrosylation in cardiovascular signaling. Circ. Res. 106, 633–646.

Lin, L., Cao, S., Yu, L., Cui, J., Hamilton, W.J., et al., 2000. Up-regulation of base excision repair activity for 8-2'deoxyhydroxyl guanosine in the mouse brain after forebrain ischemia-reperfusion. J. Neurochem. 74, 101−108.

Liu, J., Zhou, X., Li, Q., Zhou, S.M., Hu, B., et al., 2017. Role of phosphorylated HDAC4 in stroke-induced angiogenesis. Biomed. Res. Int. 2017, 2957538.

Liu, X., Wu, Z., Hayashi, Y., Nakanishi, H., 2012. Age-dependent neuroinflammatory responses and deficits in long-term potentiation in the hippocampus during systemic inflammation. Neuroscience 216, 133−142.

Liu, X.S., Zou, H., Slaughter, C., Wang, X.D., 1997. DFF: a heterodimeric protein that functions downstream of caspase-3 to trigger DNA fragmentation during apoptosis. Cell 89, 175−184.

Liu, Z., Chopp, M., 2015. Astrocytes, therapeutic targets for neuroprotection and neurorestoration in ischemic stroke. Prog. Neurobiol. 144, 103−120.

Loerch, P.M., Lu, T., Dakin, K.A., Vann, J.M., Isaacs, A., et al., 2008. Evolution of the aging brain transcriptome and synaptic regulation. PLoS One 3 (10), e3329.

Lu, T., Pan, Y., Kao, S.Y., Li, C., Kohane, I., Chan, J., et al., 2004. Gene regulation and DNA damage in the ageing human brain. Nature 429, 883−891.

Lu, Y., Li, Q., Liu, Y.Y., Sun, K., Fan, J.Y., et al., 2015. Inhibitory effect of caffeic acid on ADP-induced thrombus formation and platelet activation involves mitogen-activated protein kinases. Sci. Rep. 5, 13824.

Lucke-Wold, B.P., Turner, R.C., Logsdon, A.F., Simpkins, J.W., Alkon, D.L., et al., 2015. Common mechanisms of Alzheimer's Disease and ischemic stroke: the role of protein kinase C in the progression of age-related neurodegeneration. J. Alzheimers Dis. 43, 711−724.

Macas, J., Nern, C., Plate, K.H., Momma, S., 2006. Increased generation of neuronal progenitors after ischemic injury in the aged adult human forebrain. J. Neurosci. 26, 13114−13119.

Marcheselli, V.L., Hong, S., Lukiw, W.J., Tian, X.H., Gronert, K., et al., 2003. Novel docosanoids inhibit brain ischemia-reperfusion-mediated leukocyte infiltration and pro-inflammatory gene expression. J. Biol. Chem. 278, 43807−43817.

Marchesi, C., Paradis, P., Schiffrin, E.L., 2008. Role of the renin-angiotensin system in vascular inflammation. Trends Pharmacol. Sci. 29, 367−374.

Mark, R.J., Lovell, M.A., Markesbery, W.R., Uchida, K., Mattson, M.P., 1997. A role for 4-hydroxynonenal, an aldehydic product of lipid peroxidation, in disruption of ion homeostasis and neuronal death induced by amyloid β-peptide. J. Neurochem. 68, 255−264.

Massa, S.M., Longo, F.M., Zuo, J., Wang, S., Chen, J., et al., 1995. Cloning of ratgrp75, an hsp70-family member, and its expression in normal and ischemic brain. J. Neurosci. Res. 40, 807−819.

Mattson, M.P., Meffert, M.K., 2006. Roles for NF-kappaB in nerve cell survival, plasticity, and disease. Cell Death Differ. 13, 852−860.

Mattson, M.P., Duan, W., Pedersen, W.A., Culmsee, C., 2001. Neurodegenerative disorders and ischemic brain diseases. Apoptosis 6, 69−81.

McAfoose, J., Baune, B.T., 2009. Evidence for a cytokine model of cognitive function. Neurosci. Biobehav. Rev. 33, 355−366.

McCann, S.K., Dusting, G.J., Roulston, C.L., 2008. Early increase of Nox4 NADPH oxidase and superoxide generation following endothelin-1-induced stroke in conscious rats. J. Neurosci. Res. 86, 2524−2534.

McColl, B.W., Allan, S.M., Rothwell, N.J., 2009. Systemic infection, inflammation and acute ischemic stroke. Neuroscience 158, 1049−1061.

Mead, E.L., Mosley, A., Eaton, S., Dobson, L., Heales, S.J., et al., 2012. Microglial neurotransmitter receptors trigger superoxide production in microglia, consequences for microglial-neuronal interactions. J. Neurochem. 121, 287−301.

Mehta, S.L., Manhas, N., Raghubir, R., 2007. Molecular targets in cerebral ischemia for developing novel therapeutics. Brain Res. Rev. 54, 34–66.

Meisel, A., Harms, C., Yildirim, F., Bösel, J., Kronenberg, G., Harms, U., et al., 2006. Inhibition of histone deacetylation protects wild-type but not gelsolin-deficient neurons from oxygen/glucose deprivation. J. Neurochem. 98, 1019–1031.

Meisel, C., Schwab, J., Prass, K., Meisel, A., Dirnagl, U., 2005. Central nervous system injury-induced immune deficiency syndrome. Nat. Rev. Neurosci. 6, 775–786.

Millán, M., Arenillas, J., 2006. Gene expression in cerebral ischemia: a new approach for neuroprotection. Cerebrovasc. Dis. 21 (Suppl. 2), 30–37.

Miller, A.A., Dusting, G.J., Roulston, C.L., Sobey, C.G., 2006. NADPH-oxidase activity is elevated in penumbral and non-ischemic cerebral arteries following stroke. Brain Res. 1111, 111–116.

Miller, D.W., 1999. Immunobiology of the blood-brain barrier. J. Neurovirol. 5, 570–578.

Minami, M., Satoh, M., 2003. Chemokines and their receptors in the brain: pathophysiological roles in ischemic brain injury. Life Sci. 74, 321–327.

Mori, E., Del Zoppo, G., et al., 1992. Inhibition of polymorphonuclear leukocyte adherence suppresses no-reflow after focal cerebral ischemia in baboons. Stroke 23, 712–718.

Morrison, J.H., Baxter, M.G., 2012. The aging cortical synapse: hallmarks and implications for cognitive decline. Nat. Rev. Neurosci. 13, 240–250.

Mozaffarian, D., Benjamin, E.J., Go, A.S., Arnett, D.K., Blaha, M.J., et al., 2015. Heart disease and stroke statistics--2015 update: a report from the American Heart Association. Circulation 131, e29–e322.

Murk, K., Blanco Suarez, E.M., Cockbill, L.M., Banks, P., Hanley, J.G., 2013. The antagonistic modulation of Arp2/3 activity by N-WASP, WAVE2 and PICK1 defines dynamic changes in astrocyte morphology. J. Cell Sci. 126, 3873–3883.

Nagai, M., Re, D.B., Nagata, T., Chalazonitis, A., Jessell, T.M., et al., 2007. Astrocytes expressing ALS-linked mutated SOD1 release factors selectively toxic to motor neurons. Nat. Neurosci. 10, 615–622.

Nakamura, T., Lipton, S.A., 2009. According to GOSPEL: filling in the GAP(DH) of NO-mediated neurotoxicity. Neuron 63, 3–6.

Nito, C., Kamada, H., Endo, H., Niizuma, K., Myer, D.J., et al., 2008. Role of the p38 mitogen-activated protein kinase/cytosolic phospholipase A_2 signaling pathway in blood-brain barrier disruption after focal cerebral ischemia and reperfusion. J. Cereb. Blood Flow Metab. 28, 1686–1696.

Ooboshi, H., Ibayashi, S., Shichita, T., Kumai, Y., Takada, J., et al., 2005. Postischemic gene transfer of interleukin-10 protects against both focal and global brain ischemia. Circulation 111, 913–919.

Ouyang, Y.B., Voloboueva, L.A., Xu, L.J., Giffard, R.G., 2007. Selective dysfunction of hippocampal CA1 astrocytes contributes to delayed neuronal damage after transient forebrain ischemia. J. Neurosci. 27, 4253–4260.

Ouyang, Y.B., Xu, L., Lu, Y., Sun, X., Yue, S., Xiong, X.X., et al., 2013a. Astrocyte-enriched miR-29a targets PUMA and reduces neuronal vulnerability to forebrain ischemia. Glia 61, 1784–1794.

Ouyang, Y.B., Stary, C.M., Yang, G.Y., Giffard, R., 2013b. microRNAs: innovative targets for cerebral ischemia and stroke. Curr. Drug Targets 14, 90–101.

Ouyang, Y.B., Xu, L., Liu, S., Giffard, R.G., 2014. Role of astrocytes in delayed neuronal death: GLT-1 and its novel regulation by microRNAs. Adv. Neurobiol. 11, 171–188.

Pacher, P., Beckman, J.S., Liaudet, L., 2007. Nitric oxide and peroxynitrite in health and disease. Physiol. Rev. 87, 315–424.

Pallebage-Gamarallage, M., Takechi, R., Lam, V., Elahy, M., Mamo, J., 2015. Pharmacological modulation of dietary lipid-induced cerebral capillary dysfunction: considerations for reducing risk for Alzheimer's disease. Crit. Rev. Clin. Lab. Sci. 18, 1–18.

Pantoni, L., Sarti, C., Inzitari, D., 1998. Cytokines and cell adhesion molecules in cerebral ischemia experimental bases and therapeutic perspectives. Arterioscler. Thromb. Vasc. Biol. 18, 503–513.

Parkhurst, C.N., Yang, G., Ninan, I., Savas, J.N., Yates III, J.R., et al., 2013. Microglia promote learning-dependent synapse formation through brain-derived neurotrophic factor. Cell 155, 1596–1609.

Pascual, O., Ben Achour, S., Rostaing, P., Triller, A., Bessis, A., 2012. Microglia activation triggers astrocyte-mediated modulation of excitatory neurotransmission. Proc. Natl. Acad. Sci. USA. 109, E197–E205.

Patel, A.R., Ritzel, R., McCullough, L.D., Liu, F., 2013. Microglia and ischemic stroke: a double-edged sword. Int. J. Physiol. Pathophysiol. Pharmacol. 5, 73–90.

Pekny, M., Nilsson, M., 2005. Astrocyte activation and reactive gliosis. Glia 50, 427–434.

Peng, S., Zhao, S., Yan, F., Cheng, J., Huang, L., Chen, H., et al., 2015. HDAC2 selectively regulates FOXO3a-mediated gene transcription during oxidative stress-induced neuronal cell death. J. Neurosci. 35, 1250–1259.

Perera, M.N., Ma, H.K., Arakawa, S., Howells, D.W., Markus, R., et al., 2006. Inflammation following stroke. J. Clin. Neurosci. 13, 1–8.

Phillis, J.W., Horrocks, L.A., Farooqui, A.A., 2006. Cyclooxygenases, lipoxygenases, and epoxygenases in CNS: their role and involvement in neurological disorders. Brain Res. Rev. 52, 201–243.

Pirmoradi, M., Jemel, B., Gallagher, A., Tremblay, J., D'Hondt, F., et al., 2016. Verbal memory and verbal fluency tasks used for language localization and lateralization during magnetoencephalography. Epilepsy Res. 119, 1–9.

Pizzi, M., Sarnico, I., Lanzillotta, A., Battistin, L., Spano, P., 2009. Post-ischemic brain damage: NF-kappaB dimer heterogeneity as a molecular determinant of neuron vulnerability. FASEB J. 276, 27–35.

Plate, K.H., 1999. Mechanisms of angiogenesis in the brain. J. Neuropathol. Exp. Neurol. 58, 313–320.

Pluta, R., Kocki, J., Maciejewski, R., Ułamek-Kozioł, M., Jabłoński, M., et al., 2012. Ischemia signalling to Alzheimer-related genes. Folia Neuropathol. 50, 322–329.

Pluta, R., Jabłoński, M., Ułamek-Kozioł, M., Kocki, J., Brzozowska, J., et al., 2013a. Sporadic Alzheimer's disease begins as episodes of brain Ischemia and ischemically dysregulated Alzheimer's disease genes. Mol. Neurobiol. 48, 500–515.

Pluta, R., Furmaga-Jabłońska, W., Maciejewski, R., Ułamek-Kozioł, M., Jabłoński, M., 2013b. Brain ischemia activates β- and γ-secretase cleavage of amyloid precursor protein: significance in sporadic Alzheimer's disease. Mol. Neurobiol. 47, 425–434.

Pocernich, C.B., Butterfield, D.A., 2012. Elevation of glutathione as a therapeutic strategy in Alzheimer disease. Biochim. Biophys. Acta 1822, 625–630.

Prass, K., Meisel, C., Hoflich, C., Braun, J., Halle, E., et al., 2003. Stroke-induced immunodeficiency promotes spontaneous bacterial infections and is mediated by sympathetic activation reversal by poststroke T helper cell type 1-like immunostimulation. J. Exp. Med. 198, 725–736.

Raj, D.D., Jaarsma, D., Holtman, I.R., Olah, M., Ferreira, F.M., Schaafsma, W., 2014. Priming of microglia in a DNA-repair deficient model of accelerated aging. Neurobiol. Aging 35, 2147–2160.

Richter, V., Rassoul, F., Purschwitz, K., Hentschel, B., Reuter, W., et al., 2003. Circulating vascular cell adhesion molecules VCAM-1, ICAM-1, and E-selectin in dependence on aging. Gerontology 49, 293–300.

Ringman, J.M., Saver, J.L., Woolson, R.F., Clarke, W.R., Adams, H.P., 2004. Frequency, risk factors, anatomy, and course of unilateral neglect in an acute stroke cohort. Neurology 63, 468–474.

Risau, W., 1997. Mechanisms of angiogenesis. Nature 386, 671–674.

Rossi, A.G., Sawatzky, D.A., Walker, A., Ward, C., Sheldrake, T.A., et al., 2006. Cyclin-dependent kinase inhibitors enhance the resolution of inflammation by promoting inflammatory cell apoptosis. Nat. Med. 12, 1056−1064.

Rossi, D.J., Brady, J.D., Mohr, C., 2007. Astrocyte metabolism and signaling during brain ischemia. Nat. Neurosci. 10, 1377−1386.

Rothwell, N.J., Relton, J.K., 1993. Involvement of cytokines in acute neurodegeneration in the CNS. Neurosci. Biobehav. Rev. 17, 217−227.

Roussel, B.D., Kruppa, A.J., Miranda, E., Crowther, D.C., Lomas, D.A., Marciniak, S.J., 2013. Endoplasmic reticulum dysfunction in neurological disease. Lancet Neurol. 12, 105−118.

Russo, I., Barlati, S., Bosetti, F., 2011. Effects of neuroinflammation on the regenerative capacity of brain stem cells. J. Neurochem. 116, 947−956.

Ryu, H., Lee, J., Olofsson, B.A., Mwidau, A., Dedeoglu, A., Escudero, M., et al., 2014. Histone deacetylase inhibitors prevent oxidative neuronal death independent of expanded polyglutamine repeats via an Sp1-dependent pathway. Brain Res. Bull. 102, 15−21.

Saijo, K., Glass, C.K., 2011. Microglial cell origin and phenotypes in health and disease. Nat. Rev. Immunol. 11, 775−787.

Santello, M., Volterra, A., 2012. TNFalpha in synaptic function: switching gears. Trends Neurosci. 35, 638−647.

Sarnico, I., Lanzillotta, A., Boroni, F., Benarese, M., Alghisi, M., et al., 2009. NF-kappaB p50/RelA and c-Rel-containing dimers: opposite regulators of neuron vulnerability to ischaemia. J. Neurochem. 108, 475−485.

Save-Pédebos, J., Pinabiaux, C., Dorfmuller, G., Sorbets, S.F., Delalande, O., et al., 2016. The development of pragmatic skills in children after hemispherotomy: contribution from left and right hemispheres. Epilepsy Behav. 55, 139−145.

Savitz, S.I., Malhotra, S., Gupta, G., Rosenbaum, D.M., 2003. Cell transplants offer promise for stroke recovery. J. Cardiovasc. Nurs. 18, 57−61.

Savitz, S.I., Dinsmore, J.H., Wechsler, L.R., Rosenbaum, D.M., Caplan, L.R., 2004. Cell therapy for stroke. NeuroRx 1, 406−414.

Schuh, A.F., Rieder, C.M., Rizzi, L., Chaves, M., Roriz-Cruz, M., 2011. Mechanisms of brain aging regulation by insulin: implications for neurodegeneration in late-onset Alzheimer's disease. ISRN Neurol. 2011, 306905.

Schwarzer, C., Barnikol-Watanabe, S., Thinnes, F.P., Hilschmann, N., 2002. Voltage-dependent anion-selective channel (VDAC) interacts with the dynein light chain Tctex1 and the heat-shock protein PBP74. Int. J. Biochem. Cell Biol. 34, 1059−1070.

Selkoe, D.J., Hardy, J., 2016. The amyloid hypothesis of Alzheimer's disease at 25 years. EMBO Mol. Med. 8, 595−608.

Serhan, C.N., 2009. Systems approach to inflammation resolution: identification of novel anti-inflammatory and pro-resolving mediators. J. Thromb. Haemost. 7 (Suppl. 1), 44−48.

Serhan, C.N., 2010. Novel lipid mediators and resolution mechanisms in acute inflammation: to resolve or not? Am. J. Pathol. 177, 1576−1591.

Serhan, C.N., Chiang, N., Van Dyke, T.E., 2008. Resolving inflammation: dual anti-inflammatory and pro-resolution lipid mediators. Nat. Rev. Immunol. 8, 349−361.

Shankar, G.M., Li, S., Mehta, T.H., Garcia-Munoz, A., Shepardson, N.E., et al., 2008. Amyloid β-protein dimers isolated directly from Alzheimer brains impair synaptic plasticity and memory. Nat. Med. 14, 837−842.

Sharma, S., Yang, B., Xi, X., Grotta, J.C., Aronowski, J., Savitz, S.I., 2011. IL-10 directly protects cortical neurons by activating PI-3 kinase and STAT-3 pathways. Brain Res. 1373, 189−194.

Simundic, A.M., Basic, V., Topic, E., Demarin, V., Vrkic, N., et al., 2004. Soluble adhesion molecules in acute ischemic stroke. Clin. Invest. Med. 27, 86−92.

Smith, W.S., 2004. Pathophysiology of focal cerebral ischemia: a therapeutic perspective. J. Vasc. Interv. Radiol. 15, S3–S12.

Sorensen, E.N., Burgreen, G.W., Wagner, W.R., Antaki, J.F., 1999. Computational simulation of platelet deposition and activation: I. Model development and properties. Ann. Biomed. Eng. 27, 436–448.

Stellwagen, D., Malenka, R.C., 2006. Synaptic scaling mediated by glial TNF-alpha. Nature 440, 1054–1059.

Strbian, D., Durukan, A., Pitkonen, M., Marinkovic, I., Tatlisumak, E., et al., 2008. The blood–brain barrier is continuously open for several weeks following transient focal cerebral ischemia. Neuroscience 153, 175–181.

Sugawara, T., Fujimura, M., Noshita, N., Kim, G.W., Saito, A., et al., 2004. Neuronal death/survival signaling pathways in cerebral ischemia. NeuroRx 1, 17–25.

Sun, G.Y., Horrocks, L.A., Farooqui, A.A., 2007. The roles of NADPH oxidase and phospholipases A_2 in oxidative and inflammatory responses in neurodegenerative diseases. J. Neurochem. 103, 1–16.

Sun, J.-H., Tan, L., Yu, J.-T., 2014. Post-stroke cognitive impairment: epidemiology, mechanisms and management. Ann. Transl. Med. 2, 80.

Suzuki, H., Hayashi, T., Tojo, S.J., Kitagawa, H., Kimura, K., et al., 1999. Anti-P-selectin antibody attenuates rat brain ischemic injury. Neurosci. Lett. 265, 163–166.

Szpak, G.M., Lechowicz, W., Lewandowska, E., Bertrand, E., Wierzba-Bobrowicz, T., et al., 1999. Border zone neovascularization in cerebral ischemic infarct. Folia Neuropathol. 37, 264–268.

Takada, J., Ooboshi, H., Ago, T., Kitazono, T., Yao, H., Kadomatsu, K., et al., 2005. Postischemic gene transfer of midkine, a neurotrophic factor, protects against focal brain ischemia. Gene Ther. 12, 487–493.

Takechi, R., Galloway, S., Pallebage-Gamarallage, M.M.S., et al., 2010. Dietary fats, cerebrovasculature integrity and Alzheimer's disease risk. Prog. Lipid Res. 49, 159–170.

Taoufik, E., Probert, L., 2008. Ischemic neuronal damage. Curr. Pharm. Des. 14, 3565–3573.

Taurin, S., Seyrantepe, V., Orlov, S.N., Tremblay, T.L., Thibault, P., et al., 2002. Proteome analysis and functional expression identify mortalin as an antiapoptotic gene induced by elevation of [Na +]i/[K +]i ratio in cultured vascular smooth muscle cells. Circ. Res. 91, 915–922.

Terao, Y., Ohta, H., Oda, A., Nakagaito, Y., Kiyota, Y., Shintani, Y., 2009. Macrophage inflammatory protein-3alpha plays a key role in the inflammatory cascade in rat focal cerebral ischemia. Neurosci. Res. 64, 75–82.

Tian, L., Rauvala, H., Gahmberg, C.G., 2009. Neuronal regulation of immune responses in the central nervous system. Trends Immunol. 30, 91–99.

Tiozzo, E., Youbi, M., Dave, K., Perez-Pinzon, M., Rundek, T., et al., 2015. Aerobic, resistance and cognitive exercise training poststroke. Stroke 2015 (46), 2012–2016.

Turrens, J.F., 1997. Superoxide production by the mitochondrial respiratory chain. Biosci. Rep. 17, 3–8.

Tuttolomondo, A., Di Raimondo, D., di Sciacca, R., Pinto, A., Licata, G., 2008. Inflammatory cytokines in acute ischemic stroke. Curr. Pharm. Des. 14, 3574–3589.

Urra, X., Cervera, A., Villamor, N., Planas, A.M., Chamorro, A., 2009. Harms and benefits of lymphocyte subpopulations in patients with acute stroke. Neuroscience 158, 1174–1183.

Van Exel, E., Gussekloo, J., De Craen, A., Bootsma-Van Der Wiel, A., et al., 2002. Inflammation and stroke the Leiden 85-Plus Study. Stroke 33, 1135–1138.

Voos, W., Martin, H., Krimmer, T., Pfanner, N., 1999. Mechanisms of protein translocation into mitochondria. Biochim. Biophys. Acta 1422, 235–254.

Walsh, D.M., Hartley, D.M., Condron, M.M., Selkoe, D.J., Teplow, D.B., 2001. In vitro studies of amyloid β-protein fibril assembly and toxicity provide clues to the aetiology of Flemish variant (Ala692-- > Gly) Alzheimer's disease. Biochem. J. 355, 869–877.

Wang, Q., Tang, X.N., Yenari, M.A., 2007. The inflammatory response in stroke. J. Neuroimmunol. 184, 53–68.

Wang, B., Zhu, X., Kim, Y., Li, J., Huang, S., Saleem, S., et al., 2012a. Histone deacetylase inhibition activates transcription factor Nrf2 and protects against cerebral ischemic damage. Free Radic. Biol. Med. 52, 928–936.

Wang, X., Mao, X., Xie, L., Sun, F., Greenberg, D.A., et al., 2012b. Conditional depletion of neurogenesis inhibits long-term recovery after experimental stroke in mice. PLoS One 7, e38932.

Webster, K.A., Graham, R.M., Thompson, J.W., Spiga, M.G., Frazier, D.P., et al., 2006. Redox stress and the contributions of BH3-only proteins to infarction. Antioxid. Redox Signal. 8, 1667–1676.

Wen, Y.D., Zhang, H.L., Oin, Z.H., 2006. Inflammatory mechanism in ischemic neuronal injury. Neurosci. Bull. 22, 171–182.

Wood, P.L., 1998. Neuroinflammation: Mechanisms and Management. Humana Press, Totowa, NJ.

Wu, W.T., Jamiolkowski, M.A., Wagner, W.R., Aubry, N., Massoudi, M., et al., 2017. Multi-constituent simulation of thrombus deposition. Sci. Rep. 7, 42720.

Yagita, Y., Sakoda, S., Kitagawa, K., 2008. Gene expression in brain ischemia. Brain Nerve 60, 1347–1355.

Yakubov, E., Gottlieb, M., Gil, S., Dinerman, P., Fuchs, P., et al., 2004. Overexpression of genes in the CA1 hippocampus region of adult rat following episodes of global ischemia. Mol. Brain Res. 127, 10–25.

Yang, Y., Qin, X., Liu, S., Li, J., Zhu, X., Gao, T., et al., 2011. Peroxisome proliferator-activated receptor γ is inhibited by histone deacetylase 4 in cortical neurons under oxidative stress. J. Neurochem. 118, 429–439.

Yankner, A., Lu, T., Bruce, L.P., 2008. The aging brain. Annu. Rev. Pathol. Mech. Dis. 3, 41–66.

Yano, K., Kawasaki, K., Hattori, T., Tawara, S., Toshima, Y., et al., 2008. Demonstration of elevation and localization of Rho-kinase activity in the brain of a rat model of cerebral infarction. Eur. J. Pharmacol. 594, 77–83.

Yarchoan, M., Xie, S.X., Kling, M.A., Toledo, J.B., Wolk, D.A., et al., 2012. Cerebrovascular atherosclerosis correlates with Alzheimer pathology in neurodegenerative dementias. Brain 135, 3749–3756.

Yilmaz, G., Granger, D.N., 2008. Cell adhesion molecules and ischemic stroke. Neurol. Res. 30, 783–793.

Zeier, Z., Madorsky, I., Xu, Y., Ogle, W.O., Notterpek, L., Foster, T.C., 2011. Gene expression in the hippocampus: regionally specific effects of aging and caloric restriction. Mech. Ageing Dev. 132, 8–19.

Zhang, J.-M., An, J., 2007. Cytokines, inflammation and pain. Int. Anesthesiol. Clin. 45, 27.

Zipser, B.D., Johanson, C.E., Gonzalez, L., et al., 2007. Microvascular injury and blood-brain barrier leakage in Alzheimer's disease. Neurobiol. Aging 28, 977–986.

Potential Neuroprotective Strategies for Ischemic Injuries

INTRODUCTION

Stroke constitutes one of the major causes leading to disability and death worldwide. Stroke is a highly dynamic multifactorial metabolic insult caused by severe reduction or blockade in cerebral blood flow (CBF) due to the formation of a clot (thrombus). This blockade not only reduces oxygen and glucose delivery to the brain, but also results in the breakdown of blood—brain barrier (BBB) and build-up of potentially toxic products in brain (Moskowitz et al., 2010; Farooqui, 2010). Two types of strokes have been reported to occur in human population namely ischemic stroke and hemorrhagic stroke are caused by the bursting of the blood vessels. In the Western world, most strokes are ischemic, whereas in Asian countries majorities of strokes are of hemorrhagic in origin. Approximately 12% of strokes are hemorrhagic, whereas the remaining 88% are ischemic and result from occlusion of a cerebral artery (either thrombolic or embolic).

Stroke survivors have more than twice the risk of another stroke and subsequently developing dementia compared with people who have never had a stroke (Patel et al., 2002). For instance, a stroke localized on the left hemisphere promotes disturbance in language and comprehension, which reduce the ability to communicate (Pirmoradi et al., 2016). In contrast, when stroke affects the right hemisphere, the intuitive thinking, reasoning, solving problems as well as the perception, judgment and the visual—spatial functions may be impaired (Cumming et al., 2013; Sun et al., 2014; Tiozzo et al., 2015; Save-Pédebos et al., 2016). It makes stroke patients difficult to locate objects, walk up or down stairs or get dressed. Consequently, cognitive disorders are one of the strongest predictor of the inability to return to work, that contribute to the socioeconomic burden of stroke (Kauranen et al., 2013). As stated in

Ischemic and Traumatic Brain and Spinal Cord Injuries
DOI: https://doi.org/10.1016/B978-0-12-813596-9.00003-1

Chapter 2, Molecular Aspects of Ischemic Injury, stroke-mediated brain damage not only involves excitotoxicity, oxidative stress, apoptosis, and neuroinflammation, but also activation of glial cells and infiltration of leukocytes (Moskowitz et al., 2010; Farooqui, 2010). These processes trigger the onset of abnormal signal transduction pathways that ultimately cause irreversible neuronal injury in the ischemic core of the infarct within minutes of the onset of cerebral ischemia (Moskowitz et al., 2010). In contrast, the area that surrounds the core (penumbra) signifies brain tissue which remains partially perfused—usually through collateral vessels—and which degenerates in a more delayed fashion involving prominent apoptotic cell death (Hara and Snyder, 2007). The visualization of the penumbra has been made possible using modern magnetic resonance imaging and positron emission tomography techniques (Guadagno et al., 2004). Importantly, many investigators believe that cell death in the penumbra can be prevented with suitable neuroprotective drugs. At the molecular level, stroke is accompanied by the influx of Ca^{2+}, release of glutamate, overactivation of glutamate receptors, increase in levels of free fatty acids, generation of high levels of eicosanoids and platelet activating factor due to the activation of phospholipases A_2 (PLA_2), phospholipase C (PLC), cyclooxygenases (COXs), lipoxygenases (LOXs) with increase in expression and secretion of cytokines and chemokines (Moskowitz et al., 2010; Farooqui, 2010). PLA_2 and COX-1 and COX-2, and LOXs contribute to the breakdown of neural membrane phospholipid. Matrix metalloproteinases (MMPs) are involved in the breakdown of the microvascular basal lamina, which results in the disruption of the BBB (Heo et al., 1999). These changes are most prominent in the core infarct, where neuronal damage is maximal. Other enzymes along with MMP-9 play an important role in the progression of the cerebral infarct. Major cytokines, which contribute to neuroinflammation are interleukins (IL-1, IL-6, and IL-10) and TNF-α. Cytokines are not only responsible for the stimulation of PLA_2 and COXs, but also for the initiation and regulation of the inflammatory response and play an important role in leukocyte infiltration into the ischemic regions of the brain (Kaushal and Schlichter, 2008). Cytokines and chemokines also upregulate cellular adhesion molecules (CAMs). CAMs promote the adhesion and migration of the leukocytes. Leukocytes roll on the endothelial surface and then adhere to them. The interactions between leukocytes and the vascular endothelial cells are mediated by three proteins: the selectins, the immunoglobulin gene superfamily, and the integrins. Selectins E and P are not only upregulated, but also play an important role in leukocyte rolling and recruitment during the early stages of ischemic injury (Zhang et al., 1998). It is also revealed that β2-integrins (CD11/CD18) along with ICAM-1, and P-selectin also contribute to the recruitment of platelets in the postischemic cerebral microvasculature (Yilmaz and Granger, 2010). Immunoblockade or genetic deletion of these adhesion molecules has been shown to reduce infarct volume, edema, behavioral deficits, and/ or mortality in different animal models of ischemic stroke. Emerging evidence on the role of signaling pathways (e.g., CD40/CD40L, Notch-1) and immune cells in the regulation of ischemia—reperfusion induced leukocyte recruitment in the cerebral microvasculature offers novel targets for controlling inflammation in stroke (Moskowitz et al., 2010; Farooqui, 2010). In addition to above neurochemical changes at the cellular level following stroke, neural circuits are also disrupted due to shifts in the excitation—inhibition balance in neural networks. In the setting of a long-term depression of inhibitory signals, cortical hyperexcitability peaks several weeks after stroke, though it can persist for months (Buchkremer-Ratzmann et al., 1996).

POTENTIAL TREATMENT STRATEGIES FOR ISCHEMIC INJURIES

Stroke is not only a leading cause of serious and long-term physical, emotional, and social disabilities, but also produces lots of financial difficulties to patients, their family and friends. Despite of these social and financial issues, current established therapies for ischemic stroke are limited. Stroke is now seen as a medical emergency. Its patients must be admitted to the hospital for treatment and rehabilitation. Thus, stroke is a complex clinical condition, which requires health professionals to bring together their collective knowledge and specialized skills for the benefit of stroke survivors. Neurosurgery is required to treat the bleeding in the hemorrhagic stroke. Functional recovery after stroke has been observed in both human and animal studies (Sharma and Cohen, 2010; Calautti and Baron, 2003). After stroke-mediated neural injury, the brain undergoes reorganization and rewiring and this can occur in areas adjacent or remotely connected to the infarct (Murphy and Corbett, 2009). Significant turnover of dendritic spines and axonal sprouting in the periinfarct zone after stroke has been reported to occur in the brain and these changes in dendritic spines and axonal sprouting are correlated with improved functional outcome (Murphy and Corbett, 2009). Cortical remapping during stroke recovery is accompanied by the development of prolonged sensory responses and new structural circuits in the periinfarct and connected cortical areas, such as premotor, motor, and somatosensory cortex (Murphy and Corbett, 2009). Sprouting of axons is an activity-dependent process (Carmichael and Chesselet, 2002; Carmichael, 2003), and increasing neuronal activity can result in release of neurotrophins, such as nerve growth factor (NGF) and brain-derived neurotrophic factor (BDNF), which are known to improve recovery by enhancing axonal sprouting and dendritic branching (Zhu et al., 2011). In addition, studies on axonal sprouting transcriptome after stroke have indicated that there occurs a molecular growth program that regulates the axonal sprouting processes (Li et al., 2010). This axonal growth transcriptome may potentially provide important information, which may mediate repair and recovery after stroke. Some of these candidates have recently been demonstrated as important regulators of poststroke axonal sprouting, including ephrin-A5, which inhibits axonal sprouting (Overman et al., 2012), and growth and differentiation factor 10, which promotes axonal sprouting (Li et al., 2015) penumbra, the salvageable surrounding tissue around the ischemic core which can be treated with neuroprotective agents (Astrup et al. 1981).

Effective pharmacological treatment of stroke patients is obstructed by the BBB and reduced blood supply to ischemic brain tissue, facing repeated translational failure in recent 20 years. The pharmacological treatment of ischemic stroke treatment involves the use of (1) thrombolytic drugs, (2) neuroprotective drugs, (3) anticoagulation drugs, (4) catheter-based interventions, and (5) perfusion/reperfusion enhancers (Fagan et al., 1999) to improve cerebral blood circulation. Thus, for ischemic stroke, current interventional treatment regimens mainly include blood pressure management, anticoagulation therapy, defibrinogen therapy, and pharmacotherapy to improve cerebral blood circulation. In addition to above-mentioned therapeutic approaches, the use of hypothermia and hyperbaric oxygen therapy (HBOT) is another potent therapeutic approach to reduce experimental ischemic brain injury. Mild hypothermia (33°C) is also used for neuroprotection during neurovascular surgery (Wang et al., 2014c). Mild to moderate hypothermia not only prevents microvascular basal lamina antigen loss in experimental focal cerebral ischemia (Hamann et al., 2004) and reduces infarct volume and BBB breakdown following tissue plasminogen activator (tPA) treatment in the mouse (Tang et al., 2013; Cechmanek et al., 2015), but also diminishes oxidative DNA damage and prodeath signaling events after cerebral ischemia (Ji et al., 2007). Hypothermia also produces a lasting inhibitory effect on activation of astrogliosis (Zgavc et al., 2012). HBOT, is a nondrug and noninvasive therapeutic approach, which has been used for the treatment of stroke since 1960s. HBOT has been reported to be a safe and beneficial treatment strategy, which produces beneficial effects after stroke although some controversies still exist (Ding et al., 2014). It is well known that neural cells rely exclusively on aerobic metabolism and need a high levels of oxygen and glucose to produce adequate ATP for neuronal signal transduction. Hyperbaric

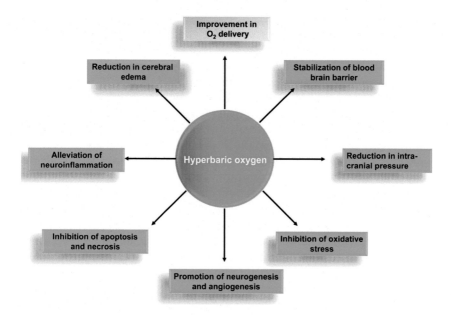

FIGURE 3.1   Beneficial effects of hyperbaric oxygen on the brain.

oxygen treatment results in improvement in O_2 delivery, BBB protection and stabilization, alleviation of neuroinflammation, reduction in cerebral edema, reduction in intracranial pressure, decrease in oxidative stress and apoptosis, increase in neurogenesis and angiogenesis promoting vascular and neural regeneration (Wang et al., 2014a) (Fig. 3.1). However, HBOT in human stroke is still not sufficiently evidence based, due to the insufficient randomized double-blind controlled clinical studies. To date, there are no uniform criteria for the dose and session duration of HBOT in different strokes.

THROMBOLYTIC DRUGS FOR THE TREATMENT OF STROKE

To date, the only effective thrombolytic drug approved for acute ischemic stroke in the United States and Canada is tPA (Schwammenthal et al., 2006). In addition to thrombolysis, antiplatelet therapies such as aspirin and glycoprotein IIb-IIIa inhibitors (clopidogrel) or anticoagulants (heparin) have been used in the prevention/treatment of acute ischemic stroke. As stated in Chapter 1, Classification and Molecular Aspects of Neurotraumatic Diseases: Similarities and

Differences With Neurodegenerative and Neuropsychiatric Diseases, and Chapter 2, Molecular Aspects of Ischemic Injury, stroke (cerebral ischemia) produces an infarct, which has a core that contains irreversibly damaged cells and an area surrounding the core called penumbra. This area contains viable neurons that can be salvaged through neuroprotective strategies. Prompt treatment with clot-dissolving (thrombolytic) medications (alteplase (Activase), streptokinase (Streptase), tPA, and urokinase (Kinlytic)) can restore blood flow before major brain damage can occur. This may allow patient to make a good recovery from the stroke (Schwammenthal et al., 2006). However, tPA needs to be applied within 3 hours of symptom onset, decreasing the availability of treatment to the majority of patients in need (Khaja and Grotta, 2007). Antiadhesion agents have been reported to widen the therapeutic window for thrombolytic therapy in these experimental models. As stated in Chapter 2, Molecular Aspects of Ischemic Injury, blood clot is formed from the aggregation of activated platelets onto fibrin meshes. Thrombolytic drugs act by activating plasminogen, which is cleaved into a product called plasmin. Plasmin is a proteolytic enzyme, which acts on the fibrin meshes to break it down to fibrin products. This process leads to the lysis of the clot. Plasmin is extremely short lived; it is quickly inactivated by α_2-antiplasmin, an abundant inhibitor that restricts the action of plasmin to the vicinity of the clot (Aoki, 2005; Gallimore, 2006). However, tPA has been reported to promote serious bleeding in the brain, which can be fatal (Wardlaw et al., 2014). Many investigations have indicated that in addition to serious bleeding in the brain, tPA also produces many undesirable side effects, such as hemodynamic perturbations, disruption of the BBB, and the damage to the extracellular matrix (Gravanis and Tsirka, 2008) (Fig. 3.2). In addition, tPA also induces brain edema and recruitment and activation of inflammatory cells such as microglia and nonneural cells of the systemic circulation. tPA-induced changes in plasminogen activating system play important roles in BBB regulation (Medcalf and Lawrence, 2016). This regulation of BBB typically involves MMPs, tissue inhibitors of metalloproteinases, and low-density lipoprotein receptor-related protein/alpha 2-macroglobulin receptor (LRPs) (Fig. 3.2). The participation of above systems involves the modulation of tPA activity by neuroserpin, a tPA modulating agent (Lebeurrier et al., 2005), critical signaling systems, i.e., tyrosine kinase (Su et al., 2008), and Rho kinase pathways (Niego et al., 2012), and receptors, i.e., LRP-1 (Yepes et al., 2003; Samson et al., 2008), and PDGFRα (Fredriksson et al., 2004, 2017) in the central nervous system (CNS) have been identified by various groups to participate in this new frontier of plasminogen activation biology. Based on signal transduction processes, it is proposed that tPA-mediated BBB breakdown promotes serious secondary hemorrhage (Ortolano and Spuch, 2013;

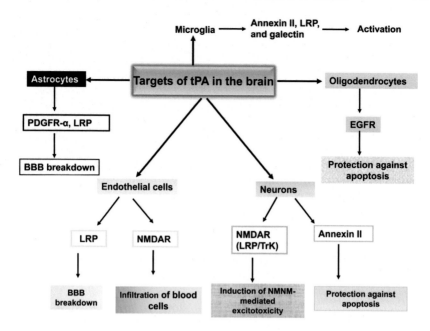

FIGURE 3.2 Neurochemical targets of tPA in the brain. *BBB*, blood—brain barrier; *EGFR*, epidermal growth factor receptor; *LRP*, LDL receptor—related protein; *NMDAR*, N-methyl-D-aspartate receptor; *PDGF-α*, platelet-derived growth factor-α; *tPA*, tissue plasminogen activator; *TrK*, tyrosine receptor kinase.

Medcalf and Lawrence, 2016). This mechanism of tPA action explains not only the induction of serious bleeding in the brain, but also the modulation of permeability of the neurovascular unit in physiological conditions as well as pathological conditions such as ischemic stroke, vascular dementia, and traumatic brain injury (Ortolano and Spuch, 2013; Medcalf and Lawrence, 2016). In spite of above-mentioned complications, tPA is the only FDA-approved medication, which restores CBF to the penumbra (Alberts, 1999). However, tPA can also promote serious bleeding in the brain, which can be fatal (Wardlaw et al., 2014). tPA therapy has now been evaluated in many randomized trials in acute ischemic stroke. tPA has been licensed for use within 3 hours of stroke in the United States and Canada, and within 4.5 hours in most European countries (Alberts, 1999; Fernandes and Umasankar, 2016). tPA does not produce any effect on infarct core, but it revitalizes the penumbra by restoring blood flow. Guidelines recommended that thrombolysis should be delivered by a clinical team with suitable training and experience and in a setting with appropriate facilities (Steiner et al., 2014; Swain et al., 2008). However, only 8% of all ischemic stroke patients are eligible for treatment with tPA (Kleindorfer et al. 2004). Investigators have also developed device to remove thrombus (MERCI retriever) (Smith et al., 2008; Tenser et al., 2011). This procedure is performed by carefully inserting and passing a special device from a blood vessel in the leg all the way into the blood vessel in the brain where the blood clot is located. The MERCI retriever captures the clot and pulls it out of the body, thus facilitating blood flow to the affected brain area (Smith, 2006; Kim et al., 2006; Tenser et al., 2011). Hyperoxia may be another powerful neuroprotective strategy to salvage acutely ischemic brain tissue and extend the time window for acute stroke treatment (Singhal, 2006, 2007). Although, earlier trials have not given satisfactory results but new studies indicate that hyperbaric and even normobaric oxygen therapy can be effective if used appropriately, and raises possibility of using hyperoxia to extend the narrow therapeutic time window for stroke thrombolysis (Singhal, 2006).

NEUROPROTECTIVE DRUGS FOR THE TREATMENT OF STROKE IN ANIMAL MODELS

Majority of stroke patients display a slow evolution of brain injury (2−6 hours) that occurs in penumbra. This "evolving injury" is a realistic target for therapeutic intervention, with the goal of blocking the progression of detrimental changes that normally occur following the acute ischemic event. Preventing or reducing this delayed neuronal damage may not only improve neurological outcome, but also promote recovery from ischemic injury. Thus investigators are making attempts to protect injured neurons from delayed ischemic injury. Studies in animal models of stroke indicate a period of at least 4 hours after onset of complete ischemia in the ischemic penumbra. In humans, the ischemic injury may be less, and the time window may be longer, but human patients are older and have other pathological conditions that may limit benefit (Zivin, 1998; Cheng et al., 2004). Neuroimaging is an important procedure, which is used for the early diagnosis of stroke in human patients. It yields essential information regarding human brain integrity, a key factor in determining the therapeutic agent. However, widespread use of neuroimaging in overall management of acute stroke is still heavily debated and remains still controversial (Dubey et al., 2013). Although, clinical treatments have improved in the acute time window, long-term therapeutics remain very much limited. Damage to complex neural cell circuits by ischemic stroke makes restoration of neuronal function after stroke very difficult. New therapeutic approaches, include not only neuroprotection by newly discovered drugs, but also neural cell transplantation or stimulation, focus on reestablishing damaged neural cell circuits through multiple mechanisms to improve circuit plasticity and remodeling. There has been remarkable development in the understanding of stroke pathophysiology and therapeutic strategies for ischemic stroke in animal models, but no drug has been approved by FDA for the neuroprotection therapy in humans. Neuroprotection is defined as strategy, or combination of strategies, that may result in salvaging, recovering, or regenerating neural cells in the brain for performing normal function. The goal of neuroprotection strategies is to limit neurodegeneration after ischemic injury. A major aim of neuroprotection strategies is to maintain the highest possible integrity of cellular interactions in the brain resulting in normal neuronal function. Current studies have indicated that the term neuroprotection is simply not enough for clinical success, and rather the focus needs to shift from neuroprotection to cerebroprotection. The term cerebroprotection includes glial cells and the vasculature (neurovascular unit) (del Zoppo, 2010). It should be noted that glial cells outnumber neurons and play an integral role not only in maintaining homeostasis in the healthy brain, but also in protecting neurons from ischemia. Neuroprotectants are agents intervene or halt the progression of neuronal injury in the ischemic penumbra. In humans, the cerebral ischemia may be less complete, and the time window may be longer, but human patients also tend to be older, with comorbidities that may limit benefit. This may limit successful neuroprotection with the short window (3−6 hours) of opportunity for active intervention (Zivin, 1998). Various neuroprotective agents have reached phase III efficacy trials in focal ischemic stroke animal models, but none has proven effective, despite successful preceding animal studies (Cheng et al., 2004).

As stated in Chapter 2, Molecular Aspects of Ischemic Injury, pathophysiology of stroke is a multifactorial process involving: energy failure, loss of cell ion homeostasis, acidosis, Ca^{2+}-influx, excitotoxicity, free radical or ROS generation along with mitochondrial dysfunction, increased production of arachidonic acid-derived products, increased expression of cytokine-mediated cytotoxicity, complement activation, disruption of the BBB, activation of glial cells, and infiltration of leukocyte (Moskowitz et al., 2010; Farooqui, 2010). Excessive glutamate receptor stimulation also results in increased nitric oxide generation which can be detrimental to cells as nitric oxide interacts with superoxide to form the toxic molecule peroxynitrite (Farooqui, 2010) (Fig. 3.3). This metabolite acts by nitrosylating specific neuronal proteins. This process leads to protein misfolding, ER stress, and mitochondrial impairment (Yang et al., 2015) supporting the view that ischemic injury is accompanied by necrotic cell death in the ischemic-core regions (Van Cruchten and Van Den Broeck, 2002; Broughton et al., 2009). Necrotic cell death is characterized by initial cellular and organelle swelling, subsequent disruption of nuclear, organelle, and plasma membranes, disintegration of nuclear structure and cytoplasmic organelles with extrusion of cell contents into the extracellular space (Van Cruchten and Van Den Broeck,

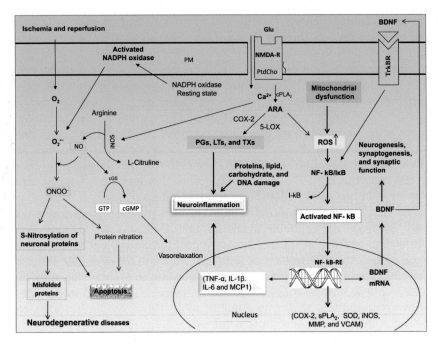

FIGURE 3.3 Pathways associated with generation of ROS and RNS in cerebral ischemia. *ARA*, arachidonic acid; *BDNF*, brain-derived neurotrophic factor; *cGMP*, cyclic guanosine monophosphate; *COX-2*, cyclooxygenase-2; *cPLA₂*, cytosolic phospholipase A$_2$; *Glu*, glutamate; *GTP*, guanosine-5′-triphosphate; *IL-1β*, interleukin-1β; *IL-6*, interleukin-6; *5-LOX*, 5-lipoxygenase; *LTs*, leukotrienes; *MCP1*, monocyte chemoattractant protein 1; *NF-κB*, nuclear factor kappa-light-chain-enhancer of activated B cells; *NMDAR*, N-methyl-D-aspartate receptor; *NOS*, nitric oxide synthase; *O₂*, superoxide; *ONOO⁻*, peroxynitrite; *PGs*, prostaglandins; *RNS*, reactive nitrogen species; *ROS*, reactive oxygen species; *sGC*, soluble guanylyl cyclase; *TNF-α*, tumor necrosis factor-α; *TrK*, tyrosine receptor kinase; *TXs*, thromboxanes.

2002; Broughton et al., 2009). As stated earlier, neuroprotective agents can be used to salvage neurons in the ischemic penumbra, a region in which neurons die by apoptotic cell death due to the activation of the intrinsic and extrinsic pathways (Anrather and Iadecola, 2016). It is becoming increasingly evident that in the ischemic penumbra neuronal apoptosis occurs several hours or days after the onset of stroke. Neurons undergoing apoptosis are dismantled from within in an organized way that minimizes damage and disruption to neighboring cells (Broughton et al., 2009).

Ideal therapeutic agents for the treatment of cerebral ischemic injury may require either a single drug that can act on multiple targets, or a combination of multiple drugs that provide better protection in addition to tPA treatment. Several neuroprotective agents have reached phase III efficacy trials, but have shown mixed results. They include N-methyl-D-aspartate (NMDA) receptor antagonists, calcium channel blockers, citicoline (CDP-choline), the free radical scavenger tirilazad, anti-intercellular adhesion molecule-1 (ICAM-1) antibody, GM_1 ganglioside, clomethiazole, a sedative and muscle relaxant, and fosphenytoin, and piracetam, a nootropic drug. However, despite the development of over 1000 compounds that have been proven effective in animal models of stroke, none has demonstrated efficacy in patients over 100 clinical trials (Green, 2008). Analysis of data presented on the Addis Insight Database (1995–2015) indicates that evaluation of 430 potential stroke medication results in discontinuation of 300 medications (70%) from the market, about 70 (17%) are undergoing preclinical assessment, 40 (9%) are in various phases of clinical trials, and only 19 (4%) have reached the market (Chen and Wang, 2016). The failure of these clinical trials raises significant concerns about neuroprotection strategies alone as a therapeutic intervention for the treatment of ischemic injury in humans. At the present time, neuroprotection strategies are focused on injured neurons and the neurotoxic environment induced by the ischemic injury. The complex processes that are induced by postischemic injury events require the targeting of not only neurons, but also nonneuronal cells (glial, endothelial, and inflammatory cells) along with alterations in axons and white matter. An ideal neuroprotective drug should be chronically active and well tolerated. They should be able to cross the BBB, have regional specificity, and should be able to reach the site where neurodegenerative process is taking place. Although, neural cells in the ischemic penumbra can be protected through neuroprotective intervention strategies much later postischemic injury than the ischemic core, future interventions should be designed to target multiple cell types involved in maintaining the integrity of neural and nonneural cells in penumbra (Barone, 2009). The concept of neuroprotection has been reported to be promising in experimental studies, but has failed to translate into clinical success. There are many reasons for this failure including the heterogeneity of human stroke and the lack of methodological agreement between preclinical and clinical studies. Furthermore, the temporal heterogeneity and complexity of ischemic events make the single neuroprotective agent-mediated intervention of ischemic injury very complex. This is tempting to speculate that multiple cellular mechanisms should be targeted for the successful treatment of ischemic injury. At present, there is no treatment of stroke in humans. However, attempts are underway to develop potential therapies for stroke in animal models.

Potential Therapies for the Treatment of Stroke

Stroke-mediated brain damage is a multifactorial process. It involves multiple signal transduction pathways. An ideal ischemic injury treatment may require either a single drug that can act on multiple targets, or a combination of multiple drug therapy to attain better neuroprotection. At present, drugs to treat stroke-mediated brain damage are not available. However, several neuroprotective agents have provided positive results in animal models. These drugs include NMDA receptor antagonists, calcium channel blockers, citicoline (CDP-choline), GM1 ganglioside, statins, omega-3 fatty acids, minocycline, polyarginine, picroside, and curcumin. The failure of these clinical trials in humans raises significant concerns about neuroprotection strategies in humans. At the present time, neuroprotection strategies are focused on injured neurons and the neurotoxic environment produced by the ischemic injury. The complex processes that are induced by postischemic injury events require the targeting of not only neurons, but also nonneuronal cells (glial, endothelial, and inflammatory cells) along with alterations in axons and white matter. An ideal neuroprotective drug for stroke should be chronically active and well tolerated. It should be able to cross the BBB, have regional specificity, and should be able to reach the site where neurodegenerative process is taking place. In addition, steps should be taken to target stroke-mediated white matter injury, a process that has been virtually ignored in animal model clinical trials and needs to be monitored more systematically in the treatment of stroke in humans (Ho et al., 2005; Wen and Sachdev, 2004). This is tempting to suggest that multiple cellular mechanisms should be targeted for the successful treatment of ischemic injury.

N-METHYL-D-ASPARTATE RECEPTOR ANTAGONISTS AND STROKE THERAPY

Although, the rationale behind using NMDA receptor antagonists for ischemic injury sounds perfect, many NMDA antagonists produce behavioral and physiological side effects (Farooqui et al., 2008). Earlier NMDA antagonists include drugs like MK 801, selfotel, dextrorphan, dextromethorphan, aptiganel (Cerestat), Eliprodil, and Ifenprodil (Fig. 3.4). These drugs do not promote neuroprotection neither in animal models nor in human patients. In humans, these NMDA and α-amino-3-hydroxy-5-methyl-4-isoxazolepropionic acid (AMPA) antagonists reduce infarct volume in animal models, but produce adverse clinical and behavioral effects (paranoia, hallucinations, agitation, confusion, paranoia, somnolence, severe motor retardation, and catatonia) regardless of the molecular mechanism of action (Schäbitz et al., 2000; Labiche and Grotta, 2004; Kawasaki-Yatsugi et al., 2000). Several clinical trials of NMDA and AMPA antagonists have been terminated prematurely. Memantine (Namenda or Ebixa) is a derivative of amantadine and noncompetitive NMDA receptor antagonist (Fig. 3.4). Memantine binds to NMDARs with a low-micromolar IC_{50} value. Furthermore, it exhibits

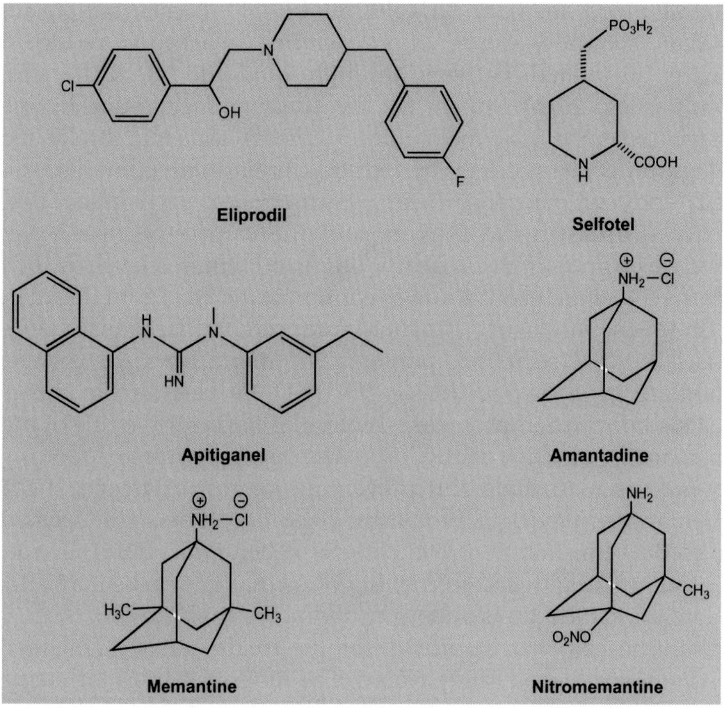

FIGURE 3.4   Chemical structures of glutamate antagonists.

poor selectivity among NMDARs subtypes, with under micromolar IC_{50} values for NR2A, NR2B, NR2C, and NR2D receptors expressed in *Xenopus* oocytes (Parsons et al., 1999). Memantine is known to produce neuroprotective effects against neuroinflammation (Willard et al., 2000), and oxidative stress (Figueiredo et al., 2013; Liu et al., 2013). Generation of NO and formation of peroxynitrite in ischemic injury (Fig. 3.3) may lead to nitrosylation as well as nitration of proteins on cysteine and tyrosine residues of protein, respectively. These processes may contribute to apoptotic cell death. A derivative of memantine called nitromemantine contains a nitro group that has been tethered to the memantine moiety, thus serving not only as an open-channel blocker of NMDA receptor, but also as an NO donor. In this manner, a nitromemantine provides increased blockade of hyperactivated NMDARs through S-nitrosylation promoting more neuroprotection to the degenerating neurons (Nakamura and Lipton, 2016). In addition, memantine not only blocks Kv1.3 potassium channels, inhibits CD3-antibody- and alloantigen-induced proliferation, but also suppresses chemokine-mediated migration of peripheral blood T cells of healthy donors. Furthermore, memantine treatment results in a profound depletion of peripheral blood memory CD45RO + CD4 + T cells supporting the view that standard doses of memantine markedly reduce T-cell responses in treated patients through blockade of Kv1.3 channels (Lowinus et al., 2016). Studies on the effect of memantine in ischemic rats have indicated that memantine prevents ischemic stroke induced neurological deficits not only by reducing brain infarct, but also decreasing ATP-induced neuronal death. Furthermore, memantine not only markedly suppresses the activation of the calpain-caspase-3 pathway and decreases apoptotic cell death, but also increases levels of BDNF, a growth factor, which contribute synaptic plasticity in rats (Picada et al., 2011). In mouse model of permanent focal cerebral ischemia, memantine decreases MMP-9 secretion, prevents the degradation of collagen IV, and inhibits postsynaptic density-95 (PSD-95) cleavage in the mouse brain. This information provides a molecular basis for the role of memantine in reducing reactive astrogliosis, decreasing neuronal apoptosis, and improving vascularization and preventing neuronal damage, suggesting that memantine may be a promising drug for recovery of sensory and motor cortical function in stroke patients (Chen et al., 2016). In addition, the clinical availability and tolerability of memantine make it an attractive candidate for clinical translation (López-Valdés et al., 2014).

Memantine has been approved for the treatment of Alzheimer' disease (AD). It has a good safety record. The molecular basis for memantine efficacy in neurological disorders is at least in part due to the improvement of overactivation of NMDA receptor that causes excessive Ca^{2+} influx through the receptor's associated ion channel and subsequent free radical formation (Farooqui, 2017). Few clinical trials have been performed on stroke patients using memantine. It is shown that 60 mg daily doses of memantine (20 mg TID) can be beneficial for neurologic function improvement of patients with ischemic stroke (Kafi et al., 2014).

CALCIUM CHANNEL BLOCKERS AND STROKE THERAPY

Hypertension is one of the most common chronic diseases and is an important risk factor for ischemic stroke. Hypertension not only results in the bursting of a blood vessel, but also accelerates the narrowing of arteries in the brain to cause a stroke which, if not lethal, can result in many catastrophic complications such as paralysis, aphasia, and coma. The damage to the brain cannot be repaired, so the only rational approach is prevention of hypertension, which is now considered as a major risk factor for the development of stroke. Calcium channel blockers exert potent antihypertensive action and are widely used as a first line antihypertensive drug with few contraindications (Chobanian et al.,

2003). They have been reported to prevent the entry of calcium ions into the ischemic neurons. Calcium channel blockers do not antagonize the effect of calcium ions but facilitate the dilation of arteries. They also exert dilator action on vascular smooth muscle cells by inhibiting calcium entry through L-type calcium channels. Recently, novel types of calcium channel blockers have been developed that express unique characteristics. Thus certain calcium channel blockers manifest blocking activity on N- (cilnidipine) and/or T- (mibefradil and efonidipine) type calcium channels as well as L-type channels, and it is surmised that these properties produce additional benefits associated with reductions in cardiovascular and cerebrovascular events and brain and renal injury. USDA approved calcium channel blockers such as nisoldipine (Sular), nifedipine (Adalat, Procardia), nicardipine (Cardene), isradipine (Dynacirc), nimodipine (Nimotop), felodipine (Plendil), amlodipine (Norvasc), diltiazem (Cardizem), and verapamil (Calan, Isoptin) for the treatment of hypertension (Fig. 3.5). Calcium channel blockers have been widely used for the treatment of hypertension and slow the onset of cerebrovascular and cardiovascular events. More than 80% of acute stroke patients have high blood pressure. Several small randomized trials have assessed the efficacy of CBF with calcium channel blockers in acute ischemic stroke (Chen and Yang, 2013; Sare et al., 2009).

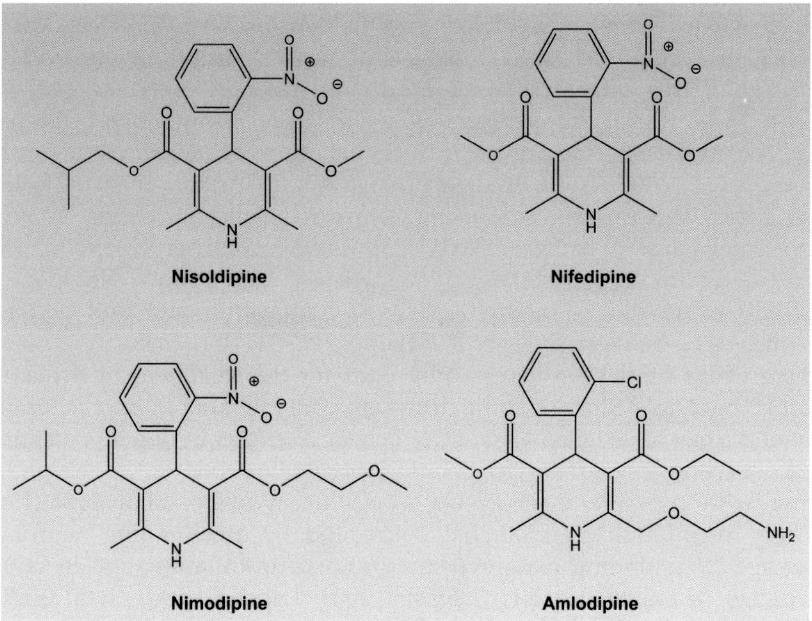

FIGURE 3.5   Chemical structures of some calcium channel blockers.

Overall, these studies demonstrate no change in cerebral perfusion. Calcium channel blockers do not alter outcome after ischemic stroke in 29 trials with 7665 patients (Sare et al., 2009). Although, the mechanism of calcium channel blocker's action in cerebral ischemia is still unclear, major mechanisms of their actions may include normalization of blood pressure and their antioxidative properties (Papademetriou and Doumas, 2009). Control of hypertension with calcium channel blockers in principle should decrease the risk of first and recurrent stroke. The most common side effects of calcium channel blockers are slow heart rate, constipation, nausea, edema, headache, drowsiness, and dizziness.

FREE RADICAL SCAVENGERS AND STROKE THERAPY

As stated in Chapter 2, Molecular Aspects of Ischemic Injury, ischemic stroke is accompanied by overproduction of reactive oxygen species (ROS) and reactive nitrogen species (RNS). Overproduction of ROS results in an imbalance in production of oxidizing chemical species and their effective removal by protective antioxidants and scavenger enzymes. Oxidative stress not only damages neural cell components such as lipids, proteins, and DNA, but also promotes neural cell death not only due to increase in intensity of oxidative stress and neuroinflammation, but also due to the development of brain edema. The molecular mechanism associated with the neuroprotective effects of free radical scavengers depends on several factors including antioxidant activity of free radical scavengers, downregulation of NF-κB activity (Shen et al., 2003), suppression of genes (proinflammatory cytokines and chemokines), induction and stabilization of synapses (Gilgun-Sherki et al., 2006; Wang et al., 2006). For successful treatment of ischemic stroke, the free radical scavenger must have ability to cross the BBB and enter injured neuronal cells, and induce neuroprotective effects (Gilgun-Sherki et al., 2006). Examples of free radical scavengers include edaravone (3-methyl-1-phenyl-2-pyrazolin-5-one) and ebselen (2-phenyl-1,2-benzisoselenazol-3(2H)-one; PZ-51, DR-3305) (Fig. 3.6). These drugs have been successfully used for the treatment of stroke in animal models. Although, these drugs are well tolerated in human stroke patients, they have failed to produce beneficial effects in human patients.

Edaravone or 3-methyl-1-phenyl-2-pyrazolin-5-one is a lipophilic drug with multiple mechanisms of action. It exerts neuroprotective effects by inhibiting endothelial injury and by ameliorating neuronal damage by inhibiting oxidative stress and neuroinflammation in brain ischemia in animal models (Higashi, 2009; Lapchak and Zivin, 2009). Edaravone can also act not only by quenching hydroxyl radicals and inhibiting lipid peroxidation, but also by reducing brain edema (Lee et al., 2010). Edaravone has been approved in Japan for the treatment of

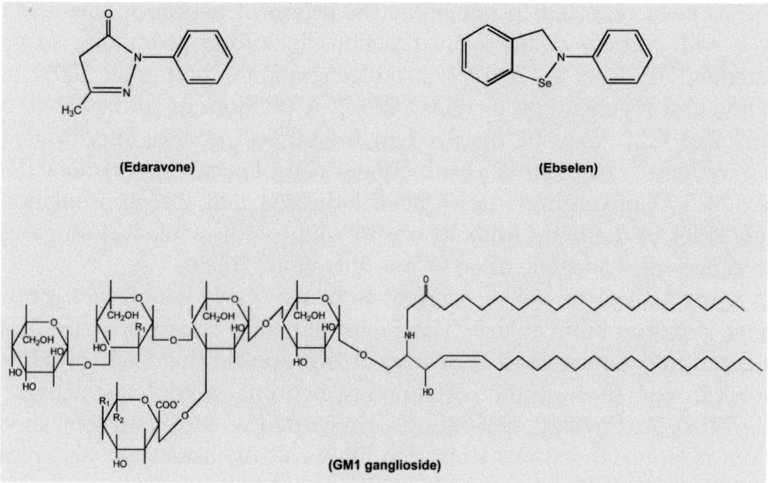

FIGURE 3.6   Chemical structures of edaravone, ebselen, and GM₁ ganglioside.

acute brain infarction within 24 hours after the onset of ischemia. However, according to Mitsubishi Tanabe Pharma Corp, edaravone should not be administered to the elderly patients who have complications of chronic renal dysfunction or dehydration (Nakase et al., 2014).

The organoselenium drug ebselen (2-phenyl-1,2-benzisoselenazol-3 (2H)-one; PZ-51, DR-3305) produces a wide range of biomedical effects that are predominantly due to its interference with redox systems catalyzed by selenoenzymes, e.g., glutathione peroxidase and thioredoxin reductase. Ebselen catalyzes several essential reactions for the protection of cellular components from oxidative and free radical damage (Noguchi, 2016). Based on many in vitro and in vivo studies, several mechanisms have been proposed to explain the biochemical actions of ebselen in health and diseases. Ebselen modulates metalloproteins, enzymatic cofactors, gene expression, epigenetics, antioxidant defenses, and immune systems (Azad and Tomar, 2014). Owing to these properties, ebselen is currently under clinical trials for the prevention of stroke. Ebselen produces neuroprotective effects in a rat transient middle cerebral artery occlusion (MCAo) model when given before the start of ischemia, but not when the insult is severe.

GM₁ GANGLIOSIDE AND STROKE THERAPY

Gangliosides are sialic acid-containing glycosphingolipids (Fig. 3.6). It is enriched in neuronal and glial cell membranes. GM₁ ganglioside is an important component of lipid rafts and is crucial for brain development and plasticity. Exogenous ganglioside can not only cross BBB, but can also act as a neurotrophic factor (Haughey et al., 2010; Gao et al., 2012).

GM$_1$ has been reported to potentiate the action of neurotrophins and display a wide variety of the brain functions including promoting survival, differentiation (Yu et al., 2010), neurodegeneration (Ohmi et al., 2009), axon stability, and regeneration (Schnaar, 2010). A plethora of studies have suggested that GM$_1$ may be involved in the stroke process, specifically the orchestration of cell death and subsequent neurological dysfunctions (Rong et al., 2013). Converging studies have indicated that the accumulation of gangliosides in the brain leads to neurite outgrowth, while lack of gangliosides causes neurodegeneration (Yamashita et al., 2005).

In a rat MCAo model of cerebral ischemia, GM$_1$ ganglioside protects against ischemic brain injury. The molecular mechanism of neuroprotection is not fully understood. However, it is proposed that GM$_1$ ganglioside may act in part through the regulation of neuronal autophagic activity (Li et al., 2016). Autophagy (self-eating) is regarded as a cell survival mechanism in response to various stress conditions. Ganglioside may also protect from ischemic injury by activating Trks receptors and stimulating BDNF secretion (Jiang et al., 2016). These processes may induce neuritogenesis.

STATINS AND STROKE THERAPY

Statins are potent cholesterol-lowering drugs (Fig. 3.7) that act by inhibiting 3-hydroxy-3-methylglutaryl coenzyme A reductase inhibitors

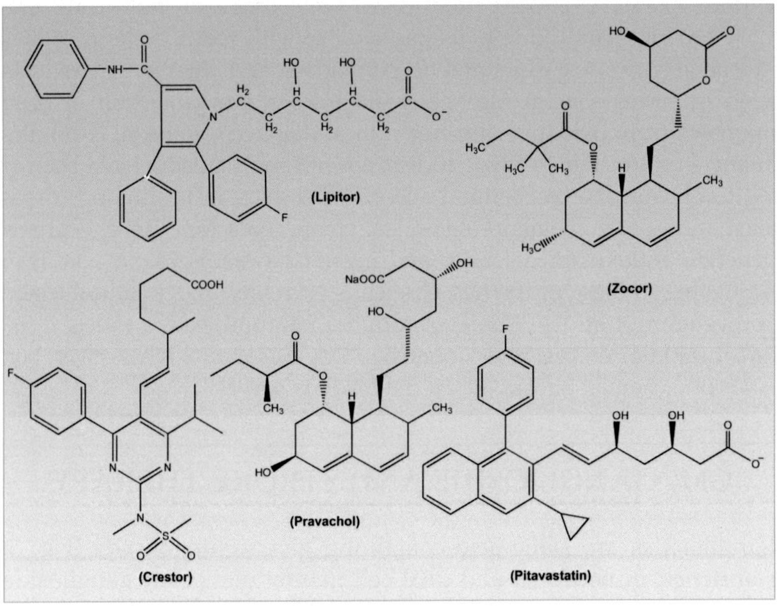

FIGURE 3.7   Chemical structures of statins.

(HMG-CoA reductase) (Endres, 2005). They are widely prescribed to reduce low-density lipoprotein (LDL)-cholesterol concentrations and can reduce cardiac events by 20%–35% (Heart Protection Study, 2002). In addition to lipid-lowering effect, statins also produce antiinflammatory, antioxidant, and antithrombotic effects. Statins also promote clot lysis, endothelial nitric oxide synthetase upregulation, plaque stabilization, LDL oxidation reduction, and angiogenesis (Fig. 3.8) (Kureishi et al., 2000; Asahi et al., 2005; Jain and Ridker, 2005; Moon et al., 2014; Zhao et al., 2014). These pleiotropic effects are potentially beneficial for acute ischemia of the brain and heart. In addition, animal experiments have shown angiogenesis, neurogenesis, and synaptogenesis in acute cerebral ischemia (Chen et al., 2003) supporting the view that statins are potentially neurorestorative as well as neuroprotective in acute cerebral ischemia (Moon et al., 2014; Zhao et al., 2014). Two randomized trials— Stroke Prevention by Aggressive Reduction in Cholesterol Levels (SPARCL) and Justification for the Use of Statin in Prevention: an Intervention Trial Evaluating Rosuvastatin (JUPITER)—have indicated that high doses of statins reduce the risk of cerebrovascular events (Amarenco et al., 2006; Ridker et al., 2008). It is expected that ongoing trials such as NeuSTART II, EUREKA may provide more valuable safety and efficacy information of statins therapy in acute ischemic stroke (Hoe Heo, 2018). Furthermore, treatment with statins either before or early after cerebral arterial occlusion has been proved to associate with reduced infarct volume and improved neurological function in animal models (Prinz et al., 2008). In several large clinical trials, the effects of statins on stroke prevention and treatment have also been well established (Mihaylova et al., 2012). Based on the results of these trials, the

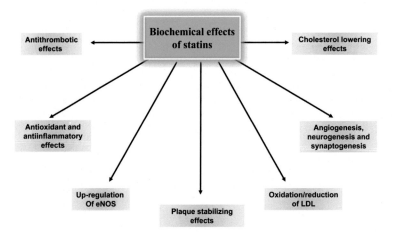

FIGURE 3.8 Biochemical effects of statins.

American Heart Association/American Stroke Association recently recommended the use of statins in patients who have suffered ischemic stroke or transient ischemic attack (Adams et al., 2008). It is reported that improved clinical outcomes observed with statin trials may be not only due to facilitated recanalization, collateral perfusion enhancement, but also due to statin-mediated plaque-stabilizing, antiplatelet aggregation, and antiinflammatory effects, with evidence of the occurrence of atherosclerotic plaque regression and reverse remodeling in patients (Lima et al., 2004; Zhao et al., 2014). Statins have different chemical and commercial names (Table 3.1), but their IC50 values for HMG-CoA reductase are not very different. In recent years, statins have surpassed other pharmacologic medicine in the reduction of the incidence of stroke and total mortality (Topol, 2004).

Although many people treated with statins do well, no drug is without potential for adverse effects. Adverse effects of statins include constipation, peripheral neuropathy, liver and kidney damage, headache, and rhabdomyolysis (Fig. 3.9). As stated earlier, statins inhibit the enzyme HMG-CoA reductase in mevalonate pathway (Moon et al., 2014; Zhao et al., 2014). This pathway generates a range of other products in addition to cholesterol, such as coenzyme Q10, heme-A, and isoprenylated proteins (Moon et al., 2014; Zhao et al., 2014), which play important roles in cell biology and human physiology and potential relevance to benefits as well as risks of statins (Zhao et al., 2014). The most common adverse effect of statin is muscle pain and weakness. This

TABLE 3.1   Statins, Their Commercial Names and IC50 Values

Generic name	Trademark	IC50 for HMG-CoA Reductase (nM)	Reference
Atorvastatin	Lipitor	8.00	Amarenco et al. (2006); Endres (2005)
Cerivastatin	Lipobay, Baycol	10.00	Rajanikant et al. (2007); Vaughan (2003)
Fluvastatin	LescolRXL	28.00	Endres (2005); Vaughan (2003)
Mevastatin	Compactin	23.00	Amarenco (2005); Vaughan (2003)
Rosuvastatin	Crestor	5.00	Endres (2005); Vaughan (2003)
Simvastatin	Zocor, Lipex	–	Endres (2005); Vaughan (2003)
Ezetimibe + Simvastatin	Vytorin	–	Endres (2005); Vaughan (2003)

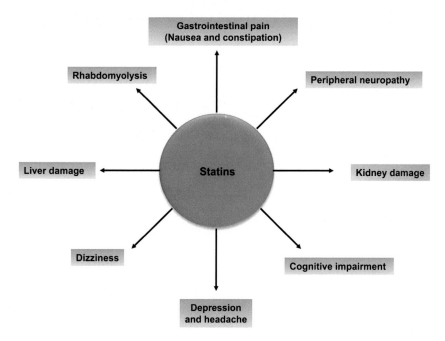

FIGURE 3.9 Side effects of statins in cardiovascular and cerebrovascular systems.

condition is called as rhabdomyolysis, a clinical syndrome that comprises destruction of skeletal muscle with outflow of intracellular muscle content into the bloodstream. These contents include potassium, phosphate, purines, enzymes (such as creatine kinase, aldolase, lactate dehydrogenase, and aspartate transferase), urate, and myoglobin (Brancaccio et al., 2010). In some individuals ($\sim 10\%$ of patients) statin treatment results in the depletion of CoQ10, a nutrient that supports muscle function. During cholesterol synthesis, statins inhibit synthesis of farnesyl pyrophosphate, a metabolite, which is an intermediate in the synthesis of ubiquinone or CoQ10. This fact, plus the role of CoQ10 in mitochondrial energy production, has resulted in the hypothesis that statin-induced CoQ10 deficiency may contribute to the pathogenesis of statin myopathy. This hypothesis is supported by studies that indicate the relationship between statin therapy and lower plasma ubiquinone level (Chu et al., 2006). Several risk factors have been identified, including advanced age, family history of myopathy, and statin dose; many cases manifest only after patients are administered an interacting medication (e.g., azole antifungals, cimetidine, clarithromycin, erythromycin, and cyclosporine) (Ahmad, 2014). Collective evidence suggests that there is insufficient evidence to prove the etiologic role of CoQ10 deficiency in statin-associated myopathy and that large double blind well-designed clinical trials are required to address this issue.

OMEGA-3 FATTY ACIDS AND STROKE THERAPY

Western diet is rich in omega-6 (ω-6 fatty acids) (mainly arachidonic acid) due to the consumption of vegetable oils. This diet increases levels of ω-6 fatty acids in various tissues including brain. The enzymic oxidation of ω-6 fatty acids not only results in the production of prostaglandins (PGs), leukotrienes (LTs), thromboxanes (TXs), and lipoxins (Fig. 3.10), but also upregulates the expression of proinflammatory cytokines and chemokines (TNF-α, IL1β, and IL-6) (Farooqui, 2014). These metabolites, cytokines, and chemokines promote neuroinflammation and oxidative stress. Although, inflammation is a neuroprotective mechanism, too much inflammation following stroke can be very harmful (Farooqui et al., 2007; Farooqui, 2014). Under normal conditions, the resolution phase of neuroinflammation is a highly coordinated process, which is involved in restoration of original tissue homeostasis. Following ischemic injury, brain fails to maintain the neuronal microenvironment due to the breakdown of BBB, a specialized barrier between blood and brain mainly consisting of specific endothelial cells, tight liner sheets formed by astrocytic end-feet and pericytes, and tight junctions. The disruption of BBB may cause the infiltration of various blood-borne immune cells into the ischemic brain from disrupted vessels.

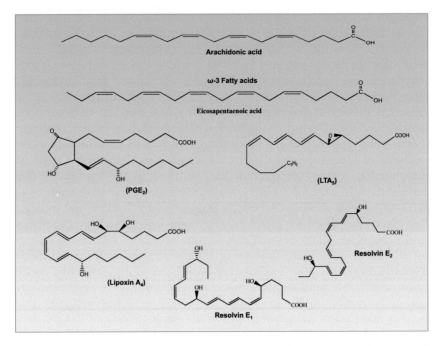

FIGURE 3.10 Chemical structures of arachidonic acid and eicosapentaenoic acid-derived lipid mediators.

These infiltrating immune cells and the injured brain cells produce more inflammatory mediators, which not only exaggerate brain edema or directly promote the death of brain cells in the penumbra, but may also promote the clearing of necrotic debris. Resolution of neuroinflammation is controlled by proresolving lipid mediators (lipoxins, resolvins, and neuroprotectins) that not only terminates leukocyte trafficking to the inflamed site and reversal of vascular permeability, but are also involved in the removal of inflammatory leukocytes, exudates and fibrin. In contrast, the consumption of Mediterranean diet, which is enriched in ω-3 fatty acids (eicosapentaenoic acid (EPA) and docosahexaenoic acid) generates resolvins E, resolvins D, neuroprotectins, and maresins (Fig. 3.11). These metabolites produce antiinflammatory, antithrombotic, antiarrhythmic, hypolipidemic, vasodilatory, and immunosuppressive effects (Simopoulos, 2006; Farooqui, 2009). Several studies have indicated that ω-3 fatty acids produce neuroprotective effects against ischemic brain damage in rat model of ischemia (Cao et al., 2007; Strokin et al., 2006; Bas et al., 2007; Belayev et al., 2011; Hong et al., 2014; Berressem et al., 2016). The consumption and administration of DHA promote CBF, inhibit $cPLA_2$, COX, and LOX activities, and reduce levels of brain postischemic prostaglandins, thromboxanes, and leukotrienes (Farooqui, 2014). In addition, consumption of DHA may produce several other beneficial effects. DHA not only decreases in BBB disruption and reduces brain edema (Hossain et al., 1998; Hong et al.,

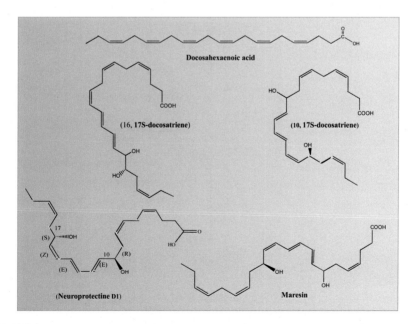

FIGURE 3.11 Chemical structures of docosahexaenoic acid-derived lipid mediators.

2015), but also has antioxidant properties (Hossain et al., 1999). At the cellular level, DHA salvages neurons and astrocytes within the infarcted areas (Belayev et al., 2009, 2011). DHA rescues more neurons by protecting astrocytes, which have a critical role in the maintenance and protection of neurons through secretion of growth and neurotrophic factors. Also DHA downregulates activation of microglia in the infarcted regions (Belayev et al., 2011) supporting the view that by affecting all neural cell types, DHA not only improves behavior, but reduces total infarct volume. At the molecular level, DHA retards production of inflammatory cytokines and chemokines by antagonizing the metabolism of arachidonic acid and its downstream metabolites through the downregulation of NF-κB, a transcription factor, which upregulates the expression of proinflammatory cytokines and chemokines. In addition, DHA treatment potentiates the synthesis of neuroprotectin D_1 (NPD$_1$), a lipid mediator derived from 15-lipoxygenase catalyzed oxidation of DHA in the penumbra 3 days after MCAo. NPD$_1$ also upregulates the antiapoptotic Bcl-2 proteins (Bcl-2 and bclxL), and decreases the expression of the proapoptotic proteins (Bax and Bad) (Bazan, 2005) (Fig. 3.12). NPD$_1$ blocks reperfusion-induced leukocyte infiltration, proinflammatory signaling, and infarct size. NPD$_1$ not only inhibits cytokine-mediated

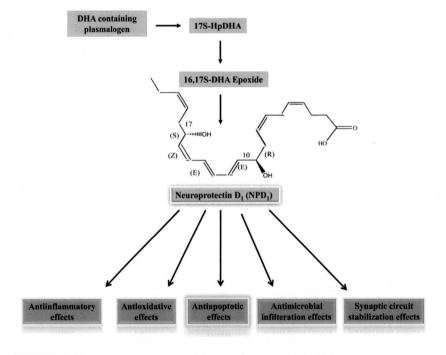

FIGURE 3.12   Synthesis and roles of neuroprotection D in the brain tissue.

cyclooxygenase-2 expression, but also promotes homeostatic regulation of the integrity of neural cells particularly during oxidative stress, and this protective signaling may be relevant to neural cell survival following ischemic injury (Bazan, 2009). These processes strengthen the survival mechanisms through ERK-mediated and/or Bcl-2-mediated prosurvival cascade.

Resolvins are another group of proresolving and antiinflammatory lipid mediator of ω-3 fatty acid metabolism that have neuroprotective effects (Serhan, 2005a,b; Bazan, 2005, 2007, 2009). DHA is metabolized to resolvin D series (RvD$_1$, RvD$_2$, RvD$_3$, RvD$_4$, RvD$_5$, and RvD$_6$), whereas EPA is converted to resolvin E series (RvE$_1$ and RvE$_2$) (Fig. 3.10). Like resolvin D series metabolite, RvE series blocks the activation of NF-κB by TNF-α (Arita et al., 2007). It is reported that RvE$_1$ binds to BLT$_1$ as a partial agonist and locally dampens the BLT$_1$-mediated signals on leukocytes along with other receptors (e.g., ChemR23-mediated counterregulatory actions) to mediate the resolution of inflammation (Arita et al., 2006, 2007).

The neuroprotective effects of ω-3 fatty acids involve not only retardation of the oxidative stress, but also enhancement in the expression of nuclear factor E2-related factor 2 (Nrf2)/heme oxygenase-1 (HO-1) (Ueda et al., 2013) (Fig. 3.13). At the molecular level, the molecular mechanism of Nrf2 stimulation involves the stimulation of Nrf2/HO-1 signaling pathway by ω-3 fatty acid-derived 4-hydroxyhexanal (4-HHE), which acts as an effective Nrf2 inducer. This pathway reduces ischemic injury by activating Nrf2 and increasing HO-1 production (Chang et al., 2013; Zhang et al., 2014a,b). It is well known that under normal conditions Nrf2 resides in the cytoplasm in the form of a complex with Kelch-like ECH-associated protein 1 (Keap1). In ischemic injury-mediated oxidative stress, 4-HHE interacts with the cysteine residues of Keap1. These interactions promote the dissociation of Nrf2 from Keap1 (Zhang et al., 2014a,b). Nrf2 then translocates from cytoplasm into the nucleus, where it binds with antioxidant responsive element, and induces the expression of phase II enzymes (Wakabayashi et al., 2004). In addition, increase in the expression of Nrf2 and HO-1 also inhibits the activation of microglia and suppresses the expression of proinflammatory cytokine (Kobayashi et al., 2004). Converging evidence suggests DHA-mediated neuroprotection against cerebral ischemic stroke may involve not only improvement in neuronal defense capacity, but inhibition of cellular inflammatory mechanisms by increasing the expression of Nrf2 and HO-1 (Xue et al., 2012).

CITICOLINE (CDP-CHOLINE) AND STROKE THERAPY

Cytidine-5'-diphosphocholine (citicoline or CDP-choline) (Fig. 3.14), an intermediate in the biosynthesis of phosphatidylcholine, has shown beneficial effects in a number of CNS injury models including cerebral

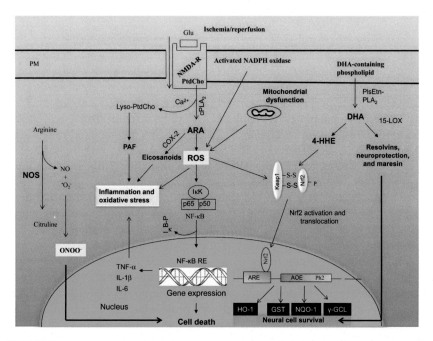

FIGURE 3.13   Diagram showing the activation of Nrf2/HO-1 signaling pathway and release and translocation of Nrf2 to the nucleus following ischemia/reperfusion-mediated oxidative stress. *ARA*, arachidonic acid; *ARE*, antioxidant response element; *COX*, cyclooxygenase; *cPLA₂*, cytosolic phospholipase A₂; *DHA*, docosahexaenoic acid; *γ-GCL*, γ-glutamate-cysteine ligase; *4-HHE*, 4-hydroxyhexanal; *HO-1*, hemeoxygenase; *IL-1β*, interleukin-1beta; *IL-6*, interleukin-6; *Keap1*, Kelch-like ECH-associated protein 1; *15-LOX*, 15-lipoxygenase; *lyso-PtdCho*, lysophosphatidylcholine; *NF-κB*, nuclear factor-kappa B; *NF-κB-RE*, nuclear factor-kappa B response element; *NMDAR*, N-methyl-D-aspartate receptors; *NO*, nitric oxide; *NQO1*, NAD(P)H:quinone oxidoreductase-1; *Nrf2*, nuclear factor-erythroid 2-related factor 2; *ONOO⁻*, peroxynitrite; *PAF*, platelet activating factor; *PM*, plasma membrane; *PtdCho*, phosphatidylcholine; *ROS*, reactive oxygen species; *TNF-α*, tumor necrosis factor-alpha.

ischemia. Citicoline is composed of two molecules: cytidine and choline. Cytidine and choline separately pass through the BBB, enter brain cells, and act as substrates for intracellular synthesis of CDP-choline (Savci and Wurtman, 1995; Secades and Lorenzo, 2006). Citicoline is the only neuroprotectant that has proved efficacy in patients with moderate to severe stroke. However, the precise mechanism by which citicoline is neuroprotective is not fully known. However, it is proposed that citicoline may act by stabilizing neural cell membranes (Savci and Wurtman, 1995; Plataras et al., 2003), attenuating glutamate-mediated excitotoxicity (Hurtado et al., 2005), oxidative stress (Adibhatla et al., 2004, 2006), apoptosis (Secades and Lorenzo, 2006; Takasaki et al., 2011), and endothelial barrier dysfunction (Ma et al., 2013). CDP-choline may also act by

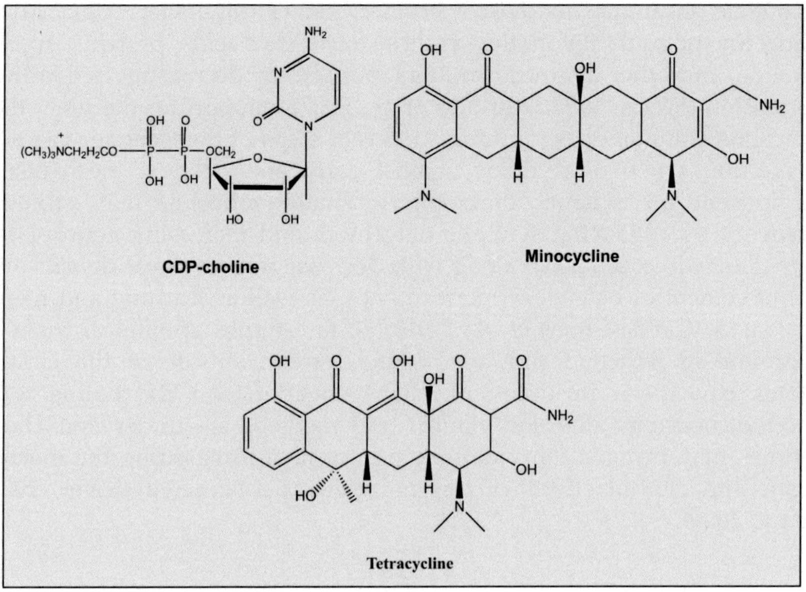

FIGURE 3.14 Chemical structures of CDP-choline, minocycline, and tetracycline.

increasing the level of acetylcholine and dopamine as well as decreasing infarct volume in animal model with cerebral ischemia (Alvarez-Sabín and Román, 2011, 2013). Citicoline may reduce free fatty acid release and recover the activities of mitochondrial ATPase and membrane Na^+/K^+ ATPase to alleviate brain damage (Plataras et al., 2003). Transient MCAo-mediated brain injury is accompanied by the increase in expression of secretory PLA_2 ($sPLA_2$)-IIA messenger RNA (mRNA) and protein levels, PtdCho-PLC activity, and PLD2 protein expression following reperfusion (Adibhatla et al., 2006). CDP-choline treatment attenuates PLA_2 activity, $sPLA_2$-IIA mRNA and protein levels, and PtdCho-PLC activity, but has no effect on PLD2 protein expression. MCAo produces decrease in CTP:phosphocholine cytidylyltransferase (CCT) activity and CCTalpha protein and CDP-choline partially restores CCT activity (Adibhatla et al., 2006). No changes are observed in cytosolic PLA_2 or calcium-independent PLA_2 activities. Citicoline treatment also attenuates the infarction volume by $55 \pm 5\%$ after 1 hour of MCAo and 1 day of reperfusion. These studies suggest that CDP-choline restores PtdCho levels by differentially affecting $sPLA_2$-IIA, PtdCho-PLC, and CCTalpha after transient focal cerebral ischemia (Adibhatla et al., 2006). Caspase activity is activated in human stroke (Rosell et al., 2008) and citicoline has been reported to decrease the release of damaging caspase activation products (Krupinski et al., 2002) by inhibiting apoptosis in animal models of brain ischemia (Montaner et al., 2011). Citicoline not only favors the synthesis of nucleic acids, proteins, acetylcholine, and other neurotransmitters, but also by decreasing free radical formation (Weiss, 1995; Hurtado et al., 2007), supporting the view that citicoline simultaneously inhibits different steps of the ischemic cascade protecting the injured tissue against early and delayed mechanisms responsible for ischemic brain injury. Finally, citicoline may promote recovery by enhancing synaptic outgrowth and increasing neuroplasticity (Hurtado et al., 2007) along with decrease in neurologic deficits and improvement of behavioral performance, as well as learning and memory tasks (García-Cobos et al., 2010). So far studies on clinical trials of citicoline in ischemic and hemorrhagic stroke outside of the United States have been unsuccessful. Reinvestigation of CDP-choline with modern neuroimaging and clinical trial methods are underway. These studies may provide more definitive information regarding the mechanistic and clinical effects of this neurotherapeutic agent (Saver, 2008; Clark, 2009).

MINOCYCLINE AND STROKE THERAPY

Minocycline is a semisynthetic tetracycline (Fig. 3.14). It has a high oral bioavailability, excellent penetration into the brain and is well tolerated in humans (Buller et al., 2009). These properties make minocycline ideal therapeutic agent for neurological disorders. Minocycline produces neuroprotective effects in several animal models of brain ischemia. Thus in a focal cerebral ischemia model, minocycline inhibits enzymes that contribute to inflammation such as the inducible form of nitric oxide synthase (iNOS) and Interleukin-1beta-Converting Enzyme (ICE-1), suppresses apoptosis, and reduces microglial activation (Yrjänheikki et al., 1998). Minocycline also reduces ischemia/reperfusion injury by inhibiting MMPs and reducing the activation of microglial cells (Fig. 3.15). Minocycline treatment also reduces infarct size and intracerebral hemorrhage leading to improved neurobehavioral outcome in response to minocycline (Garrido-Mesa et al., 2013; Liao et al., 2013). In addition, minocycline not only blocks the adhesion of leukocytes to cerebrovascular endothelial cells and reduces TNF-α production in the brain after lipopolysaccharides treatment, but also mediates antiinflammatory effects to block neuroinflammation (Garrido-Mesa et al., 2013). Furthermore, it is also shown that minocycline enhances the phosphorylation/activation of Akt and phosphorylation/inactivation of glycogen synthase kinase-3beta (GSK-3β) supporting the view that PtdIns 3K/Akt and GSK-3β pathway may also contribute to the neuroprotective effect

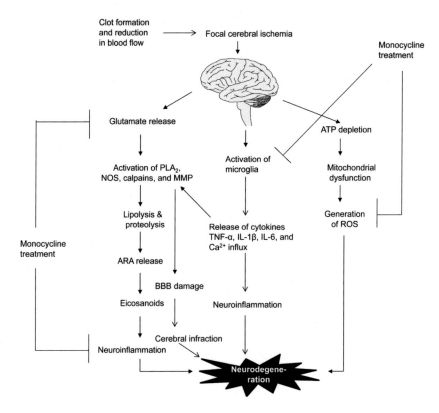

FIGURE 3.15   Targets for minocycline action.

of minocycline. More recently, minocycline has been shown to be a potent inhibitor of poly-(ADP)ribose polymerase by acting as a mimetic of the essential cofactor, NADH (Alano et al., 2006) and secretory phospholipase A_2 (Dalm et al., 2010). Converging evidence suggests that beneficial effects of minocycline have short-term neuroprotective effects during subacute stage of stroke through the reduction of neuroinflammation, suppression of free radical production, and attenuation of apoptosis. Later investigations have indicated that minocycline may induce neurovascular remodeling by inhibiting angiogenesis in vessels of ischemic brain regions for 3 weeks (Yang et al., 2015). Collectively, these studies suggest that minocycline produces neuroprotective effects in multiple mechanism in several animal models and three human trials not only due to the reduction in apoptosis, neuroinflammation, and infarct size, but also in retardation in vascular injury.

POLYARGININE AND STROKE THERAPY

It is becoming increasingly evident that cell-penetrating peptides (CPPs) such as Arg-9, penetratin, and TAT-D not only facilitate the delivery of normally nonpermeable cargos such as other peptides, proteins, nucleic acids, or drugs into cells, but also produce neuroprotective effects in cortical neuronal cultures following exposure to glutamic acid, kainic acid, or in vitro ischemia (oxygen–glucose deprivation) (Meloni et al., 2014). Thus Arg-9, penetratin, and TAT-D display consistently high level of neuroprotective activity in both the glutamic acid (IC50: 0.78, 3.4, 13.9 µM) and kainic acid (IC50: 0.81, 2.0, 6.2 µM) injury models, while the use of Pep-1 has been ineffective (Meloni et al., 2014). Similarly, polyarginine and arginine-rich peptides also produce potent neuroprotective properties in in vitro injury models that mimic the effects of stroke (Meloni et al., 2014, 2015a,b). Moreover, treatment with polyarginine peptides (R9, R12, and R18) significantly reduces infarct volume in a MCAo stroke model (Meloni et al., 2015a, 2016a,b). Based on these in vitro and in vivo observations, it is proposed that arginine-rich peptides including "neuroprotective peptides" fused to arginine-rich CPPs (TAT-NR2B9c and TAT-JNKI-1) represent a new class of neuroprotective agents (Aarts et al., 2002; Borsellol et al., 2003). The presence of arginine residues is critical for neuroprotective activity. Detailed investigations have indicated that R18 is effective neuroprotective agent over an even wider therapeutic window (60 minutes) and broader dose range (100–1000 nmol/kg). In addition, R18 is more effective than the extensively characterized neuroprotective peptide, TAT-NR2B9c. Treatment with R18 (H-RRRRRRRRRRRRRRRRRR-OH), as well as to a lesser extent TAT-NR2B9c (H-YRKKRRQRRR-KLSSIESDV-OH, also known as NA-1), results in some functional recovery as assessed by behavioral tests, but not to statistically significant levels, which most likely reflects the severity of the stroke model used coupled with the relatively small numbers of animals in the study (Milani et al., 2016a,b). Based on this information a phase III clinical trial has been planned on stroke patients (Field randomization of NA-1 therapy in early αresponders. http://www.strokecenter.org/).

PICROSIDE AND STROKE THERAPY

Picroside 2 is an iridoid glucoside, which is extracted from the roots of the plant *Picrorhiza scrophulariiflora* (*Scrophulariaceae*) (Fig. 3.16). This plant grows in a high altitude in certain regions of Tibet and China. The roots of this plant are used in traditional Chinese medicine for a number

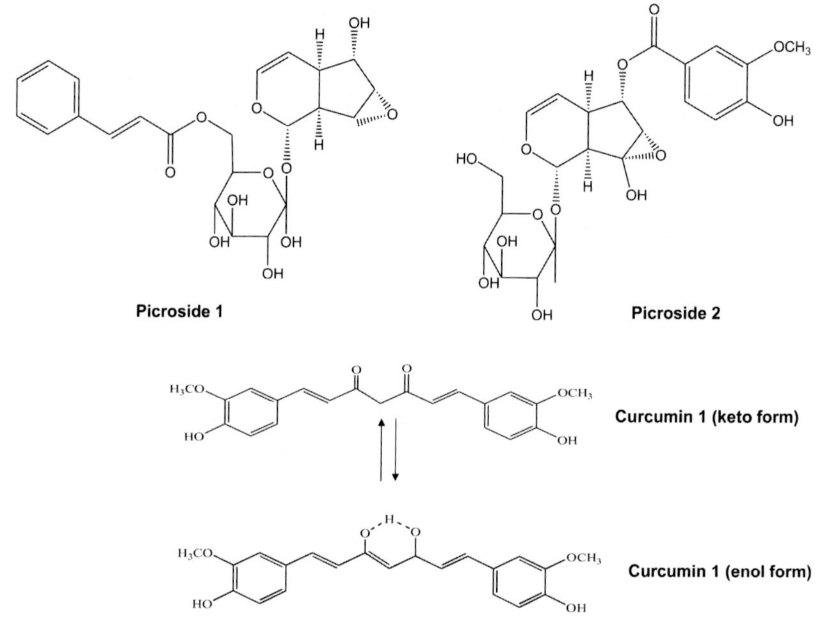

FIGURE 3.16   Chemical structures of picroside 1 and 2 and curcumin.

of disease conditions (Li et al., 1998). It has been traditionally used to treat liver diseases, upper respiratory tract diseases, dyspepsia, chronic diarrhea, and scorpion sting due to its neuroprotective (Li et al., 2007), antiapoptotic, anticholestatic, antioxidant, antiinflammation, immune-modulating activities (Liu et al., 2007; He et al., 2009). Picroside 2 enhances NGF-induced PC12 cell axon growth, reduces H_2O_2-induced PC12 cell damage, and improves cell survival in vitro (Tao et al., 2003; Guo et al., 2007, 2016). Studies on neuroprotective effects of picroside 2 in animal models of stroke in rats have indicated that treatment with the picroside extract inhibits apoptotic cell death in ischemic penumbra following MCAo/reperfusion (MCAo/R) (Yin et al., 2005). It is also reported that picroside 2 inhibits the expressions of NFκB and IκB following MCAo/R in rats (Li et al., 2010). Based on above-mentioned studies, it is suggested that picroside 2 not only acts by downregulating the expressions of TLR4, NFκB, and TNFα to inhibiting apoptosis and neuroinflammation, but also by inhibiting COX-2 expression and MEK-ERK1/2 activities following MCAo/R-mediated injury (Wang et al., 2015). Modulation of above-mentioned signal transduction pathways improves the neurobehavioral function of rats (Guo et al., 2016).

MICRORNA AND STROKE THERAPY

MicroRNAs (miRNAs) are composed of a group of endogenous and noncoding small RNAs (approximately 22 nucleotides long) which control expression of complementary target mRNAs. miRNAs are not only involved in the regulation of gene expression at the posttranscriptional level, but are also associated with cell proliferation, differentiation, and apoptosis (Guan et al., 2010; Gallego et al., 2012; Cheng et al., 2013). Due to their ability to simultaneously modulate the fate of different genes, these molecules are particularly well suited to act as key regulators during immune cell differentiation and activation, and their dysfunction can contribute to pathological conditions associated with neuroinflammation. In addition, miRNAs not only play important role in the differentiation of progenitor cells into microglia, but alterations in expression of several miRNAs have been observed in ischemic injury, AD, and multiple sclerosis. miRNA have several features such as stability in bodily fluids (plasma, serum, urine, saliva, milk, and cerebrospinal fluid (CSF)), role in pathogenesis of disease, and the ability to be detected early in the disease course, hence strongly advocating the use of miRNA as disease biomarkers and new therapeutic targets (Siegel et al., 2012). After processing by endonucleases (Cheng et al., 2013), the resultant single-stranded miRNAs combine with other macromolecules to form RNA-induced silencing complexes (RISC). These RISCs target complementary mRNA strands for degradation, altering cellular function (Cheng et al., 2013). In the brain miRNA are key regulators of different biological functions including synaptic plasticity and neurogenesis, where they channelize the cellular physiology toward neuronal differentiation. Also, they can indirectly influence neurogenesis by regulating the proliferation and self-renewal of neural stem cells (NSCc) (Grasso et al., 2014).

Initial studies in MCAo rat model have indicated that circulating miR-124 (a brain-specific miRNA) can be a potential biomarker for diagnosis of cerebral ischemia. The plasma miR-124 levels are significantly increased after MCAo and peaked at 24 hours (up to 150-fold compared to sham-operated controls), which demonstrated the potential of brain-specific miRNAs to serve as biomarkers of tissue injury (Laterza et al., 2009; Weng et al., 2011). Other studies have indicated that in similar animal models of stroke, circulating miR-125b, miR-27, miR-422a, miR-488, and miR-627 are also increased after the onset of ischemic stroke (Sepramaniam et al., 2014). Furthermore, levels of miR-290 are elevated at 24 hours after reperfusion (Jeyaseelan et al., 2008). miR-10a, miR-182, miR-200b, and miR-298 are increased in both blood and brain 24 hours following ischemia/reperfusion (Liu et al., 2010). It is also reported that in vivo inhibition of miR-155 after experimental mouse ischemia supports brain microvasculature in the periinfarct area, reduces brain tissue damage, and improves the animal functional recovery (Caballero-Garrido et al., 2015). In addition, miR-155 inhibition after distal middle cerebral artery occlusion results in alterations of several cytokine/chemokine gene expression (Caballero-Garrido et al., 2015), suggesting a possible role of miR-155 in postischemic inflammation. miR-155 is expressed in hematopoietic cells (including B cells, T cells, monocytes, and granulocytes), endothelial cells, microglia, and astrocytes (Butovsky et al., 2015; Elton et al., 2013). All these cell types are able to express and secrete pro- and antiinflammatory molecules and, thus, actively participate in the inflammation process. Therefore it is proposed that systemic in vivo inhibition of miR-155 may significantly affect the poststroke inflammatory response.

Testing of miRNAs by microarray and real-time PCR analyses in human subjects has indicated that levels of circulating hsa-miR-106b-5P and hsa-miR-4306 are increased, whereas hsa-miR-320e and hsa-miR-320d are decreased in plasma suggesting these miRNAs may be used as novel biomarkers for the early detection of acute stroke in humans (Wang et al., 2014a; Rink and Khanna, 2011). Another study has indicated that presence of miRNA can be used to determine the severity of stroke and involvement of miRNA in the regulation of inflammatory responses. The results show that serum miR-124, miR-9, and miR-219 are suppressed in acute ischemic stroke, which promote and support neuroinflammation and brain injury (Liu et al., 2015). It also reported that circulating miR-30a and miR-126 levels are markedly downregulated in all patients with ischemic stroke until 24 weeks. Circulating levels of let-7b are reduced in patients with large-vessel atherosclerosis than healthy controls, whereas levels of let-7b are increased in patients with other kinds of ischemic stroke until 24 weeks. These circulating miRNAs returned to normal 48 weeks after symptom onset. Investigations with other acute ischemic stroke patients have indicated that miR-122, miR-148a, let-7i, miR-19a, miR-320d, and miR-4429 are decreased and miR-363 and miR-487b are increased compared to vascular risk factor controls. It is proposed that the presence of these miRNAs may be related to the regulation of leukocyte gene expression in ischemic stroke including pathways involved in immune activation, leukocyte extravasation, and thrombosis (Jickling et al., 2014). Collective evidence suggests that miRNA profile changes in both brain and peripheral blood are important. However, a further exploration is necessary to clarify the time course of expression and to correlate miRNA changes with the severity of stroke.

CURCUMIN AND STROKE THERAPY

Curcumin ($C_{21}H_{20}O_6$) or diferuloylmethane (*bis*-α,β-unsaturated β-diketone) (Fig. 3.16) is a hydrophobic polyphenolic compound (mol mass of 368.38) present in the Indian spice turmeric (curry powder). It is derived from the rhizomes of *Curcuma longa*, which belongs to family Zingiberaceae (Anand et al., 2008; Goel et al., 2008; Farooqui, 2016). It has been used for centuries in Chinese traditional medicine and Indian medicine (Ayurvedic medicine) systems as a nociceptive, antiinflammatory, and antishock drug to relieve pain and inflammation in muscles (Anand et al., 2008; Goel et al., 2008; Farooqui, 2016) and for the treatment of many pathological conditions, such as rheumatism, digestive and inflammatory disorders, intermittent fevers, urinary discharges, leukoderma and amenorrhea as part of traditional medicine (Anand et al., 2008; Goel et al., 2008; Farooqui, 2016). Turmeric products have been declared as safe not only by the FDA (http://www.accessdata.fda.gov/scripts/fcn/gras_notices/GRN000460.pdf) in the United States, and the Natural Health Products Directorate of Canada, but also by the Joint Expert Committee of the Food and Agriculture Organization/World Health Organization (FAO/WHO). Thus curcumin is a safe and nontoxic compound, which exhibits a wide range of pharmacological activities, such as antiinflammatory, antioxidant, anticarcinogenic, antimutagenic, anticoagulant, antifertility, antidiabetic, antibacterial, antifungal, antiprotozoal, antiviral, antifibrotic, antivenom, antiulcer, hypotensive, and hypocholesteremic activities (Anand et al., 2008; Aggarwal et al., 2014). Curcumin reduces oxidative damage and improves cognitive functions related to aging process. A single injection of curcumin 30 minutes after focal cerebral ischemic /reperfusion injury in rats produces beneficial effects by decreasing infarct volume, improving neurological deficit, and reducing mortality in a dose-dependent manner (Jiang et al., 2007). Curcumin also induce vascular protective effects in persons at risk for stroke (Ovbiagele, 2008; Farooqui, 2016). Collective evidence suggests that stroke preventive properties of curcumin can be attributed to: (1) neuroprotection via free radical scavenging, inhibiting nitric oxide synthase and lipid peroxidation (Strimpakos and Sharma, 2008); (2) antiinflammatory property by suppressing the production of IL-1, IL-8, and TNF-α (Strimpakos and Sharma, 2008); (3) antilipidemic property by lowering cholesterol and boosting up HDL (Soni and Kuttan, 1992); and (4) antiaggregation property by inhibiting platelet aggregation and inducing platelet aggregation factor (Strimpakos and Sharma, 2008). The ability of curcumin to cross BBB also favors its selection over other therapeutic agents/molecules during cerebral stroke (Tsai et al., 2011). The therapeutic efficacy of curcumin in MCAo models of rat and mice has been explored and it is reported that curcumin protects from cerebral ischemia not only due to its antiinflammatory, antilipidemic, antioxidative, and antiapoptotic properties (Strimpakos and Sharma, 2008; Tyagi et al. 2012), but also due to the activation of Notch signaling pathway leading to the stimulation of neurogenesis (Liu et al., 2016). The antiinflammatory effects of curcumin in cerebral ischemia are mediated through its ability to inhibit not only COX-2, but also 5-LOX. These important enzymes mediate inflammatory processes by generating prostaglandins, leukotrienes, and thromboxanes (Rao, 2007; de Alcantara et al., 2016). In cultured astrocytes, curcumin significantly inhibits iNOS expression. Curcumin induces its effects not only by preventing peroxynitrite-mediated BBB alterations, but also by decreasing lipid peroxidation-mediated damage, preventing glial cell activation, and retarding apoptotic cell death (Jiang et al., 2007). It is well known that phosphatidylinositol 3-kinase (PtdIns 3K)/ Akt pathway plays a crucial role in neural cell survival, which are driven by growth factors (Farooqui, 2016). Furthermore, the Akt phosphorylation promote the translocation of nuclear factor-erythroid 2-related factor 2(Nrf2), its downstream transcription factor, to the nucleus which could induce expression of genes encoding phase II drug-metabolizing enzymes such as NAD(P)H:quinone oxidoreductase-1(NQO1), glutathione S-transferase (GST), aldoketo-reductase(AR), hemeoxygenase-1(HO-1), and so on. It is also reported that curcumin upregulates AR expression via Nrf2 in a PtdIns 3K/Akt-dependent manner against oxidative stress damage in vascular smooth muscle as well as neural cells (Kang et al., 2007; Scapagnini et al., 2006; Yang et al., 2009; Wu et al., 2013). Collective evidence suggests that neuroprotective activities of curcumin in cerebral ischemia are due to its antioxidant, antiinflammatory, and antiapoptotic activities (Zhao et al., 2010; Farooqui, 2016).

P53 AND STROKE THERAPY

p53 is a transcription factor, which is critical for activation or suppression of multiple genes (Riley et al., 2008). It upregulated in cerebral ischemia (Li et al., 2015). Involvement of p53 in ischemic injury is not only supported by the observation that p53 knockout mice are protected from ischemic injury (Crumrine et al., 1994). In addition, treatment with p35 inhibitor (Pifithrin-alpha, PFT-α) reduces damage induced by ischemic stroke (Culmsee et al., 2003). Thus administration of PFT-α starting from the first day after MCAo promotes not only neurogenesis and angiogenesis, but also reduces infarct volume and enhances behavioral outcomes at 7 days after MCAo in rats supporting the view PFT-α administration may improve stroke outcome. In addition, PFT-α also promotes the survival of grafted NSCs and improves functional recovery in the stroke model (Lei et al., 2013). The molecular mechanisms of neuroprotective action of PFT-α are not known. However, it is suggested that PFT-α acts by promoting neurogenesis and angiogenesis through the vascular endothelial growth factor (VEGF) signal pathway in a MCAo model, suggesting a new potential mechanism of PFT-α for stroke treatment, highlighting a key target of p53 as a mediator of brain repair for a disorder frequently difficult to treat after its occurrence (Zhang et al., 2016a,b).

Most survivors of ischemic stroke remain physically disabled and require prolonged rehabilitation (Clarke and Forster, 2015). However, some stroke victims achieve almost full neurological recovery (95%) supporting the view that the human brain has mechanism(s) to defend against ischemic injury. Studies on rat model of cerebral ischemia have indicated that endogenous neuroprotective mechanism(s) involve activation of α7 nicotinic acetylcholine receptors (nAChRs). These receptors are not only expressed in the brain, but also in peripheral and CNS immune cells. The activation of α7 nAChRs on these cells suppresses inflammatory processes (Kalkman and Feuerbach, 2016). Since neuroinflammation is closely associated with neurological disorders (Farooqui, 2014), specific α7 nAChR agonists can produce therapeutic effects. Based on this information, α7 nAChR agonists have been used to treat rats with less severe ischemic injury. Intranasal administration of α7 nAChR agonist significantly augments ischemic injury. Furthermore, inhibitors of calcium/calmodulin-dependent kinase-II also produce neuroprotective effects (Sun et al., 2017).

VACCINE AND STROKE THERAPY

Immunotherapy for the treatment of stroke has attracted considerable scientific attention. As stated in Chapter 2, Molecular Aspects of Ischemic Injury, many signaling pathways are altered after cerebral ischemic insult. Blocking certain deleterious pathways may delay the damage to brain tissue and even widen the time window for revascularization therapy. The interaction of antibodies with cytotoxic molecules and their receptors may maintain neural cell viability or delay neurodegeneration following ischemia/reperfusion. Current investigations of stroke immunotherapy include active immunization by inoculation with peptides and passive immunization by direct injection of antibody into the animals. Many molecules have been targeted for stroke therapy, and a number of antibodies have been developed. These molecules are primarily found on the neural cell membranes or in the extracellular space where they are accessible to the antibodies. Stroke vaccine have been developed for Nogo-A, NR1 subunit of the NMDA receptor, selectin E, and angiotensin II peptide (Caroni and Schwab, 1988; During et al., 2000; Wakayama et al., 2017). Treatment of stroke stricken (unilateral distal permanent MCAo) aged rats with anti-Nogo-A results in improved performance on the reference memory portion of the Morris water maze task. However, this improved performance does not correlate with structural changes in the hippocampal neurons (Gillani et al., 2010). Similarly, an adenoassociated virus vaccine generating autoantibodies has been used to target NR1 subunit of the NMDA receptor. This single dose of vaccine produces neuroprotective effects in a MCAo stroke model in rats at 1−5 months following vaccination (During et al., 2000). In another study, a nasal spray is used for delivering a protein (E-selectin) that, under normal circumstances, is associated with inflammation of the cells that line the inner walls of blood vessels of hypertensive, genetically stroke-prone rats (Takeda et al., 2002). Neuroinflammation not only plays an important role in stroke, but also makes cerebral blood vessels more vulnerable to formation of a clot. Exposing rats to E-selectin programs its lymphocytes to monitor the blood vessel lining for the inflammatory protein, when these lymphocytes detect E-selectin, they produce mediators that prevent inflammation. Thus nasal instillation of E-selectin, which is specifically expressed on activated endothelium, potently prevents the development of ischemic and hemorrhagic strokes in spontaneously hypertensive stroke-prone rats with untreated hypertension (Takeda et al., 2002). These vaccines have no effect on blood pressure indicating their beneficial effects are not linked to reduction of high blood pressure. While these vaccines produce neuroprotective effects in rats by reducing brain damage, clinical trials for several antibodies have failed due to poor patient outcomes (During et al., 2000; Takeda et al., 2002).

STEM CELL THERAPY FOR STROKE

Stem cell therapy is a novel procedure for the treatment of stroke. Stem cell transplant studies in animal models of ischemic stroke have shown that stem cells transplanted into the brain can lead to functional improvement (Chopp and Li, 2002). Various cell types have been used to improve function and the recovery after stroke, including embryonic stem cells (ESCs), immortalized pluripotent stem cells (iPSCs), neural stem/progenitor cells, and nonneuronal adult stem cells such as mesenchymal stem cells (MSCs) and bone marrow mononuclear cells (MNCs). Most clinical trials involving patients with stroke have used adult stem cells, such as MSCs, MNCs, and NSCs. The International Cellular Medicine Society classifies culture-expanded autologous MSCs as a clinical cell line, unlike ESCs, iPSCs, and genetically modified stem cells. MSCs can migrate into damaged brain regions (tropism) and self-renew, reportedly without inducing tumorogenesis. Sufficient numbers of MSCs can be easily obtained within several weeks of culture expansion. Based on animal model studies, several clinical trials of stem cell therapy have been conducted in patients with stroke since 2005, including studies using MSCs, bone marrow MNCs, and neural stem/progenitor cells. In addition, several clinical trials of the use of adult stem cells to treat ischemic stroke are ongoing (Bang, 2016). Stem cells, which are pluripotential cells, can differentiate into neural lineages to replace lost neurons. They not only provide the delivery of BDNF or glial-derived neurotrophic factor (GDNF) to the penumbra and enhance vasculogenesis, but also promote survival, migration, and differentiation of the endogenous precursor cells after stroke (Hicks and Jolkkonen, 2009) enhancing neurogenesis, angiogenesis, and synaptogenesis (Bang, 2016). In vitro studies have indicated that phosphatidyl-inositide 3-kinase (PtdIns 3K) pathway is necessary for the survival of both neurons and NSCs which are essential for endogenous neurogenesis (Tang et al., 2015; Bokara et al., 2016). Activated PtdIns 3K phosphorylates Akt, which is a downstream effector. Phosphorylated Akt not only affects mouse double minute 2 homolog (MDM2), nuclear factor kappa-light-chain-enhancer of activated B cells (NF-kB), but also modulates endothelial nitric oxide synthase (eNOS), mammalian target of rapamycin (mTOR), and S6 kinase and inhibits Forkhead box O (FOXO), BAD, and glycogen synthase kinase (GSK)-3β. All of these signals contribute to the protection and neurogenesis of NSCs (Koh and Lo, 2015). Besides trophic factors, stem cells may release extracellular vesicles to deliver functional proteins and miRNAs to NSCs or neuronal cells (Lai et al., 2011). In addition, stem cells may also exert their actions by attenuating neuroinflammation (Kim et al., 2009), reducing scar thickness (which may interfere with the recovery process) (Shen et al., 2007), enhancing autophagy (Shin et al., 2014), and normalizing microenvironmental/metabolic profiles (Paik et al., 2009) in the damaged area of the brain. However, there are still problems associated with true neuronal substitution using cell replacement to restore neuronal function after stroke (Dihné et al., 2011). The primary limitations of current stem cell therapies include (1) the limited source of engraftable stem cells, (2) the presence of optimal time window for stem cell therapies, (3) inherited limitation of stem cells in terms of growth, trophic support, and differentiation potential, and (4) possible transplanted cell-mediated adverse effects, such as tumor formation (Bang et al., 2016). Very little is known about the molecular mechanisms contributing to homing of stem cells in humans and discovery of the molecular pathways that facilitate the homing of stem cells into the ischemic areas. These molecular pathways may facilitate the development of new treatment regimens, perhaps using small molecules, designed to enhance endogenous mobilization of stem cells in the chronic stroke. For maximal functional recovery, however, regenerative therapy may need to follow combinatorial approaches, which may not only include cell replacement, trophic support, protection from oxidative stress/inflammation, but also the neutralization of the growth-inhibitory components for endogenous neuronal stem cells (Chang et al., 2007). Thus understanding the exact molecular basis of stem cell plasticity in relation to local ischemic signals may offer new insights to permit better management of stroke and other ischemic disorders. All together, a number of studies support the view that potential of systemic delivery of stem cells is a novel therapeutic approach for stroke. Although, stem cell transplantation is an important development for stroke therapy, only few studies have been performed using a single dose and at a single time point poststroke (Yu et al., 2009). Due to the rapid degeneration and low survival rate of neurons at the damage or injury site and partial behavioral recovery, new strategies are needed to improve the quality and beneficial effects of stem cell transplantation in stroke. Enhanced recovery from stroke is mostly associated with a reduction in apoptosis in a recent metaanalysis evaluating preclinical stem cell studies (Janowski et al., 2010). In addition, in stroke-mediated brain damage stem cells may play role as a local or systemic immunoregulators. This process may also contribute to their ability to improve stroke recovery by decreasing inflammatory effects (Horie et al., 2011). NSCs and bone marrow-derived stem cells augment poststroke plasticity through upregulation of synapse formation, dendritic branching, and axonal connections (Andres et al., 2011). Stem cells may not only enhance angiogenesis, but also promote BBB repair, which may contribute to improvement in recovery process (Horie et al., 2011). Although, small numbers of transplanted cells may integrate into tissue, the extent of behavioral improvement does not appear to correlate with the number of cells. Additionally, the timing of synapse formation does not always correlate with functional improvement (Englund et al., 2002). Given the complex pathophysiology of stroke, the importance of timing on the effects of factors, and the balance of signals in the pathways of recovery as described earlier, it is essential to better understand the mechanisms of improvement following stem cell therapy in order to translate these discoveries to clinical applications. Thus long-term studies are required to determine whether the stem cell-mediated enhanced recovery can be sustained and translate into beneficial behavioral and functional outcome (Chang et al., 2007; Yu et al., 2009). There is a possibility that stem cell transplantation may initiate tumorigenesis in brain that may be fetal for recovering stroke patients. Thus additional preclinical studies are warranted to reveal the optimal stem transplant regimen that is safe and efficacious prior to proceeding to large-scale clinical application of these cells for stroke therapy (Yu et al., 2009).

EXOSOMES AND STROKE THERAPY

Exosomes are endosome-derived small membrane vesicles, approximately 30–100 nm in diameter, and are released into extracellular fluids by cells in all living systems (Lai and Breakefield, 2012; György et al., 2015). They are present in biofluids such as blood and the CSF (György et al., 2015). Exosomes carry proteins, lipids, and genetic materials and play essential roles in intercellular communication by transferring their cargo between source and target cells under physiological and pathophysiological conditions (Lai and Breakefield, 2012; György et al., 2015). Recovery from stroke-mediated injury is orchestrated by a set of highly interactive processes (angiogenesis, neurogenesis, oligodendrogenesis, synaptogenesis, and axonal outgrowth) involving the neurovascular unit and NSCs (Zhang and Chopp, 2009). During stroke recovery, ischemic brain undergoes a series of remodeling events, which result in limited spontaneous functional recovery (Nudo, 2007). Relatively quiescent cerebral endothelial cells in preexisting blood vessels are activated by stroke-mediated injury. This activation of endothelial cells leads to angiogenesis in experimental stroke models and human ischemic brain (Zhang et al., 2000). In addition to cerebral endothelial cells, circulating endothelial progenitor cells are also involved in the generation of new blood vessels (Zhang et al., 2002). Stroke-induced angiogenesis not only occurs in the periinfarct regions, but also in the ventricular/subventricular zone (V/SVZ) of the lateral ventricles, a neurogenic region (Zhang et al., 2014a,b). Stroke-induced angiogenesis is a multistep process that involves endothelial cell proliferation, migration, tube formation, branching, and anastomosis (Carmeliet, 2000). VEGF and VEGF receptor 2 (VEGFR2) initiate angiogenesis, and angiopoietins 1 and 2 and their receptor, Tie2, are involved in maturation, stabilization, and remodeling of vessels (Yancopoulos et al., 1998). Treatment with VEGF 24 hours after stroke enhances angiogenesis (Jin et al., 2002). At early stages of recovery, angiogenic vessels are permeable, but new vessels become less leaky and functional when they mature (Zhang et al., 2000; Plate, 1999). It is suggested that increase in angiogenesis is highly associated with improved neurological outcomes (Zhang and Chopp, 2009).

Similarly, neurogenesis, which occurs throughout adulthood in the SVZ and the subgranular zone of the dentate gyrus in the hippocampus of the brain can promote migration of stem cells into the ischemic penumbra of the striatum and cerebral cortex (Tobin et al., 2014) resulting in generation of new neurons, which can replace damaged or lost neurons. This neurogenic response, however, is generally considered too weak to yield enough neurons for compensation and recovery of lost neurocytes and their functions (Kreuzberg et al., 2010). Exosome-mediated neurogenesis may provide some success in supplying neural stem/progenitor cells (NSCs/NPCs) to replace the injured neural cells after acute stroke (Abe et al., 2012). It should be noted that these observations are preliminary and there are multiple unanswered questions and challenges in the development of exosome therapy for stroke. These questions include the following: (1) identification of the cellular signals by which the ischemic brain is able to affect the content and quantity of exosomes released by brain parenchymal cells and by remote organs, (2) understanding how exosomal cargo affects expression of endogenous genes and proteins in recipient cells of injured brain, (3) delineation of the specific cell types that are targeted by brain parenchymal cell–derived exosomes, and (4) knowledge of the effects of sex, age, and comorbidity on the cellular generation of exosomes and their cargo and the effect of sex, age, and comorbidity in response to exosome treatment after stroke (Zhang and Chopp, 2009).

PREVENTION OF STROKE THROUGH THE MODULATION OF RISK FACTORS

Above discussion clearly indicates that neuroprotective therapy has either failed or has provided limited benefits, clinicians have therefore focused on preventive strategies to limit its first onset and recurrence of stroke. Prevention begins with awareness of risk factors by patients and clinicians. According to The American Stroke Association and American Heart Association guidelines, as mentioned in Chapter 1, Classification and Molecular Aspects of Neurotraumatic Diseases: Similarities and Differences With Neurodegenerative and Neuropsychiatric Diseases, there are two types of risk factors for stroke: nonmodifiable and modifiable or potentially modifiable (Rincon and Sacco, 2008; Romero et al., 2008). Nonmodifiable risk factors include age, sex, low birth weight, race/ethnicity, and genetic factors. Well-documented and modifiable risk factors include hypertension, exposure to cigarette smoke, diabetes, atrial fibrillation and certain other cardiac conditions, dyslipidemia, carotid artery stenosis, sickle cell disease, postmenopausal hormone therapy, poor diet, physical inactivity, and obesity and body fat distribution (Rincon and Sacco, 2008). Less well-documented or potentially modifiable risk factors include the metabolic syndrome, alcohol abuse, drug abuse, oral contraceptive use, sleep-disordered breathing, migraine headache, hyperhomocysteinemia, elevated lipoprotein(a), elevated lipoprotein-associated phospholipase, hypercoagulability, inflammation, and infection (Rincon and Sacco, 2008). These guidelines not only provide comprehensive and timely evidence-based recommendations on the prevention of ischemic stroke among survivors of stroke or transient ischemic attack, but also guide healthcare providers a potential explanation for the causes of stroke in an individual patient to select therapies that reduce the risk of recurrent events and other vascular events (Rincon and Sacco, 2008; Romero, 2007; Romero et al., 2008). Current stroke prevention strategies include high blood pressure (hypertension) control and retarding the formation of blood clots using drugs such as aspirin and warfarin.

SELECTION OF DIET AND STROKE

In order to protect the aging population from stroke, it is crucial to explore methods that may retard or slow the molecular cascade associated with oxidative stress, excitotoxicity, and neuroinflammation. Diet enriched in antioxidants and antiinflammatory components may lower the risk of stroke. These components are present in the Mediterranean diet. Components of Mediterranean diet include vegetables, legumes, fruits, whole grains, fish, olive oil, fresh garlic, low levels of dairy products (cheese and yogurt), nuts, and modest intake of red wine (Farooqui, 2012). Fruits and vegetables are enriched in vitamins, carotenoids, flavonoids, fiber, potassium, magnesium, and other minerals. These components prevent age-related neurologic dysfunction not only by preventing free radical damage and neuroinflammation but also by protecting the body from age-dependent cognitive decline and increasing longevity (Farooqui, 2010, 2012). Oleuropein and oleocanthal are olive oil components. Oleocanthal inhibits COX, but also induces antioxidant effects in the brain (Qosa et al., 2015; Abuznait et al., 2013). In addition, both oleuropein and oleocanthal produce antiinflammatory effects. Similarly, consumption of fish in Mediterranean diet provides DHA and EPA, which are metabolized to resolvins, neuroprotectins, and maresins (Farooqui, 2009; Farooqui and Farooqui, 2009). Red wine contains resveratrol. Resveratrol not only produces cardioprotective, anticancer, antiinflammatory, and antioxidant properties, but also increases life span of yeast, worms, flies, and rodents (Baur et al., 2006).

Garlic (*Allium sativum*) contains several organosulfur compounds, such as, allicin, alliin, diallyl sulfide, diallyl disulfide, diallyl trisulfide, S-allylcysteine (SAC), dithiins, ajoene, methyl allyl disulfide, methyl allyl trisulfide, 2-vinyl-1,3-dithiin, 3-vinyl-1,2-dithiin (Fig. 3.3) (Rybak et al., 2004). These are lipophilic thioesters derived from oxidized allicin, which are synthesized when garlic cloves are crushed. Garlic preparations induce their effects via different antioxidant mechanisms such as their ability to (1) scavenge ROS and RNS, (2) increase enzymic and nonenzymic antioxidants levels, and (3) inhibition of some prooxidant enzymes (xanthine oxidase, cyclooxygenase, and NADPH oxidase) (Sun et al., 2007). Collective evidence suggests that individual components of the Mediterranean diet (tyrosol, hydroxytyrosol, oleocanthal, resveratrol, alliin, docosahexaenoic and eicosapentaenoic acids) produce beneficial effects in animal models of stroke by inhibiting oxidative stress, neuroinflammation, normalizing mitochondrial dysfunction, improving endothelial function, and increasing cognitive function (Farooqui, 2010). Furthermore, nitrate, which is present in vegetables and fruits is metabolized into nitrite and nitric oxide. It not only improves endothelial function, reduces blood pressure, but also increases regional perfusion in the brain. In addition, dietary nitrate promotes cognitive performance and prefrontal cortex CBF parameters in healthy adults supporting the view that dietary nitrate can produce beneficial effects on brain function (Jones, 2014; Wightman et al., 2015). A number of recent cross-sectional and prospective studies have indicated that consumption of Mediterranean diet significantly decreases cognitive dysfunction and mortality in 182 men and women aged 70 years (Trichopoulou et al., 1995). This study has been recently extended to larger population in Greece (more than 22,000 adults) displaying a significant reduction in total mortality with greater adherence to the traditional Mediterranean diet (Trichopoulou et al., 2003). The exact molecular mechanisms associated with increased longevity are not understood. However, it is suggested that long-term consumption of Mediterranean diet increases the longevity through maintenance of the telomeres length and prevention of brain atrophy (López-Miranda et al., 2012; Boccardi et al., 2013; Mosconi et al., 2014).

PHYSICAL EXERCISE AND STROKE

In the brain, exercise produces both acute and long-term changes, such as increased levels of various neurotrophic factors or enhanced cognition. The molecular mechanisms associated with exercise-induced changes in the brain are not fully understood. However, it is proposed that physical exercise produces increase in metabolic activity leading to neuroadaptive and neuroprotective changes in brain (Trejo et al., 2002). This regular exercise-mediated neuroadaptations result in beneficial effects on stroke and other neurological disorders (Dishman et al., 2006). Furthermore, chronic voluntary physical activity not only reduces hypertension and decreases chances of heart failure, but also decreases elevated sympathetic nervous system activity. Studies on in vivo and in vitro models of stroke have indicated that exercise enhances cardiorespiratory fitness, muscular endurance, and functional recovery of stroke patients resulting in a higher quality of life (Macko et al., 2005; Marsden et al., 2013). Brain uses several proteins and signaling pathways to protect neurons against ischemic injury (Farooqui, 2010). These include neurotrophic factors (BDNF, GDNF, and VEGF), nuclear factor erythroid-related factor 2 (Nrf2), protein chaperones (heat shock protein 70, Hsp70), and glucose regulated protein 78 (GRP78); antioxidant enzymes (heme oxygenase-1), and the regulator of mitochondrial biogenesis PGC-1α. The increase in expression and production of abovementioned factors not only protects neurons from stroke-mediated neuronal injury, but also increases the rate of neurogenesis in rodents (Lee et al., 2002; Kernie and Parent, 2010). Nrf2 is a transcription factor that regulates a group of antioxidant genes that act to remove ROS through sequential enzymatic reactions (Nguyen et al., 2009). Studies in animal models of stroke have indicated that increasing Nrf2 activity is highly neuroprotective stroke-mediated neuronal damage (Johnson et al., 2008) Thus administration of *tert*-butylhydroquinone (*t*BHQ), a well-known Nrf2 inducer significantly improves sensorimotor and histological outcome in two models of I/R in rats and mice (Shih et al., 2005). It is also reported that Nrf2 activation before stroke salvages the cortical penumbra but not the stroke core following ischemic injury. In addition, treadmill exercise the expression of heat shock proteins (Hsp 70 and Hsp 27) in rats (Hayes et al., 2008; Hamilton et al., 2003; Rane et al., 2003). Overexpression of inducible Hsp 70 has been reported to provide protection from cerebral ischemia both in animal stroke models. As a molecular chaperone Hsp 70 not only interacts with NF-κB to exert antiinflammatory effect, but also facilitates optimal folding of nascent and denatured proteins during normal as well as stressful circumstances. Hsp 70 regulates apoptotic cell death by interfering with apoptosis inducing factor, as well as increasing levels of antiapoptotic proteins, such as the Bcl-2 family. The expression of Hsp 27 is also increased following ischemic injury. It is also reported that Hsp 27 produces neuroprotective effects by interacting with the Akt (PKB) signaling pathway. Hsp 27 forms a complex with Akt (Rane et al., 2003).

These interactions promote survival via a series of signal transduction events that lead to the inhibition of apoptosis, via the phosphorylation and inactivation of Bad. Collective evidence suggests that exercise produces beneficial effects in animal models of stroke (Yang et al., 2003). Little information is available on the effects of exercise in patients with stroke. Based on few human studies, it is suggested that exercise produces multiple beneficial effects in patients with stroke.

TRANSCRANIAL MAGNETIC STIMULATION STUDIES IN STROKE

Transcranial magnetic stimulation (TMS) has been used to study the interhemispheric interaction in stroke patients. The paired pulse stimulus protocol has been utilized among stroke patients to study interhemispheric interactions. It is shown that there is a decrease in interhemispheric inhibition from the infarcted hemisphere to noninfarcted hemisphere (Bütefisch et al., 2008). TMS provides the ability to inhibit or facilitate target region of the brain, which can be used to enhance recovery from the stroke. There have been several prior studies of stimulating premotor or motor cortex in order to manipulate interhemispheric competition and improve motor function. These studies have shown various levels of motor improvement by modulating interhemispheric balance of motor regions (Baumer et al., 2006; Wang et al., 2012). These studies give great promise for the use of TMS when there is interhemispheric imbalance such as stroke. A 3-months treatment of stroke patients with TMS results in improvement in various motor functions such as hand grip strength, keyboard tapping, and NIH stroke scale (Khedr et al., 2009). Also, cortical excitability of the stroke hemisphere is significantly increased and excitability of contralateral hemisphere is decreased which agrees with the concept of using TMS to reverse stroke-mediated imbalance in interhemispheric inhibitory function. Other studies on the use of TMS (10 days) in stroke patients along with language training have indicated that there is a significant improvement in language performance by behavioral tests (Khedr et al., 2014). However, there is no improvement in motor function as assessed by hand grip strength in this study (Khedr et al., 2014). More recently, there have been more reports on improvements in motor function in stroke patients after TMS treatment. These studies indicate that there are improvements not only in finger flexor muscle strength and Fugl-Meyer Assessment, but also in Wolf Motor Function test which is a composite measurement of speed, strength, and quality of upper extremity movement (Sung et al., 2013). A similar protocol of inhibitory

TMS contralaterally and facilitatory TMS ipsilaterally with a long-term follow up of 3 months showed long lasting improvement in motor function (Wang et al., 2014b).

OCCUPATIONAL THERAPY AND REHABILITATION AFTER STROKE

Stroke survivors face multiple challenges, such as unilateral paralysis weakness on one side of the body, alterations in coordination, balance, and movements, decline in memory or attention, cognitive and emotional functioning (anxiety or depression), vision problems, social disability, inability to walk and care, and decrease in community participation. Occupational therapy can address these challenges at all stages in the continuum of care and is an important component of the interdisciplinary care provided to stroke survivors in a variety of settings such as neurointensive care units, inpatient and outpatient rehabilitation facilities, and home care. Ischemic damage leads to dramatic alterations in the entire complex neural network within the affected area. It is well known that the cerebral cortex exhibits spontaneous phenomena of brain plasticity in response to damage (Gerloff et al., 2006; Nudo, 2007). Thus the destruction of neural networks by stroke stimulates a reorganization of the connections and this rewiring is highly sensitive to the experience following the damage (Li and Carmichael, 2006). Such plastic phenomena involve particularly the perilesional tissue in the injured hemisphere, but also the contralateral hemisphere, subcortical and spinal regions. Rehabilitation during interdisciplinary care promotes cerebral reorganization through external input or stimulus (Govender and Kalra, 2007). This reorganization can not only contribute to the release of neurotrophic factors that promotes neurogenesis, synaptogenesis, angiogenesis, dendritic arborization, and reinforcement of existing leading to the synthesis of neurotransmitters, but may also promote functionally silent synaptic connections (particularly at the periphery of core lesion). These processes may promote this reeducation process and encourage the development of lost skills, while accommodating for specific physical, cognitive, or affective impairments. Principles of motor, sensory, cognitive, and affective rehabilitation are incorporated into effective task-specific activities, and environments are adapted to create the optimum conditions for successful rehabilitation (Govender and Kalra, 2007). Very little information is available on molecular aspects of rehabilitation and effectiveness of occupational therapy after stroke (Rossini et al., 2007). However, it is proposed that rehabilitation may involve unmasking of subthreshold preexisting connections or sprouting of new fibers (Murphy and Corbett, 2009). In this context, the

GABAergic system and the extracellular matrix have been reported to play an important role in controlling these plastic phenomena. Chondroitin sulfate proteoglycans (CSPGs), a component of specialized extracellular matrix structure, surrounds the soma of GABAergic neurons. CSPGs play an important role in constraining brain plasticity and repair (Fawcett, 2015). Following ischemic injury, the degradation of Perineuronal Nets, by injections of the bacterial enzyme chondroitinase ABC, promotes sensory-motor recovery through the reactivation of neuroplasticity (Soleman et al., 2012; Gherardini et al., 2015). This observation supports the view that CSPGs degradation at the injury site may contribute to an enhanced neuroplasticity during rehabilitation (Alia et al., 2017). The term neuroplasticity defines all the modifications in the organization of neural components occurring in the brain during the entire life span of an individual (Sale et al., 2009). Such changes are thought to be highly involved in mechanisms of aging, adaptation to environment and learning. Moreover, neuronal plastic phenomena are likely to be at the basis of adaptive modifications in response to anatomical or functional deficit or brain damage (Nudo, 2006). Animal model studies have indicated that a time-limited window of neuroplasticity opens following a stroke, during which the greatest gains in recovery can occur.

Plasticity mechanisms include activity-dependent rewiring and synapse strengthening. The challenge for improving stroke recovery is to understand how to optimally engage and modify surviving neuronal networks to provide new response strategies that compensate for tissue lost to injury (Murphy and Corbett, 2009). These findings are supported by neuroimaging studies, which clearly indicate some functional reorganization, which may be the principle process responsible for recovery after stroke (Rossini et al., 2007). Although many molecular signaling pathways may be involved, BDNF signaling has emerged as a key facilitator of neuroplasticity involved in motor learning and rehabilitation after stroke (Mang et al., 2013). Thus rehabilitation strategies that optimize BDNF effects on neuroplasticity may be especially effective for improving poststroke motor function. BDNF exerts its action by interacting with TrkB receptors. Binding of BDNF to TrkB leads to the activation of various intracellular signaling pathways, including the PtdIns 3K/Akt and MAPK/ERK pathways, which are the most critical for the biological effects of BDNF (Chen et al., 2013). The PtdIns 3K/Akt pathway contributes mainly to neuroprotection (Kaplan and Miller, 2000). The MAPK pathway is involved in neuroprotection and plays a pivotal role in the mechanisms of neurogenesis and neuroplasticity (Jiang et al., 2015). Aerobic exercise as a part of rehabilitation is a valuable intervention for improving brain function (Kramer et al., 2006; Rand et al., 2010) and that these effects are mediated, in part, by upregulation of BDNF

(Cotman et al., 2007). Thus aerobic exercise induced increases in BDNF can promote motor learning-related neuroplasticity after stroke. Nevertheless, the basic processes that drive neuroplasticity, such as BDNF signaling, are dependent on the expression of genes. As a result, genetic variation can modulate an individual's response to motor rehabilitation training, aerobic exercise training, and overall motor recovery after stroke (Pearson-Fuhrhop and Cramer, 2010). It is also suggested that different postischemic interventions like physiotherapy, occupational therapy, speech therapy, and electrical stimulation may further support and facilitate more functional reorganization and regeneration in the damaged brain (Aichner et al., 2002). Converging evidence suggests that rehabilitation after stroke is an active process beginning during hospitalization, progressing to a systematic program of rehabilitation services, and continuing after the individual returns home.

CONCLUSION

Stroke is a complex neurological disorder that involves multiple pathological factors, including excitotoxicity, oxidative stress, neuroinflammation, and gene expression. Present-day neuroprotection strategies have failed to promote the cellular, biochemical, and metabolic recovery. Most trials for the treatment of stroke are targeted using one neuroprotectant (drug) against one specific mechanism, namely, oxidative damage have failed. Since the pathogenesis of ischemic injury involves multiple factors, the use of a cocktail of neuroprotectants (free radical scavengers and antiinflammatory agents) at the earliest stages of ischemic injury may be required to stop or slow brain damage. In addition, present-day neuroprotectant therapy is essentially restricted to prevent or limit neuronal damage in penumbra.

The use of NSCs may provide the possibility of two new approaches: the transplantation of stem cells or the recruitment of endogenous stem cells for generating new neurons by means of proliferation/differentiation factors. In the latter approach, key regulators of stem cell survival, proliferation, and differentiation into neurons are proteins called "neurotrophic factors." Endogenous neurotrophic factors are actually produced in the penumbra, but this process is evidently insufficient or inadequate for providing the endogenous stem cells with the proper cues to correctly proliferate, differentiate into neurons, and migrate in the correct position to restore function. Therefore modulating the levels of neurotrophic factors in penumbra areas through stem cell transplantation represents a new approach for the stroke therapy. Since a large number of neuroprotectants have failed in clinical trials and stem cell therapy for stroke is in initial stages, prevention has become an important strategy to limit the onset and recurrence of stroke. Targets for prevention include modifiable risk factors such as hypertension, diabetes mellitus, dyslipidemia, cigarette smoking, obesity, alcohol use, and physical inactivity. Brain functional imaging studies show that partial recovery from strokes during rehabilitation is associated with a marked reorganization of the activation patterns of specific brain structures. Development of neuroimaging techniques has allowed the understanding of brain physiology during the stroke recovery process to provide a solid rationale for development of rehabilitation protocols, which can provide maximum benefit for stroke patients. Through neuroimaging, it will be possible to design, optimize, and synchronize functional training of brain regions ascribed to those areas innately undergoing neuronal plasticity change responsible for stroke recovery.

References

Aarts, M., Liu, Y., Liu, L., Besshoh, S., Arundine, M., et al., 2002. Treatment of ischemic brain damage by perturbing NMDA receptor-PSD-95 protein interactions. Science 298, 846–850.

Abe, K., Yamashita, T., Takizawa, S., Kuroda, S., Kinouchi, H., et al., 2012. Stem cell therapy for cerebral ischemia: from basic science to clinical applications. J. Cereb. Blood Flow Metab. 32, 1317–1331.

Abuznait, A.H., Qosa, H., Busnena, B.A., El Sayed, K.A., Kaddoumi, A., 2013. Olive-oil-derived oleocanthal enhances β-amyloid clearance as a potential neuroprotective mechanism against Alzheimer's disease: in vitro and in vivo studies. ACS Chem. Neurosci. 4, 973–982.

Adams, R.J., Albers, G., Alberts, M.J., Benavente, O., Furie, K., Goldstein, L.B., et al., 2008. Update to the AHA/ASA recommendations for the prevention of stroke in patients with stroke and transient ischemic attack. Stroke 39, 1647–1652.

Adibhatla, R.M., Hatcher, J.F., Dempsey, R.J., 2004. Cytidine-5'-diphosphocholine affects CTP-phosphocholine cytidylyltransferase and lyso-phosphatidylcholine after transient brain ischemia. J. Neurosci. Res. 76, 390–396.

Adibhatla, R.M., Hatcher, J.F., Larsen, E.C., Chen, X., Sun, D., et al., 2006. CDP-choline significantly restores phosphatidylcholine levels by differentially affecting phospholipase A_2 and CTP: phosphocholine cytidylyltransferase after stroke. J. Biol. Chem. 281, 6718–6725.

Aggarwal, B.B., Deb, L., Prasad, S., 2014. Curcumin differs from tetrahydrocurcumin for molecular targets, signaling pathways and cellular responses. Molecules 20, 185–205.

Ahmad, Z., 2014. Statin intolerance. Am. J. Cardiol. 113, 1765–1771.

Aichner, F., Adelwohrer, C., Haring, H.P., 2002. Rehabilitation approaches to stroke. J. Neural. Transm. Suppl. 63, 59–73.

Alberts, M.J., 1999. Diagnosis and treatment of ischemic stroke. Am. J. Med. 106, 211–221.

Alia, C., Spalletti, C., Lai, S., Panarese, A., Lamola, G., et al., 2017. Neuroplastic changes following brain ischemia and their contribution to stroke recovery: novel approaches in neurorehabilitation. Front. Cell. Neurosci. 11, 76.

Alvarez-Sabín, J., Román, G.C., 2011. Citicoline in vascular cognitive impairment and vascular dementia after stroke. Stroke 42 (1 Suppl.), S40–S43.

Alvarez-Sabín, J., Román, G.C., 2013. The role of citicoline in neuroprotection and neurorepair in ischemic stroke. Brain Sci. 3, 1395–1414.

Alano, C.C., Kauppinen, T.M., Valls, A.V., Swanson, R.A., 2006. Minocycline inhibits poly (ADP-ribose) polymerase-1 at nanomolar concentrations. Proc. Natl. Acad. Sci. 103, 9685–9690.

Amarenco, P., 2005. Cryptogenic stroke, aortic arch atheroma, patent foramen ovale, and the risk of stroke. Cerebrovasc Dis 20 (Suppl. 2), 68–74.

Amarenco, P., Bogousslavsky, J., Callahan 3rd, A., Goldstein, L.B., Hennerici, M., et al., 2006. High-dose atorvastatin after stroke or transient ischemic attack. N. Engl. J. Med. 355, 549–559.

Anand, P., Thomas, S.G., Kunnumakkara, A.B., Sundaram, C., Harikumar, K.B., et al., 2008. Biological activities of curcumin and its analogues (Congeners) made by man and Mother Nature. Biochem. Pharmacol. 76, 1590–1611.

Andres, R.H., Horie, N., Slikker, W., Keren-Gill, H., Zhan, K., et al., 2011. Human neural stem cells enhance structural plasticity and axonal transport in the ischaemic brain. Brain 134, 1777–1789.

Anrather, J., Iadecola, C., 2016. Inflammation and stroke: an overview. Neurotherapeutics 13, 661–670.

Aoki, N., 2005. Discovery of α_2-plasmin inhibitor and its congenital deficiency. J. Thromb. Haemostat. 3, 623–631.

Arita, M., Oh, S.F., Chonan, T., Hong, S., Elangovan, S., et al., 2006. Metabolic inactivation of resolvin E_1 and stabilization of its anti-inflammatory actions. J. Biol. Chem. 281, 22847–22854.

Arita, M., Ohira, T., Sun, Y.P., Elangovan, S., Chiang, N., et al., 2007. Resolvin E1 selectively interacts with leukotriene B_4 receptor BLT_1 and ChemR23 to regulate inflammation. J. Immunol. 178, 3912–3917.

Asahi, M., Huang, Z., Thomas, S., Yoshimura, S., Sumii, T., et al., 2005. Protective effects of statins involving both eNOS and tPA in focal cerebral ischemia. J. Cereb. Blood Flow Metab. 25, 722–729.

Astrup, J., Siesjo, B.K., Symon, L., 1981. Thresholds in cerebral ischemia – the ischemic penumbra. Stroke 12, 723–725.

Azad, G.K., Tomar, R.S., 2014. Ebselen, a promising antioxidant drug: mechanisms of action and targets of biological pathways. Mol. Biol. Rep. 41, 4865–4879.

Bang, O.Y., 2016. Clinical trials of adult stem cell therapy in patients with ischemic stroke. J. Clin. Neurol. 12, 14–20.

Bang, O.Y., Kim, E.H., Cha, J.M., Moon, G.J., 2016. Adult stem cell therapy for stroke: challenges and progress. J. Stroke 18, 256–266.

Barone, F.C., 2009. Ischemic stroke intervention requires mixed cellular protection of the penumbra. Curr. Opin. Invest. Drugs 10, 220–223.

Bas, O., Songur, A., Sahin, O., Mollaoglu, H., Ozen, O.A., et al., 2007. The protective effect of fish n-3 fatty acids on cerebral ischemia in rat hippocampus. Neurochem. Int. 50, 548–554.

Baumer, T., Bock, F., Koch, G., Lange, R., Rothwell, J.C., et al., 2006. Magnetic stimulation of human premotor or motor cortex produces interhemispheric facilitation through distinct pathways. J. Physiol. 572, 857–868.

Baur, J.A., Pearson, K.J., Price, N.L., 2006. Resveratrol improves health and survival of mice on a high-calorie diet. Nature 444, 337–342.

Bazan, N.G., 2005. Neuroprotectin D_1 (NPD_1): a DHA-derived mediator that protects brain and retina against cell injury-induced oxidative stress. Brain Pathol. 15, 159–166.

Bazan, N.G., 2007. Omega-3 fatty acids, pro-inflammatory signaling and neuroprotection. Curr. Opin. Clin. Nutr. Metab. Care 10, 136–141.

Bazan, N.G., 2009. Neuroprotectin D_1-mediated anti-inflammatory and survival signaling in stroke, retinal degenerations and Alzheimer's disease. J. Lipid Res 50 (Suppl), S400–S405.

Belayev, L., Khoutorova, L., Atkins, K.D., Bazan, N.G., 2009. Robust docosahexaenoic acid-mediated neuroprotection in a rat Model of transient focal cerebral ischemia. Stroke 40, 3121–3126.

Belayev, L., Khoutorova, L., Atkins, K.D., Eady, T.N., Hong, S., et al., 2011. Docosahexaenoic acid therapy of experimental ischemic stroke. Transl. Stroke Res. 2, 33–41.

Berressem, D., Koch, K., Franke, N., Klein, J., Eckert, G.P., 2016. Intravenous treatment with a long-chain omega-3 lipid emulsion provides neuroprotection in a murine model of Ischemic stroke – a pilot study. PLoS One 11, e0167329.

Boccardi, V., Esposito, A., Rizzo, M.R., Marfella, R., Barbieri, M., et al., 2013. Mediterranean diet, telomere maintenance and health status among elderly. PLoS One 8, e62781.

Bokara, K.K., Kim, J.H., Kim, J.Y., Lee, J.E., 2016. Transfection of arginine decarboxylase gene increases the neuronal differentiation of neural progenitor cells. Stem Cell Res. 17, 256–265.

Borsellol, T., Clarkel, P.G.H., Hirt, L., Vercelli, A., Repici, M., et al., 2003. A peptide inhibitor of c-Jun N-terminal kinase protects against excitotoxicity and cerebral ischemia. Nat. Med. 9, 1180–1186.

Brancaccio, P., Lippi, G., Maffulli, N., 2010. Biochemical markers of muscular damage. Clin. Chem. Lab. Med. 48, 757–767.

Broughton, B.R.S., Reutens, D.C., Sobey, C.G., 2009. Apoptotic mechanisms after cerebral ischemia. Stroke 40, E331–E339.

Buchkremer-Ratzmann, I., August, M., Hagemann, G., Witte, O.W., 1996. Electrophysiological transcortical diaschisis after cortical photothrombosis in rat brain. Stroke 27, 1105–1111.

Buller, K.M., Carty, M.L., Reinebrant, H.E., Wixey, J.A., 2009. Minocycline: a neuroprotective agent for hypoxic-ischemic brain injury in the neonate. J. Neurosci. Res. 87, 599–608.

Bütefisch, C.M., Wessling, M., Netz, J., Seitz, R.J., Hömberg, V., 2008. Relationship between interhemispheric inhibition and motor cortex excitability in subacute stroke patients. Neurorehabil. Neural Repair 22, 4–21.

Butovsky, O., Jedrychowski, M.P., Cialic, R., Krasemann, S., Murugaiyan, G., et al., 2015. Targeting miR-155 restores abnormal microglia and attenuates disease in SOD1 mice. Ann. Neurol. 77, 75–99.

Caballero-Garrido, E., Pena-Philippides, J.C., Lordkipanidze, T., Bragin, D., Yang, Y., et al., 2015. In vivo inhibition of miR-155 promotes recovery after experimental mouse stroke. J. Neurosci. 35, 12446–12464.

Calautti, C., Baron, J.-C., 2003. Functional neuroimaging studies of motor recovery after stroke in adults: a review. Stroke 34, 1553–1566.

Cao, D., Yang, B., Hou, L., et al., 2007. Chronic daily administration of ethyl docosahexaenoate protects against gerbil brain ischemic damage through reduction of arachidonic acid liberation and accumulation. J. Nutr. Biochem 18, 297–304.

Carmeliet, P., 2000. VEGF gene therapy: stimulating angiogenesis or angioma-genesis? Nat. Med. 6, 1102–1103.

Carmichael, S.T., 2003. Plasticity of cortical projections after stroke. Neuroscientist 9, 64–75.

Carmichael, S.T., Chesselet, M.-F., 2002. Synchronous neuronal activity is a signal for axonal sprouting after cortical lesions in the adult. J. Neurosci. 22, 6062–6070.

Caroni, P., Schwab, M.E., 1988. Antibody against myelin-associated inhibitor of neurite growth neutralizes nonpermissive substrate properties of CNS white matter. Neuron 1, 85–96.

Cechmanek, B.K., Tuor, U.I., Rushforth, D., Barber, P.A., 2015. Very mild hypothermia (35 degrees c) postischemia reduces infarct volume and blood/brain barrier breakdown following tPA treatment in the mouse. Ther. Hypothermia Temp. Manag. 5, 203–208.

Chang, C.-Y., Kuan, Y.-H., Li, J.-R., Chen, W.Y., Ou, Y., et al., 2013. Docosahexaenoic acid reduces cellular inflammatory response following permanent focal cerebral ischemia in rats. J. Nutr. Biochem. 24, 2127–2137.

Chang, Y.C., Shyu, W.C., Lin, S.Z., Li, H., 2007. Regenerative therapy for stroke. Cell Transplant. 16, 171–181.

Chen, A., Xiong, L.J., Tong, Y., Mao, M., 2013. The neuroprotective roles of BDNF in hypoxic ischemic brain injury. Biomed. Rep. 1, 167–176.

Chen, G.J., Yang, M.S., 2013. The effects of calcium channel blockers in the prevention of stroke in adults with hypertension: a meta-analysis of data from 273,543 participants in 31 randomized controlled trials. PLoS One 8, e57854.

Chen, J., Zhang, Z.G., Li, Y., Wang, Y., Wang, L., Jiang, H., et al., 2003. Statins induce angiogenesis, neurogenesis, and synaptogenesis after stroke. Ann. Neurol. 53, 743–751.

Chen, X., Wang, K., 2016. The fate of medications evaluated for ischemic stroke pharmacotherapy over the period 1995–2015. Acta Pharm. Sin. B 6, 522–530.

Chen, Z.Z., Yang, D.D., Zhao, Z., Yan, H., Ji, J., et al., 2016. Memantine mediates neuroprotection via regulating neurovascular unit in a mouse model of focal cerebral ischemia. Life Sci. 150, 8–14.

Cheng, Y.D., Al-Khoury, L., Zivin, J.A., 2004. Neuroprotection for Ischemic stroke: two decades of success and failure. NeuroRx 1, 36–45.

Cheng, L., Quek, C.Y., Sun, X., Bellingham, S.A., Hill, A.F., 2013. The detection of microRNA associated with Alzheimer's disease in biological fluids using next-generation sequencing technologies. Front. Genet. 4, 150.

Chobanian, A.V., Bakris, G.L., Black, H.R., Cushman, W.C., Green, L.A., et al., 2003. Seventh report of the Joint National Committee on Prevention, Detection, Evaluation, and Treatment of High Blood Pressure. Hypertension 42, 1206–1252.

Chopp, M., Li, Y., 2002. Treatment of neural injury with marrow stromal cells. Lancet Neurol. 1, 92–100.

Chu, C.S., Kou, H.S., Lee, C., Lee, K.T., Chen, S.H., et al., 2006. Effect of atorvastatin withdrawal on circulating coenzyme Q10 concentration in patients with hypercholesterolemia. Biofactors 28, 177–184.

Clark, W.M., 2009. Efficacy of citicoline as an acute stroke treatment. Expert Opin. Pharmacother. 10, 839–846.

Clarke, D.J., Forster, A., 2015. Improving post-stroke recovery: the role of the multidisciplinary health care team. J. Multidiscip. Healthc. 8, 433–442.

Cotman, C.W., Berchtold, N.C., Christie, L.A., 2007. Exercise builds brain health: key roles of growth factor cascades and inflammation. Trends Neurosci. 30, 464–472.

Crumrine, R.C., Thomas, A.L., Morgan, P.F., 1994. Attenuation of p53 expression protects against focal ischemic damage in transgenic mice. J. Cereb. Blood Flow Metab. 14, 887–891.

Culmsee, C., Siewe, J., Junker, V., Retiounskaia, M., Schwarz, S., et al., 2003. Reciprocal inhibition of p53 and nuclear factor-kappaB transcriptional activities determines cell survival or death in neurons. J. Neurosci. 23, 8586–8595.

Cumming, T.B., Marshall, R.S., Lazar, R.M., 2013. Stroke, cognitive deficits and rehabilitation: still an incomplete picture. Int. J. Stroke 8, 38–45.

Dalm, D., Palm, G.J., Aleksandrov, A., Simonson, T., Hinrichs, W., 2010. Nonantibiotic properties of tetracyclines: structural basis for inhibition of secretory phospholipase A_2. J. Mol. Biol. 398, 83–96.

de Alcantara, G.F., Simoses-neto, E., da Cruz, G.N., Norbre, M., Neves, K.R., et al., 2016. Curcumin reverses neurochemical, histological and immuno-histochemical alterations in the model of global brain ischemia. J. Trad. Complement. Med. 267, 156–171.

del Zoppo, G.J., 2010. The neurovascular unit in the setting of stroke. J. Intern. Med. 267, 156–1571.

Dihné, M., Hartung, H.P., Seitz, R.J., 2011. Restoring neuronal function after stroke by cell replacement: anatomic and functional considerations. Stroke 42, 2342–2350.

Ding, Z., Tong, W.C., Lu, X.X., Peng, H.P., 2014. Hyperbaric oxygen therapy in acute ischemic stroke: a review. Interv. Neurol. 2, 201–211.

Dishman, R.K., Berthoud, H.R., Booth, F.W., Cotman, C.W., Edgerton, V.R., et al., 2006. Neurobiology of exercise. Obesity (Silver Spring) 14, 345–356.

Dubey, P., Pandey, S., Moonis, G., 2013. Acute stroke imaging: recent updates. Stroke Res. Treat 2013, 767212.

During, M.J., Symes, C.W., Lawlor, P.A., Lin, J., Dunning, J., et al., 2000. An oral vaccine against NMDAR1 with efficacy in experimental stroke and epilepsy. Science 287, 1453–1460.

Elton, T.S., Selemon, H., Elton, S.M., Parinandi, N.L., 2013. Regulation of the MIR155 host gene in physiological and pathological processes. Gene 532, 1–12.

Endres, M., 2005. Statins and stroke. J. Cereb. Blood Flow Metab. 25, 1093–1110.

Englund, U., Bjorklund, A., Wictorin, K., Lindvall, O., Kokaia, M., 2002. Grafted neural stem cells develop into functional pyramidal neurons and integrate into host cortical circuitry. Proc. Natl. Acad. Sci. U.S.A. 99, 17089–17094.

Fagan, S.C., Bowes, M.P., Berri, S.A., Zivin, J.A., 1999. Combination treatment for acute ischemic stroke: a ray of hope? J. Stroke Cerebrovasc. Dis. 8, 359–367.

Farooqui, A.A., 2009. Beneficial Effects of Fish oil on Human Brain. Springer, New York, NY.

Farooqui, A.A., 2010. Neurochemical Aspects of Neurotraumatic and Neurodegenerative Diseases. Springer, New York, NY.

Farooqui, A.A., 2012. Phytochemical, Signal Transduction and Neurological Disorders. Springer, New York, NY.

Farooqui, A.A., 2014. Inflammation and Oxidative stress in Neurological Disorders. Springer International Publishing, Switzerland.

Farooqui, A.A., 2016. Therapeutic Potentials of Curcumin for Alzheimer Disease. Springer International Publishing, Switzerland.

Farooqui, A.A., 2017. Neurochemical Aspects of Alzheimer's Disease: Risk Factors, Pathogenesis, Biomarkers, and Potential Treatment Strategies. Academic Press, London, San Diego, CA.

Farooqui, A.A., Horrocks, L.A., Farooqui, T., 2007. Modulation of inflammation in brain: a matter of fat. J. Neurochem. 101, 577–599.

Farooqui, A.A., Ong, W.Y., Horrocks, L.A., 2008. Neurochemical Aspects of Excitotoxicity. Springer, New York, NY.

Farooqui, T., Farooqui, A.A., 2009. Aging: an important factor for the pathogenesis of neurodegenerative diseases. Mech. Ageing Dev. 130, 203–215.

Fawcett, J.W., 2015. The extracellular matrix in plasticity and regeneration after CNS injury and neurodegenerative disease. Prog. Brain Res. 218, 213–226.

Fernandes, D., Umasankar, U., 2016. Improving door to needle time in patients for thrombolysis. BMJ Qual. Improv. Rep. 5, pii: u212969.

Figueiredo, C.P., Clarke, J.R., Ledo, J.H., Ribeiro, F.C., Costa, C.V., et al., 2013. Memantine rescues transient cognitive impairment caused by high-molecular-weight aβ oligomers but not the persistent impairment induced by low-molecular-weight oligomers. J. Neurosci. 33, 9626−9634.

Fredriksson, L., Li, H., Fieber, C., Li, X., Eriksson, U., 2004. Tissue plasminogen activator is a potent activator of PDGF-CC. EMBO J. 23, 3793−3802.

Fredriksson, L., Lawrence, D.A., Medcalf, R.L., 2017. tPA modulation of the blood-brain barrier: a unifying explanation for the pleiotropic effects of tPA in the CNS. Semin. Thromb. Hemostat. 43, 154−168.

Gallego, J.A., Gordon, M.L., Claycomb, K., Bhatt, M., Lencz, T., et al., 2012. In vivo microRNA detection and quantitation in cerebrospinal fluid. J. Mol. Neurosci. 47, 243−248.

Gallimore, M.J., 2006. More on: discovery of alpha2-plasmin inhibitor and its congenital deficiency. J. Thromb. Haemost 4, 284−285.

Gao, L., Jiang, T., Guo, J., Liu, Y., Cui, G., Gu, L., et al., 2012. Inhibition of autophagy contributes to ischemic postconditioning-induced neuroprotection against focal cerebral ischemia in rats. PLoS One 7, e46092.

García-Cobos, R., Frank-Garcia, A., Gutiérrez-Fernández, M., Díez-Tejedor, E., 2010. Citicoline, use in cognitive decline: vascular and degenerative. J. Neurol. Sci. 299, 188−192.

Garrido-Mesa, N., Zarzuelo, A., Gálvez, J., 2013. Minocycline: far beyond an antibiotic. Br. J. Pharmacol. 169, 337−352.

Gerloff, C., Bushara, K., Sailer, A., Wassermann, E.M., Chen, R., et al., 2006. Multimodal imaging of brain reorganization in motor areas of the contralesional hemisphere of well recovered patients after capsular stroke. Brain 129, 791−808.

Gherardini, L., Gennaro, M., Pizzorusso, T., 2015. Perilesional treatment with chondroitinase ABC and motor training promote functional recovery after stroke in rats. Cereb. Cortex 25, 202−212.

Gilgun-Sherki, Y., Melamed, E., Offen, D., 2006. Anti-inflammatory drugs in the treatment of neurodegenerative diseases: current state. Curr. Pharm. Design 12, 3509−3519.

Gillani, R.L., Tsai, S.Y., Wallace, D.G., O'Brien, T.E., Arhebamen, E., et al., 2010. Cognitive recovery in the aged rat after stroke and Anti-Nogo-A immunotherapy. Behav. Brain Res. 208, 415−424.

Goel, A., Kunnumakkara, A.B., Aggarwal, B.B., 2008. Curcumin as "Curcumin": from kitchen to clinic. Biochem. Pharmacol. 75, 787−809.

Govender, P., Kalra, L., 2007. Benefits of occupational therapy in stroke rehabilitation. Expert Rev. Neurother. 7, 1013−1019.

Grasso, M., Piscopo, P., Confaloni, A., Denti, M.A., 2014. Circulating miRNAs as biomarkers for neurodegenerative disorders. Molecules 19, 6891−6910.

Guadagno, J.V., Donnan, G.A., Markus, R., Gillard, J.H., Baron, J.C., 2004. Imaging the ischemic penumbra. Curr. Opin. Neurol. 17, 61−67.

Gravanis, I., Tsirka, S.E., 2008. Tissue-type plasminogen activator as a therapeutic target in stroke. Expert Opin. Ther. Targets 12, 159−170.

Green, A.R., 2008. Pharmacological approaches to acute ischaemic stroke: reperfusion certainly, neuroprotection possibly. Br. J. Pharmacol. 153 (Suppl. 1), S332−S338.

Guan, Y., Mizoguchi, M., Yoshimoto, K., Hata, N., Shono, T., et al., 2010. MiRNA-196 is upregulated in glioblastoma but not in anaplastic astrocytoma and has prognostic significance. Clin. Cancer Res. 16, 4289−4297.

Guo, M.C., Cao, Y., Liu, J.W., 2007. Protective effects of picroside 2 on glutamate injury of PC12 cells. Chin. J. Clin. Pharmacol. Ther. 12, 440−443.

Guo, Y., Xu, X., Li, Q., Li, Z., Du, F., 2016. Anti-inflammation effects of picroside 2 in cerebral ischemic injury rats. Behav. Brain Funct. 6, 43.

György, B., Hung, M.E., Breakefield, X.O., Leonard, J.N., 2015. Therapeutic applications of extracellular vesicles: clinical promise and open questions. Annu. Rev. Pharmacol. Toxicol 55, 439–464.

Hamann, G.F., Burggraf, D., Martens, H.K., Liebetrau, M., Jager, G., et al., 2004. Mild to moderate hypothermia prevents microvascular basal lamina antigen loss in experimental focal cerebral ischemia. Stroke 35, 764–769.

Hamilton, K.L., Staib, J.L., Phillips, T., Hess, A., Lennon, S.L., et al., 2003. Exercise, antioxidants, and HSP 72: protection against myocardial ischemia/reperfusion. Free Radic. Biol. Med. 34, 800–809.

Hara, M.R., Snyder, S.H., 2007. Cell signaling and neuronal death. Annu. Rev. Pharmacol. Toxicol. 47, 117–141.

Haughey, N.J., Bandaru, V.V., Bae, M., Mattson, M.P., 2010. Roles for dysfunctional sphingolipid metabolism in Alzheimer's disease neuropathogenesis. Biochim. Biophys. Acta 1801, 878–886.

Hayes, K., Sprague, S., Guo, M., Davis, W., Friedman, A., et al., 2008. Forced, not voluntary, exercise effectively induces neuroprotection in stroke. Acta Neuropathol. 115, 289–296.

He, L.J., Liang, M., Hou, F.F., Guo, Z.J., Xie, D., Zhang, X., 2009. Ethanol extraction of *Picrorhiza scrophulariiflora* prevents renal injury in experimental diabetes via anti-inflammation action. J. Endocrinol. 200, 347–355.

Heart Protection Study Collaborative G, 2002. MRC/BHF Heart Protection Study of cholesterol lowering with simvastatin in 20,536 high-risk individuals: a randomised placebo-controlled trial. Lancet 360, 7–22.

Ho, P.W., Reutens, D.C., Phan, T.G., Wright, P.M., Markus, R., et al., 2005. Is white matter involved in patients entered into typical trials of neuroprotection? Stroke 36, 2742–2744.

Heo, J.H., Lucero, J., Abumiya, T., Koziol, J.A., Copeland, B.R., et al., 1999. Matrix metalloproteinases increase very early during experimental focal cerebral ischemia. J. Cereb. Blood Flow Metab. 19, 624–633.

Higashi, Y., 2009. Edaravone for the treatment of acute cerebral infarction: role of endothelium-derived nitric oxide and oxidative stress. Expert Opin. Pharmacother. 10, 323–331.

Hicks, A., Jolkkonen, J., 2009. Challenges and possibilities of intravascular cell therapy in stroke. Acta Neurobiol. Exp. (Wars) 69, 1–11.

Hoe Heo, J. (Principal Investigator). The Effect of Very Early Use of Rosuvastatin in Preventing Recurrence of Ischemic Stroke: EUREKA. NCT01364220 Clinical Trial 2018. From the Stroke Center Clinical Trials Registry: <http://www.strokecenter.org/trials/clini-calstudies/the-effects-of-very-early-use-of-rosuvastatin-inpreventing-recurrence-of-ischemic-stroke> (accessed 24.08.12.).

Hong, S.H., Belayev, L., Khoutorova, L., Obenaus, A., Bazan, N.G., 2014. Docosahexaenoic acid confers enduring neuroprotection in experimental stroke. J. Neurol. Sci. 338, 135–141.

Hong, S.H., Khoutorova, L., Bazan, N.G., Belayev, L., 2015. Docosahexaenoic acid improves behavior and attenuates blood–brain barrier injury induced by focal cerebral ischemia in rats. Exp. Transl. Stroke Med. 7, 3.

Horie, N., Pereira, M.P., Niizuma, K., Sun, G., Keren-Gill, H., et al., 2011. Transplanted stem cell-secreted VEGF effects post-stroke recovery, inflammation, and vascular repair. Stem Cells 29, 274–285.

Hossain, M.S., Hashimoto, M., Masumura, S., 1998. Influence of docosahexaenoic acid on cerebral lipid peroxide level in aged rats with and without hypercholesterolemia. Neurosci. Lett 244, 157–160.

Hossain, M.S., Hashimoto, M., Gamoh, S., Masumura, S., 1999. Antioxidative effects of docosahexaenoic acid in the cerebrum versus cerebellum and brainstem of aged hypercholesterolemic rats. J. Neurochem 72, 1133–1138.

Hurtado, O., Moro, M.A., Cárdenas, A., Sánchez, V., Fernández-Tomé, P., Leza, J.C., et al., 2005. Neuroprotection afforded by prior citicoline administration in experimental brain ischemia: effects on glutamate transport. Neurobiol. Dis 18, 336–345.

Hurtado, O., Cárdenas, A., Pradillo, J.M., Morales, J.R., Ortego, F., Sobrino, T., et al., 2007. A chronic treatment with CDP-choline improves functional recovery and increases neuronal plasticity after experimental stroke. Neurobiol. Dis. 26, 105–111.

Jain, M.K., Ridker, P.M., 2005. Anti-inflammatory effects of statins: clinical evidence and basic mechanisms. Nat. Rev. Drug Discov. 4, 977–987.

Janowski, M., Walczak, P., Date, I., 2010. Intravenous route of cell delivery for treatment of neurological disorders: a meta-analysis of preclinical results. Stem Cells Dev. 19, 5–16.

Jeyaseelan, K., Lim, K.Y., Armugam, A., 2008. MicroRNA expression in the blood and brain of rats subjected to transient focal ischemia by middle cerebral artery occlusion. Stroke 39, 959–966.

Ji, X., Luo, Y., Ling, F., Stetler, R.A., Lan, J., et al., 2007. Mild hypothermia diminishes oxidative DNA damage and pro-death signaling events after cerebral ischemia: a mechanism for neuroprotection. Front Biosci. 12, 1737–1747.

Jiang, J., Wang, W., Sun, Y., Hu, M., Li, F., Zhu, D.Y., 2007. Neuroprotective effect of curcumin on focal cerebral ischemic rats by preventing blood-brain barrier damage. Eur. J. Pharmacol. 561, 54–62.

Jiang, P., Zhu, T., Xia, Z., Gao, F., Gu, W., et al., 2015. Inhibition of MAPK/ERK signaling blocks hippocampal neurogenesis and impairs cognitive performance in prenatally infected neonatal rats. Eur. Arch. Psychiatry Clin. Neurosci. 265, 497–509.

Jiang, B., Song, L., Wang, C.N., Zhang, W., Huang, C., Tong, et al., 2016. Antidepressant-like effects of GM1 ganglioside involving the BDNF signaling cascade in mice. Int. J. Neuropsychopharmacol. 19, pii: pyw046.

Jickling, G.C., Ander, B.P., Zhan, X., et al., 2014. microRNA expression in peripheral blood cells following acute ischemic stroke and their predicted gene targets. PLoS One 9, e99283.

Jin, K., Zhu, Y., Sun, Y., Mao, X.O., Xie, L., et al., 2002. Vascular endothelial growth factor (VEGF) stimulates neurogenesis in vitro and in vivo. Proc. Natl. Acad. Sci. U.S.A. 99, 11946–11950.

Johnson, J.A., Johnson, D.A., Kraft, A.D., Calkins, M.J., Jakel, R.J., 2008. The Nrf2-ARE pathway: an indicator and modulator of oxidative stress in neurodegeneration. Ann. N. Y. Acad. Sci. 1147, 61–69.

Jones, A.M., 2014. Dietary nitrate supplementation and exercise performance. Sports Med. 44 (Suppl. 1), S35–S45.

Kafi, H., Salamzadeh, J., Beladimoghadam, N., Sistanizad, M., Kouchek, M., 2014. Study of the neuroprotective effects of memantine in patients with mild to moderate ischemic stroke. Iran. J. Pharm. Res. 13, 591–598.

Kalkman, H.O., Feuerbach, D., 2016. Modulatory effects of $\alpha7$ nAChRs on the immune system and its relevance for CNS disorders. Cell Mol. Life Sci. 73, 2511–2530.

Kang, E.S., Woo, I.S., Kim, H.J., Eun, S.Y., Paek, K.S., et al., 2007. Up-regulation of aldose reductase expression mediated by phosphatidylinositol 3-kinase/Akt and Nrf2 is involved in the protective effect of curcumin against oxidative damage. Free Radic. Biol. Med. 43, 535–545.

Kaplan, D.R., Miller, F.D., 2000. Neurotrophin signal transduction in the nervous system. Curr. Opin. Neurobiol. 70, 381–391.

Kauranen, T., Turunen, K., Laari, S., Mustanoja, S., Baumann, P., et al., 2013. The severity of cognitive deficits predicts return to work after a first-ever ischaemic stroke. J. Neurol. Neurosurg. Psychiatry 84, 316−321.

Kaushal, V., Schlichter, L.C., 2008. Mechanisms of microglia-mediated neurotoxicity in a new model of the stroke penumbra. J. Neurosci. 28, 2221−2230.

Kawasaki-Yatsugi, S., Ichiki, C., Yatsugi, S., Takahashi, M., Shimizu-Sasamata, M., et al., 2000. Neuroprotective effects of an AMPA receptor antagonist YM872 in a rat transient middle cerebral artery occlusion model. Neuropharmacology 39, 211−217.

Kernie, S.G., Parent, J.M., 2010. Forebrain neurogenesis after focal Ischemic and traumatic brain injury. Neurobiol. Dis. 37, 267−274.

Khaja, A.M., Grotta, J.C., 2007. Established treatments for acute ischaemic stroke. Lancet 27, 319−330.

Khedr, E.M., Abdel-Fadeil, M.R., Farghali, A., Qaid, M., 2009. Role of 1 and 3 Hz repetitive transcranial magnetic stimulation on motor function recovery after acute ischaemic stroke. Eur. J. Neurol. 16, 1323−1330.

Khedr, E.M., Abo El-Fetoh, N., Ali, A.M., El-Hammady, D.H., Khalifa, H., et al., 2014. Dual-hemisphere repetitive transcranial magnetic stimulation for rehabilitation of poststroke aphasia: a randomized, double-blind clinical trial. Neurorehabil. Neural Repair 28, 740−750.

Kim, D., Jahan, R., Starkman, S., Abolian, A., Kidwell, C.S., et al., 2006. Endovascular mechanical clot retrieval in a broad ischemic stroke cohort. AJNR Am. J. Neuroradiol. 27, 2048−2052.

Kim, Y.J., Park, H.J., Lee, G., Bang, O.Y., Ahn, Y.H., et al., 2009. Neuroprotective effects of human mesenchymal stem cells on dopaminergic neurons through anti-inflammatory action. Glia 57, 13−23.

Kleindorfer, D., Kissela, B., Schneider, A., Woo, D., Khoury, J., et al., 2004. Eligibility for recombinant tissue plasminogen activator in acute ischemic stroke: a population-based study. Stroke 35, e27−e29.

Kobayashi, A., Kang, M.-I., Okawa, H., Ohtsuji, M., Zenke, Y., et al., 2004. Oxidative stress sensor Keap1 functions as an adaptor for Cul3-based E3 ligase to regulate proteasomal degradation of Nrf2. Mol. Cell. Biol. 24, 7130−7139.

Koh, S.H., Lo, E.H., 2015. The role of the PI3K pathway in the regeneration of the damaged brain by neural stem cells after cerebral infarction. J. Clin. Neurol. 11, 297−304.

Kramer, A.F., Erickson, K.I., Colcombe, S.J., 2006. Exercise, cognition, and the aging brain. J. Appl. Physiol. 101, 1237−1242.

Kreuzberg, M., Kanov, E., Timofeev, O., Schwaninger, M., Monyer, H., et al., 2010. Increased subventricular zone-derived cortical neurogenesis after ischemic lesion. Exp. Neurol. 226, 90−99.

Krupinski, J., Ferrer, I., Barrachina, M., Secades, J.J., Mercadal, J., et al., 2002. CDP-choline reduces pro-caspase and cleaved caspase-3 expression, nuclear DNA fragmentation, and specific PARP-cleaved products of caspase activation following middle cerebral artery occlusion in the rat. Neuropharmacology 42, 846−854.

Kureishi, Y., Luo, Z., Shiojima, I., Bialik, A., Fulton, D., Lefer, D.J., et al., 2000. The HMG-CoA reductase inhibitor simvastatin activates the protein kinase Akt and promotes angiogenesis in normocholesterolemic animals. Nat. Med. 6, 1004−1010.

Labiche, L.A., Grotta, J.C., 2004. Clinical trials for cytoprotection in stroke. NeuroRx 1, 46−70.

Lai, C.P., Breakefield, X.O., 2012. Role of exosomes/microvesicles in the nervous system and use in emerging therapies. Front Physiol 3, 228.

Lai, R.C., Chen, T.S., Lim, S.K., 2011. Mesenchymal stem cell exosome: a novel stem cell-based therapy for cardiovascular disease. Regen. Med. 6, 481−492.

Lapchak, P.A., Zivin, J.A., 2009. The lipophilic multifunctional antioxidant edaravone (radicut) improves behavior following embolic strokes in rabbits: a combination therapy study with tissue plasminogen activator. Exp. Neurol. 215, 95−100.

Laterza, O.F., Lim, L., Garrett-Engele, P.W., et al., 2009. Plasma microRNAs as sensitive and specific biomarkers of tissue injury. Clin. Chem. 55, 1977−1983.

Lebeurrier, N., Liot, G., Lopez-Atalaya, J.P., Orset, C., Fernandez-Monreal, M., et al., 2005. The brain-specific tissue-type plasminogen activator inhibitor, neuroserpin, protects neurons against excitotoxicity both in vitro and in vivo. Mol. Cell. Neurosci. 30, 552−558.

Lee, B.J., Egi, Y., van Leyen, K., Lo, E.H., Arai, K., 2010. Edaravone, a free radical scavenger, protects components of the neurovascular unit against oxidative stress in vitro. Brain Res. 1307, 22−27.

Lee, J., Duan, W., Mattson, M.P., 2002. Evidence that brain-derived neurotrophic factor is required for basal neurogenesis and mediates, in part, the enhancement of neurogenesis by dietary restriction in the hippocampus of adult mice. J. Neurochem. 82, 1367−1375.

Lei, X.H., Zhao, D., Li, Y.L., Li, X.F., Sun, X., et al., 2013. Pifithrin-alpha enhances the survival of transplanted neural stem cells in stroke rats by inhibiting p53 nuclear translocation. CNS Neurosci. Ther. 19, 109−116.

Li, J.X., Li, P., Tezuka, Y., Namba, T., Kadota, S., 1998. Three phenylethanoid glycosides and an iridoid glycoside from *Picrorhiza scrophulariiflora*. Phytochemistry 48, 537−542.

Li, S., Carmichael, S.T., 2006. Growth-associated gene and protein expression in the region of axonal sprouting in the aged brain after stroke. Neurobiol. Dis. 23, 362−373.

Li, T., Liu, J.W., Zhang, X.D., Guo, M.C., Ji, G., 2007. The neuroprotective effect of picroside 2 from hu-huang-lian against oxidtive stress. Am. J. Chin. Med. 35, 681−691.

Li, Z., Xu, X.Y., Shen, W., Guo, Y.L., 2010. The interferring effects of picroside II on the expressions of NF-κB and I-κB following cerebral ischemia reperfusion injury in rats. Chin. Pharmacol. Bull. 26, 56−59.

Li, X., Gu, S., Ling, Y., Shen, C., Cao, X., et al., 2015a. p53 inhibition provides a pivotal protective effect against ischemia-reperfusion injury *in vitro* via mTOR signaling. Brain Res. 1605, 31−38.

Li, L., Tian, J., Long, M.K., Chen, Y., Lu, J., et al., 2016. Protection against experimental stroke by ganglioside GM1 is associated with the inhibition of autophagy. PLoS One 11, e0144219.

Liao, T.V., Forehand, C.C., Hess, D.C., Fagan, S.C., 2013. Minocycline repurposing in critical illness: focus on stroke. Curr. Top. Med. Chem. 13, 2283−2290.

Lima, J.A., Desai, M.Y., Steen, H., Warren, W.P., Gautam, S., et al., 2004. Statin-induced cholesterol lowering and plaque regression after 6 months of magnetic resonance imaging-monitored therapy. Circulation 110, 2336−2341.

Liu, D.-Z., Tian, Y., Ander, B.P., et al., 2010. Brain and blood microRNA expression profiling of ischemic stroke, intracerebral hemorrhage, and kainate seizures. J. Cereb. Blood Flow Metab. 30, 92−101.

Liu, J.W., Yu, Y.J., Zheng, P.Y., Zhang, X.D., Li, T., Cao, Y., et al., 2007. Synergistic protective effect of picroside 2 and NGF on PC12 cells against oxidative stress induced by H_2O_2. Pharmacol. Rep. 59, 573−579.

Liu, S., Cao, Y., Qu, M., Zhang, Z., Feng, L., et al., 2016. Curcumin protects against stroke and increases levels of Notch intracellular domain. Neurol. Res. 38, 553−559.

Liu, W., Xu, Z., Deng, Y., Xu, B., Wei, Y., et al., 2013. Protective effects of memantine against methylmercury-induced glutamate dyshomeostasis and oxidative stress in rat cerebral cortex. Neurotox. Res. 24, 320−337.

Liu, Y.P., Zhang, J.J., Han, R.F., Liu, H.X., Sun, D., et al., 2015. Downregulation of serum brain specific microRNA is associated with inflammation and infarct volume in acute ischemic stroke. J. Clin. Neurosci. 22, 291–295.

López-Valdés, H.E., Clarkson, A.N., Ao, Y., Charles, A.C., Carmichael, S.T., et al., 2014. Memantine enhances recovery from stroke. Stroke 45, 2093–2100.

López-Miranda, V., Soto-Montenegro, M.L., Vera, G., Herradón, E., Desco, M., et al., 2012. Resveratrol: a neuroprotective polyphenol in the Mediterranean diet. Rev. Neurol. 54, 349–356.

Lowinus, T., Bose, T., Busse, S., Busse, M., Reinhold, D., Schraven, B., et al., 2016. Immunomodulation by memantine in therapy of Alzheimer's disease is mediated through inhibition of Kv1.3 channels and T cell responsiveness. Oncotarget 7, 53797–53807.

Ma, X., Zhang, H., Pan, Q., et al., 2013. Hypoxia/aglycemia-induced endothelial barrier dysfunction and tight junction protein down-regulation can be ameliorated by Citicolone. PLoS One 8, e82604.

Macko, R.F., Ivey, F.M., Forrester, L.W., Hanley, D., Sorkin, J.D., et al., 2005. Treadmill exercise rehabilitation improves ambulatory function and cardiovascular fitness in patients with chronic stroke: a randomized, controlled trial. Stroke 36, 2206–2211.

Mang, C.S., Campbell, K.L., Ross, C.J., Boyd, L.A., 2013. Promoting neuroplasticity for motor rehabilitation after stroke: considering the effects of aerobic exercise and genetic variation on brain-derived neurotrophic factor. Phys. Ther. 93, 1707–1716.

Marsden, D.L., Dunn, A., Callister, R., Levi, C.R., Spratt, N.J., 2013. Characteristics of exercise training interventions to improve cardiorespiratory fitness after stroke: a systematic review with meta-analysis. Neurorehabil. Neural Repair 27, 775–788.

Medcalf, R.L., Lawrence, D.A., 2016. Editorial: The role of the plasminogen activating system in neurobiology. Front. Cell. Neurosci. 10, 222.

Meloni, B.P., Craig, A.J., Milech, N., Hopkins, R.M., Watt, P.M., et al., 2014. The neuroprotective efficacy of cell-penetrating peptides TAT, penetratin, Arg-9, and Pep-1 in glutamic acid, kainic acid, and in vitro ischemia injury models using primary cortical neuronal cultures. Cell. Mol. Neurobiol. 34, 173–181.

Meloni, B.P., Brookes, L.M., Clark, V.W., et al., 2015a. Poly-arginine and arginine-rich peptides are neuroprotective in stroke models. J. Cereb. Blood Flow Metab. 35, 993–1004.

Meloni, B.P., Milani, D., Edwards, A.B., et al., 2015b. Neuroprotective peptides fused to arginine-rich cell penetrating peptides: neuroprotective mechanism likely mediated by peptide endocytic properties. Pharmacol. Ther. 153, 36–54.

Mihaylova, B., Emberson, J., Blackwell, L., Keech, A., Simes, J., et al., 2012. The effects of lowering LDL cholesterol with statin therapy in people at low risk of vascular disease: meta-analysis of individual data from 27 randomised trials. Lancet. 380, 581–590.

Milani, D., Clark, V.W., Cross, J.L., Anderton, R.S., Knuckey, N.W., et al., 2016a. Poly-arginine peptides reduce infarct volume in a permanent middle cerebral artery rat stroke model. BMC Neurosci. 17, 1–8.

Milani, D., Knuckey, N.W., Anderton, R.S., Cross, J.L., Meloni, B.P., 2016b. The R18 polyarginine peptide is more effective than the TAT-NR2B9c (NA-1) peptide when administered 60 minutes after permanent middle cerebral artery occlusion in the rat. Stroke Res. Treat. 2016, 237271.

Montaner, J., Mendioroz, M., Ribó, M., Delgado, P., Quintana, M., et al., 2011. A panel of biomarkers including caspase-3 and D-dimer may differentiate acute stroke from stroke-mimicking conditions in the emergency department. J. Intern. Med. 270, 166–174.

Moon, G.J., Kim, S.J., Cho, Y.H., Ryoo, S., Bang, O.Y., 2014. Antioxidant effects of statins in patients with atherosclerotic cerebrovascular disease. J. Clin. Neurol. 10, 140–147.

Mosconi, L., Murray, J., Tsui, W.H., Li, Y., Davies, M., et al., 2014. Mediterranean diet and magnetic resonance imaging-assessed brain atrophy in cognitively normal individuals at risk for Alzheimer's disease. J. Prev. Alzheimers Dis 1, 23–32.

Moskowitz, M.A., Lo, E.H., Iadecola, C., 2010. The science of stroke: mechanisms in search of treatments. Neuron 67, 181–198.

Murphy, T.H., Corbett, D., 2009. Plasticity during stroke recovery: from synapse to behaviour. Nat. Rev. Neurosci. 10, 861–872.

Nakamura, T., Lipton, S.A., 2016. Protein S-nitrosylation as a therapeutic target for neurodegenerative diseases. Trends Pharmacol. Sci. 37, 73–84.

Nakase, T., Sasaki, M., Suzuki, A., 2014. Edaravone, a free radical scavenger, can effect on the inflammatory biomarkers in acute ischemic stroke patients. J. Neurol. Disord. 2, 167.

Nguyen, T., Nioi, P., Pickett, C.B., 2009. The nrf2-antioxidant response element signaling pathway and its activation by oxidative stress. J. Biol. Chem. 284, 13291–13295.

Niego, B., Freeman, R., Puschmann, T.B., Turnley, A.M., Medcalf, R.L., 2012. t-PA-specific modulation of a human blood-brain barrier model involves plasmin-mediated activation of the Rho kinase pathway in astrocytes. Blood 119, 4752–4761.

Noguchi, N., 2016. Ebselen, a useful tool for understanding cellular redox biology and a promising drug candidate for use in human diseases. Arch. Biochem. Biophys. 595, 109–112.

Nudo, R.J., 2006. Mechanisms for recovery of motor function following cortical damage. Curr. Opin. Neurobiol. 16, 638–644.

Nudo, R.J., 2007. Postinfarct cortical plasticity and behavioral recovery. Stroke 38, 840–845.

Ohmi, Y., Tajima, O., Ohkawa, Y., Mori, A., Sugiura, Y., et al., 2009. Gangliosides play pivotal roles in the regulation of complement systems and in the maintenance of integrity in nerve tissues. Proc. Natl. Acad. Sci. U.S.A. 106, 22405–22410.

Ortolano, S., Spuch, C., 2013. tPA in the central nervous system: relations between tPA and cell surface LRPs. Recent Pat. Endocr. Metab. Immune Drug Discov. 7, 65–76.

Ovbiagele, B., 2008. Potential role of curcumin in stroke prevention. Expert Rev. Neurother. 8, 1175–1176.

Overman, J.J., Clarkson, A.N., Wanner, I.B., et al., 2012. A role for ephrin-A5 in axonal sprouting, recovery, and activity-dependent plasticity after stroke. Proc. Natl. Acad. Sci. U.S.A. 109, E2230–E2239.

Paik, M.J., Li, W.Y., Ahn, Y.H., Lee, P.H., Choi, S., et al., 2009. The free fatty acid metabolome in cerebral ischemia following human mesenchymal stem cell transplantation in rats. Clin. Chim. Acta 402, 25–30.

Papademetriou, V., Doumas, M., 2009. Treatment strategies to prevent stroke: focus on optimal lipid and blood pressure control. Expert Opin. Pharmacother. 10, 955–966.

Parsons, C.G., Danysz, W., Bartmann, A., Spielmanns, P., Frankiewicz, T., et al., 1999. Amino-alkyl-cyclohexanes are novel uncompetitive NMDA receptor antagonists with strong voltage-dependency and fast blocking kinetics: in vitro and in vivo characterization. Neuropharmacology 38, 85–108.

Patel, M.D., Coshall, C., Rudd, A.G., Wolfe, C.D.A., 2002. Cognitive impairment after stroke: clinical determinants and its associations with long-term stroke outcomes. J. Am. Geriatr. Soc. 50, 700–706.

Pearson-Fuhrhop, K.M., Cramer, S.C., 2010. Genetic influences on neural plasticity. PM&R 2, S227–S240.

Picada, J., Flores, E., Cappelari, S., Pereira, P., 2011. Effects of memantine, a noncompetitive N-methyl-D-aspartate receptor antagonist, on genomic stability. Basic Clin. Pharmacol. Toxicol. 109, 413–417.

Pirmoradi, M., Jemel, B., Gallagher, A., Tremblay, J., D'Hondt, F., et al., 2016. Verbal memory and verbal fluency tasks used for language localization and lateralization during magnetoencephalography. Epilepsy Res. 119, 1–9.

Plataras, C., Angelogianni, P., Tsakiris, S., 2003. Effect of CDP-choline on hippocampal acetylcholinesterase and Na^+, K^+-ATPase in adult and aged rats. Z. Naturforsch. 58, 277–281.

Plate, K.H., 1999. Mechanisms of angiogenesis in the brain. J. Neuropathol. Exp. Neurol. 58, 313–320.

Prinz, V., Laufs, U., Gertz, K., Kronenberg, G., Balkaya, M., et al., 2008. Intravenous rosuvastatin for acute stroke treatment: an animal study. Stroke 39, 433–438.

Qosa, H., Mohamed, L.A., Batarseh, Y.S., Alqahtani, S., Ibrahim, B., et al., 2015. Extra-virgin olive oil attenuates amyloid-β and tau pathologies in the brains of TgSwDI mice. J. Nutr. Biochem. 26, 1479–1490.

Rajanikant, G.K., Zemke, D., Kassab, M., Majid, A., 2007. The therapeutic potential of statins in neurological disorders. Curr. Med. Chem. 14, 103–112.

Rand, D., Eng, J.J., Liu-Ambrose, T., Tawashy, A.E., 2010. Feasibility of a 6-month exercise and recreation program to improve executive functioning and memory in individuals with chronic stroke. Neurorehabil. Neural Repair 24, 722–729.

Rane, M.J., Pan, Y., Singh, S., Powell, D.W., Wu, R., Cummins, T., et al., 2003. Heat shock protein 27 controls apoptosis by regulating Akt activation. J. Biol. Chem. 278, 27828–27835.

Rao, C.V., 2007. Regulation of COX and LOX by curcumin. Adv. Exp. Med. Biol. 595, 213–226.

Ridker, P.M., Danielson, E., Fonseca, F.A., Genest, J., Gotto Jr, A.M., et al., 2008. Rosuvastatin to prevent vascular events in men and women with elevated C-reactive protein. N. Engl. J. Med. 359, 2195–2207.

Riley, T., Sontag, E., Chen, P., Levine, A., 2008. Transcriptional control of human p53-regulated genes. Nat. Rev. Mol. Cell Biol. 9, 402–412.

Rincon, F., Sacco, R.L., 2008. Secondary stroke prevention. J. Cardiovasc. Nurs. 23, 34–41.

Rink, C., Khanna, S., 2011. MicroRNA in ischemic stroke etiology and pathology. Physiol. Genomics 43, 521–528.

Romero, J.R., 2007. Prevention of ischemic stroke: overview of traditional risk factors. Curr. Drug Targets 8, 794–801.

Romero, J.R., Morris, J., Pikula, A., 2008. Stroke prevention: modifying risk factors. Ther. Adv. Cardiovasc. Dis. 2, 287–303.

Rong, X., Zhou, W., Xiao-Wen, C., Tao, L., Tang, J., 2013. Ganglioside GM1 reduces white matter damage in neonatal rats. Acta Neurobiol. Exp. (Wars) 73, 379–386.

Rosell, A., Cuadrado, E., Alvarez-Sabín, J., Hernández-Guillamon, M., Delgado, P., et al., 2008. Caspase-3 is related to infarct growth after human ischemic stroke. Neurosci. Lett. 430, 1–6.

Rossini, P.M., Altamura, C., Ferreri, F., Melgari, J.M., et al., 2007. Neuroimaging experimental studies on brain plasticity in recovery from stroke. Eura. Midicophys. 43, 241–254.

Rybak, M.E., Calvey, E.M., Harnly, J.M., 2004. Quantitative determination of allicin in garlic: supercritical fluid extraction and standard addition of alliin. J. Agric. Food Chem. 52, 682–687.

Sale, A., Berardi, N., Maffei, L., 2009. Enrich the environment to empower the brain. Trends Neurosci. 32, 233–239.

Samson, A.L., Nevin, S.T., Croucher, D., Niego, B., Daniel, P.B., et al., 2008. Tissue-type plasminogen activator requires a co-receptor to enhance NMDA receptor function. J. Neurochem. 107, 1091–1101.

Sare, G.M., Geeganage, C., Bath, P.M., 2009. High blood pressure in acute oschaemic stroke-broadening therapeutic horizons. Cerebrovasc. Dis. 1, 156−161.

Savci, V., Wurtman, R.J., 1995. Effect of cytidine on membrane phospholipid synthesis in rat striatal slices. J. Neurochem. 64, 378−384.

Save-Pédebos, J., Pinabiaux, C., Dorfmuller, G., Sorbets, S.F., Delalande, O., et al., 2016. The development of pragmatic skills in children after hemispherotomy: contribution from left and right hemispheres. Epilepsy Behav. 55, 139−145.

Saver, J.L., 2008. Citicoline: update on a promising and widely available agent for neuroprotection and neurorepair. Rev. Neurol. Dis. 5, 167−177.

Schäbitz, W.R., Li, F., Fisher, M., 2000. The N-methyl-D-aspartate antagonist CNS 1102 protects cerebral gray and white matter from ischemic injury following temporary focal ischemia in rats. Stroke 31, 1709−1714.

Scapagnini, G., Colombrita, C., Amadio, M., D'Agata, V., Arcelli, E., et al., 2006. Curcumin activates defensive genes and protects neurons against oxidative stress. Antioxid. Redox Signal. 8, 395−403.

Schnaar, R.L., 2010. Brain gangliosides in axon-myelin stability and axon regeneration. FEBS Lett. 584, 1741−1747.

Schwammenthal, Y., Tsabari, R., Bakon, M., Orion, D., Merzeliak, O., Tanne, D., 2006. Thrombolysis in acute stroke. Isr. Med. Assoc. J. 8, 784−787.

Secades, J.J., Lorenzo, J.L., 2006. Citicoline: pharmacological and clinical review, 2006 update. Methods Find Exp. Clin. Pharmacol. 28 (Suppl. B), 1−56.

Sepramaniam, S., Tan, J.-R., Tan, K.-S., et al., 2014. Circulating microRNAs as biomarkers of acute stroke. Int. J. Mol. Sci. 15, 1418−1432.

Serhan, C.N., 2005a. Novel ω-3-derived local mediators in anti-inflammation and resolution. Pharmacol. Ther. 105, 7−21.

Serhan, C.N., 2005b. Novel eicosanoid and docosanoid mediators: resolvins, docosatrienes, and neuroprotectins. Curr. Opin. Clin. Nutr. Metab. Care 8, 115−121.

Sharma, N., Cohen, L.G., 2010. Recovery of motor function after stroke. Dev. Psychobiol. 54, 254−262.

Shen, L.H., Li, Y., Chen, J., Zacharek, A., Gao, Q., et al., 2007. Therapeutic benefit of bone marrow stromal cells administered 1 month after stroke. J. Cereb. Blood Flow Metab. 27, 6−13.

Shen, W.H., Zhang, C.Y., Zhang, G.Y., 2003. Antioxidants attenuate reperfusion injury after global brain ischemia through inhibiting nuclear factor-kappa B activity in rats. Acta Pharmacol. Sin. 24, 1125−1130.

Shih, A.Y., Li, P., Murphy, T.H., 2005. A small molecule inducible Nrf2-mediated antioxidant response provides effective prophylaxis against cerebral ischemia in vivo. J. Neurosci. 25, 10321−10335.

Shin, J.Y., Park, H.J., Kim, H.N., Oh, S.H., Bae, J.S., et al., 2014. Mesenchymal stem cells enhance autophagy and increase β-amyloid clearance in Alzheimer disease models. Autophagy 10, 32−44.

Siegel, S.R., Mackenzie, J., Chaplin, G., Jablonski, N.G., Griffiths, L., 2012. Circulating microRNAs involved in multiple sclerosis. Mol. Biol. Rep. 39, 6219−6225.

Simopoulos, A.P., 2006. Evolutionary aspects of diet, the omega-6/omega-3 ratio and genetic variation: nutritional implications for chronic diseases. Biomed. Pharmacother. 60, 502−507.

Singhal, A.B., 2006. Oxygen therapy in stroke: past, present, and future. Int. J. Stroke. 1, 191−200.

Singhal, A.B., 2007. A review of oxygen therapy in ischemic stroke. Neurol. Res. 29, 173−183.

Smith, W.S., 2006. Safety of mechanical thrombectomy and intravenous tissue plasminogen activator in acute ischemic stroke. Results of the multi Mechanical Embolus Removal in Cerebral Ischemia (MERCI) trial, part I. AJNR Am. J. Neuroradiol. 27, 1177−1182.

Smith, W.S., Sung, G., Saver, J., Budzik, R., Duckwiler, G., et al., 2008. Mechanical thrombectomy for acute ischemic stroke: final results of the Multi MERCI trial. Stroke 39, 1205–1212.

Soleman, S., Yip, P.K., Duricki, D.A., Moon, L.D.F., 2012. Delayed treatment with chondroitinase ABC promotes sensorimotor recovery and plasticity after stroke in aged rats. Brain 135, 1210–1223.

Soni, K.B., Kuttan, R., 1992. Effect of oral curcumin administration on serum peroxides and cholesterol levels in human volunteers. Indian J. Physiol. Pharmacol. 36, 273–275.

Steiner, T., Al-Shahi Salman, R., Ntaios, G., 2014. The European Stroke Organisation (ESO) guidelines. Int. J. Stroke 9, 838–839.

Strimpakos, A.S., Sharma, R.A., 2008. Curcumin: preventive and therapeutic properties in laboratory studies and clinical trials. Antioxid. Redox Signal. 10, 511–545.

Strokin, M., Chechneva, O., Reymann, K.G., Reiser, G., 2006. Neuroprotection of rat hippocampal slices exposed to oxygen-glucose deprivation by enrichment with docosahexaenoic acid and by inhibition of hydrolysis of docosahexaenoic acid-containing phospholipids by calcium independent phospholipase A_2. Neuroscience 140, 547–553.

Su, E.J., Fredriksson, L., Geyer, M., Folestad, E., Cale, J., et al., 2008. Activation of PDGF-CC by tissue plasminogen activator impairs blood-brain barrier integrity during ischemic stroke. Nat. Med. 14, 731–737.

Sun, G.Y., Horrocks, L.A., Farooqui, A.A., 2007. The roles of NADPH oxidase and phospholipases A_2 in oxidative and inflammatory responses in neurodegenerative diseases. J. Neurochem. 103, 1–16.

Sun, F., Johnson, S.R., Jin, K., Uteshev, V.V., 2017. Boosting endogenous resistance of brain to ischemia. Mol. Neurobiol. 54, 2045–2059.

Sun, J.-H., Tan, L., Yu, J.-T., 2014. Post-stroke cognitive impairment: epidemiology, mechanisms and management. Ann. Transl. Med. 2, 80.

Sung, W.H., Wang, C.P., Chou, C.L., Chen, Y.C., Chang, Y.C., et al., 2013. Efficacy of coupling inhibitory and facilitatory repetitive transcranial magnetic stimulation to enhance motor recovery in hemiplegic stroke patients. Stroke 44, 1375–1382.

Swain, S., Turner, C., Tyrrell, P., Rudd, A., 2008. Recognition and management of transient ischaemic attack. BMJ 337, 291–293.

Takasaki, K., Uchida, K., Fujikawa, R., et al., 2011. Neuroprotective effects of citidine-5-diphosphocholine on impaired spatial memory in a rat model of cerebrovascular dementia. J. Pharmacol. Sci. 116, 232–237.

Takeda, H., Spatz, M., Ruetzler, C., McCarron, R., Becker, K., et al., 2002. Induction of mucosal tolerance to E-selectin prevents ischemic and hemorrhagic stroke in spontaneously hypertensive genetically stroke-prone rats. Stroke 33, 2156–2163.

Tang, G., Dong, X., Huang, X., Huang, X.J., Liu, H., et al., 2015. A natural diarylheptanoid promotes neuronal differentiation via activating ERK and PI3K-Akt dependent pathways. Neuroscience 303, 389–401.

Tang, X.N., Liu, L., Koike, M.A., Yenari, M.A., 2013. Mild hypothermia reduces tissue plasminogen activator-related hemorrhage and blood brain barrier disruption after experimental stroke. Ther. Hypothermia Temp. Manag. 3, 74–83.

Tao, Y.W., Liu, J.W., Wei, D.Z., Su, W., Zhou, W.Y., 2003. Protective effect of picroside 2 on the damage of culture PC12 cells in vitro. Chin. J. Clin. Pharmacol. Ther. 8, 27–30.

Tenser, M.S., Amar, A.P., Mack, W.J., 2011. Mechanical thrombectomy for acute ischemic stroke using the MERCI retriever and penumbra aspiration systems. World Neurosurg. 76 (6 Suppl.), S16–S23.

Tiozzo, E., Youbi, M., Dave, K., Perez-Pinzon, M., Rundek, T., et al., 2015. Aerobic, resistance and cognitive exercise training post stroke. Stroke 46, 2012–2016.

Tobin, M.K., Bonds, J.A., Minshall, R.D., Pelligrino, D.A., Testai, F.D., et al., 2014. Neurogenesis and inflammation after ischemic stroke: what is known and where we go from here. J. Cereb. Blood Flow Metab. 34, 1573–1584.

Topol, E.J., 2004. Intensive statin therapy − a sea change in cardiovascular prevention. N. Engl. J. Med. 350, 1562−1564.

Trejo, J.L., Carro, E., Nunez, A., Torres-Aleman, I., 2002. Sedentary life impairs self-reparative processes in the brain: the role of serum insulin-like growth factor-I. Rev. Neurosci. 13, 365−374.

Trichopoulou, A., Kouris-Blazos, A., Wahlqvist, M.L., et al., 1995. Diet and overall survival in elderly people. BMJ 311, 1457−1460.

Trichopoulou, A., Costacou, T., Bamia, C., Trichopoulos, D., 2003. Adherence to a Mediterranean diet and survival in a Greek population. N. Engl. J. Med. 348, 2599−2608.

Tsai, Y.M., Chien, C.F., Lin, L.C., Tsai, T.H., 2011. Curcumin and its nano-formulation: the kinetics of tissue distribution and blood-brain barrier penetration. Int. J. Pharm. 416, 331−338.

Tyagi, N., Qipshidze, N., Munjal, C., Vacek, J.C., Metreveli, N., et al., 2012. Tetrahydrocurcumin ameliorates homocysteinylated cytochrome-c mediated autophagy in hyperhomocysteinemia mice after cerebral ischemia. J. Mol. Neurosci. 47, 128−138.

Ueda, M., Inaba, T., Nito, C., Kamiya, N., Katayama, Y., 2013. Therapeutic impact of eicosapentaenoic acid on ischemic brain damage following transient focal cerebral ischemia in rats. Brain Res. 1519, 95−104.

Van Cruchten, S., Van Den Broeck, W., 2002. Morphological and biochemical aspects of apoptosis, oncosis and necrosis. Anat. Histol. Embryol. 31, 214−223.

Vaughan, C.J., 2003. Prevention of stroke and dementia with statins: effects beyond lipid lowering. Am. J. Cardiol. 91, 23B−29B.

Wakabayashi, N., Dinkova-Kostova, A.T., Holtzclaw, W.D., Kang, M.I., Kobayashi, A., et al., 2004. Protection against electrophile and oxidant stress by induction of the phase 2 response: fate of cysteines of the Keap1 sensor modified by inducers. Proc. Natl. Acad. Sci. U.S.A. 101, 2040−2045.

Wakayama, K., Shimamura, M., Suzuki, J.I., Watanabe, R., Koriyama, H., et al., 2017. Angiotensin II peptide vaccine protects ischemic brain through reducing oxidative stress. Stroke 48, 1362−1368.

Wang, J.Y., Wen, L.L., Huang, Y.N., Chen, Y.T., Ku, M.C., 2006. Dual effects of antioxidants in neurodegeneration: Direct neuroprotection against oxidative stress and indirect protection via suppression of glia-mediated inflammation. Curr. Pharmaceut. Design 12, 3521−3533.

Wang, R.Y., Tseng, H.Y., Liao, K.K., Wang, C.J., Lai, K.L., et al., 2012. rTMS combined with task-oriented training to improve symmetry of interhemispheric corticomotor excitability and gait performance after stroke: a randomized trial. Neurorehabil. Neural Repair 26, 222−230.

Wang, W.H., Guan, S., Zhang, L.Y., Lei, S., Zeng, Y.J., 2014a. Circulating microRNAs as novel potential biomarkers for early diagnosis of acute stroke in humans. J. Stroke Cerebrovas. Dis. 23, 2607−2613.

Wang, C.P., Tsai, P.Y., Yang, T.F., Yang, K.Y., Wang, C.C., 2014b. Differential effect of conditioning sequences in coupling inhibitory/facilitatory repetitive transcranial magnetic stimulation for poststroke motor recovery. CNS Neurosci. Ther. 20, 355−363.

Wang, Y., Chen, D., Chen, G., 2014c. Hyperbaric oxygen therapy applied research in traumatic brain injury: from mechanisms to clinical investigation. Med. Gas Res. 4, 18.

Wang, T., Zhai, L., Zhang, H., Zhao, L., Guo, Y., 2015. Picroside II Inhibits the MEK-ERK1/2-COX2 Signal Pathway to Prevent Cerebral Ischemic Injury in Rats. J. Mol. Neurosci. 57, 335−351.

Wardlaw, J.M., Murray, V., Berge, E., del Zoppo, G.J., 2014. Thrombolysis for acute ischaemic stroke. Cochrane Database Syst. Rev. CD000213.

Weiss, G.B., 1995. Metabolism and actions of CDP-choline as an endogenous compound and administered exogenously as citicoline. Life Sci. 56, 637–660.

Wen, W., Sachdev, P.S., 2004. Extent and distribution of white matter hyperintensities in stroke patients: the Sydney stroke study. Stroke 35, 2813–2819.

Weng, H., Shen, C., Hirokawa, G., et al., 2011. Plasma miR-124 as a biomarker for cerebral infarction. Biomed. Res. 32, 135–141.

Wightman, E.L., Haskell-Ramsay, C.F., Thompson, K.G., Blackwell, J.R., Winyard, P.G., et al., 2015. Dietary nitrate modulates cerebral blood flow parameters and cognitive performance in humans: a double-blind, placebo-controlled, crossover investigation. Physiol. Behav. 149, 149–158.

Willard, L.B., Hauss-Wegrzyniak, B., Danysz, W., Wenk, G.L., 2000. The cytotoxicity of chronic neuroinflammation upon basal forebrain cholinergic neurons of rats can be attenuated by glutamatergic antagonism or cyclooxygenase-2 inhibition. Exp. Brain Res. 134, 58–65.

Wu, J., Li, Q., Wang, X., Yu, S., Li, L., et al., 2013. Neuroprotection by curcumin in ischemic brain injury involves the Akt/Nrf2 pathway. PLoS One 8, e59843.

Xue, B., Yang, Z., Wang, X., Shi, H., 2012. Omega-3 polyunsaturated fatty acids antagonize macrophage inflammation via activation of AMPK/SIRT1 pathway. PLoS One 7, e45990.

Yamashita, T., Wu, Y.P., Sandhoff, R., Werth, N., Mizukami, H., et al., 2005. Interruption of ganglioside synthesis produces central nervous system degeneration and altered axon-glial interactions. Proc. Natl. Acad. Sci. U.S.A. 102, 2725–2730.

Yancopoulos, G.D., Klagsbrun, M., Folkman, J., 1998. Vasculogenesis, angiogenesis, and growth factors: ephrins enter the fray at the border. Cell 93, 661–664.

Yang, C., Zhang, X., Fan, H., Liu, Y., 2009. Curcumin upregulates transcription factor Nrf2, HO-1 expression and protects rat brains against focal ischemia. Brain Res. 1282, 133–141.

Yang, L., Calay, E.S., Fan, J., Arduini, A., Kunz, R.C., et al., 2015. S-Nitrosylation links obesity-associated inflammation to endoplasmic reticulum dysfunction. Science 349, 500–506.

Yang, Y.R., Wang, R.Y., Wang, P.S., Yu, S.M., 2003. Treadmill training effects on neurological outcome after middle cerebral artery occlusion in rats. Can. J. Neurol. Sci. 30, 252–258.

Yepes, M., Sandkvist, M., Moore, E.G., Bugge, T.H., Strickland, D.K., et al., 2003. Tissue-type plasminogen activator induces opening of the blood-brain barrier via the LDL receptor-related protein. J. Clin. Invest. 112, 1533–1540.

Yilmaz, G., Granger, D.N., 2010. Leukocyte recruitment and ischemic brain injury. Neuromol. Med. 12, 193–204.

Yin, J.J., Zhang, W., Du, F., 2005. Effects of extraction of Huhuanglian on apoptosis and Bcl-2 gene in penumbra area in ischemia reperfusion rats. Shandong J. Tradit. Chin. Med. 24, 364–366.

Yrjänheikki, J., Keinänen, R., Pellikka, M., Hökfelt, T., Koistinaho, J., 1998. Tetracyclines inhibit microglial activation and are neuroprotective in global brain ischemia. Proc. Natl. Acad. Sci. U.S.A. 95, 15769–157674.

Yu, G., Borlongan, C.V., Stahl, C.E., Hess, D.C., Ou, Y., et al., 2009. Systemic delivery of umbilical cord blood cells for stroke therapy: a review. Restor. Neurol. Neurosci. 27, 41–54.

Yu, R.K., Suzuki, Y., Yanagisawa, M., 2010. Membrane glycolipids in stem cells. FEBS Lett. 584, 1694–1699.

Zgavc, T., Ceulemans, A.G., Hachimi-Idrissi, S., Kooijman, R., Sarre, S., et al., 2012. The neuroprotective effect of post ischemic brief mild hypothermic treatment correlates with apoptosis, but not with gliosis in endothelin-1 treated rats. BMC Neurosci. 13, 105.

Zhang, R., Chopp, M., Zhang, Z., Jiang, N., 1998. The expression of P- and E-selectins in three models of middle cerebral artery occlusion. Brain Res. 785, 207–214.

Zhang, M., Wang, S., Mao, L., Leak, R.K., Shi, Y., et al., 2014a. Omega-3 fatty acids protect the brain against ischemic injury by activating Nrf2 and upregulating heme oxygenase 1. J. Neurosci. 34, 1903–1915.

Zhang, R.L., Chopp, M., Roberts, C., Liu, X., Wei, M., et al., 2014b. Stroke increases neural stem cells and angiogenesis in the neurogenic niche of the adult mouse. PLoS One 9, e113972.

Zhang, P., Lei, X., Sun, Y., Zhang, H., Chang, L., et al., 2016a. Regenerative repair of Pifithrin-α in cerebral ischemia via VEGF dependent manner. Sci. Rep. 6, 26295.

Zhang, Y., Chopp, M., Zhang, Z.G., Katakowski, M., Xin, H., et al., 2016b. Systemic administration of cell-free exosomes generated by human bone marrow derived mesenchymal stem cells cultured under 2D and 3D conditions improves functional recovery in rats after traumatic brain injury. Neurochem. Int. S0197-0186 (16), 30251-0.

Zhang, Z.G., Chopp, M., 2009. Neurorestorative therapies for stroke: underlying mechanisms and translation to the clinic. Lancet Neurol. 8, 491–500.

Zhang, Z.G., Zhang, L., Jiang, Q., Zhang, R., Davies, K., et al., 2000. VEGF enhances angiogenesis and promotes blood-brain barrier leakage in the ischemic brain. J. Clin. Invest. 106, 829–838.

Zhang, Z.G., Zhang, L., Jiang, Q., Chopp, M., 2002. Bone marrow-derived endothelial progenitor cells participate in cerebral neovascularization after focal cerebral ischemia in the adult mouse. Circ. Res. 90, 284–288.

Zhao, J., Yu, S., Zheng, W., Feng, G., Luo, G., et al., 2010. Curcumin improves outcomes and attenuates focal cerebral ischemic injury via antiapoptotic mechanisms in rats. Neurochem. Res. 35, 374–379.

Zhao, J., Zhang, X., Dong, L., Wen, Y., Cui, L., 2014. The many roles of statins in ischemic stroke. Curr. Neuropharmacol. 12, 564–574.

Zhu, J.M., Zhao, Y.Y., Chen, S.D., Zhang, W.H., Lou, L., Jin, X., 2011. Functional recovery after transplantation of neural stem cells modified by brain-derived neurotrophic factor in rats with cerebral ischaemia. J. Int. Med. Res. 39, 488–498.

Zivin, J.A., 1998. Factors determining the therapeutic window for stroke. Neurology 50, 599–603.

Molecular Aspects of Spinal Cord Injury

INTRODUCTION

Spinal cord injury (SCI) is a devastating medical emergency that results from severe physical trauma to the spine. SCI affects 1.3 million North Americans. It results in devastating physical, social, and vocational impairments. SCI produces tissue damage that results in the loss of motor and sensory functions, the extent of which is related both to the neurologic level and neurologic completeness of injury. As stated in Chapter 1, Classification and Molecular Aspects of Neurotraumatic Diseases: Similarities and Differences With Neurodegenerative and Neuropsychiatric Diseases, several experimental animal models of SCI have been developed, including contusion, compression, distraction, dislocation, transection, laceration, and crush in a variety of species (Young, 2002). These systems produce highly stereotypical injuries and minimize heterogeneity in severity, timing of injury, genetic background, and environmental exposure. While elimination of inter-animal variability likely enhances detection of the effects of putative therapeutic interventions, it does not fully reflect the diverse injury characteristics that complicate naturally occurring SCI (Jeffery et al., 2006).

The spinal cord at the time of injury may be subjected to hyperbending, overstretching, twisting, or laceration (Bauchet et al., 2009). SCI induces autodestructive changes, which consists of two broadly defined events: a primary injury, attributable to the mechanical insult itself, and a secondary injury, attributable to the series of systemic and local neurochemical and pathophysiological changes that occur in spinal cord after the SCI (Klussmann and Martin-Villalba, 2005). The primary injury occurs instantaneously and beyond therapeutic management. In contrast, the secondary injury develops over the hours and days after primary SCI around the injury core, causing behavioral and functional impairments. The secondary injury phase can be in turn classified into three different subphases such as acute phase (2 hours to 2 days), sub-acute phase (days to weeks), and chronic phase (months to years) (Norenberg et al., 2004; Rowland et al., 2008). One of the earliest events in the primary phase of SCI is the disruption of the blood—spinal cord barrier by a mechanical force that destroys neural tissue and tears neuronal and endothelial cell membranes (Profyris et al., 2004). This not only disturbs the microenvironment of the spinal cord but also alters vascular permeability, facilitates the entry of peripheral immune cells, and exposes the adjacent noninjured tissue to potentially noxious molecules (Losey et al., 2014). In addition, the primary SCI also disrupts of local blood supply leading to dramatic changes in spinal cord volume (Ahuja et al., 2016). In contrast, secondary SCI damage involves a cascade of vascular, biochemical, and cellular event leading to many histological and neurochemical alterations such as induction of ischemia, edema, hemorrhage, and inflammation, proapoptotic signaling, increase in excitatory amino acids, the release of proteases, and the formation of nitric oxide and free radicals (superoxide and hydroxyl radicals) in early stages. These neurochemical alterations are supported not only by the activation of neurons, astrocytes, microglial cells, and demyelination involving oligodendrocytes but also by the modulation of leukocyte infiltration and activation of macrophages and vascular endothelial cells (Bramlett and Dietrich, 2004; Darian-Smith, 2009). These changes promote harsh postinjury microenvironment.

Pathophysiology of SCI also involves apoptosis, a programmed cell death, which occurs in spinal cord many days and even weeks after SCI, especially in oligodendrocytes of the cord white matter leading to demyelination and further dysfunction (Sastry and Rao, 2000). Mechanistically, oligodendrocyte death appears to be related to the death receptor Fas (Casha et al., 2001, 2005). Administration of soluble Fas (Ackery et al., 2006) has a protective effect on SCI associated demyelination. SCI also triggers a systemic, neurogenic immune depression syndrome characterized by a rapid and drastic decrease of CD14 + monocytes, CD3 + T-lymphocytes, and CD19 + B-lymphocytes and MHC class II (HLA-Dr)$^{+}$ cells within 24 hours reaching minimum levels within the first week (Riegger et al., 2009). This suggests that SCI is associated with an early onset of immune suppression and secondary immune deficiency syndrome (SCI-IDS). In addition, SCI also results in the synthesis of autoantibodies that bind nuclear antigens including DNA and RNA (Ankeny and Popovich, 2009). Collectively these studies suggest that secondary event associated with SCI involves interactions among excitotoxicity (a process by which high levels of glutamate induce neurodegeneration), oxidative stress (a process involving cytotoxic consequences initiated and caused by oxygen free radicals), and neuroinflammation (a neuroprotective mechanism whose prolonged presence is injurious to neurons) (Farooqui et al., 2007; Farooqui and Horrocks, 2007, 2009). In SCI, the induction of excitotoxicity, oxidative stress, and neuroinflammation is supported by neurochemical changes in ion homeostasis (Ca^{2+} influx), cellular redox, induction of mitochondrial dysfunction, alterations in PLA_2, COX-2, NOS, Caspases, and calpains, expression of neurodestructive and neuroprotective genes, and changes in neurotrophic factor expression (Fig. 4.1). In addition, SCI also triggers an early and prolonged release of proinflammatory cytokines (TNF-α, interleukin-1β, IL-6) and chemokines (MCP-1). In addition, transient alterations are observed in subunit populations of the transcription factor nuclear factor-kappa B (NF-κB), which plays a key role in regulating the expression of proinflammatory cytokines and chemokines (Fig. 4.1) (Farooqui and Horrocks, 2009).

As the SCI lesions mature into the chronic phase, the activation of astrocytes promotes glial scarring. Reactive astrocytes secrete a plethora of both growth promoting and inhibitory factors after SCI. However, the production of inhibitory components surpasses the growth stimulating factors, thus causing inhibitory effects. In severe cases of SCI, astrogliosis promotes the formation of irreversible glial scarring that acts as

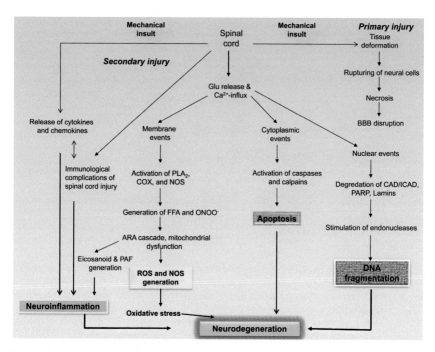

FIGURE 4.1   Diagram showing neurochemical changes associated with primary and secondary events in SCI.

regeneration barrier due to the expression of inhibitory components such as chondroitin sulfate proteoglycans (CSPGs) (Karimi-Abdolrezaee and Billakanti, 2012). At the molecular level, inhibition of regeneration involves myelin glycoproteins (MAG) and its receptor (MAG receptor), Nogo, and its receptor (NgR1), and the neurotrophin receptor p75^{NTR}, and CSPGs. These factors are modulated by the Rho-ROCK (rho-associated protein kinase) pathway to inhibit neurite outgrowth by signaling growth cone collapse through effector kinases (Fig. 4.2) (Forgione and Fehlings, 2014). Activation of RhoA/Rho kinase results in growth cone collapse and neurite retraction. Inhibition of RhoA/Rho kinase not only improves axon regeneration, remyelination, and functional recovery but also regulates the cytoskeleton. There are two essential components of Rho/ROCK signaling pathway: Rho-A and Rho-associated kinase1 and 2 (ROCK$_1$ and ROCK$_2$) (Hou et al., 2015; Jia et al., 2016). Rho GTPases are important regulators of the actin cytoskeleton and thereby control the adhesive and migratory behaviors of cells (Govek et al., 2005).

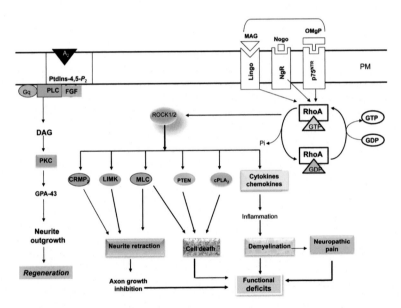

FIGURE 4.2   Neurochemical changes associated with functional deficits and regeneration in SCI. PtdIns-4,5-P_2, Phosphatidylinositol 4,5-bisphosphate; PLC, phospholipase C; Lingo, specific transmembrane protein that binds NgR1 and p75^{NTR}; NgR, Nogo receptor; OMgP, oligodendrocytemyelin glycoprotein; p75^{NTR}, low-affinity neurotrophin receptor p75; DAG, diacylglycerol; GDI, Rho—GDP dissociation inhibitor; ROCK, serine/threonine kinases; PKC, protein kinase C; GAP-43, growth associated protein-43; GTP, guanosine 5'-triphosphate; GDP, guanosine 5'-diphosphate; cPLA$_2$, cytosolic phospholipase A$_2$; LIMK, LIM kinase; MLC, myosin light chain; PTEN, phosphatase and tensin homologue; and CRMP2, collapsing response mediator protein-2.

Among various Rho GTPases, Cdc42, Rac, and Rho-A have been shown to participate in regulating the growth of neural axons; Cdc42 and Rac regulate the actin to promote axon growth and stability (Nobes and Hall, 1995). Rho-A activates the downstream signaling molecule, $ROCK_2$, and then triggers a series of reactions that cause the growth cone to collapse and retraction that result in limited regeneration of neural axons (Dickson, 2001). The inhibition of regeneration results in significant functional deficits, and depending on the severity of injury, and may contribute to permanent paralysis or loss of senses distal to the site of injury. There is a relationship between RhoA/Rho kinase and cytosolic phospholipase A_2 ($cPLA_2$), a lipase that contributes to neuroinflammation, oxidative stress, and cell death, in contusive SCI model (Wu et al., 2017). Inhibition of RhoA, Rho kinase, and $cPLA_2$ significantly reduces TNF-α/glutamate-mediated cell death. Inhibition of RhoA and Rho kinase not only downregulates $cPLA_2$ activation but also reduces the release of arachidonic acid (Wu et al., 2017). The immunofluorescence staining studies have indicated that $ROCK_1$ and $ROCK_2$ are colocalized with $cPLA_2$ in neuronal cytoplasm. Interestingly, co-immunoprecipitation (Co-IP) assay show that $ROCK_1$ or $ROCK_2$ bond directly with $cPLA_2$ and phospho-$cPLA_2$. Rho kinase inhibitor Y27632 significantly decreases $cPLA_2$ activation and expression and reduces SCI-mediated apoptosis at and close to the lesion site. Taken together, these results suggest that RhoA/Rho kinase promote neuronal death through the regulation of $cPLA_2$ activation (Wu et al., 2017).

In addition, 40% of SCI patients develop persistent neuropathic pain, which has a detrimental impact on the patient's quality of life and is a major specific healthcare problem in its own right. In addition, optimal spinal cord regeneration also involves a heightened internal growth state and the presence of mediators, which overcome inhibitory influences to guide axons to appropriate targets to the injured neuronal populations, without effecting noninjured populations. Furthermore, functional recovery after SCI also requires locomotion and other movement for the re-establishment of movement patterning, growth, and connection of multiple neuronal populations. Secondary injury also involves onset of Wallerian degeneration, development of cysts, syrinx, and schwannosis in later stages of SCI (Norenberg et al., 2004). Angiogenic responses and remodeling of vascular structure also contribute to the development of secondary injury. It is well acknowledged that effective restraint of secondary injury plays a fundamental role in minimizing neurodegeneration and significantly improves functional recovery after SCI.

The functional consequences of SCI not only depend on the level but also on completeness of the injury. Thus, the effect of SCI on loss of motor and non-motor function depends on the site of the injury. Nerves controlled by spinal cord segments below the injury site often lose their connections due to changes in descending motor pathways and ascending sensory pathways resulting in disruption of the body—brain communication. Trauma to cervical segments of the spinal cord reproduces decrease in motor and/or sensory function not only in the upper and lower limbs but also in the trunk causing tetraplegia or quadriplegia. In contrast, trauma to thoracic, lumbar, or sacral segments spares upper limb function but affects the lower limbs and trunk to varying degrees resulting in paraplegia (Kirshblum et al., 2011). The completeness of the injury is another determinant of SCI-mediated dysfunction. It is well known that SCIs can be classified as either complete or incomplete. Complete SCI represents an absence of motor and sensory function in S4—S5 segments (i.e., no sacral sparing), whereas in incomplete SCI there is preservation of some motor and/or sensory function below the level of injury. The incompleteness of SCI can be further classified into mild, medium, severe types based on the amount of function preserved in patients. Collective evidence suggests that SCI is accompanied by the massive cell death, including loss of neurons, astrocytes, and oligodendrocytes, and almost no functional recovery in mammals' spinal cord.

SCI produces marked changes in the brain. Thus, SCI results in extensive long-term reorganization of the cerebral cortex (Freund et al., 2011). Furthermore, complete thoracic SCI patients show a decrease in grey matter volume in primary motor cortex that is consistent with neuronal loss and/or atrophy (Wrigley et al., 2009). Prospective longitudinal MRI studies also indicate that SCI produces progressive reduction in grey matter volume not only in the sensorimotor cortex but also in the regions not directly connected to the injury site, such as cerebellar cortex, medial prefrontal, and anterior cingulate cortices that are critical for the processing of emotional relevant information and the modulation of attentional states (Wrigley et al., 2009; Freund et al., 2013). Collective evidence suggests that SCI induces progressive and widespread changes in the brain (Faden et al., 2016). These SCI-induced changes in the brain are reflected in form of impairment of spatial and retention memory and depressive-like behavior in rats and mice model of SCI. Thus, SCI produces impairment in the Morris water maze, Y-maze, novel objective recognition, sucrose preference, and tail suspension tests (Wu et al., 2014a, 2014b) and support the view that SCI may cause physiological changes in the brain. These changes can be modified by inhibiting the posttraumatic neuroinflammatory response (Faden et al., 2016).

Apart from local injury within the spinal cord, SCI patients (depending on the level and severity of the SCI) also develop many complications, which are characterized by multiple organ dysfunction or failure (Lazzaro et al., 2013). Thus, SCI patients develop neurogenic pain, depression, lung injury, cardiovascular disease, liver damage, kidney dysfunction, urinary tract infection, and increase in susceptibility to pathologic infection (Fig. 4.3). Disturbances in urinary and gastrointestinal systems contribute to sexual dysfunction. In addition, frequent complications of cervical and high thoracic SCI also include neurogenic shock, bradyarrhythmias, hypotension, ectopic beats, abnormal temperature control, and disturbance of sweating, vasodilatation, and autonomic dysreflexia (Hagen, 2015). Autonomic dysreflexia is an abrupt, uncontrolled sympathetic response, induced by stimuli below the level of injury. These symptoms may be mild such as skin rash or slight headache but can cause severe hypertension, cerebral hemorrhage, and death (Hagen, 2015). Disturbance of respiratory function is frequently associated with tetraplegia, and a primary cause of both short- and long-term morbidity and mortality is pulmonary complications. Due to physical inactivity and altered hemostasis, patients with SCI have a higher risk of venous thromboembolism and pressure ulcers. Spasticity and pain are frequent complications that need to be addressed. The psychological stress associated with SCI may contribute to anxiety and depression. These pathologic conditions hinder functional recovery, which can not only affect quality of life but can also be life threatening. Mechanisms contributing to SCI-mediated pathological conditions are not fully understood. However, several lines of evidences indicate that SCI not only triggers postinjury systemic inflammation due to increase

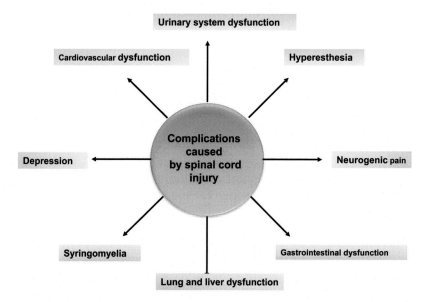

FIGURE 4.3 Complications caused by SCI.

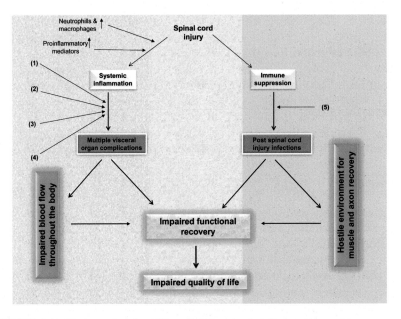

FIGURE 4.4   Diagram showing SCI-mediated systemic inflammation and immune suppression impairing the quality of life. (1) Neutrophil/macrophage infiltration; (2) microglial/astrocyte activation; (3) activation of MPO/ iNOS/COX-2; (4) Activation of NF-κB; (5) and decrease in cells involved in innate and adaptive immunity.

in circulation of immune cells and proinflammatory mediators leading to persistence of an inflammatory microenvironment that contributes to organ dysfunction but also promotes immune suppression resulting in impaired responsiveness to pathogen infection (Fig. 4.4) (Sun et al., 2016). It is proposed that interactions between systemic inflammation and immune suppression may not only produce impaired functional recovery but also affects the quality of life in SCI patients (Sun et al., 2016). Converging evidence suggests that the pathophysiology of SCI involves the shearing of neural cell membranes and axons, disruption of the blood–spinal cord barrier, induction of excitotoxicity, oxidative stress, and inflammation, stimulation of Ca^{2+}-dependent enzymes, induction of necrotic and apoptotic neural cell death, immune cell transmigration, and myelin degradation (Table 4.1).

NECROSIS, APOPTOSIS, AND AUTOPHAGY IN SCI

Apoptosis and necrosis are two basic mechanisms of neural cell death that occur in SCI (Farooqui, 2009). As stated above, in primary injury mechanical trauma to spinal card ruptures neuronal membranes

TABLE 4.1   Neurochemical Consequences of SCI

Parameters	Effect	Reference
Excitotoxicity	Increased	Farooqui (2009)
Oxidative stress	Increased	Farooqui (2009)
Inflammation	Increased	Farooqui (2009)
Activities of Ca^{2+}-dependent enzymes	Increased	Farooqui (2009)
Levels of pain inducing mediators	Increased	Farooqui (2009)
Levels of transcription factors	Increased	Farooqui (2009)
Immunogenic function	Decreased	Sun et al. (2016)
Growth factors	Increased	Farooqui (2009)

TABLE 4.2   Morphological and Neurochemical Features of Necrosis and Apoptosis

Characteristics	Apoptosis	Necrosis
Stimuli	Physiological	Pathological
Nature	Controlled process	Uncontrolled process
Energy requirement	Energy required (active)	Energy not required (passive)
Morphology	Nuclear fragmentation	Nuclear dissolution
Membrane integrity	Loss of membrane asymmetry	Loss of membrane integrity
Levels of Ca^{2+}	Low until late in apoptosis	Early increase in Ca^{2+}
Inflammation	Absent	Present
Phagocytosis	Present	Absent
Cell involved	Individual or small group of cells	Large group of cells
Lysosomal enzyme release	Absent	Present
Effect of cycloheximide	Protection	No effect

and releases of intracellular components that induce inflammatory reaction. Necrosis is a passive process characterized by the lethal disruption of cell structure and activity (Table 4.2). It involves mitochondrial damage, rapid loss of ATP, sudden loss of ion homeostasis, and induction of ROS. Necrosis occurs early after SCI at the site of injury and adjacent segments. It is considered harmful because it promotes and aggravates secondary injury and interferes with axonal regeneration. Necrosis in SCI may also lead to an unfavorable environment for intralesional implants. In contrast, apoptosis is an active process, where neurochemical changes occur in an orderly fashion (Table 4.2). In contrast, apoptosis is characterized by the activation of cell signaling involving direct involvement of the mitochondria and the subsequent activation of a proteolytic cascade involving executioner caspases (Farooqui, 2009). Apoptotic cell death is not only accompanied by caspase activation, cell shrinkage, chromatin condensation, DNA fragmentation, and laddering but also by the loss of plasma membrane phospholipid asymmetry (externalization of phosphatidylserine residues) and the release of cytochrome c from mitochondria (Farooqui, 2009). Plasma membrane and other subcellular organelles such as mitochondria and endoplasmic reticulum (ER) remain active during apoptosis. In SCI, apoptotic cell death is observed in both neurons and oligodendrocytes and is prominent in the white matter, in which Wallerian degeneration can be simultaneously observed. In a rat spinal contusion model of SCI, acute oligodendrocyte loss can be detected within 15 minutes postinjury with continual loss occurring for 4 hours (Liu et al., 1997). Similarly, in a mouse SCI model, oligodendrocyte numbers is decreased within 24 hours and steadily declined by 3—7 days postinjury (Lytle and Wrathall, 2007). A time course study in rat SCI has revealed that apoptosis occurs as early as 4 hours post injury and can be observed in decreasing numbers as late as 3 weeks after SCI (Keane et al., 2006). After SCI, caspase activation occurs in neurons at the injury site within hours, and in oligodendrocytes adjacent to, and distant from, the injury site over a period of days. The long-term neurological deficits after SCI may be due in part to widespread apoptosis of neurons and oligodendroglia in regions distant from and relatively unaffected by the initial injury (Keane et al., 2006). Collectively these studies indicate that neuronal death along with prolonged oligodendrocyte apoptosis after SCI may be a common phenomenon across multiple injury models in mammals.

Autophagy is a major pathway for bulk cytosolic degradation and efficient turnover under stress. It plays an important role in maintaining cellular homeostasis by degrading and recycling damaged organelles, toxic agents, and long-lived, unwanted proteins through an autophagosomal—lysosomal pathway (Shin et al., 2016). Autophagy involves three steps: formation of autophagosomes, fusion of autophagosomes with lysosomes, and degradation in the autolysosomes (Glick et al., 2010). It is becoming increasingly evident that autophagy can act as a prosurvival mechanism via regulating the neural cells death in SCI (Lipinski et al., 2015). The molecular mechanism associated with this process is not fully understood. However, it is suggested that autophagy depresses neuronal cell death by promoting the elimination of toxic proteins and damaged mitochondria (mitophagy) (Yu et al., 2013). It is also reported that Beclin 1, a Bcl-2-interacting protein, is known to be a promoter of autophagy (Kanno et al., 2009; Liu et al., 2015). The increased expression of Beclin 1 starts from 4 hours, peaked at 3 days, and lasted for at least 21 days in a hemisection model of SCI in mice. The Beclin 1 expression has been observed in neurons, astrocytes, and oligodendrocytes. The nuclei in the Beclin 1 expressing cells have round morphology, which is normally observed in autophagic cell death. This is in contrast to apoptotic nuclei, which show fragmentation of DNA. It is suggested that autophagic changes are closely associated with the onset of SCI in the mice spinal cord (Kanno et al., 2009).

CONTRIBUTION OF EXCITOTOXICITY IN SCI

Excitotoxicity is the pathological mechanism that produces neuronal injury and death through the overactivation of glutamate receptors such as the N-methyl-D-aspartate (NMDA) receptor and α-amino-3-hydroxy-5-methyl-4-isoxazole propionate (AMPA) receptor. The induction of excitotoxicity is accompanied by Ca^{2+}-influx and activation of calcium-dependent enzymes (Farooqui and Horrocks, 1991). Ca^{2+}-dependent enzymes include phospholipase A_2 (PLA_2), cyclooxygenase-2 (COX-2), lipoxygenases (LOX), calpains, nitric oxide synthase (NOS), calcineurin, MAP kinase, matrix metalloproteinase (MMP), caspases, and poly(ADP-ribose) polymerase (PARP) (Bao et al., 2009; Ray et al., 2003a; Ray et al., 2003b; Knoblach et al., 2005; McEwen and Springer, 2005; Lee et al., 2009; Gris et al., 2008). Within 15 minutes after SCI, glutamate levels at the epicenter and surrounding regions increase six times higher than physiological levels due to the overstimulation of glutamate receptors and a massive increase of intracellular Ca^{2+} and Na^+. This Ca^{2+}-influx stimulates the above-mentioned Ca^{2+}-dependent enzymes (Weber, 2004). Moreover, the augmented expressions of genes related to neurotransmitter receptors (NMDA, AMPA, Ach, GABA, Glur, and Kainate) increase demyelination and oligodendrocyte destruction (Nesic et al., 2002; Cox et al., 2015).

Excitotoxicity also promotes mitochondrial dysfunction, a process, which subsequently results in the generation of reactive oxygen species (ROS). ROS include superoxide anions ($O_2^{\bullet-}$), hydroxyl ($^{\bullet}OH$), and peroxyl radicals ($ROO^{\bullet}$), and hydrogen peroxide, which are generated as by-product of oxidative metabolism, in which energy activation and electron reduction are involved. Nitric oxide (NO) is another reactive species that is generated by the mitochondria during the breakdown of arginine to citrulline by a family of NADPH-dependent enzymes called mitochondrial nitric oxide synthases (mtNOS). Superoxide ($O_2^{\bullet-}$) and nitric oxide ($NO^{\bullet}$) react with each other and produce peroxynitrite $ONOO^-$), a toxic reaction product that produces apoptotic cell death (Park et al., 2004; Farooqui et al., 2008; Farooqui, 2009). SCI increases the concentration of NO$^{\bullet}$ three to five times more than baseline levels and reaches its peak at 12 hours. The elevated NO$^{\bullet}$ concentration not only induces cell damage and lipid peroxidation but also increases vascular permeability and promotes edema (Sharma et al., 1996). Collective evidence suggests that NO$^{\bullet}$ participates in the development of the excessive glutamate and calcium levels that induce excitotoxicity (Dawson et al., 1994).

Increased degradation of neural membrane glycerophospholipid, accumulation of oxygenated arachidonic acid metabolites including prostaglandins (PGs), leukotrienes (LTs), and thromboxanes (TXs), along with abnormal ion homeostasis, changes in redox status, cytoskeletal degradation, induction of extrinsic and intrinsic apoptotic pathways, and lack of energy generation are closely associated with neural cell injury in SCI (Park et al., 2004; Farooqui, 2009). PG and LTs function as immune cell chemoattractants, vasodilators, inducers of oxidative stress, and modulators of neurosensory processing. Furthermore, the acute increase in prostaglandins, leukotrienes, and TXs after experimental SCI remains elevated for several months posttrauma (Dulin et al., 2013). In addition, the accumulation of ROS may promote the migration of NF-κB to the nucleus, where NF-κB interacts with NF-κB-RE, which promote the expression of proinflammatory cytokines (TNF-IL-α, IL-1β, and IL-6) and chemokine. Proinflammatory eicosanoids and proinflammatory cytokines and chemokine facilitate the induction of neuroinflammation during the secondary phase following SCI (Farooqui and Horrocks, 2009). Neuroinflammation not only plays an important role in glial scar formation, cytotoxicity, and sensitization of neural pathways but also contributes to regeneration of injured CNS axons (Benowitz and Popovich, 2011), suggesting the importance of complexity of the inflammatory response within the injured spinal cord. It is also reported that peripheral immune cells and activated microglia are present within the spinal cord up to 1 year after injury (Beck et al., 2010; Byrnes et al., 2011). This raises the possibility that neuroinflammation following SCI may not be transient but may in fact continue into the chronic phase of injury.

High levels of glutamate also produce damage to glial cells in the spinal cord through mechanism that does not involve glutamate receptor activation but rather glutamate uptake (Matute et al., 2006). High concentration of glutamate interferes with cystine/glutamate antiporter, which normally transports cystine into the cell. Inhibition of cystine uptake leads to a decrease in the level of intracellular cystine and its reduction product cysteine, with a consequent decrease in glutathione synthesis, accumulation of cellular oxidants, and eventual cell death (Matute et al., 2006). Collective evidence suggests that excitotoxic damage in SCI involves not only interactions among excitotoxicity and oxidative glutamate toxicity but also mitochondrial dysfunction, decrease in ATP levels, and changes in neural cell redox (Farooqui and Horrocks, 1991; Farooqui and Horrocks, 1991). SCI also results in increased expression of receptor for advanced glycation end products (RAGE). Upregulation of RAGE protein expression in spinal cord tissue can be observed at 12 hours after SCI and continued at 2 and 5 days. In RAGE-deficient mice locomotor recovery can be improved and lesion pathology can be reduced after SCI. RAGE deficiency in mice attenuates apoptosis after SCI by inhibiting p53/Bax/caspase-3 pathway. RAGE deficiency in mice not only retards inflammation after SCI but also reduces myeloperoxidase activity. Furthermore, RAGE deficiency in mice exposed to SCI suppress the upregulation of inducible nitric oxide synthase (iNOS) and gp91-phox and attenuated oxidative and nitrosative stresses, marked by reduction in the synthesis of malondialdehyde, ROS, peroxynitrite ($OONO^-$), and 3-nitrotyrosine. SCI in RAGE-deficient mice also may retard glial scar at the injury site and decreases the expression of glial fibrillary acidic protein (GFAP). These data indicate that the RAGE plays an important role in the development of SCI (Guo et al., 2014)

CHANGES IN ENZYMIC ACTIVITIES IN SCI

SCI produces alterations in activities of many enzymes related to phospholipids and protein metabolism such as phospholipases A_2 ($cPLA_2$, $sPLA_2$) calpains, NOSs, cyclooxygenases, lipoxygenases, calcineurin, and caspases, and MMPs. Activation of isoforms of PLA_2, cyclooxygenase-2, and lipoxygenase contribute to the production of eicosanoids and other nonenzymic arachidonic acid—derived products, such as 4-hydroxynonenal and isoprotane (Farooqui and Horrocks, 2009). Activation of calpains contributes to the degradation of cytoskeleton proteins (spectrin and MAP2). Activation of NOS promotes the generation of NO and the synthesis of peroxynitrite, and finally activation of caspases in SCI is associated with apoptotic cell death (Farooqui and Horrocks, 2009) (Fig. 4.5).

It is well known rat and monkey spinal cord contains calcium-dependent cytosolic phospholipase A_2 ($cPLA_2$) activity. At the cellular level, dense immunoreactivity is present in motor neurons from cervical, thoracic, lumbar, and sacral regions (Ong et al., 1999). Traumatic injury to spinal cord stimulates activities of lipases and phospholipases (Liu et al., 2006). SCI significantly stimulates $cPLA_2$ activity and its expression in injured spinal cord. This increase in $cPLA_2$ activity can be blocked by the PLA_2 inhibitor, mepacrine (Liu et al., 2006). At the injury site, PLA_2

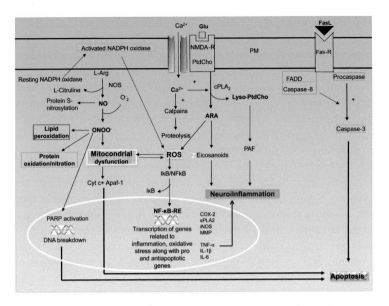

FIGURE 4.5 Involvement of Fas and NMDA receptors in apoptotic and necrotic cell death. FasL, Fas ligand; Fas-R, Fas receptor; PtdCho, phosphatidylcholine; cPLA$_2$, cytosolic phospholipase A$_2$; ARA, arachidonic acid; Arg, Arginine; O$_2^-$, superoxide; ONOO$^-$, peroxynitrite; lyso-PtdCho, lyso-phosphatidylcholine; PAF, platelet activating factor; Cytc, cytochrome c; Apaf-1, apoptosome complex with apoptosis activating factor-1; and poly (ADP)ribose polymerase (PARP); secretory phospholipase (sPLA$_2$); cyclooxygenase-2 (COX-2); NF-κB-RE, nuclear factor κB-response element; I-κB, inhibitory subunit of NF-κB.

product, arachidonic acid is metabolized into proinflammatory metabolite such as prostaglandin E$_2$ (PGE$_2$), which not only facilitates macrophage and microglial recruitment but also increases local blood flow and enhances vascular permeability and proinflammatory cytokine expression (Amar and Levy, 1999). Furthermore, intravenous injection of cPLA$_2$ inhibitor, arachidonyl trifluoromethyl ketone (AACOCF$_3$) not only produces neuroprotective effects but also improves locomotion parameter (Huang et al., 2009).

Annexin A1 (ANXA1), a family of structurally related calcium- and phospholipid-binding and PLA$_2$ inhibitory protein, is known to facilitate antiinflammatory action of glucocorticoids. SCI upregulates the expression of Annexins I, II, and V in the injured spinal cord. Thus, Annexin I expression increases at 3 days after SCI, peaks at 7 days, start to decline at 14 days, and return to the baseline level at and beyond 28 days postinjury (Liu et al., 2004). Similarly, the expression of Annexin II begins to increase at 3 days, reaches its maximal level at 14 days, remain at a high level up to 28 days, and then decline to the basal level by

56 days after injury. Annexin V expression start to elevate at day 3, reaches its maximal level at day 7 and remain at this level until 56 days after injury. Reverse transcriptasepolymerase chain reaction (RT-PCR) studies confirm the expression of all three annexins at the mRNA level after SCI. Injections of ANXA1 (Ac 2-26) into the acutely injured spinal cord prevent SCI-induced increase in PLA_2 and myeloperoxidase activities (Liu et al., 2007). These studies along with electrophysiologic measures support the view that ANXA1 has a neuroprotective effect in SCI (Liu et al., 2004; Liu et al., 2007).

ACTIVATION OF COX-2 IN SCI

SCI stimulates the activity and expression of cyclooxygenase-2 (COX-2) and synthesis of prostaglandins is increased 2 hours following injury (Resnick et al., 1998). COX-2 levels peak at 48 hours following traumatic SCI. Levels of PGs and LTs remain markedly elevated 9 months after SCI, indicating that proinflammatory signaling is present even after prolonged periods postinjury. To gain a better understanding of the global metabolic changes within the chronically injured spinal cord, metabolomic screening studies have been performed to identify biochemical metabolites that are altered during chronic SCI. It is reported that in a proinflammatory and pro-oxidative environment within the chronically injured spinal cord levels of proinflammatory arachidonic acid metabolite remain high in the chronic phase of SCI. Selective inhibition of COX-2 activity with SC58125 or licofelone not only results neuroprotection from SCI but also improve locomotion patterns in the injured animals. Reverse transcriptasepolymerase chain reaction (RT-PCR) studies reveal that COX-2 transcription in the spinal cord starts to increase within 30 minutes, peaks at 3 hours after SCI (Adachi et al., 2005; Cicero and Laghi, 2007).

ACTIVATION OF NOS IN SCI

NO is a diffusible molecule, which is generated during the conversion of arginine to citrulline. It plays an important role in the pathophysiology of SCI (Chatzipanteli et al., 2002; Marsala et al., 2007). The conversion of arginine to citrulline is catalyzed by NOS. NO is not only involved in a wide variety of physiological processes, such as immune modulation, neurotransmission, hormone release, and vasodilation (Calabrese et al., 2007), but persistently elevated levels of NO may produce neurodestructive effects in the spinal cord. Many forms of NOS are present in brain and spinal cord. They include neuronal NOS (nNOS, Type I), endothelial NOS (eNOS, Type III), and inducible NOS (iNOS, Type II). Whereas nNOS and eNOS are calcium-dependent, constitutively expressed enzymes, iNOS is calcium-independent and is largely expressed by cells of the innate immune system, in response to cell damage and proinflammatory cytokines (Marsala et al., 2007). As stated above, SCI is accompanied by the generation of superoxide and nitric oxide. NO combines with the superoxide radical to form the highly reactive oxidizing agent, peroxynitrite. This molecule is highly apoptogenic. It damages nucleic acids, essential intracellular proteins, inactivates membrane lipoproteins, and lipids (Chatzipanteli et al., 2002; Marsala et al., 2007). Oxidative and nitrosative stresses cause by the production of superoxide radicals, nitric oxide and peroxynitrite result in the activation of poly(ADP-ribose) polymerase (PARP), a nuclear enzyme implicated in DNA repair. Marked PARP activation results not only in energetic depletion but also in apoptotic cell death. Peroxynitrite may also contribute to myelin as well as axonal damage following SCI (Xiong et al., 2007; Ashki et al., 2008).

3-Nitrotyrosine (3-NT) is a specific marker for peroxynitrite-mediated damage. It rapidly accumulates at all time points and is significantly increased in injured rats compared with sham rats after SCI. Accumulation of 3-NT is accompanied by significant increase in the levels of protein oxidation-related protein carbonyl and lipid peroxidation product, 4-hydroxynonenal (4-HNE). Highest increases in 3-NT and 4-HNE are seen at 24 hours postinjury (Xiong et al., 2007). Based on these results, it is proposed that activation of calpain is most likely linked to peroxynitrite-mediated secondary oxidative damage (Xiong et al., 2007). Studies on peroxynitrite-mediated damage in SCI are supported by the effect of ww-85, a metalloporphyrinic peroxynitrite decomposition catalyst. Ww-85 significantly improves the recovery of limb function in a dose-dependent manner. These results demonstrate that ww-85 treatment reduces the development of inflammation and tissue injury associated with spinal cord trauma (Genovese et al., 2009a).

ACTIVATION OF CALCINEURIN IN SCI

Calcineurin, a serine/threonine phosphatase, is modulated by cellular Ca^{2+} and calmodulin, a Ca^{2+}-binding protein, which occurs as a complex with Bcl-2 in various regions of rat and mouse brain and spinal cord. Activation of the caspase-3 apoptotic cascade in SCI is regulated, in part, by calcineurin-induced BAD dephosphorylation (Springer et al.,

2000). The activity of calcineurin 1 is significantly increased in spinal cord of rats with SCI (Wang et al., 2016). Knocking down of calcineurin 1 markedly promotes the structural and functional recovery in the spinal cord, as illustrated by the decrease of lesion volume and combined behavioral score scores. Downregulation of calcineurin 1 not only blocks the increase in proinflammatory cytokines, including IL-1β and TNF-α, but also inhibits the increase of TUNEL-positive cell numbers and caspases 3 and 9 activities. In addition, SCI also decreases the consumption of oxygen rate and increases the expression of glucose-regulated protein 78 (GRP78) and phosphorylation of protein kinase RNA-like ER kinase (PERK) in rats. Moreover, knockdown of calcineurin 1 ameliorates oxidative stress in rats with SCI, decreases of TBA reactive substances and GSSG content, and increases of glutathione level. Collective evidence suggests that calcineurin 1 play an important role in SCI through regulation of various pathological processes (Wang et al., 2016).

ACTIVATION OF MMPs IN SCI

MMPs are a family of at least 24 mammalian extracellular zinc-dependent endopeptidases that degrade the extracellular matrix and other extracellular proteins in the basement membrane (Malemud, 2006). These enzymes contribute to both injury and repair mechanisms in brain and spinal cord. In brain and SCI, MMPs, including MMP-9 (gelatinase B), contribute to early secondary pathogenesis by disrupting the blood—brain/spinal cord barrier and promoting inflammation, oxidative stress, and demyelination (Hsu et al., 2006).

Three members of the MMP family, MMP-2, MMP-9, and MMP-12, are transiently upregulated in the spinal cord wound following SCI (Hsu et al., 2006; Hsu et al., 2008; Yu et al., 2008). The expression of MMP-12 is increased 189-fold over normal levels (Wells et al., 2003). SCI studies in wild-type (WT) and MMP-12 null mice indicate that these mice show significant improvement in functional recovery compared with WT controls.

Unlesioned human spinal cord show very low MMP immunoreactivity. The involvement of MMP-1, -2, -9, and -12 has been reported in the posttraumatic events after human SCI (Buss et al., 2007). With an expression pattern, MMPs are similar to experimental studies in animals. MMPs are mainly expressed during the first weeks after SCI and are most likely associated with the destructive inflammatory events of protein breakdown and phagocytosis carried out by infiltrating neutrophils and macrophages, as well as being involved in enhanced permeability of the blood—spinal cord barrier (Buss et al., 2007). Collective evidence suggests that MMPs play a key role in abnormal vascular permeability and inflammation within the first 3 days after SCI, and that blockade of MMPs during this critical period attenuates these vascular events and leads to improved locomotor recovery. As stated above, SCI is also accompanied by glial scar formation. The glial scar not only imposes a physical barrier to regenerative axons but also produces inhibitory molecules, such as CSPGs, which chemically block the regrowth of injured axons across the lesion (McKeon et al.,1999; Barnabe-Heider et al., 2010), leading to the failure of functional recovery (Goldshmit et al., 2014). Despite its detrimental role in the injured spinal cord, the glial scar may benefit wound healing by preventing inflammatory cells and harmful substances in the lesion core from spreading out, thereby protecting the originally uninjured tissue from secondary injuries (Faulkner et al., 2004). Formation of the glial scar involves the migration of astrocytes toward the injury site. MMP-9 and MMP-2 are two proteases that modulate the migration of astrocytes through their ability to degrade constituents of the extracellular matrix. These enzymes are promising therapeutic target to reduce glial scar formation during wound healing after SCI (Hsu et al., 2008). Collective evidence suggests that MMPs contribute to the pathogenesis of SCI, and their inhibitors may not only decrease pain and apoptotic cell death but also reduce glial scar formation leading to better recovery process.

ACTIVATION OF POLY (ADP-RIBOSE) POLYMERASE IN SCI

PARP is a DNA-binding protein that is primarily activated by nicks in the DNA molecule. Upon binding to DNA breaks, activated PARP hydrolyzes NAD^+ into nicotinamide and ADP-ribose and promotes the polymerization of the ADP-ribose on nuclear acceptor proteins including histones, transcription factors, and PARP itself. Marked activation of PARP-1 results in neuronal death through mechanisms that involve NAD^+ depletion and release of apoptosis inducing factor from the mitochondria (Fig. 4.5) (Kauppinen and Swanson, 2007).

Stimulation of PARP activity in SCI increases poly(ADP-ribose) (PAR) immunoreactivity at the injury site in the injured spinal cord (Genovese et al., 2005). Although, the molecular mechanism of PARP-mediated spinal cord damage is not fully defined, the generation of peroxynitrite is known to mediate overactivation of PARP resulting in the depletion of NAD^+ and ATP, and the release of apoptosis inducing factor from the mitochondria leading to cell death in traumatic situations (Fig. 4.5). PARP also upregulates numerous proinflammatory genes and adhesion molecules through the activation of NF-κB and AP-1 (Komjati et al., 2005), supporting the view that PARP is closely associated with the pathogenesis of SCI (Genovese et al., 2005; Genovese and Cuzzocrea, 2008).

ACTIVATION OF CASPASES IN SCI

Caspases, a family of aspartate-specific cysteine proteases, play an important role in the initiation and execution of apoptotic cell death (Creagh et al., 2003; Cohen, 1997). Caspases are expressed as inactive proenzymes (zymogens) that become active during apoptotic cell death. Among 14 caspases, caspase-3 is the major effector of neuronal apoptosis mediated by a variety of stimuli as well as traumatic injuries (Fig. 4.5). Caspases not only breakdown other downstream caspases but also use variety of other enzymes, cytokines, cytoskeletal, and nuclear, and cell cycle regulatory proteins as their substrate (Cohen, 1997; Ray et al., 2003a; Ray et al., 2003b). Their activities in brain and spinal cord are modulated by members of Bcl-2 family and certain cellular proteins (cIAPs), which act as inhibitors of apoptosis.

Caspases contribute apoptotic cell death in experimental SCI (Yakovlev et al., 2005). Determination of caspase activity in injured spinal cord indicates that Caspases 3, 8, and 9 are activated from 1 to 72 hours after SCI. A time-dependent study on the distribution of cells containing activated caspase-3 at 4 hours, 1 day, 2 days, 4 days, and 8 days following SCI in rats indicates that numerous caspase-3–positive cells are observed at 4 hours and 1 day postinjury and colocalized most often with CC1, a marker for oligodendroglia. Both markers disappear near the injury epicenter over the next several days. Activated caspase-3 is again present in the injured spinal cord on Postoperative Day 8, which coincided with a reemergence of CC1-positive cells. Many of these CC1-positive cells again colocalized activated caspase-3. NeuN-positive neurons of the dorsal horn are occasionally immunopositive for activated caspase-3 at early time points. OX42-positive microglia/macrophages rarely contained activated caspase-3. These results indicate a biphasic pattern of caspase-3 activation during the first 8 days postinjury, suggesting that at least two mechanisms activate caspase-3 following SCI (Springer et al., 2000; McEwen and Springer, 2005). Involvement of caspase-3 in the pathogenesis of SCI is supported by studies on the effect of caspase inhibitors. Thus, intrathecal injection of the pan-caspase inhibitor, Boc-Asp (OMe)-fluoromethylketone (Boc-d-fmk) and treatment with N-benzyloxycarbonyl-Asp-Glu-Val-Asp-fluoromethyl ketone (z-DEVD-fmk), a selective caspase 3 inhibitor, improves locomotion function after SCI (Yakovlev et al., 2005; Barut et al., 2005; Citron et al., 2008).

ACTIVATION OF CALPAINS AND OTHER PROTEASES IN SCI

Calpains are a family of calcium-dependent nonlysosomal cysteine proteases that are widely expressed in brain and spinal cord tissues. Calpains have been implicated in degradation of cytoskeleton and neurodegeneration at the site of SCI and its penumbra (Ray et al., 2003a; Ray et al., 2003b). Inhibiting calpain expression with the cell-permeable, irreversible cysteine protease inhibitor E-64-d can prevent apoptosis and restore transcription of proteolipid protein and myelin basic protein genes, which indicates the therapeutic efficacy of E-64-d for treatment of SCI (Ray et al., 2000; Ray et al., 2011). These enzymes have been implicated in cell death in SCI (Ray et al., 2003b). As stated above, caspases are the main cysteine proteases for execution of apoptosis, and these enzymes are activated in apoptotic death of neurons and glial cells in SCI (Ray et al., 2003b). Experimental use of selective and cell permeable inhibitors of caspases demonstrates neuroptective effects in SCI (Barut et al., 2005). Cathepsins, the lysosomal acidic proteases, also contribute to the pathogenesis and neurodegeneration in SCI. There are more than a dozen of cathepsins, which are mostly cysteine proteases and only a few are aspartyl and serine proteases. Cathepsin B (a cysteine protease) and Cathepsin D (an aspartyl protease) are known to cause pathogenesis in SCI (Banik et al., 1986). Therefore, inhibition of these cathepsins may be a therapeutic option in SCI.

ACTIVATION OF PROINFLAMMATORY CYTOKINES AND CHEMOKINES IN SCI

Cytokines and chemokines are a large family of small signaling proteins and peptides, which are not only associated with intercellular communication that are normally involved in the immune response and its modulation but also induce pleiotropic effects such as cellular communication through autocrine, paracrine, or endocrine mechanisms, cellular growth, survival, and differentiation (Wilson et al., 2002). Cytokines and chemokines include interleukins (IL-1, IL-2, IL-6, and IL-12), interferons (IFN-γ), tumor necrosis factor (TNF-α), tumor growth factors (TGF-α and TGF-β), colony stimulating factors, and monocyte chemoattractant protein-1 (MCP-1) (Sun et al., 2004; Kim et al., 2001). Expression and levels of cytokines and chemokines are very low in normal spinal cord and brain. SCI induces significant increases in the synthesis of multiple cytokines, including TNF-α, interleukin-6 (IL-6), IL-1β (Yang et al., 2004; Farooqui and Horrocks, 2009). Macrophages and neutrophils, astrocytes, and microglial cells are the major sources of cytokines and chemokines. Increased immunoreactivities of TNF-α, IL-1β, and IL-6 are detected in neurons 30 minutes after SCI, and in neurons and microglia 5 hours after injury, but the expression of these proinflammatory cytokines is short-lived and declines sharply to baseline by 2 days after injury. As early as 30 minutes after SCI, activated microglial cells are detected along with axonal swellings at the injury site. In addition, axons are surrounded by microglial processes. Numerous neutrophils appear in the injured cord 1 day after injury and then their number declines dramatically, whereas macrophages progressively increase after Day 1 (Yang et al., 2004). These observations suggest not only the upregulation in expression of TNF-α, IL-1β, and IL-6 but also increase in their transport across the blood–spinal cord barrier. The increase in TNFα occurs before other cytokines in SCI. TNF-α and IL-1β have been reported to contribute to oligodendrocyte death when the latter are placed in co-culture with both astrocytes and microglia. Both cytokines inhibit glutamate transporters in astrocytes and thus expose oligodendrocytes to an excessive glutamate concentration. It is important to note that antagonists of AMPA/kainate glutamate receptors such as NBQX (2,3-dioxo-6-nitro-7-sulfamoilbenzo(f)quinoxalina) and CNQX (6-cyano-7-nitroquinoxaline-2,3-dione) can retard IL-1β toxicity towards oligodendrocytes (Takahashi et al., 2003). It is important to note that TNF-α is the principal promoter of Wallerian degeneration because it activates resident Schwann cells in the peripheral nervous system and facilitates macrophage recruitment into the injury site (Feldman, 2008). These macrophages also release proteases, free radicals, and cytokines (Esposito and Cuzzocrea, 2011). Similar to the facts stated above, the extracellular expression of TNF-α (Esposito and Cuzzocrea, 2011) in the surrounding white matter was detected 3 hours posterior to contusion SCI, with a peak that took place from Days 1 to 3 (Lee et al., 2010). The majority of cytokines induce their effects by interacting with specific cell surface receptors. The binding between cytokines and their receptors triggers intracellular signaling and activates transcription factors such as AP-1 and NF-$\kappa\beta$ (Dinarello, 2007) leading to the modulation of inflammation, myelin destruction, apoptotic neuronal cell death, and astrocytic toxicity. Cytokine are also capable of stimulating neurite outgrowth, secretion of growth factors, and tissue remodeling (Pan and Kastin, 2008; Chi et al., 2008). Cytokines produce their effect by modulating a number of signaling pathways, including phosphatases, kinases, phospholipases, sphingomyelinases, oxygen radicals, and transcription factors (Jupp et al., 2003; Gomes-Leal et al., 2004). SCI induces the TNF-α mediated activation of NF-κB (Xu et al., 1998; Bethea et al., 1998), which in turn modulates the transcription of other proinflammatory cytokines, chemokines, and proinflammatory enzymes, such as isoforms PLA_2, COX-2, iNOS, SMase, and MMP. These enzymes further intensify SCI.

Like cytokines, chemokines induce specific actions in the immune system. Chemokines are essential for trafficking of leukocytes in both physiological and pathological conditions (Ubogu et al., 2006). CXCL12, also known as stromal-derived growth factor 1 or SDF-1, can act through two G-coupled receptors, CXCR4 and CXCR7. CXCL12 and its receptor CXCR4 play multiple roles both in the immune and nervous systems. CXCL12 is a highly efficacious chemoattractant for lymphocytes and monocytes but not neutrophils (Bleul et al., 1996). CXCR4 signaling is required for the migration of neuronal precursors, axon guidance/path finding and maintenance of neural progenitor cells. Chemokines are released in response to trauma (Lee et al., 2000). MCP-1 mRNA is present in the normal spinal cord. Levels of MCP-1 mRNA are increased 1 hour after SCI, peaks at 24 hours, and returned to a low level by Day 14. MCP-1 is expressed by astrocytes that surround white matter. In addition, MIP-1α mRNA is present in the normal spinal cord, where it is increased at 1 hour after SCI, peaks from 3 to 6 hours, decreases by day 1, remains unchanged until day 7, and returned to a low level by day 14. Another study indicates that the chemokines, MCP-1, MIP-1, MIP-1α, MIP-2, and IP-10 are expressed locally at 30 minutes with a peak at 6 hours after SCI. It is worth mentioning that chemokines are present 24 days after injury—at lower levels—in contrast with the rest of the cytokines (Rice et al., 2007). Collective evidence suggests that secondary injury is orchestrated by the expression of specific genes, in particular those of signaling proteins such as cytokines and chemokines. The balance between the proinflammatory and antiinflammatory effects of cytokines and chemokines plays an important role in the progression and outcome of the SCI-mediated degenerative process. Most of these cytokines have a dual role in a range between beneficial and injurious, depending on the time and the cell implicated in secondary injury after SCI. The excessive and uncontrolled inflammatory response after SCI enhances the damage to the spinal cord, which suppresses the regenerative effects of antiinflammatory cytokines and chemokines (Farooqui and Horrocks, 2009).

FAS/CD-95 RECEPTOR-LIGAND SYSTEM IN SCI

The Fas/CD95 receptor-ligand system plays an important role in apoptotic cell death after SCI (Casha et al., 2005; Yu et al., 2009) (Fig. 4.5). SCI promotes the translocation of FasL and Fas into membrane raft microdomains where Fas binds with the adaptor proteins Fas-associated death domain (FADD), caspase-8, cellular FLIP long form (cFLIPL), and caspase-3. These components form a death-inducing signaling complex (DISC). SCI also facilitates the expression of Fas in clusters around the nucleus in both neurons and astrocytes in the injured spinal cord (Casha et al., 2005; Yu et al., 2009). The formation of the DISC signaling platform induces a rapid activation of initiator caspase-8 and effector caspase-3, and the modification of signaling intermediates such as FADD and cFLIP(L). This observation suggests that FasL/Fas-mediated signaling after SCI is similar to Fas-induced cellular apoptosis (Casha et al., 2005; Yu et al., 2009). Although, it is generally believed that Fas activation mediates apoptotic cell death predominantly through the extrinsic pathway, involvement of intrinsic mitochondrial signaling in Fas-induced apoptosis after SCI has also been reported (Yu et al., 2009). FAS-deficient mice not only show reduction in apoptotic cell death in neurons but also exhibit improved locomotor recovery, axonal sparing, and preservation of oligodendrocytes and myelin. FAS-deficient mice do not show a significant increase in surviving neurons in the spinal cord at 6 weeks after injury, supporting the involvement of other cell death mechanisms for neurodegeneration in SCI (Casha et al., 2005).

ACTIVATION OF TRANSCRIPTION FACTORS IN SCI

It is well known that transcription factors are involved in the regulation of gene expression that bind to the promoter elements upstream of genes and either promote or block transcription. Through this process they modulate gene expression. Transcription factors consist of two essential functional domains: a DNA-binding domain and an activator domain. The DNA-binding domain consists of amino acids that recognize specific DNA bases near the start of transcription. Transcription factors not only interact with RNA polymerase but also bind to other transcription factors and cis-acting DNA sequences. SCI induces changes in several transcription factors, including NF-κB, AP-1 and members of STAT family (Fig. 4.6) (Xu et al., 1998; Bethea et al., 1998; Rafati et al., 2008).

NF-κB IN SCI

SCI produces transient activation of activator protein-1 (AP-1) and nuclear factor kappa B (NF-κB) in animal models. Activation of these factors play an important role in are activated in modulation of inflammation (Rafati et al., 2008; Barnes and Karin, 1997; Karin et al., 1997;

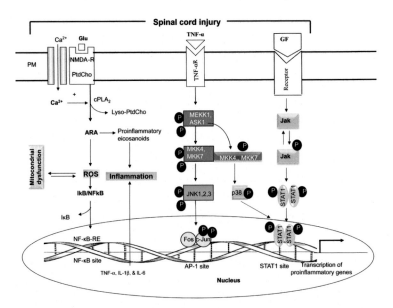

FIGURE 4.6   Activation of transcription factors (NF-κB, AP-1, anf STAT) following SCI. PM, plasma membrane; PtdCho, phosphatidylcholine; cPLA$_2$, cytosolic phospholipase A$_2$; ARA, arachidonic acid; Lyso-PtdCho, lyso-phosphatidylcholine; NF-κB-RE, nuclear factor κB-response element; I-κB, inhibitory subunit of NF-κB; JNK, c-Jun N-terminal kinase; AP-1, activator protein-1; JaK, Janus kinase; MAPK, mitogen activated protein kinases; MEKK1, MEK kinase 1; ASK1, apoptosis signal-regulating kinase 1; MKK4, MAPK kinases 4.

Bethea et al., 1998). AP-1 is a dimer composed of various Fos and Jun family proteins (Chiu et al., 1988). Immunostaining show an increase in the expression of the Fos-B and c-Jun components of AP-1 in the injured cord (Xu et al., 1998). These constituent components of AP-1 are not only present in the cytosol but are also found in nuclei (Xu et al., 1998), suggesting their migration to the nucleus to control gene expression. The specificity of SCI-induced AP-1 activation has been confirmed by an antisense strategy directed at c-fos that blocked AP-1 activation after SCI (Xu et al., 1998). Like AP-1, NF-κB is also present in the inactive form (complexed with the inhibitor IκB-α) in the cytosol. Following SCI, ROS-mediated activation of NF-κB results in translocation of free NF-κB to the nucleus, where it binds to NF-κB-RE and initiate the expression of proinflammatory cytokines, chemokines, and enzymes. NF-κB and AP-1 not only act individually but can also produce synergistic effects in expression of proinflammatory proteins such as cytokines and adhesion molecules, proinflammatory enzymes including iNOS and inducible cyclooxygenase II, and proinflammatory proteases (Barnes and Karin, 1997; Karin et al., 1997). In rat model of SCI, AP-1 binding activity is increased after SCI, starting at 1 hour, peaking at 8 hours, and declining to basal levels by 7 days (Xu et al., 1998). Similarly, SCI is also accompanied by increase in NF-κB binding activity, which peaks between 1 and 3 days postinjury (Xu et al., 1998). Posttraumatic inflammatory reaction involves the activation of AP-1, and NF-κB is a protracted process that lasts for days to weeks. The time course of AP-1 and NF-kB activation in is compatible. NF-κB inactivation in astrocytes results in improved functional recovery following SCI. This not only correlates with reduction in expression of proinflammatory mediators and CSPGs but also with increased white matter preservation (Brambilla et al., 2005). It is proposed that inactivation of astrocytic NF-κB creates a more permissive environment for axonal sprouting and regeneration. Detailed investigations on transgenic mice (GFAP-IκBα-dn) in which NF-κβ is specifically inactivated in astrocytes by overexpression of a truncated form of the inhibitor IκBα (IκBα-dn) under the control of the GFAP promoter (Brambilla et al., 2005). It is reported that blocking NF-κB activation in astrocytes results in reduced expression of cytokines and chemokines such as CXCL10, CCL2 and transforming growth factor beta, and in a smaller lesion volume and increased white matter sparing along with a significant improvement in locomotor function following SCI (Brambilla et al., 2005). Further studies have demonstrated that inhibition of astroglial NF-κB promotes axonal sparing and sprouting of supraspinal and propriospinal axons, which are essential for locomotion (Brambilla et al., 2005; Brambilla et al., 2009).

PEROXISOME PROLIFERATOR ACTIVATOR ACTIVATED RECEPTOR IN SCI

It is well recognized that SCI contribute the loss of bone minerals (Jiang et al., 2007) inducing osteoporosis, a well-known secondary complication of SCI (Garland, 1988). Shortly after the SCI, sublesional bone density and mass decline rapidly and linearly. This profound bone loss occurs in 2 phases: (1) rapid, acute bone loss that plateaus between 12 and 36 months post-injury and (2) chronic, ongoing bone loss that is more gradual in nature (Jiang et al., 2006). Based on the rodent studies, it is suggested that rapid bone loss in the acute phase of SCI is due to increased osteocyte production of sclerostin in response to the abrupt loss of mechanical loading (Lin et al., 2009). The molecular mechanism associated with SCI-mediated osteoporosis is not fully understood. However, it is proposed that peroxisome proliferator activated receptor (PPARs) family members may be involved in this process. Among PPAR family members (PPAR-α, PPAR-γ, and PPAR-δ) (Drew et al., 2005). PPAR-α contribute to the modulation of inflammatory processes associated with SCI (Genovese et al., 2009b). In contrast, PPAR-γ is an inducer of adipogenesis, and PPAR-γ insufficiency results in the enhancement of osteogenesis and suppression of adipogenesis in mice (Akune et al., 2004). It is also reported that elevation in PPAR-γ levels can promote adipogenesis in pluripotent mesenchymal cells in vitro (Rzonca et al., 2004) suggesting that PPAR-γ levels play a dominant suppressive influence on osteogenesis. In contrast, canonical Wnt signaling enhances osteoblast differentiation. It is also demonstrated that the mechanical unloading produces a decrease in Wnt/beta-catenin signaling activity (Lin et al., 2009). Sclerostin, a Wnt signaling pathway antagonist produced by osteocytes, is a potent inhibitor of bone formation, and circulating sclerostin has been found to be elevated in short-term SCI patients (≤ 5 years after injury) (Battaglino et al., 2012). Taken together, these findings can explain the imbalance between adipogenesis and osteoblastogenesis after SCI and can explain the induction of osteoporosis following SCI.

SIGNAL TRANSDUCTION AND TRANSCRIPTION-3 (STATE3) IN SCI

It is well known that astrocytes respond to SCI through the activation of a variety of different potential signaling pathways such as the activation of cAMP, MAP kinases, NF-κB, and Jak-STATs. These pathways are closely associated with cellular hypertrophy, migration, proliferation, and scar formation (Silver and Miller, 2004). Information on the involvement of NF-κB in SCI has been described above. Jak-STAT is a generic name for intracellular signaling pathways involving the activation of two families of proteins: the Janus kinase (JAK), which consist of four tyrosine kinases (Jak1, Jak2, Jak3, and TYK2), and the signal transducer and activator of transcription (STAT) containing seven transcription factors (STAT1, STAT2, STAT3, STAT4, STAT5A, STAT5B, and STAT6). The Jak-STAT pathway is an efficient and highly regulated system mainly dedicated to the regulation of gene expression. This pathway is associated with the activation of a receptor by growth factors or cytokines. These interactions lead to the activation of Jak. Jak phosphorylates STATs, which then dimerizes. The STAT dimer migrates to the nucleus where it binds to the DNA and regulates transcription (Fig. 4.6). The control of activity of this pathway involves different mechanisms including regulation of the phosphorylation state of Jak and STAT by phosphatases, or of the Jak kinase activity by SOCS (suppressor of cytokine signaling). Activation of different components of the Jak–STAT pathway is observed in mammalian SCI. Thus, an increase in the levels of cytokines (Pineau and Lacroix, 2007; Slaets et al., 2014) or increase in phosphorylation of Signal transduction and transcription-3 (pSTAT3) (Herrmann et al., 2008), and elevation in SOCS3 (Park et al., 2014) have been reported to be involved in SCI. Moreover, functional studies have demonstrated that STAT3 is necessary for astrocyte response in glial scar formation, which in turn contains the inflammatory response and aids axon regeneration (Herrmann et al., 2008; Wanner et al., 2013). In addition, gain-of-function studies have also indicated that the Jak−STAT pathway improves axon regeneration and collateral sprouting, enhancing motor recovery (Jin et al., 2015; Lang et al., 2013). Collectively these studies suggest that STAT3 signaling is a critical regulator of certain aspects of reactive astrogliosis and scar formation. This may restrict the spread of inflammatory cells after SCI.

GENE TRANSCRIPTION IN SCI

SCI leads to induction and/or suppression of many genes, the interplay of which governs the neuronal death and subsequent loss of motor function (Song et al., 2001; Bareyre and Schwab, 2003). Early stages of SCI induce potent upregulation of genes associated with transcription and inflammation along with the downregulation of genes modulating expression of structural proteins and proteins involved in neurotransmission. Later stages of SCI involve the upregulation of genes responsible for the modulation of growth factors, axonal guidance factors, extracellular matrix molecules, and angiogenic factors. These genes have been implicated in repair, recovery, and survival processes after SCI (Bareyre and Schwab, 2003). In addition, upregulation of immediate early genes, gene regulation of heat-shock proteins (Hsp-70), and proinflammatory genes (IL-6) have also been reported to occur after SCI. In SCI, induction of Hsp has beneficial effects. These proteins are expressed by acutely stressed microglial, endothelial, and ependymal cells. They assist in the protection of motor neurons and to prevent chronic inflammation after SCI (Reddy et al., 2008). Hsps promote cell survival by preventing mitochondrial outer membrane permeabilization or apoptosome formation as well as via regulation of Akt and JNK activities (Beere, 2005). This up- and downregulation of gene transcription persists for many hours (more than 24 hours), after SCI (Song et al., 2001). In addition, SCI also affects genes involved in cell cycle (gadd45a, c-myc, cyclin D1 and cdk4, pcna, cyclin G, Rb, and E2F5) (Di Giovanni et al., 2003). Microarray studies have also unveiled the short-and long-term responses to SCI at the molecular level. These studies have identified rapid expression of immediate early genes after SCI, followed by genes associated with inflammation, oxidative stress, DNA damage, and cell cycle (Hayashi et al., 2000; Pan et al., 2002). Transcription factors, particularly those involved in cell damage and death, including nuclear factor kappa B, c-JUN, and SOCS 3, were also observed to be upregulated (Carmel et al., 2001). Several of the above findings have been proven by using experimental methods (Pan et al., 2002); thus, data from DNA microarray analysis can be reliable and useful for discovering novel targets for neuroprotective or restorative therapeutic approaches. In addition, microRNAs (miRNAs) that can posttranscriptionally regulate the entire set of genes exhibited altered expression following traumatic SCI (Liu et al., 2009). Previous studies have suggested that miRNAs may act as mediators of neural plasticity (Kosik, 2006) and possibly be involvement in neurodegeneration (Schaefer et al., 2007). Collective evidence suggests that transcription of various genes after SCI not only modulates oxidative stress and inflammation but also controls neurotransmitter dysfunction, ionic imbalance, and redox status in the injured spinal cord.

GROWTH FACTORS IN SCI

Neurotrophins are critical for the survival of neurons not only during development but also after acute neural trauma. Astroglial cells respond to SCI and become reactive and forming scar, a physical and chemical barrier to axonal regeneration. Astrocytic response involves well-described morphological alterations and less characterized functional changes. The functional consequences of astrocyte reactivity seem to depend on the molecular pathway involved and may result in the enhancement of several neuroprotective and neurotrophic functions. Epidermal growth factor (EGF) receptor is upregulated in astrocytes after SCI and facilitates resting astrocyte transformation into reactive astrocytes (Table 4.2). EGF receptor inhibitors enhance axon regeneration promote recovery after SCI. The signaling pathways associated with above processes involves mTOR pathway, a key regulator of astrocyte physiology (Codeluppi et al., 2009). mTOR pathway integrates signals from multiple upstream pathways, including insulin, insulin-like growth factor-1 (IGF-1), and IGF-2 and mitogens. mTOR also functions as a sensor of nutrients, energy status, and cellular redox. These processes occur through Akt-mediated phosphorylation of the GTPase-activating protein Tuberin, which blocks Tuberin's ability to inhibit the small GTPase Rheb. Indeed, Rheb is necessary for EGF-dependent mTOR activation in spinal cord astrocytes. The astrocytic growth and EGF-dependent chemoattraction are blocked by the mTOR-selective drug rapamycin (Codeluppi et al., 2009). In ischemic model of SCI, elevation in levels of activated EGF receptor and mTOR signaling occurs in reactive astrocytes in vivo. Furthermore, increased Rheb expression likely contributes to mTOR activation in the injured spinal cord. Treatment of injured rats with rapamycin shows reduced signs of reactive gliosis, suggesting that rapamycin can be used to promote more permissive environment for axon regeneration (Codeluppi et al., 2009). Like the expression of EGF in SCI, unilateral hemisection and contusion injury to adult rat spinal cord causes increased expression of fibroblast growth factor (FGF) and FGF-binding protein (FGF-BP) (Tassi et al., 2007) (Table 4.2). Increase in expression of FGF-BP occurs at all postinjury time points peaking at Day 4, a time when injury-mediated increase in levels of FGF2 levels has been reported to be maximal. Although, the molecular mechanism associated with the involvement of FGF-BP/FGF2 is not fully understood. However, FGF-BP is known to enhance FGF2-induced protein tyrosine phosphorylation and AKT/PKB activation. All together, these results indicate that FGF-BP is an early response gene after SCI and that its upregulation in regenerating spinal cord tissue may be associated with enhancing the initial FGF2-mediated neurotrophic effects after SCI. Similarly, SCI also increases the expression of thrombospondin-1 (TSP-1) and TGF-β in the injured segment of rat spinal cord. After 12 hours, levels of TSP-1 increase more rapidly and dramatically than TGF-β levels in the injured segment. Elevations in TSP-1 and TGF-β concentrations persist for 24 hours after injury (Wang et al., 2009). Vascular endothelial growth factor (VEGF), a potent mitogen for endothelial cells, plays an important role in vessel outgrowth, arterial and venous differentiation, and vascular remodeling, and patterning involved in angiogenesis. Three major isoforms of VEGF (VEGF120, VEGF188, and VEGF164) are known to occur in vascular system. They differ from each other in their solubility (VEGF120 is freely soluble and VEGF188 is completely matrix-bound, while VEGF164 has intermediate properties) and receptor binding properties. SCI decreases the levels of VEGF165 and other VEGF isoforms at the lesion epicenter 1 day after injury, which was maintained up to 1 month after injury, indicating that VEGF may be associated with the pathophysiology of SCI (Herrera et al., 2009) (Table 4.2).

In addition, SCI markedly effects the expression of several members of neurotrophin family including nerve growth factor, brain-derived neurotrophic factor (BDNF), and neurotrophin-3 (NT-3). All these neurotrophins are significantly reduced in the injured spinal cord, as early as 6 hours after the induction of the contusion (Hajebrahimi et al., 2008). The expression of other neurotrophin receptors (high-affinity Trk receptors) is severely reduced after the contusion. The expression of TrkA and TrkC is completely blocked after injury along with decrease in expression of TrkB receptor. In contrast to expression of Trk receptors, the expression of p75^{NTR} receptor is significantly upregulated after SCI. p75^{NTR} cooperates with TrkA to promote survival. Detailed investigations on the role of the p75^{NTR} in a clip compression model of SCI in p75^{NTR} null mice with an exon III mutation indicate that compared to the functionally deficient p75^{NTR} mice, p75^{NTR} mice functional show an increase in caspase-9 activation at 3 days after SCI. No differences in the activation of the effector caspases (caspase-3 and caspase-6) are observed in the spinal cord lesion at 7 days following SCI (Chu et al., 2007). SCI produces an increase in terminal deoxynucleotidyl transferase-mediated dUTP nick-end (TUNEL)−positive cell death in p75NTR-deficient mice at the injury site at 7 days after SCI. Double labeling with TUNEL and cell-specific markers indicates that the deficiency of p75^{NTR} increases the extent of neuronal but not oligodendroglial cell death at the injury site. This selective loss of neuronal cells after SCI is accompanied by a decrease in levels of microtubule-associated protein 2 in the p75^{NTR} null mice. Furthermore, the WT mice show a dramatic improvement in survival and enhancement in locomotor recovery at 8 weeks after SCI when compared with the p75^{NTR} null mice (Chu et al., 2007). Also at 8 weeks, more neurons present at the injury site of WT mice when compared with p75^{NTR} null mice, supporting the view that p75^{NTR} receptor is an integral part of neuronal cell survival in compressive/contusive SCI (Chu et al., 2007).

NEUROPATHIC PAIN IN SCI

Pain is an unpleasant sensory experience induced by noxious stimuli. SCI patients suffer from pain, which can be categorized into nociceptive and neuropathic type. Neuropathic pains result from damage to the spinal cord, and nociceptive pains are caused by the unusual demands an SCI places on the upper limbs. Neuropathic pain is spontaneous and persistent. It is characterized by a range of abnormally evoked responses, e.g., allodynia (pain evoked by normally non-noxious stimuli) and hyperalgesia (an increased response to noxious stimuli). Neuropathic pain following SCI is usually present at or below the level of injury (Yiu and He, 2006; Dijkers et al., 2009). Neuropathic pain following SCI is caused by damage to or dysfunction of the nervous system, whereas nociceptive pain is caused by damage to non-neural tissue either musculoskeletal due to bone, joint, muscle trauma or inflammation, mechanical instability, or muscle spasm. Pain of visceral origin may develop for instance due to renal calculus, bowel, sphincter dysfunction, headache related to autonomic dysreflexia and secondary overuse syndromes (Siddall, 2009; Finnerup et al., 2014). Neuropathic pain above the level of injury is often induced by concomitant compressive radiculopathies or sometimes by complex regional pain syndromes. Neuropathic pain at the level of injury is caused by nerve-root compression development of complications such as syringomyelia or SCI itself, whereas neuropathic pain below the level of injury is produced by spinal cord trauma or disease. At the cellular level, interactions between dorsal horn sensory neurons and microglia modulate the intensity of pain. Thus, experimental SCI is accompanied by chronic activation of microglial cells (Hains and Waxman, 2006; McKay et al., 2007; Zhao et al., 2007a). Selective inhibition of microglial cell activation and signaling results in a return to the resting morphological phenotype as well as reductions in electrophysiologic and behavioral concomitants of pain (Hains and Waxman, 2006; Zhao et al., 2007a; Zhao et al., 2007b). The molecular mechanism associated with neuropathic pain is not fully understood. However, it is proposed that neuroinflammation, which is mediated by PGE_2 and proinflammatory cytokines and chemokines, plays an important role in establishing and maintaining neuropathic pain. The production and release PGE2 are regulated by pERK1/2 MAP kinase (Zhao et al., 2007a). This is mechanistically different than from peripheral nerve injury where microglia play a role in the initiation phase of pain. Accumulating evidence also indicates that several chemokines are upregulated after SCI and contribute to the pathogenesis of neuropathic pain via different forms of neuron–glia interaction in the spinal cord (Zhang et al., 2017). For example, chemokine CX3CL1 is expressed in primary afferents and spinal neurons. It induces microglial activation via microglial receptor CX3CR1 (neuron-to-microglia signaling). In addition, CCL2 and CXCL1 are expressed in spinal astrocytes and act on CCR2 and CXCR2 in spinal neurons to increase excitatory synaptic transmission (astrocyte-to-neuron signaling). Finally, CXCL13 is highly upregulated in spinal neurons after spinal nerve ligation and induces spinal astrocyte activation via receptor CXCR5 (neuron-to-astrocyte signaling) (Zhang et al., 2017). In addition, endogenous IL-1β in neuropathic rats enhances the release of glutamate from the primary afferent terminals leading to overactivation of glutamate receptors and increase in expression of proinflammatory cytokines, such as IL-1β in the spinal cord dorsal horn. These processes may also contribute to the pathogenesis of neuropathic pain (Yan and Weng, 2013).

INTERPLAY AMONG EXCITOTOXICITY, OXIDATIVE STRESS, AND INFLAMMATION IN SCI

It is well known that excitotoxicity, oxidative stress, and inflammation play an important role in the pathogenesis of SCI. Thus, neurodegeneration in SCI is a coordinated multistep process that involves cross talk among excitotoxicity, oxidative stress, and neuroinflammation. The effect of this cross talk among excitotoxicity, oxidative stress, and neuroinflammation may be synergistic or cumulative. Terminally differentiated neurons may commit to death in response to abnormal signal transduction processes initiated by the interplay among excitotoxicity, oxidative stress, and inflammation (Farooqui et al., 2007). Initially, the coordinated interplay among excitotoxicity, oxidative stress, and neuroinflammation in SCI may cause abnormalities in motor and cognitive performance. An enhanced rate (upregulation) of interplay among excitotoxicity, oxidative stress, and neuroinflammation may contribute to increased rate of neurodegeneration in SCI. It is proposed that cross talk among excitotoxicity, oxidative stress, and neuroinflammation may be a common mechanism of neural cell damage in acute neurotraumatic diseases, which includes SCI, TBI, and stroke (Farooqui and Horrocks, 2007; Farooqui. 2009; Farooqui and Horrocks, 2009). Environmental factors such as diet (enrichment of ω-6 fatty acids) and life style (lack of exercise and sleep) may also play a prominent role in modulating the interplay among excitotoxicity, oxidative stress, and neuroinflammation. Thus, long- and short-term locomotor activity of moderate intensity induce stimuli sufficient to recruit a majority of spinal cells to increased BDNF synthesis, suggesting that continuous tuning of pro-BDNF and BDNF levels permits spinal networks to undergo trophic modulation without requiring changes in TrkB mRNA supply. In SCI, neurons die rapidly, a matter of hours to days, because of the sudden lack of oxygen, decrease in ATP level, sudden collapse of ion gradients, and the rapid upregulation of interplay among excitotoxicity, oxidative stress, and neuroinflammation. In contrast, in neurodegenerative diseases, oxygen, nutrients, and ATP continue to be available to the nerve cells, and ionic homeostasis is maintained to a limited extent. The interplay among excitotoxicity, oxidative stress, and neuroinflammation occurs at a slow rate, resulting in a neurodegenerative process that takes several years to develop (Farooqui, 2009).

CONCLUSION

SCI is an irreversible neurological condition that causes damage to myelinated fiber tracts that carry sensation and motor signals to and from the brain. SCI involves contribution of primary and secondary injury mechanisms. The primary injury is accompanied by the disruption of the blood–spinal cord barrier by a mechanical force, which tears neuronal and endothelial cell membranes. Primary injury not only disturbs the microenvironment of the spinal cord but also exposes the adjacent noninjured tissue to potentially noxious molecules. In contrast, secondary injury involves a cascade of vascular, biochemical, and cellular events leading to induction of ischemia, edema, hemorrhage, induction of excitotoxicity, oxidative stress, and inflammation. These processes involves high levels of ROS, activation of calcium-dependent enzymes (PLA$_2$, COX-2, NOS, calpains, caspases, and MMP), activation of transcription factors, and increased expression of proinflammatory cytokines and chemokines. Neurodegeneration in SCI involves both necrotic and apoptotic neural cell death. Necrotic cell death occurs in the primary phase of SCI, whereas in secondary injury neuronal and oligodendrocytic cell death occurs via apoptosis. This type of cell death involves the mitochondrial dysfunction and release of cytochrome c, activation of caspases, and ultimately induction of nuclear DNA condensation and fragmentation. Following SCI, apoptotic cell death continues, and scarring and demyelination accompany Wallerian degeneration. These processes are reflected in a general failure of normal neural functions and a stage of signal shock that lasts for several days in experimental SCI.

References

Ackery, A., Robins, S., Fehlings, M.G., 2006. Inhibition of Fas-mediated apoptosis through administration of soluble Fas receptor improves functional outcome and reduces posttraumatic axonal degeneration after acute spinal cord injury. J. Neurotrauma 23, 604−616.

Adachi, K., Yimin, Y., Satake, K., Matsuyama, Y., Ishiguro, N., et al., 2005. Localization of cyclooxygenase-2 induced following traumatic spinal cord injury. Neurosci. Res. 51, 73−80.

Ahuja, C.S., Martin, A.R., Fehlings, M., 2016. Recent advances in managing a spinal cord injury secondary to trauma. F1000Res 5, pii: F1000 Faculty Rev-1017.

Akune, T., Ohba, S., Kamekura, S., et al., 2004. PPARgamma insufficiency enhances osteogenesis through osteoblast formation from bone marrow progenitors. J. Clin. Invest. 113, 846−855.

Ankeny, D.P., Popovich, P.G., 2009. Mechanisms and implications of adaptive immune responses after traumatic spinal cord injury. Neuroscience 158, 1112−1121.

Amar, A.P., Levy, M.L., 1999. Pathogenesis and pharmacological strategies for mitigating secondary damage in acute spinal cord injury. Neurosurgery 44, 1027−1039.

Ashki, N., Hayes, K.C., Bao, F., 2008. The peroxynitrite donor 3-morpholinosydnonimine induces reversible changes in electrophysiological properties of neurons of the guinea-pig spinal cord. Neuroscience 156, 107−117.

Banik, N.L., Hogan, E.L., Powers, J.M., Smith, K.P., 1986. Proteolytic enzymes in experimental spinal cord injury. J. Neurol. Sci. 73, 245−256.

Bao, F., Bailey, C.S., Gurr, K.R., Bailey, S.I., Rosas-Arellano, M.P., et al., 2009. Increased oxidative activity in human blood neutrophils and monocytes after spinal cord injury. Exp. Neurol. 215, 308−316.

Bareyre, F.M., Schwab, M.E., 2003. Inflammation, degeneration and regeneration in the injured spinal cord: insights from DNA microarrays. Trends Neurosci. 26, 555−563.

Barnabe-Heider, F., Goritz, C., Sabelstrom, H., Takebayashi, H., Pfrieger, F.W., Meletis, K., Frisen, J., 2010. Origin of new glial cells in intact and injured adult spinal cord. Cell Stem Cell 7, 470–482.

Barnes, P.J., Karin, M., 1997. Nuclear factor-kappaB: a pivotal transcription factor in chronic inflammatory diseases. N. Engl. J. Med. 336, 1066–1071.

Barut, S., Unlu, Y.A., Karaoglan, A., Tuncdemir, M., Dagistanli, F.K., Ozturk, M., Colak, A., 2005. The neuroprotective effects of z-DEVD.fmk, a caspase-3 inhibitor, on traumatic spinal cord injury in rats. Surg. Neurol. 64, 213–220.

Battaglino, R.A., Sudhakar, S., Lazzari, A., Garshick, E., Zafonte, R., et al., 2012. Circulating sclerostin is elevated in short-term and reduced in long-term SCI. Bone 51, 600–605.

Bauchet, L., Lonjon, N., Perrin, F.-E., Gilbert, C., Privat, A., Fattal, C., 2009. Strategies for spinal cord repair after injury: a review of the literature and information. Ann. Phys. Rehab. Med. 52, 330–351.

Beck, K.D., Nguyen, H.X., Galvan, M.D., Salazar, D.L., Woodruff, T.M., Anderson, A.J., 2010. Quantitative analysis of cellular inflammation after traumatic spinal cord injury: evidence for a multiphasic inflammatory response in the acute to chronic environment. Brain 133, 433–447.

Beere, H.M., 2005. Death versus survival: functional interaction between the apoptotic and stress-inducible heat shock protein pathways. J. Clin. Invest. 115, 2633–2639.

Benowitz, L.I., Popovich, P.G., 2011. Inflammation and axon regeneration. Curr. Opin. Neurol. 24, 577–583.

Bethea, J.R., Castro, M., Keane, R.W., Lee, T.T., Dietrich, W.D., et al., 1998. Traumatic spinal cord injury induces nuclear factor-κB activation. J. Neurosci. 18, 3251–3260.

Bleul, C.C., Fuhlbrigge, R.C., Casasnovas, J.M., Aiuti, A., Springer, T.A., 1996. A highly efficacious lymphocyte chemoattractant, stromal cell-derived factor 1 (SDF-1). J. Exp. Med. 184, 1101–1109.

Brambilla, R., Bracchi-Ricard, V., Hu, W.H., Frydel, B., Bramwell, A., et al., 2005. Inhibition of astroglial nuclear factor kappaB reduces inflammation and improves functional recovery after spinal cord injury. J. Exp. Med. 202, 145–156.

Brambilla, R., Hurtado, A., Persaud, T., Esham, K., Pearse, D.D., et al., 2009. Transgenic inhibition of astroglial NF-kappaB leads to increased axonal sparing and sprouting following spinal cord injury. J. Neurochem. 110, 765–778.

Bramlett, H.M., Dietrich, W.D., 2004. Pathophysiology of cerebral ischemia and brain trauma: similarities and differences. J. Cereb. Blood Flow Metab. 24, 133–150.

Buss, A., Pech, K., Kakulas, B.A., Martin, D., Schoenen, J., et al., 2007. Matrix metalloproteinases and their inhibitors in human traumatic spinal cord injury. BMC Neurol. 26, 7–17.

Byrnes, K.R., Washington, P.M., Knoblach, S.M., Hoffman, E., Faden, A.I., 2011. Delayed inflammatory mRNA and protein expression after spinal cord injury. J Neuroinflamm. 8, 130.

Calabrese, V., Mancuso, C., Calvani, M., Rizzarelli, E., Butterfield, D.A., et al., 2007. Nitric oxide in the central nervous system: neuroprotection versus neurotoxicity. Nat. Rev. Neurosci. 8, 766–775.

Carmel, J.B., Galante, A., Soteropoulos, P., Tolias, P., Recce, M., et al., 2001. Gene expression profiling of acute spinal cord injury reveals spreading inflammatory signals and neuron loss. Physiol. Genomics 7, 201–213.

Casha, S., Yu, W.R., Fehlings, M.G., 2001. Oligodendroglial apoptosis occurs along degenerating axons and is associated with FAS and p75 expression following spinal cord injury in the rat. Neuroscience 103, 203–218.

Casha, S., Yu, W.R., Fehlings, M.G., 2005. FAS deficiency reduces apoptosis, spares axons and improves function after spinal cord injury. Exp. Neurol. 196, 390–400.

Chatzipanteli, K., Garcia, R., Marcillo, A.E., Loor, K.E., Kraydieh, S., et al., 2002. Temporal and segmental distribution of constitutive and inducible nitric oxide synthases after traumatic spinal cord injury: effect of aminoguanidine treatment. J. Neurotrauma 19, 639–651.

Chi, L.-Y., Yu, J., Zhu, H., Li, X.-G., Zhu, S.-G., et al., 2008. The dual role of tumor necrosis factor-alpha in the pathophysiology of spinal cord injury,". Neurosci. Lett 438, 174–179.

Chiu, R., Boyle, W.J., Meek, J., Smeal, T., Hunter, T., et al., 1988. The c-Fos protein interacts with c-Jun/AP-1 to stimulate transcription of AP-1 responsive genes. Cell 54, 541–552.

Chu, G.K., Yu, W., Fehlings, M.G., 2007. The p75 neurotrophin receptor is essential for neuronal cell survival and improvement of functional recovery after spinal cord injury. Neuroscience 148, 668–682.

Cicero, A.F., Laghi, L., 2007. Activity and potential role of licofelone in the management of osteoarthritis. Clin. Interv. Aging 2, 73–79.

Citron, B.A., Arnold, P.M., Haynes, N.G., Ameenuddin, S., Farooque, M., et al., 2008. Neuroprotective effects of caspase-3 inhibition on functional recovery and tissue sparing after acute spinal cord injury. Spine 33, 2269–2277.

Codeluppi, S., Svensson, C.I., Hefferan, M.P., Valencia, F., Silldorff, M.D., et al., 2009. The Rheb-mTOR pathway is upregulated in reactive astrocytes of the injured spinal cord. J. Neurosci. 29, 1093–1104.

Cohen, G.M., 1997. Caspases: the executioners of apoptosis. Biochem. J. 326, 1–16.

Cox, A., Varma, A., Banik, N., 2015. Recent advances in the pharmacologic treatment of spinal cord injury. Metab. Brain Dis. 30, 473–482.

Creagh, E.M., Conroy, H., Martin, S.J., 2003. Caspase-activation pathways in apoptosis and immunity. Immunol. Rev. 193, 10–21.

Darian-Smith, C., 2009. Synaptic plasticity, neurogenesis, and functional recovery after spinal cord injury. Neuroscientist 15, 149–165.

Dawson, T.M., Zhang, J., Dawson, V.L., Snyder, S.H., 1994. Nitric oxide: cellular regulation and neuronal injury. In: Neural Regeneration chapter 30. Elsevier BV, pp. 365–369.

Dickson, B.J., 2001. Rho GTPases in growth cone guidance. Curr. Opin. Neurobiol. 11, 103–110.

Di Giovanni, S., Knoblach, S.M., Brandoli, C., Aden, S.A., Hoffman, E.P., et al., 2003. Gene profiling in spinal cord injury shows role of cell cycle in neuronal death. Ann. Neurol. 53, 454–468.

Dijkers, M., Bryce, T., Zanca, J., 2009. Prevalence of chronic pain after traumatic spinal cord injury: a systematic review. J. Rehabil. Res. Dev. 46, 13–29.

Dinarello, C.A., 2007. Historical insights into cytokines. Eur. J. Immunol. 37 (supplement 1), S34–S45.

Drew, P.D., Storer, P.D., Xu, J., Chavis, J.A., 2005. Hormone regulation of microglial cell activation: relevance to multiple sclerosis. Brain Res. Rev. 48, 322–327.

Dulin, J.N., Karoly, E.D., Wang, Y., Strobel, H.W., Grill, R.J., 2013. Licofelone modulates neuroinflammation and attenuates mechanical hypersensitivity in the chronic phase of spinal cord injury. J. Neurosci. 33, 652–664.

Esposito, E., Cuzzocrea, S., 2011. Anti-TNF therapy in the injured spinal cord. Trends Pharmacol. Sci. 32, 107–115.

Faden, A.I., Wu, J., Stoica, B.A., Loane, D.J., 2016. Progressive inflammation-mediated neurodegeneration after traumatic brain or spinal cord injury. Br. J. Pharmacol 173, 681–691.

Farooqui, A.A., 2009. Hot Topics in Neural membrane Lipidology. Springer, New York.

Farooqui, A.A., Horrocks, L.A., 1991. Excitatory amino acid receptors, neural membrane phospholipid metabolism and neurological disorders. Brain Res. Rev. 16, 171–191.

Farooqui, A.A., Horrocks, L.A., 2007. Glycerophospholipids in Brain. Springer, New York.

Farooqui, A.A., Horrocks, L.A., Farooqui, T., 2007. Modulation of inflammation in brain: a matter of fat. J. Neurochem. 101, 577–599.

Farooqui, A.A., Ong, W.Y., Horrocks, L.A., 2008. Neurochemical Aspects of Excitotoxicity. Springer, New York.

Farooqui, A.A., Horrocks, L.A., 2009. Glutamate and cytokine-mediated alterations of phospholipids in head injury and spinal cord trauma. In: Banik, N.K., Ray, S.K. (Eds.), Handbook of Neurochemistry and Molecular Neurobiology, Vol. 24. Springer, New York, pp. 71–89.

Faulkner, J.R., Herrmann, J.E., Woo, M.J., Tansey, K.E., Doan, N.B., et al., 2004. Reactive astrocytes protect tissue and preserve function after spinal cord injury. J Neurosci. 24, 2143–2155.

Feldman, A.M., 2008. TNF alpha—still a therapeutic target. Clin. Transl. Sci. 1, 145.

Finnerup, N.B., Norrbrink, C., Trok, K., Piehl, F., Johannesen, I.L., et al., 2014. Phenotypes and predictors of pain following traumatic spinal cord injury: a prospective study. J. Pain 15, 40–48.

Forgione, N., Fehlings, M.G., 2014. Rho-ROCK inhibition in the treatment of spinal cord injury. World Neurosurg. 82, e535–e539.

Freund, P., Weiskopf, N., Ward, N.S., Hutton, C., Gall, A., et al., 2011. Disability, atrophy and cortical reorganization following spinal cord injury. Brain 134, 1610–1622.

Freund, P., Weiskopf, N., Ashburner, J., Wolf, K., Sutter, R., et al., 2013. MRI investigation of the sensorimotor cortex and the corticospinal tract after acute spinal cord injury: a prospective longitudinal study. Lancet Neurol. 12, 873–881.

Garland, D.E., 1988. Clinical observations on fractures and heterotopic ossification in the spinal cord and traumatic brain injured populations. Clin. Orthop. Relat. Res. 86–101.

Genovese, T., Cuzzocrea, S., 2008. Role of free radicals and poly(ADP-ribose)polymerase-1 in the development of spinal cord injury: new potential therapeutic targets. Curr. Med. Chem. 43, 763–780.

Genovese, T., Mazzon, E., Esposito, E., Di Paola, R., Bramanti, P., et al., 2005. Inhibitors of poly(ADP-ribose) polymerase modulate signal transduction pathways and secondary damage in experimental spinal cord trauma. J. Pharmacol. Exp. Ther. 312, 449–457.

Genovese, T., Mazzon, E., Esposito, E., Di Paola, R., Murthy, K., et al., 2009a. Effects of a metalloporphyrinic peroxynitrite decomposition catalyst, ww-85, in a mouse model of spinal cord injury. Free Radic. Res. 5, 1–15.

Genovese, T., Esposito, E., Mazzon, E., Crisafulli, C., Paterniti, I., et al., 2009b. PPAR-α modulate the anti-inflammatory effect of glucocorticoids in the secondary damage in experimental spinal cord trauma. Pharmacol. Res. 59, 338–350.

Glick, D., Barth, S., Macleod, K.F., 2010. Autophagy: cellular and molecular mechanisms. J. Pathol. 221, 3–12.

Goldshmit, Y., Frisca, F., Pinto, A.R., Pebay, A., Tang, J.K., et al., 2014. Fgf2 improves functional recovery-decreasing gliosis and increasing radial glia and neural progenitor cells after spinal cord injury. Brain Behav. 4, 187–200.

Gomes-Leal, W., Corkill, D.J., Freire, M.A., Picanço-Diniz, C.W., Perry, V.H., 2004. Astrocytosis, microglia activation, oligodendrocyte degeneration, and pyknosis following acute spinal cord injury. Exp. Neurol. 190, 456–467.

Govek, E.E., Newey, S.E., Van Aelst, L., 2005. The role of the Rho GTPases in neuronal development. Genes Dev. 19, 1–49.

Gris, D., Hamilton, E.F., Weaver, L.C., 2008. The systemic inflammatory response after spinal cord injury damages lungs and kidneys. Exp. Neurol. 211, 259–270.

Guo, J.D., Li, L., Shi, Y.M., Wang, H.D., Yuan, Y.L., et al., 2014. Genetic ablation of receptor for advanced glycation end products promotes functional recovery in mouse model of spinal cord injury. Mol. Cell. Biochem. 390, 215–223.

Hagen, E.M., 2015. Acute complications of spinal cord injuries. World J. Orthop. 6, 17–23.

Hains, B.C., Waxman, S.G., 2006. Activated microglia contribute to the maintenance of chronic pain after spinal cord injury. J. Neurosci. 26, 4308–4317.

Hajebrahimi, Z., Mowla, S.J., Movahedin, M., Tavallaei, M., 2008. Gene expression alterations of neurotrophins, their receptors and prohormone convertases in a rat model of spinal cord contusion. Neurosci. Lett. 441, 261–266.

Hayashi, M., Ueyama, T., Nemoto, K., Tamaki, T., Senba, E., 2000. Sequential mRNA expression for immediate early genes, cytokines and neurotrophins in spinal cord injury. J. Neurotrauma 17, 203–218.

Herrera, J.J., Nesic-Taylor, D.O., Narayana, P.A., 2009. Reduced vascular endothelial growth factor expression in contusive spinal cord injury. J. Neurotrauma 26, 995–1003.

Herrmann, J.E., Imura, T., Song, B., Oi, J., Ao, Y., et al., 2008. STAT3 is a critical regulator of astrogliosis and scar formation after spinal cord injury. J. Neurosci. 28, 7231–7243.

Hou, X.L., Chen, Y., Yin, H., Duan, W.G., 2015. Combination of fasudil and celecoxib promotes the recovery of injured spinal cord in rats better than celecoxib or fasudil alone. Neural Regen. Res. 10, 1836–1840.

Hsu, J.Y., Mckeon, R., Goussev, S., Werb, Z., Lee, J.U., et al., 2006. Matrix metalloproteinase-2 facilitates wound healing events that promote functional recovery after spinal cord injury. J. Neurosci. 26, 9841–9850.

Hsu, J.Y., Bourguignon, L.Y., Adams, C.M., Peyrollier, K., Zhang, H., et al., 2008. Matrix metalloproteinase-9 facilitates glial scar formation in the injured spinal cord. J. Neurosci. 28, 13467–13477.

Huang, W., Bhavsar, A., Ward, R.E., Hall, J.C., Priestley, J.V., et al., 2009. Arachidonyl trifluoromethyl ketone is neuroprotective after spinal cord injury. J. Neurotrauma 26, 1429–1434.

Jeffery, N.D., Smith, P.M., Lakatos, A., Ibanez, C., Ito, D., et al., 2006. Clinical canine spinal cord injury provides an opportunity to examine the issues in translating laboratory techniques into practical therapy. Spinal Cord 44, 584–593.

Jia, X.F., Ye, F., Wang, Y.B., Feng, D.X., 2016. ROCK inhibition enhances neurite outgrowth in neural stem cells by upregulating YAP expression in vitro. Neural Regen. Res. 11, 983–987.

Jiang, S.D., Dai, L.Y., Jiang, L.S., 2006. Osteoporosis after spinal cord injury. Osteoporos. Int. 17, 180–192.

Jiang, S.D., Jiang, L.S., Dai, L.Y., 2007. Changes in bone mass, bone structure, bone biomechanical properties, and bone metabolism after spinal cord injury: a 6-month longitudinal study in growing rats. Calcif. Tissue Int. 80, 167–175.

Jin, D., Liu, Y., Sun, F., Wang, X., Liu, X., et al., 2015. Restoration of skilled locomotion by sprouting corticospinal axons induced by co-deletion of PTEN and SOCS3. Nat. Commun 6, 8074.

Jupp, O.J., Vandenabeele, P., MacEwan, D.J., 2003. Distinct regulation of cytosolic phospholipase A_2 phosphorylation, translocation, proteolysis and activation by tumour necrosis factor- receptor subtypes. Biochem. J. 374, 453–461.

Kanno, H., Ozawa, H., Sekiguchi, A., Itoi, E., 2009. Spinal cord injury induces upregulation of beclin 1 and promotes autophagic cell death. Neurobiol. Dis. 33, 143–148.

Karimi-Abdolrezaee, S., Billakanti, R., 2012. Reactive astrogliosis after spinal cord injury-beneficial and detrimental effects. Mol. Neurobiol. 46, 251–264.

Karin, M., Liu, Z., Zandi, E., 1997. AP-1 function and regulation. Curr. Opin. Cell Biol. 9, 240–246.

Kauppinen, T.M., Swanson, R.A., 2007. The role of poly(ADP-ribose) polymerase-1 in CNS disease. Neuroscience 145, 1267–1272.

Keane, R.W., Davis, A.R., Dietrich, W.D., 2006. Inflammatory and apoptotic signaling after spinal cord injury. J. Neurotrauma 23, 335–344.

Kim, G.M., Xu, J., Xu, J.M., Song, S.K., Yan, P., et al., 2001. Tumor necrosis factor receptor deletion reduces nuclear factor-kappa B activation, cellular inhibitor of apoptosis protein 2 expression, and functional recovery after traumatic spinal cord injury. J. Neurosci. 21, 6617–6625.

Kirshblum, S.C., Burns, S.P., Biering-Sorensen, F., Donovan, W., Graves, D.E., et al., 2011. International standards for neurological classification of spinal cord injury. J. Spinal Cord Med. 34, 535–546.

Klussmann, S., Martin-Villalba, A., 2005. Molecular targets in spinal cord injury. J. Mol. Med. 83, 657–671.

Knoblach, S.M., Huang, X., VanGelderen, J., Calva-Cerqueira, D., Faden, A.E., 2005. Selective caspase activation may contribute to neurological dysfunction after experimental spinal cord trauma. J. Neurosci. Res. 80, 369–380.

Komjati, K., Besson, V.C., Szabo, C., 2005. Poly (adp-ribose) polymerase inhibitors as potential therapeutic agents in stroke and neurotrauma. Curr. Drug Targets CNS Neurol. Disord. 4, 179–194.

Kosik, K.S., 2006. The neuronal microRNA system. Nat. Rev. Neurosci. 7, 911–920.

Lang, C., Bradley, P.M., Jacobi, A., Kerschensteiner, M., Bareyre, F.M., 2013. STAT3 promotes corticospinal remodelling and functional recovery after spinal cord injury. EMBO Reports 2013 (1), 931–937.

Lazzaro, I., Tran, Y., Wijesuriya, N., Craig, A., 2013. Central correlates of impaired information processing in people with spinal cord injury. J. Clin. Neurophysiol. 30, 59–65.

Lee, Y.L., Bao, P., Ghirnikar, R.S., Eng, L.F., 2000. Cytokine chemokine expression in contused rat spinal cord. Neurochem. Int. 36, 417–425.

Lee, M.Y., Chen, L., Toborek, M., 2009. Nicotine attenuates iNOS expression and contributes to neuroprotection in a compressive model of spinal cord injury. J. Neurosci. Res. 87, 937–947.

Lee, S.I., Jeong, S.R., Kang, Y.M., et al., 2010. Endogenous expression of interleukin-4 regulates macrophage activation and confines cavity formation after traumatic spinal cord injury. J. Neurosci. Res. 88, 2409–2419.

Lin, C., Jiang, X., Dai, Z., Guo, X., Weng, T., et al., 2009. Sclerostin mediates bone response to mechanical unloading through antagonizing Wnt/beta-catenin signaling. J. Bone Miner. Res. 24, 1651–1661.

Lipinski, M.M., Wu, J., Faden, A.I., Sarkar, C., 2015. Function and mechanisms of autophagy in brain and spinal cord trauma. Antioxid. Redox Signal. 23, 565–577.

Liu, N., Han, S., Lu, P.H., Xu, X.M., 2004. Upregulation of annexins I, II, and V after traumatic spinal cord injury in adult rats. J. Neurosci. Res. 77, 391–401.

Liu, N.K., Zhang, Y.P., Titsworth, W.L., Jiang, X., Han, S., et al., 2006. A novel role of phospholipase A_2 in mediating spinal cord secondary injury. Ann. Neurol. 59, 606–619.

Liu, N.K., Zhang, Y.P., Han, S., Pei, J., Xu, L.Y., et al., 2007. Annexin A1 reduces inflammatory reaction and tissue damage through inhibition of phospholipase A_2 activation in adult rats following spinal cord injury. J. Neuropathol. Exp. Neurol. 66, 932–943.

Liu, N.K., Wang, X.F., Lu, Q.B., Xu, X.M., 2009. Altered microRNA expression following traumatic spinal cord injury. Exp. Neurol. 219, 424–429.

Liu, S., Sarkar, C., Dinizo, M., Faden, A.I., Koh, E.Y., et al., 2015. Disrupted autophagy after spinal cord injury is associated with ER stress and neuronal cell death. Cell Death Dis. 6, e1582.

Liu, X.Z., Xu, X.M., Hu, R., et al., 1997. Neuronal and glial apoptosis after traumatic spinal cord injury. J. Neurosci. 17, 5395–5406.

Losey, P., Young, C., Krimholtz, E., Bordet, E.R., Anthony, D.C., 2014. The role of hemorrhage following spinal-cord injury. Brain Res. 1569, 9–18.

Lytle, J.M., Wrathall, J.R., 2007. Glial cell loss, proliferation and replacement in the contused murine spinal cord. Eur. J. Neurosci. 25, 1711–1724.

Malemud, C.J., 2006. Matrix metalloproteinases (MMPs) in health and disease: an overview. Front. BioSci. 11, 1696–1701.

Marsala, J., Orendacova, J., Lukacova, N., Vanicky, I., 2007. Traumatic injury of the spinal cord and nitric oxide. Prog. Brain Res. 161, 171–183.

Matute, C., Domercq, M., Sánchez-Gómez, M.V., 2006. Glutamate-mediated glial injury: mechanisms and clinical importance. Glia 53, 212–224.

McEwen, M.L., Springer, J.E., 2005. A mapping study of caspase-3 activation following acute spinal cord contusion in rats. J. Histochem. Cytochem. 53, 809–819.

McKay, S.M., Brooks, D.J., Hu, P., McLachlan, E.M., 2007. Distinct types of microglial activation in white and grey matter of rat lumbosacral cord after mid-thoracic spinal transection. J. Neuropathol. Exp. Neurol. 66, 698–710.

McKeon, R.J., Jurynec, M.J., Buck, C.R., 1999. The chondroitin sulfate proteoglycans neurocan and phosphacan are expressed by reactive astrocytes in the chronic CNS glial scar. J. Neurosci. 19, 10778–10788.

Nesic, O., Svrakic, N.M., Xu, G.-Y., et al., 2002. DNA microarray analysis of the contused spinal cord: effect of NMDA receptor inhibition. J. Neurosci. Res. 68, 406–423. 2002.

Nobes, C.D., Hall, A., 1995. Rho, rac, and cdc42 GTPases regulate the assembly of multimolecular focal complexes associated with actin stress fibers, lamellipodia, and filopodia. Cell 81, 53–62.

Norenberg, M.D., Smith, J., Marcillo, A., 2004. The pathology of human spinal cord injury: defining the problems. J. Neurotrauma 21, 429–440.

Ong, W.Y., Horrocks, L.A., Farooqui, A.A., 1999. Immunocytochemical localization of $cPLA_2$ in rat and monkey spinal cords. J. Mol. Neurosci. 12, 123–130.

Pan, J.Z., Ni, L., Sodhi, A., Aguanno, A., Young, W., Hart, R.P., 2002. Cytokine activity contributes to induction of inflammatory cytokine mRNAs in spinal cord following contusion. J. Neurosci. Res. 68, 315–322.

Pan, W., Kastin, A.J., 2008. Cytokine transport across the injured blood-spinal cord barrier. Curr. Pharm. Des 14, 1620–1624.

Park, E., Velumian, A.A., Fehling, M.S., 2004. The role of excitotoxicity in secondary mechanisms of spinal cord injury: a review with an emphasis on the implications for white matter degeneration. J. Neurotrauma 21, 754–774.

Park, K., Lin, C., Lee, Y., 2014. Expression of Suppressor of Cytokine Signaling-3 (SOCS3) and its role in neuronal death after complete spinal cord injury. Exp. Neurol. 261, 65–75.

Pineau, I., Lacroix, S., 2007. Proinflammatory cytokine synthesis in the injured mouse spinal cord: multiphasic expression pattern and identification of the cell types involved. J. Comp. Neurol. 2007 (500), 267–285.

Profyris, C., Cheema, S.S., Zang, D., Azari, M.F., Boyle, K., et al., 2004. Degenerative and regenerative mechanisms governing spinal cord injury. Neurobiol. Dis. 15, 415–436.

Rafati, D.S., Geissler, K., Johnson, K., Unabia, G., Hulsebosch, C., et al., 2008. Nuclear factor-kappaB decoy amelioration of spinal cord injury-induced inflammation and behavior outcomes. J. Neurosci. Res. 86, 566–568.

Ray, S.K., Matzelle, D.C., Wilford, G.G., Hogan, E.L., Banik, N.L., 2000. E-64-d prevents both calpain upregulation and apoptosis in the lesion and penumbra following spinal cord injury in rats. Brain Res. 867, 80–89.

Ray, S.K., Matzelle, D.D., Sribnick, E.A., Guyton, M.K., Wingrave, J.M., et al., 2003a. Calpain inhibitor prevented apoptosis and maintained transcription of proteolipid protein and myelin basic protein genes in rat spinal cord injury. J. Chem. Neuroanat. 26, 119–124.

Ray, S.K., Hogan, E.L., Banik, N.L., 2003b. Calpain in the pathophysiology of spinal cord injury: neuroprotection with calpain inhibitors. Brain Res. Rev. 42, 169–185.

Ray, S.K., Samantaray, S., Smith, J.A., Matzelle, D.D., Das, A., et al., 2011. Inhibition of cysteine proteases in acute and chronic spinal cord injury. Neurotherapeutics 8, 180–186.

Reddy, S.J., La Marca, F., Park, P., 2008. The role of heat shock proteins in spinal cord injury. Neurosurg. Focus. 25, E4.

Resnick, D.K., Graham, S.H., Dixon, C.E., Marion, D.W., 1998. Role of cyclooxygenase 2 in acute spinal cord injury. J. Neurotrauma 15, 1005–1013.

Rice, T., Larsen, J., Rivest, S., Yong, V.W., 2007. Characterization of the early neuroinflammation after spinal cord injury in mice. J. Neuropath. Exp. Neurol. 66, 184–195.

Riegger, T., Conrad, S., Schluesener, H.J., Kaps, H.P., Badke, A., et al., 2009. Immune depression syndrome following human spinal cord injury (SCI): a pilot study. Neuroscience 158, 1194–1199.

Rowland, J.W., Hawryluk, G.W.J., Kwon, B., Fehlings, M.G., 2008. Current status of acute spinal cord injury pathophysiology and emerging therapies: promise on the horizon. Neurosurg. Focus 25, E2.

Rzonca, S.O., Suva, L.J., Gaddy, D., Montague, D.C., Lecka-Czernik, B., 2004. Bone is a target for the antidiabetic compound rosiglitazone. Endocrinology 145, 401–406.

Sastry, P.S., Rao, K.S., 2000. Apoptosis and the nervous system. J. Neurochem. 74, 1–20.

Schaefer, A., O'Carroll, D., Tan, C.L., Hillman, D., Sugimori, M., et al., 2007. Cerebellar neurodegeneration in the absence of microRNAs. J. Exp. Med. 204, 1553–1558.

Sharma, H.S., Westman, J., Olsson, Y., Alm, P., 1996. Involvement of nitric oxide in acute spinal cord injury: an immunocytochemical study using light and electron microscopy in the rat. Neurosci. Res. 24, 373–384.

Shin, H.J., Kim, H., Oh, S., Lee, J.G., Kee, M., et al., 2016. AMPK-SKP2-CARM1 signaling cascade in transcriptional regulation of autophagy. Nature 534, 553–557.

Siddall, P.J., 2009. Management of neuropathic pain following spinal cord injury: now and in the future. Spinal Cord 47, 352–359.

Silver, J., Miller, J.H., 2004. Regeneration beyond the glial scar. Nat. Rev. Neurosci. 5, 146–156.

Slaets, H., Nelissen, S., Janssens, K., Vidal, P.M., Lemmens, E., et al., 2014. Oncostatin M reduces lesion size and promotes functional recovery and neurite outgrowth after spinal cord injury. Mol. Neurobiol. 50, 1142–1151.

Song, G., Cechvala, C., Resnick, D.K., Dempsey, R.J., Rao, V.L., 2001. GeneChip analysis after acute spinal cord injury in rat. J. Neurochem. 79, 804–815.

Springer, J.E., Azbill, R.D., Nottingham, S.A., Kennedy, S.E., 2000. Calcineurin-mediated BAD dephosphorylation activates the caspase-3 apoptotic cascade in traumatic spinal cord injury. J. Neurosci. 20, 7246–7251.

Sun, D., Newman, T.A., Perry, V.H., Weller, R.O., 2004. Cytokine-induced enhancement of autoimmune inflammation in the brain and spinal cord: implications for multiple sclerosis. Neuropathol. Appl. Neurobiol. 30, 374–384.

Sun, X., Jones, Z.B., Chen, X.M., Zhou, L., So, K.F., et al., 2016. Multiple organ dysfunction and systemic inflammation after spinal cord injury: a complex relationship. J. Neuroinflamm. 13, 260.

Takahashi, J.L., Giuliani, F., Power, C., Imai, Y., Yong, V.W., 2003. Interleukin-1β promotes oligodendrocyte death through glutamate excitotoxicity. Ann. Neurol 53, 588–595.

Tassi, E., Walter, S., Aigner, A., Cabal-Manzano, R.H., 2007. Effects on neurite outgrowth and cell survival of a secreted fibroblast growth factor binding protein upregulated during spinal cord injury. Am. J. Physiol. Regul. Integr. Comp. Physiol. 293, R775–R783.

Ubogu, E.E., Cossoy, M.B., Ransohoff, R.M., 2006. The expression and function of chemokines involved in CNS inflammation. Trends Pharmacol. Sci. 27, 48–55.

Wang, G., Zhao, Y., Liu, S., Jia, J., Lu, T., 2016. Critical role of regulator of calcineurin 1 in spinal cord injury. J. Physiol. Biochem. 72, 605–613.

Wang, X., Chen, W., Liu, W., Wu, J., Shao, Y., et al., 2009. The role of thrombospondin-1 and transforming growth factor-beta after spinal cord injury in the rat. J. Clin. Neurosci. 16, 818–821.

Wanner, I.B., Anderson, M.A., Song, B., Levine, J., Fernandez, A., et al., 2013. Glial scar borders are formed by newly proliferated, elongated astrocytes that interact to corral inflammatory and fibrotic cells via STAT3-dependent mechanisms after spinal cord injury. J. Neurosci. 33, 12870–12886.

Weber, J.T., 2004. "Calcium homeostasis following traumatic neuronal injury,". Curr. Neurovasc. Res 1, 151–171.

Wells, J.E., Rice, T.K., Nuttall, R.K., Edwards, D.R., Zekki, H., et al., 2003. An adverse role for matrix metalloproteinase 12 after spinal cord injury in mice. J. Neurosci. 23, 10107–10115.

Wilson, C.J., Finch, C.E., Cohen, H.J., 2002. Cytokines and cognition—the case for a head-to-toe inflammatory paradigm. J. Am. Geriatr. Soc. 50, 2041–2056.

Wrigley, P.J., Gustin, S.M., Macey, P.M., Nash, P.G., Gandevia, S.C., et al., 2009. Anatomical changes in human motor cortex and motor pathways following complete thoracic spinal cord injury. Cereb. Cortex 19, 224–232.

Wu, J., Zhao, Z., Sabirzhanov, B., Stoica, B.A., Kumar, A., et al., 2014a. Spinal cord injury causes brain inflammation associated with cognitive and affective changes: role of cell cycle pathways. J. Neurosci. 34, 10989–11006.

Wu, J., Stoica, B.A., Luo, T., Sabirzhanov, B., Zhao, Z., et al., 2014b. Isolated spinal cord contusion in rats induces chronic brain neuroinflammation, neurodegeneration, and cognitive impairment. Cell Cycle 13, 2446–2458.

Wu, W., Chandler, L., Lu, Q., Wu, W., Eddelman, D.B., Parish, J.M., Xu, X.-M., 2017. RhoA/Rho kinase mediates neuronal death through regulating cPLA$_2$ activation. Mol. Neurobiol. 54, 6885–6895.

Xiong, Y., Rabchevsky, A.G., Hall, E.D., 2007. Role of peroxynitrite in secondary oxidative damage after spinal cord injury. J. Neurochem. 100, 639–649.

Xu, J., Fan, G.S., Chen, S.W., Wu, Y.J., Xu, X.M., Hsu, C.Y., 1998. Methylprednisolone inhibition of TNF-α expression and NF-κB activation after spinal cord injury in rats. Mol. Brain Res. 59, 135–142.

Yakovlev, A.G., Huang, X., VanGelderen, J., Calva-Cerqueira, D., Faden, A.I., 2005. Selective caspase activation may contribute to neurological dysfunction after experimental spinal cord trauma. J. Neurosci. Res. 80, 369–380.

Yan, X., Weng, H.-R., 2013. Endogenous interleukin-1β in neuropathic rats enhances glutamate release from the primary afferents in the spinal dorsal horn through coupling with presynaptic N-methyl-D-aspartic Acid receptors. J. Biol. Chem. 288, 30544–30557.

Yang, L., Blumbergs, P.C., Jones, N.R., Manavis, J., Sarvestani, G.T., et al., 2004. Early expression and cellular localization of proinflammatory cytokines interleukin-1beta, interleukin-6, and tumor necrosis factor-alpha in human traumatic spinal cord injury. Spine 29, 966–971.

Young, W., 2002. Spinal cord contusion models. Prog. Brain Res. 137, 231–255.

Yiu, G., He, Z., 2006. Glial inhibition of CNS axon regeneration. Nat. Rev. Neurosci. 7, 617–627.

Yu, F., Kamada, H., Niizuma, K., Endo, H., Chan, P.H., 2008. Induction of MMP-9 expression and endothelial injury by oxidative stress after spinal cord injury. J. Neurotrauma 25, 184–195.

Yu, W.R., Liu, T., Fehlings, T.K., Fehlings, M.G., 2009. Involvement of mitochondrial signaling pathways in the mechanism of Fas-mediated apoptosis after spinal cord injury. Eur. J. Neurosci. 29, 114–131.

Yu, D., Li, M., Ni, B., Kong, J., Zhang, Z., 2013. Induction of neuronal mitophagy in acute spinal cord injury in rats. Neurotox. Res. 24, 512–522.

Zhang, Z.J., Jiang, B.C., Gao, Y.J., 2017. Chemokines in neuron-glial cell interaction and pathogenesis of neuropathic pain. Cell Mol. Life Sci. 74 (18), 3275–3291. Available from: https://doi.org/10.1007/s00018-017-2513-1.

Zhao, P., Waxman, S.G., Hains, B.C., 2007a. Extracellular signal-regulated kinase-regulated microglia-neuron signaling by prostaglandin E2 contributes to pain after spinal cord injury. J Neurosci. 27, 2357–2368.

Zhao, P., Waxman, S.G., Hains, B.C., 2007b. Modulation of thalamic nociceptive processing after spinal cord injury through remote activation of thalamic microglia by cysteine chemokine ligand 21. J. Neurosci. 27, 8893–8902.

Potential Neuroprotective Strategies for Experimental Spinal Cord Injury

INTRODUCTION

Spinal cord injury (SCI) is a complex and devastating clinical condition, which is accompanied by the loss of motor and sensory functions below the injury site drastically decreasing the quality of life of affected individuals (Budh and Osteraker, 2007). The extent of functional losses following an SCI is largely determined by two factors: (1) the level at which the injury occurs (tetraplegia with cervical injuries or paraplegia with thoracic and lumbar injuries) and (2) the extent of tissue damage at the lesion site (complete or incomplete). Oxidative stress and neuroinflammation along with compromised energy metabolism are major contributors of neurodegeneration in SCI. Oxidative stress results in a number of detrimental effects such as lipid peroxidation, protein oxidation, and DNA damage. Lipid peroxidation not only disrupts normal structure and function of lipid bilayers surrounding both the cell itself and membrane-bound organelles but may also alter membrane permeability, transport processes, and fluidity (Farooqui and Horrocks, 2007; Catala, 2012). In addition, lipid peroxidation may ultimately result in the production of multiple aldehyde species (e.g., acrolein, malondialdehyde (MDA)), which may further contribute to toxicity associated with lipid peroxidation. Elevated markers of lipid peroxidation, including MDA, 4-hydroxynonenal (4-HNE), and acrolein, have been shown in animal models of SCI, indicating that lipid peroxidation may be an important contributor to the pathophysiology of SCI (Farooqui et al., 2004; Farooqui and Horrocks, 2009; Farooqui, 2010). ROS/RNS-mediated protein modifications include protein fragmentation, protein misfolding, protein—protein cross-linkages, production of

197

protein carbonyls, and priming of oxidized proteins for proteasomal degradation (Farooqui, 2010). In addition to lipid and protein oxidation, SCI may also induce ROS-mediated damage to DNA (Smith et al., 2013), which is accompanied by modification of DNA bases. Among all the nucleotide bases, guanine is the most susceptible to oxidative modifications due to its lowest reduction potential. Hydroxyl radicals have been shown to interact with the C4, C5, and C8 positions in the imidazole ring of guanine. Thus, formation of 8-hydroxyguanosine (8-OxoG) has been reported in a wide variety of disease states (Cooke et al., 2003). Similarly, peroxynitrite can react with guanine to form 8-nitroguanine (8-NO$_2$-G). This metabolite is considered a marker of nitrosative DNA damage (Smith et al., 2013). Unrepaired DNA damage can trigger apoptosis of neurons that is typically mediated by the ataxia telangiectasia mutated (ATM)-p53 pathway. Studies on telomere-directed DNA damage have indicated that postmitotic neurons with reduced telomerase activity are not only vulnerable to DNA damage but are also prone to apoptosis demonstrating a pivotal role for telomere maintenance in both mitotic cells and post mitotic neurons (Smith et al., 2013).

Neuroinflammation is a complex host defense mechanism that isolates the damaged neural cells from uninjured cells, destroys injured neural cells, and repairs the extracellular matrix (Farooqui, 2010, 2014). Neuroinflammation is orchestrated by microglia and astrocytes to re-establish homeostasis in the spinal cord after SCI-mediated disequilibrium of normal physiology. Neuroinflammation is mediated and maintained by the generation of high levels of proinflammatory eicosanoids (prostaglandins (PGs), leukotriens (LTs), and thromboxanes (TXs)), platelet-activating factor, and increased expression of high levels of proinflammatory cytokines (tumor necrosis factor-α (TNF-α), interleukin-1β (IL-1β), and interleukin 10 (IL-10)) and chemokines (MCP-1). High levels of proinflammatory eicosanoids; cytokines and chemokines not only overwhelm antioxidant and antiinflammatory defenses but also contribute to the development of cytotoxicity, edema, and neurodegeneration following SCI (Farooqui, 2014).

As stated in Chapter 4, Molecular Aspects of Spinal Cord Injury, SCI is accompanied by influx of extracellular Ca^{2+}, activation of phospholipase A$_2$ (PLA$_2$), nitric oxide synthase (NOS), protein kinases, and calpains along with disruption of many biochemical pathways, which result in induction apoptosis (Farooqui, 2010). After SCI, depletion of peripheral macrophages enhances axonal regeneration and improves functional recovery (Popovich et al., 1999). Administration of the antiinflammatory drug minocycline produces similar effects (Stirling et al., 2005). However, more recent studies indicate that the inflammatory response may also positively contribute to regeneration (Yong and Rivest, 2009; David and Kroner, 2011), as is exemplified by an improved behavioral outcome after SCI resulting from an increased number of monocyte-derived macrophages via adoptive transfer (Shechter et al., 2009). These observations have led to substantial controversy regarding the negative or positive effect of acute inflammation in brain and spinal cord regeneration. In contrast to mammals, adult zebrafish are capable of extensive and successful regeneration throughout their body, including their fins, heart, liver, and central nervous system (CNS) (Keightley et al., 2014). Thus, adult zebrafish retains the capacity of robust axonal regeneration and can morphologically and functionally recover from optic nerve and spinal cord injuries (Becker and Becker, 2014). Moreover, similar to the situation in mammals, an acute inflammatory response occurs after CNS injury in zebrafish, which has recently been suggested to positively contribute to the regenerative process (Kyritsis et al., 2014).

Earlier studies on the treatment of SCI with antioxidants and antiinflammatory drugs have resulted in limited beneficial effects, because injured axons within the brain and spinal cord do not regenerate spontaneously. In addition to the above changes that cause secondary tissue damage, substances inhibitory to spinal cord repair, and a barrier to axon growth (a scar) forms begin to appear. Thus, for the survival of neurons and repair of the spinal cord, neuroscientists must consider halting the spread of secondary tissue damage to save as many neurons as possible, curb inflammation, reduce scar formation, neutralize inhibitory factors, awaken nerve cells to regrow fibers, provide sustenance to surviving nerve cells, promote fiber growth across the area of injury, guide growth to appropriate areas, and enable the formation of connections. In recent years, basic science, preclinical, and clinical studies are aimed at overcoming the factors that are involved in successful recovery from SCI (Varma et al., 2013; Ahuja et al., 2016). Specifically, a major objective of current research is to manage SCI patients by retarding secondary injury, promoting regeneration, and replacing damaged spinal cord tissue (Schwab et al., 2006; Fouad and Tse, 2008; Wilson et al., 2013; Tsintou et al., 2015). To this end, many ongoing clinical trials of neuroprotective agents are underway in SCI patients (Kwon et al., 2011). Furthermore, there has been increasing interest in research on strategies to optimize conditions for the survival and the function of the grafted stem cells are needed for the treatment of SCI (Wilson et al., 2013; Guest et al., 2011; Silva et al., 2014).

NEUROCHEMICAL ASPECTS OF GLIAL SCAR FORMATION

Several factors such as myelin-associated glycoprotein (MAG), inhibitors associated with the glial scar that are induced after injury (chondroitin sulfate proteoglycans, CSPGs); and inhibitors of the axon guidance molecules (semaphorin, ephrin, slits, netrin and bone morpho-genetic proteins, BMPs) along with myelin-associated glycoprotein (Nogo) and oligodendrocyte-myelin glycoprotein (OMgp), alterations in Wnts signaling, and local inflammatory response contribute to the growth-hostile environment in the injured spinal cord tissue (Yiu and He, 2006) and this growth-hostile environment not only promote glial scar formation, but also retards the regeneration of injured neurons in the spinal cord after SCI (Filbin, 2003; McKerracher and Rosen, 2015; Pizzi and Crowe, 2007; Kwok et al., 2008; Yiu and He, 2006). In addition, SCI also promote the increase in immunolabeling of neurocan, brevican, and versican within days in injured spinal cord at the lesion site. The neurocan and verican immunolabeling peaks at 2 weeks and remain elevated from weeks to months. These molecules may also limit axonal regeneration (Jones et al., 2003).

After SCI, astrocytes become hypertrophic, undergo proliferation, migrate towards the injury site, synthesize CSPGs, a linear polysaccharide of varying length made up of the repeating disaccharide units glucuronic acid and N-acetylgalactosamine that are sulfated within the extracellular matrix, and create an irregular mesh-like barrier of inter-woven cell processes (Bartus et al., 2011; Yuan and He, 2013). The extent of sulfation in CSPGs varies dynamically not only during development, but also diseases and injury. As stated in chapter 4, main inhibitory myelin components include oligodendrocyte-myelin glycoprotein (OMgp), MAG and leukocyte common antigen-related phosphatase (LAR); transmembrane protein tyrosine phosphatase (PTPσ); Nogo receptor1/3 (NgR1/3); and $p75^{NTR}$. The converging intra-axonal inhibitory signals from these molecules activate RhoA. Subsequently, the Rho-associated coiled kinase (ROCK) is activated. ROCK not only contributes to modulation of cytoskeleton of the nerve fiber growth cone, but also induces collapse of growth cones (Schmandke et al. 2007). In addition, inhibition of RhoA/Rho kinase improves axon regeneration, remyelination and functional recovery. To determine whether RhoA/Rho kinase plays a role in neuronal death after injury. To investigate the relationship between RhoA/Rho kinase and cytosolic phospholipase A_2 (cPLA$_2$), a lipase that contribute to neuroinflammation and cell death, in vivo studies have been performed in contusive SCI model (Wu et al., 2017) and it is reported that inhibition of RhoA, Rho kinase and cPLA$_2$ significantly reduces TNF-α/glutamate-mediated cell death. Inhibition of RhoA and Rho kinase also significantly downregulates cPLA$_2$ activation. Furthermore, inhibition of RhoA and Rho kinase reduces the release of arachidonic acid. The immunofluorescence staining demonstrates that two isoforms of Rho kinase (ROCK$_1$ and ROCK$_2$), are co-localized with cPLA$_2$ in neuronal cytoplasm. Interestingly, co-immunoprecipitation (Co-IP) assay show that ROCK$_1$ or ROCK$_2$ bond directly with cPLA$_2$ and phospho-cPLA$_2$. Treatment with the Rho kinase inhibitor Y27632 significantly decreases $cPLA_2$ activation and expression and reduces SCI-mediated apoptosis at and close to the lesion site. Taken together, these results reveal a novel mechanism of RhoA/Rho kinase-mediated neuronal death through regulating $cPLA_2$ activation (Wu et 2017). Furthermore, inhibition of the Rho-cascade blocks the integration of the growth-inhibitory signal into the injured axon, resulting in propagated sprouting following axonal injury. NG2 cells (oligodendrocyte progenitors or polydendrocytes), which are typically expressed on the cell membrane contribute to scar formation by shedding their extracellular domain *via* cleavage with metalloproteinases (MMPs) (Asher et al., 2005). These cells proliferate and differentiate into oligodendrocytes and astrocytes *in vitro* as well as development of oligodendrocytes *in vivo* through Jak/STAT signaling after contusive SCI (Barres et al., 1996, Ishibashi et al., 2009). Surprisingly little is known about the cellular interactions and signaling mechanisms whereby astroglia and NG2 cells interact with each other to form scar borders or to surround other cells in the lesion core. The expression of cytokine is increased in the glial scar region after contusive SCI (Tripathi and McTigue, 2008, Zai et al., 2005) and high levels of phospho-STAT3, which is nearly undetectable in the uninjured spinal cord, are increased in NG2 cells in this region (Hesp et al., 2015, Tripathi and McTigue, 2008). It is proposed that both STAT3 and SOCS3 contribute to astroglial scar formation after SCI (Herrmann et al., 2008; Wanner et al., 2013). In addition, increase in the expression of NG2 (an integral membrane protein) in the glial scar also promote inhibition of axon regeneration (Dou and Levine, 1994). This is accompanied by fibroblast-mediated deposition of CSPGs and tenascin (Snow et al., 1990; Höke and Silver, 1996). During scar formation CSPGs and myelin glycoproteins act via the Rho-ROCK (rho-associated protein kinase) pathway to inhibit neurite outgrowth by signaling growth cone collapse through effector kinases (Fig. 5.1) (Forgione and Fehlings, 2014). This affects axon projections, guidance, extension and nerve regeneration (Liu, 2012; Teramura et al., 2012). Thus, researchers have targeted the Rho/ROCK signaling pathway in attempts to promote neural regeneration (Fujimura et al., 2011; Tan et al., 2009).

Together, induction of above mentioned mechanisms severely restricts endogenous neural circuit regeneration and oligodendrocyte remyelination at a cellular level. As stated in chapter 4, treatment of CSPGs chains with exogenous chondroitinase ABC promotes axon regeneration and reactivates neural plasticity (Kwok et al., 2008). Inhibitor of mitochondrial fission called Mdivi-1 has been reported to modulate astrocyte proliferation, astroglial scar formation, and axonal regeneration following SCI in rats (Li et al., 2016). Furthermore, Mdivi-1 reduces the expression of glial fibrillary acidic protein (GFAP) and neurocan (CSPG). Notably, immunofluorescent labeling and Nissl staining

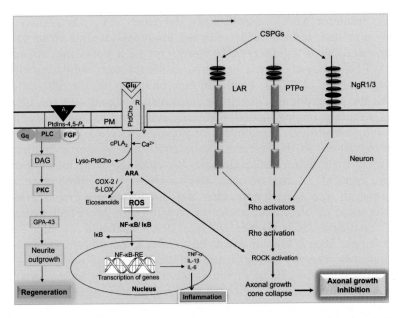

FIGURE 5.1 Inhibition of axonal growth by CSPGs and its receptors. PM, Plasma membrane; Glu, glutamate; NMDA-R, N-Methyl-D-aspartate receptor; PtdCho, phosphatidylcholine; lyso-PtdCho, lyso-phosphatidylcholine; PtdIns-4,5-P_2, Phosphatidylinositol 4,5-bisphosphate; PLC, phospholipase C; COX-2, cyclooxygenase-2; LOX, lipoxygenase; LTs, leukotriens; TXs, thromboxanes; ROS, reactive oxygen species; NF-κB-RE, nuclear factor-κB response element; LAR, leukocyte common antigen-related phosphatase; PTPσ, transmembrane protein tyrosine phosphatase; NgR1/3, Nogo receptor 1/3; small GTPase RhoA; ROCK, Rho kinase; DAG, diacylglycerol; PKC, protein kinase C; GAP-43, growth associated protein-43.

studies show that Mdivi-1 elevates the production of growth-associated protein-43 and increases neuronal survival at 4 weeks after SCI (Li et al., 2016). Finally, hematoxylin-eosin staining and behavioral evaluation of motor function indicates that Mdivi-1 also reduces cavity formation and improves motor function 4 weeks after SCI. Collectively, these studies support the view that Mdivi-1 promotes motor function after SCI not only by inhibiting astrocyte activation, retarding astroglial scar formation and contribute to axonal regeneration after SCI in rats, but also by reactivating neural plasticity (Kwok et al., 2008; Li et al., 2016).

METALLOPROTEINASES AND GLIAL SCAR FORMATION

As stated above, during glial scar formation, astrocytes migrate toward the lesion, and this process involves matrix metalloproteinases (MMPs), a family of zinc-dependent proteinases, which are associated with the degradation of components of the extracellular matrix and cleavage of cell surface receptors and adhesion molecules (Noble et al., 2002; Wells et al., 2002; Pizzi and Crowe, 2007). MMPs not only facilitate the migration of astrocytes by degrading the core protein of some CSPGs as well as other growth-inhibitory molecules such as Nogo and tenascin-C but also play an important role in blood–spinal cord barrier dysfunction, inflammation, and locomotor recovery (Noble et al., 2002; Hsu et al., 2008). Regulation of MMPs occurs at multiple levels, including transcription, proximity to the cell surface, zymogen activation, degradation/inactivation, and endogenous inhibition (Parks et al., 2004). MMP expression is generally low in the adult brain and spinal cord but is upregulated in response to various CNS injuries and diseases (Yong, 2005). SCI results in activation of MMPs, in particular gelatinase B (MMP-9). MMPs activation in the spinal cord contributes to disruption of the blood–spinal cord barrier, and the influx of leukocytes into the injured cord, as well as apoptosis (Yong, 2005). MMP-9 and MMP-2 regulate neuroinflammation and neuropathic pain following SCI. Inhibition of MMPs or the gelatinases (MMP-2 and MMP-9) results in an improvement in long-term neurological recovery and is associated with reduced glial scarring and neuropathic pain supporting the view that MMPs play a crucial role in SCIs.

Studies on MMP-9-null mice, which exhibit significantly less disruption of the blood–spinal cord barrier, attenuation of neutrophil infiltration, and significant locomotor recovery compared with wild-type mice, have indicated that MMP-9 plays a key role in abnormal vascular permeability and inflammation within the first 3 days after SCI (Noble et al., 2002). Detailed investigation on the SCI in wild-type mice expressing MMPs and MMP-9 null mice indicate that wild-type mice expressing MMPs develop a more severe glial scar and enhanced expression of CPGS supporting the existence of a more inhibitory environment for axonal regeneration/plasticity than MMP-9 null mice (Hsu et al., 2008). Treatment of MMP-9 null astrocytes and wild-type astrocytes with MMP-9 inhibitor results in impairment of astrocytes migration compared to untreated wild-type controls. MMP-9 null astrocytes show abnormalities in the actin cytoskeletal organization and function but no detectable untoward effects on proliferation, cellular viability, or adhesion (Wells et al., 2002; Hsu et al., 2008). Interestingly, MMP-2 null astrocytes show increased migration, which can be attenuated in the presence of an MMP-9 inhibitor. Collective evidence suggests that MMP-9 contributes to inhibitory glial scar formation and cytoskeleton-mediated astrocyte migration.

As stated in Chapter 4, Molecular Aspects of Spinal Cord Injury, numerous neurochemical changes in spinal cord tissue occur following SCI. There is no treatment available that restores the SCI-induced loss of function to a degree that an independent life can be guaranteed. Three fundamental strategies have been developed in animal models of SCI. They include neuroprotection (pharmacological prevention of some of the damaging intracellular cascades that lead to secondary tissue loss) to reduce the progressive secondary injury processes that occur during the first few weeks after the initial trauma. The second strategy, which is initiated not long after the trauma, aims at promoting axonal regeneration by acting on the main barrier to regeneration of lesioned axons: the glial scar (cell transplantation, genetic engineering to increase growth factors, neutralization of inhibitory factors, and reduction in scar formation). The third strategy includes the management of the sublesional spinal cord by sensorimotor stimulation and/or supply of missing key afferents as a part of rehabilitation (Bunge, 2008). The main objective of investigators in SCI field is to discover the effective combination strategies to improve outcome after SCI to the adult rat thoracic spinal cord. Combination interventions include implantation of Schwann cells (SCs) plus neuroprotective drugs (methylprednisolone sodium succinate (MPSS), monosialo-ganglioside GM_1, calpain inhibitors, ω-3 or n-3 fatty acids) (Fig. 5.2) administration of growth factors (BDNF, bFGF, EGF, GDNF, IGF-1) in various ways, olfactory ensheathing cell (OEC) implantation, chondroitinase addition, or elevation of cyclic AMP, and injection of stem/progenitor cells (Bunge, 2008). All these are known to promote behavioral and functional recovery in animal models of SCI.

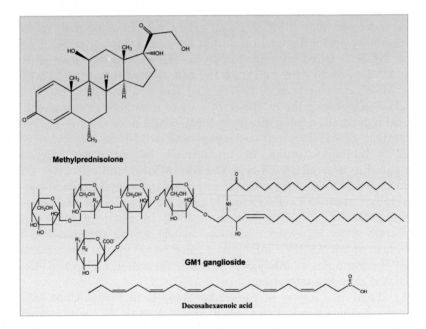

FIGURE 5.2   Chemical structures of MP, GM1 ganglioside, SJA6017, and docosahexaenoic acid.

NEUROPROTECTIVE STRATEGIES FOR SCI

Very little progress has been made on pharmacologic treatment of SCI in humans. Many treatment studies have shown no improvement on behavioral and neurologic outcome following SCI in animal models. These trials involve not only the treatment with neuroprotective agents and regeneration inducing agents but also surgery and rehabilitation care (Hawryluk et al., 2008). In neuroprotection trials involve the use of methylprednisolone (MP), thyrotropin-releasing hormone, and gangliosides. Many randomized controlled trials have been performed on the use of MPSS, monosialoganglioside (GM1), thyrotropin releasing hormone, and calpain inhibitors. The primary outcome in these trials has been negative. However, administration of MPSS within 8 hours after SCI produces some beneficial effects. A drawback of these SCI trials has been the use of therapeutic agents that block single pathway. It is well known that neurodegeneration in SCI is multifactorial process involving excitotoxicity, oxidative stress, mitochondrial dysfunction, and neuroinflammation. So, the effective therapies for SCI must include drugs that modulate multiple pathophysiological pathways associated with oxidative stress and neuroinflammation.

Regeneration involves stem cell transplantation and similar rehabilitative restorative approaches designed to optimize spontaneous regeneration by mobilizing endogenous stem cells and facilitating other cellular mechanisms of regeneration, such as axonal growth and myelination. It includes the use of pluripotent human stem cells, embryonic stem cells, and a number of adult-derived stem and progenitor cells, such as mesenchymal stem cells, SCs, OECs, and adult-derived neural precursor cells. Although current strategies to repair the subacutely injured cord appear promising, many obstacles continue to render the treatment of acute and chronic SCI challenging; therefore, more research is required on the treatment of SCI (Eftekharpour et al., 2008; Hawryluk et al., 2008).

Strategies for rehabilitation include passive exercise, active exercise with some voluntary control, and the use of neuroprostheses. These activities enhance sensorimotor recovery after SCI by promoting adaptive structural and functional plasticity while mitigating maladaptive changes at multiple levels of the neuraxis. Following SCI, the degree and extent of neuroplasticity and recovery depend not only on the level and extent of injury but also on postinjury medical and surgical care and rehabilitative interventions. Rehabilitation strategies are focused less on repairing lost connections and more on modulating neuroplasticity, which may promote regaining of neural cell function (Lynskey et al., 2008). The mechanism of plasticity and neural adaptation is not fully understood. However, basic mechanisms of plasticity include neurogenesis, programmed cell death, and activity-dependent synaptic plasticity. Repetitive stimulation of synapses may result in long-term potentiation or long-term depression of neurotransmission. These changes are associated with physical changes in dendritic spines and neuronal circuits. There are four major types of plasticity: adaptive plasticity, impaired plasticity, excessive plasticity, and the "Achilles heel" of the developing brain. Plasticity is modulated by genetic factors, such as mutations in brain-derived neuronal growth factor. Induction of neural plasticity may facilitate endogenous recovery. The reorganization of injured tissue is rapidly induced by acute injury and is likely based on unmasking of latent synapses resulting from modulation of neurotransmitters, while the long-term changes after chronic injury involve changes of synaptic efficacy modulated by long-term potentiation and axonal regeneration and sprouting (Ding et al., 2005). The functional significance of neural plasticity after SCI remains unclear. It indicates that in some situations plasticity changes can result in functional improvement, whereas in other situations they may have harmful consequences. Thus, more studies and better understanding of the molecular mechanisms of plasticity may lead to better ways of promoting useful reorganization and preventing undesirable consequences (Ding et al., 2005).

MP AND SCI

MP is a synthetic glucocorticoid hormone, which is the most commonly used antiinflammatory and antioxidant drug in the treatment of acute SCI (Bains and Hall, 2012). In the landmark, Second National Spinal Cord Injury Study (NASCIS-II) was performed with 437 participants with acute SCIs. These patients were randomized to an initial bolus of 30 mg/kg of MPSS (Fig. 5.2) followed by an infusion of 5.4 mg/kg/hour for 23 hours versus either naloxone or placebo (Bracken et al., 1990, 1992). The standard MPSS treatment protocol also requires the spine immobilization, management of neurogenic shock for perfusion and oxygenation, intravenous injection of MPSS, surgical interventions to stabilize and decompress the spinal cord, prompt anatomic alignment of the spine bony elements along with continuous intravenous injection of dopamine hydrochloride to reverse the neurogenic shock, and maintenance of normal to high blood pressure.

The molecular mechanism associated with action of MPSS is not fully understood. However, it is proposed that in animal models of SCI, MPSS acts through the modulation of the Wnt/β-catenin signaling pathway, a process that is activated following SCI (Fig. 5.3) (Lu et al., 2016). The molecular and cellular mechanisms underlying these neuroprotective effects of MPSS may be associated with a reduction in the number

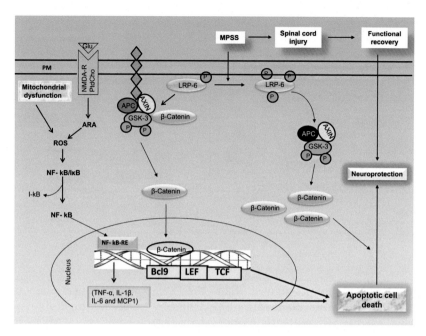

FIGURE 5.3 Hypothetical diagram showing beneficial effects of MP in SCI. PM, Plasma membrane; Glu, glutamate; NMDA-R, N-Methyl-D-aspartate receptor; PtdCho, phosphatidylcholine; ROS, reactive oxygen species; NF-κB-RE, nuclear factor-κB response element; LRP6, low-density lipoprotein receptor—related protein 6, LEF-1, lymphoid enhancer factor-1 (LEF-1); TCF, T-cell factor; Axin, scaffolding protein; APC, the tumor suppressor *adenomatous polyposis coli* gene product; GSK3, glycogen synthase kinase 3.

of apoptotic cells, which is accompanied by reduction in levels of activated caspase-3, caspase-9, and Bax protein expression, while the anti-apoptotic Bcl-2 levels are increased in the spinal cord anterior horn of MPSS-treated rats. Interestingly, MPSS further upregulates the expression levels and activation of the Wnt/β-catenin signaling pathway, including LRP-6 phosphorylation, β-catenin, and GSK3-β phosphorylation, following SCI. Collectively, these studies indicate that neuroprotective effect of MPSS involves suppression of apoptotic cell death, which may be correlated with the activation of the Wnt/β-catenin signaling pathway (Lu et al., 2016).

In recent years, however, the use of MPSS for acute SCI in human patients has become controversial due to the induction of increased risk of major complications (Fehlings et al., 2014; Hurlbert, 2014) such as gastrointestinal ulcer/bleeding, immunosuppression, and increased risk of infections (Fig. 5.4). Investigators supporting the use of MPSS for SCI argue that the evidence for MPSS administration supports modest neurological benefit although the strength of this evidence is moderate.

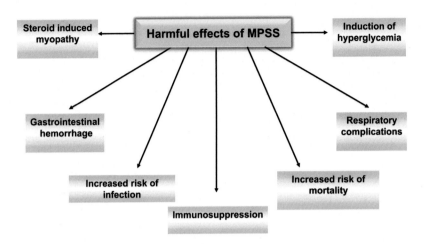

FIGURE 5.4   Harmful effects of MP in SCI.

These investigators suggest that the small neurological benefits (inhibition of neuroinflammation) mediated by MPSS administration are important for SCI patients. Critics of the administration of MPSS for acute SCI note that MPSS has never demonstrated benefit in the analysis of the primary endpoint in any study (Chappell, 2002; Bracken, 2012). In their opinion the statistical methods used in the supporting literature lack rigor and that the potential harms of MPSS outweigh any small potential neurological benefits (Chappell, 2002; Bracken, 2012). NASCIS III studies have also reached to similar conclusion. The failure of NASCIS II and III studies to show profound improvement in recoveries of SCI patients suggests that MPSS may not be a good neuroprotective agent in SCI patients. Although neuroprotective studies in human patients have failed, studies on the effect of MPSS in animal models of SCI indicate that injections of 30 mg/kg MP into rats with SCI immediately postinjury and at 1 and 2 days postinjury promote locomotor functional recovery between 2 and 6 weeks postinjury (Lu et al., 2016). Furthermore, the number of surviving motor neurons increased significantly, whereas the lesion size is significantly decreased following MP treatment at 7 days postinjury. In addition, caspase-3, caspase-9, and Bax protein expression levels and the number of apoptotic cells are reduced at 3 and 7 days postinjury, whereas Bcl-2 levels at 7 days postinjury are increased in MP-treated rats compared with saline-treated rats. At 3 and 7 days postinjury, MP treatment upregulates expression and activation of the Wnt/β-catenin signaling pathway (Lu et al., 2016). These results indicate that MP mediates its neuroprotective effects through the activation of the Wnt/β-catenin signaling pathway, which involves the increased expression of specific proteins, including low-density lipoprotein receptor—related protein-6 phosphorylation, β-catenin, and glycogen synthase kinase-3β (Lu et al., 2016). MPSS may also act by producing antiautophagic effects in neuron-like cells exposed to oxidative damage (Gao et al., 2016).

GM1 GANGLIOSIDE AND SCI

Gangliosides, sialic acid-containing glycosphingolipids, are a major component of neuronal cells and are essential for brain function. They contain sphingosine, fatty acid, and an oligosaccharide chain that varies in size from one to four or more monosaccharides (Fig. 5.2). They not only are involved in the development, differentiation, and function of nervous tissues but also play important roles in the maintenance and repair of nervous tissues (Ohmi et al., 2012).

Studies on animal models of SCI have indicated that GM1 ganglioside produces beneficial effects in SCI. In animal models of SCI, GM1 ganglioside may act not only as a membrane stabilizer, an antiexcitotoxic, and antioxidant but may also reduce neuronal edema by promoting activation of sodium, potassium, and magnesium pumps. Furthermore, it has been shown to facilitate nerve cell homeostasis by re-establishing the membrane equilibrium (Walker and Harris, 1993). In addition, it has been shown to increase the presence of endogenous neurotrophic factors. These activities diminish the destruction of neurons following trauma by increasing the plasticity of lesioned medullary circuits and hastening the recovery of the functional connections (Geisler et al., 2001a, 2001b). Administration of GM1 ganglioside produces an effective locomotive function recovery in rats (Carvalho et al., 2008). An initial small single-center phase II trial of 37 patients indicated that the administration of GM1 to SCI patients within 24 hours after injury may induce improvement in neurological recovery (Geisler et al., 1991). Subsequently, the same investigator led a multi-center Phase III trial of GM1 in acute SCI patients. Because GM1 trial was performed after the widespread acceptance of high-dose MPSS as the standard of care for acute SCI, studies on effects of GM1 were performed after 24-hour NASCIS II high-dose MP protocol (Geisler et al., 2001a; Geisler et al., 2001b). GM1 failed to show any evidence of a significant enhancement in the extent of neurological recovery over the MP therapy alone.

INHIBITORS OF CALPAINS, NOS, PLA₂ IN SCI

As stated in Chapter 4, Molecular Aspects of Spinal Cord Injury, SCI is characterized by the influx of free Ca^{2+}, which results in the stimulation of Ca^{2+}-dependent enzymes including calpains, NOSs, phospholipases A_2, protein kinase C (Farooqui, 2010). At the injury site calpains activity is markedly increased, and this activation contributes to neuronal death (Ray et al., 2003; Buki et al 2003). As stated in Chapter 4, calpain activity is modulated by calpastatin. Overactivation of calpains promotes the degradation of key cytoskeletal, membrane, and myelin proteins. Cleavage of these key proteins by calpain is an irreversible process that perturbs the integrity and stability of neural cells, leading to neuronal cell death. It is reported that calpains in conjunction with caspases and Kallikrein 6 promote neuronal apoptosis in brain and spinal cord tissues. Many cell-permeable calpain inhibitors such as calpeptin and SJA 6017 (Fig. 5.5) target the active site of calpains and have been effective against these enzymes and are under evaluation in animal models of SCI. Other calpain inhibitors (MDL-28170, N-acetyl-Leu-Leu-Met-CHO (ALLM), calpain inhibitor III (CI III) (MDL28170 and CEP-4143)) have shown to be significantly neuroprotective in animal models of SCI suggesting their therapeutic potential (Ray et al., 2003; Buki et al 2003; Schumacher et al., 2000; Moriwaki et al., 2005). Clinical trials of calpain inhibitors have not been performed in human patients with SCI.

Several isoforms of NOS have been reported to occur in brain and spinal cord (Marsala et al., 2007). The activities of endothelial NOS (eNOS)

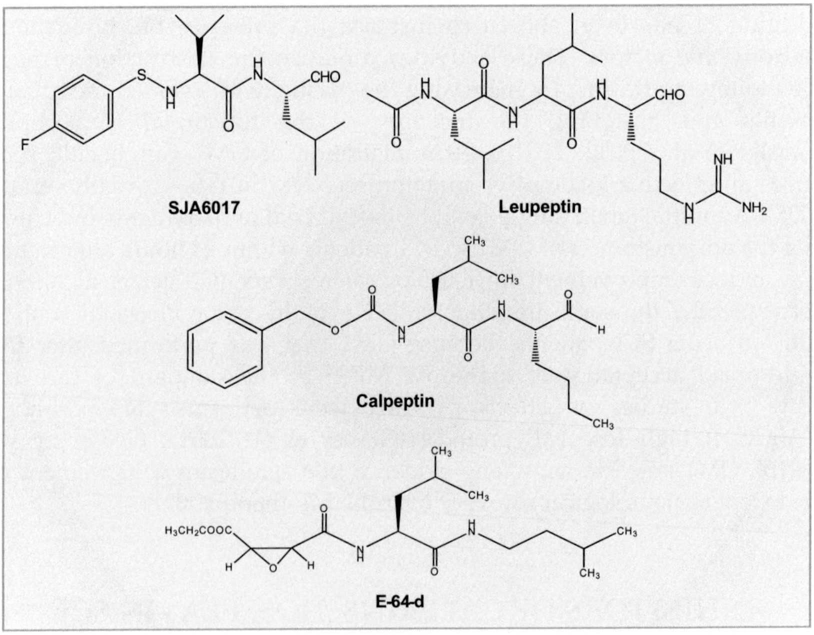

FIGURE 5.5   Chemical structures of calpain inhibitors used for SCI studies.

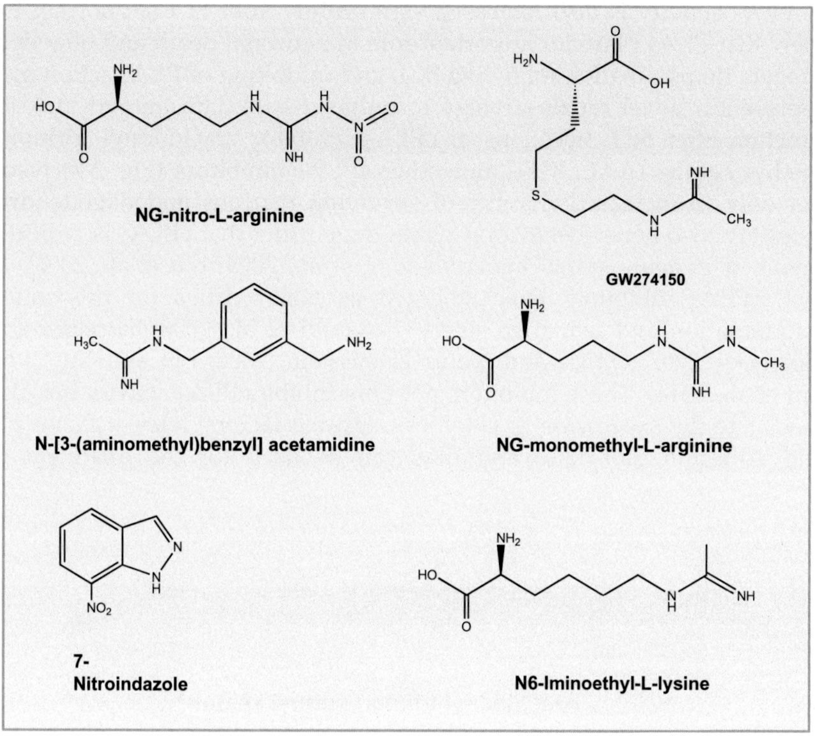

FIGURE 5.6   Chemical structures of NOS inhibitors used for SCI studies.

or neuronal NOS (nNOS) are modulated by phosphorylation, which is triggered by influx of Ca^{2+} and binding with calmodulin. In contrast, the regulation of inducible NOS (iNOS) depends on de novo synthesis of the enzyme in response to a variety of cytokines, such as TNF-α and interferon-γ. SCI produces upregulation of nNOS activity in neurons, eNOS in glial cells and vascular endothelium, and later an increase in iNOS activity has been observed in a range of cells, including infiltrating neutrophils and macrophages, activated microglia and astrocytes. Studies on expression of inducible iNOS and/or nNOS in injured spinal cords indicate that SCI dramatically increases iNOS (but not nNOS) mRNA and protein levels in microglial cells in the thoracic and lumbar regions of spinal cords. iNOS overexpression causes an increased nitrotyrosine formation, decreased number of NeuN (neuronal nuclei)-immunoreactive cells, and upregulation of inflammatory genes (Fig. 5.6) (Lee et al., 2009). As stated in Chapter 4, excessive amounts of NO in neural cells give arise to highly toxic oxidant (peroxynitrite, nitric dioxide, and nitron ion) that is associated with apoptotic and necrotic cell death in SCI. Clinical trials of NOS inhibitors in animal models and human patients have not been performed.

PLA$_2$ activity is also increased significantly after SCI supporting the view that PLA$_2$ plays an important role in neuronal death and oligodendrocyte demyelination following SCI, and inhibition of PLA$_2$ action may represent a novel repair strategy to reduce tissue damage and increase function after SCI. Injections of cPLA$_2$ inhibitor arachidonyl trifluoromethyl ketone (AACOCF$_3$) and other cPLA$_2$ inhibitors (Fig. 5.7) result not only in increased number of surviving neurons and oligodendrocytes but also better behavioral scores suggesting that cPLA$_2$ is critically involved in acute spinal injury (Huang et al., 2009; Liu et al., 2006). In fact, cPLA$_2$ inhibitors have emerged as major drugs for preventing inflammation and oxidative stress (Farooqui et al., 2006; Farooqui and Horrocks, 2007; Olivas and Noble-Haeusslein, 2006; Liu and Xu, 2010; Liu et al., 2014). These inhibitors not only inhibit cPLA$_2$ activity but also modulate the expression of cytokines, growth factors, nuclear factor-κB, and adhesion molecules and thus can be used for the treatment of

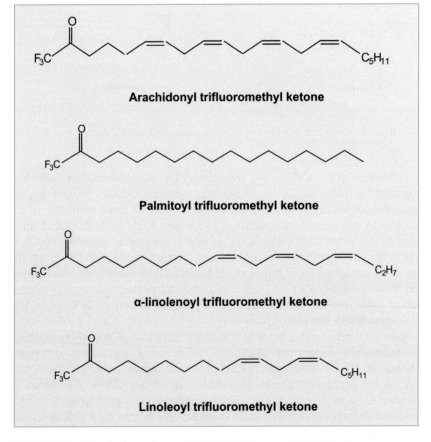

Arachidonyl trifluoromethyl ketone

Palmitoyl trifluoromethyl ketone

α-linolenoyl trifluoromethyl ketone

Linoleoyl trifluoromethyl ketone

FIGURE 5.7   Chemical structures of cPLA$_2$ inhibitors used for SCI studies.

endogenous oxidative stress and neuroinflammation in SCI animal models. Genetic deletion of $cPLA_2$ also inhibits the expression of active caspase-3 after SCI, suggesting that $cPLA_2$ activation mediates neural apoptosis. $cPLA_2^{-/-}$ mice also show significant reductions in ARA release and eicosanoid production in response to a variety of stimuli (Sapirstein and Bonventre, 2000). Collectively, these studies suggest that $cPLA_2$ contributes to neuronal injury by a direct effect on cell membranes and/or indirectly through generation of its metabolites, which are inflammatory and vasoconstrictive mediators (Farooqui and Horrocks, 2007). Clinical trials of $cPLA_2$ inhibitors in animal models and human SCI patients have not been performed.

MINOCYCLINE AND SCI

Minocycline is a lipophilic second-generation tetracycline analog (Fig. 5.8) that crosses BBB and produces neuroprotection in animal models of acute neural trauma and neurodegenerative diseases. Although, precise molecular mechanism of its action and primary target still remain elusive, recent studies indicate that minocycline may produce antiinflammatory, immunomodulatory, and neuroprotective effects.

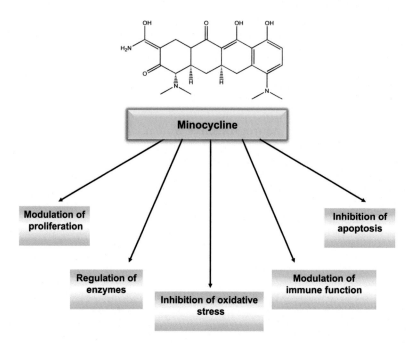

FIGURE 5.8 Chemical structures of minocycline and processes inhibited by minocycline.

These effects may involve (1) inhibitory effects on the activities of key enzymes, like iNOS, MMPs, and PLA$_2$; (2) reduction of protein tyrosine nitration because of its peroxynitrite-scavenging properties; (3) inhibition of caspase-1 and caspase-3 activation; (4) enhancement of Bcl-2-derived effects, thus protecting the cells against apoptosis; (5) reduction of p38 mitogen-activated protein kinase (MAPK) phosphorylation; and (6) inhibition of PARP-1 activity (Stirling et al., 2005; Lee et al., 2003; Festoff et al., 2006; Marchand et al., 2009; Garrido-Mesa et al., 2013). Minocycline also has the ability to bind with Ca^{2+} and Mg^{2+}, and this process may account for some of above biological activities (Fig. 5.8) (Garrido-Mesa et al., 2013). Minocycline spares white matter and increases ventral horn motor neuron survival in spinal cord adjacent to the injury site, where neurodegeneration occurs following SCI (Teng et al., 2004). Minocycline reduces the number of reactive astrocytes and augment survival of oligodendrocytes in the spared white matter. Thus, minocycline is a multifaceted therapeutic agent that has proven clinical safety and efficacy during a clinically relevant therapeutic window. It can be effective in treating acute SCI. Minocycline also inhibits microglial cell activation, reduces microglial OX-42 expression, attenuates reductions in O1- and O4-positive oligodendrocyte progenitor cells, and long-term pain phenomenon following SCI supporting the view that modulation of microglial signaling may provide a new therapeutic strategy for patients suffering from post-SCI pain (Tan et al., 2009; Moini-Zanjani et al., 2016). Cytokines and chemokines are proteins that coordinate the immune response throughout the body. The dysregulation of cytokines and chemokines is a central feature in the development of neuroinflammation, neurodegeneration, and demyelination both in the central and peripheral nervous systems and in conditions of neuropathic pain. Collective evidence suggests that minocycline produces neuroprotective and nociceptive effects in SCI not only through its antiinflammatory and antiapoptotic effects but also by inhibiting MMP-2, MMP-9, caspase-1, caspase-3, p38 MAPK, and lowering levels of cytokines and chemokines. Clinical trials of minocycline in animal models and human SCI patients have not been performed.

RILUZOLE AND SCI

Riluzole is a benzothiazole drug, which is a sodium-channel blocker (Fig. 5.9), which is approved by US Food and Drug Administration (FDA) for the treatment of amyotrophic lateral sclerosis (ALS) (Miller et al., 2007). The molecular mechanisms of action of riluzole have not

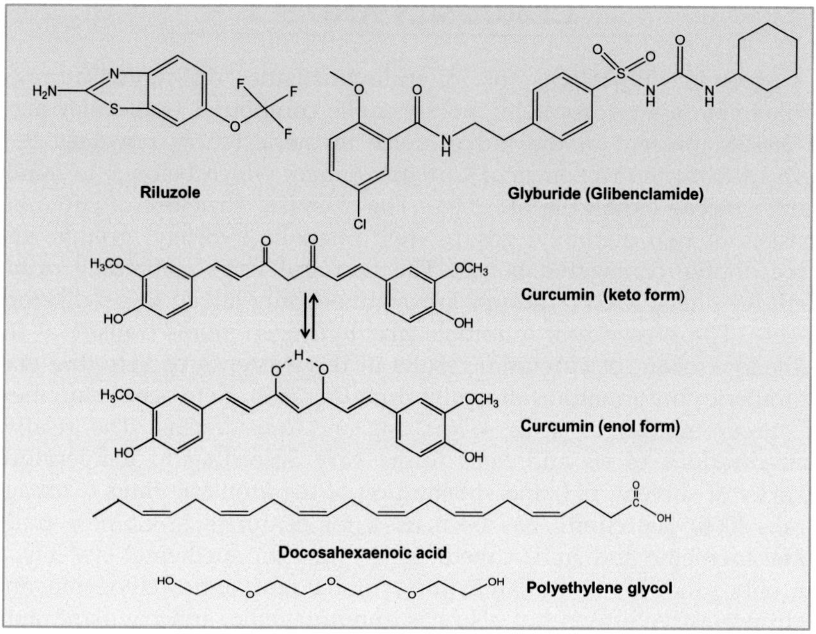

FIGURE 5.9 Chemical structures of riluzole, glyburide, curcumin, docosahexaenoic acid, and polyethylene glycol.

been fully delineated. However, it is proposed that riluzole may act on multiple molecular targets to promote and improve functional recovery. Thus, riluzole may offer neuroprotection after SCI by reducing excitotoxicity via the inhibition of presynaptic glutamate release (Coderre et al., 2007). Following experimental SCI, riluzole has been shown to be neuroprotective, leading to preserved axonal integrity through the lesion epicenter, reduced cavitation, decreased calpain activation, subsequent reduction in proteolysis of cytoskeletal substrates (Springer et al., 1997), and improved neurobehavioral outcomes. Riluzole, in combination with MPSS significantly increases in spared tissue and locomotor function following SCI (Mu et al., 2000). Finally, it is also reported that riluzole may also act by blocking Na + influx, a key early event in the pathogenesis of secondary SCI (Tator et al., 2012). In comparison to control animals, riluzole-treated animals show reduction in tissue cavitation and better preservation of white matter, motor neurons, mitochondrial function, somatosensory-evoked potentials, and locomotor scores in different studies (Springer et al., 1997). Based on these promising experimental results in animal models of SCI and an excellent safety profile in ALS, riluzole is currently in a Phase I clinical trial for the treatment of SCI.

CURCUMIN AND SCI

Curcumin ($C_{21}H_{20}O_6$) or diferuloylmethane (bis-α,β-unsaturated β-diketone) is a hydrophobic polyphenolic compound (molecular mass of 368.38) present in the Indian spice turmeric (curry powder). It is derived from the rhizomes of Curcuma longa, which belongs to family Zingiberaceae (Anand et al., 2008). The chemical structure of curcumin consists of two methoxyl groups, two phenolic hydroxyl groups, and three double conjugated bonds. The two aryl rings containing ortho-methoxy phenolic OH^- groups are symmetrically linked to a β-diketone moiety. The presence of intramolecular hydrogen atoms transfer at the β-diketone chain of curcumin results in the existence of keto and enol tautomeric conformations in equilibrium (Fig. 5.9). Keto–enol tautomers of curcumin also exist in several *cis* and *trans* forms. The relative concentrations of *cis* and *trans* forms vary according to temperature, polarity of solvent, pH, and substitution of the aromatic rings (Cornago et al., 2008). Curcumin has been used for centuries in Chinese tradi-tional medicine and Indian medicine (Ayurvedic medicine) systems. It not only produces antiinflammatory, antioxidant, anticarcinogenic, and neuroprotective effects but also has antimutagenic, anticoagulant, anti-fertility, antidiabetic, antibacterial, hypotensive, and hypocholesteremic activities (Anand et al., 2008; Aggarwal et al., 2014; Farooqui, 2016).

Curcumin produces beneficial effects in SCI not only by inhibiting oxidative stress, neuroinflammation, and apoptotic cell death but also by quenching astrocyte activation leading to significant improvements in neurologic deficit, and restoration of cellular homeostasis and normalization of redox equilibrium around the injury site (Lin et al., 2011a; Lin et al., 2011b). Curcumin not only reduces the expression of NF-κB, proinflammatory cytokines, chemokines, and the GFAP but also suppresses the reactive gliosis by inhibiting the generation of TGF-β1, TGF-β2, SOX-9, and by decreasing the deposition of chondroitin sulfate proteoglycan and improving the microenvironment for nerve growth (Sanivarapu et al., 2016). In addition, curcumin treatment decreases levels of Iba-1 (a marker for inflammatory microglia). Lastly, neurofilament-200 expression (a marker for neurons) is dramatically increased in the curcumin group, suggesting that more native neurons remains in mice treated with curcumin (Sanivarapu et al., 2016). Curcumin also inhibits the activation of signal transducer and activator of transcription-3 (STAT-3) and NF-κB in the injured spinal cord (Wang et al., 2014). As mentioned above, curcumin treatment greatly reduces the astrogliosis in SCI mice and significantly decreases the expression of IL-1β and NO, as well as the number of Iba1$^+$ inflammatory cells at the lesion site (Wang et al., 2014). Association of calcitonin gene-related peptide (CGRP) expression in improvement of neuromotor function has been recently reported (Sun and Xu, 2013). In rat models of SCI low and high doses of curcumin show increase in CGRP expression and gave superior motor function scores compared with sham and control groups (Sanivarapu et al., 2016). Converging evidence suggests that curcumin increases neuronal survival not only by inhibiting neuroinflammation and oxidative stress, but also by attenuating astrocyte reactivation along with suppression of glial scar formation (Lin et al., 2011a; Lin et al., 2011b; Wang et al., 2014; Yuan et al., 2015). Curcumin also increases tissue levels of glutathione and glutathione peroxidase and catalase, which may be beneficial for neuronal survival (Cemil et al., 2010). Clinical trials of curcumin in animal models and human SCI patients have not been performed.

DANTROLENE AND SCI

Dantrolene (DNT), a long-acting muscle relaxant (Fig. 5.4), which acts through ryanodine receptors (RyRs) and abolishes excitation−contraction coupling in muscle cells. RyRs are associated with the release of intracellular Ca^{2+}, and this release can be blocked by DNT. This large increase of intracellular Ca^{2+} activates proteases, such as calpains and caspases, which trigger apoptosis. Based on electrophysiological studies, it is suggested that injurious effects of Ca^{2+} in white matter injury may be mediated by RyRs (Thorell et al., 2002). DNT also produces neuroprotective effects through its antioxidant and antiapoptotic properties. Treatment of SCI in rat model results in significant improvement in DNT-treated rats, 24 hours after SCI, with respect to control. SCI-mediated increase in the lipid peroxidation, decrease in enzymic or nonenzymic endogenous antioxidative defense systems, and increase in apoptotic cell numbers can be prevented by DNT. DNT treatment not only blocks lipid peroxidation but also significantly decreases the apoptotic cell death following SCI (Aslan et al., 2009). In addition, DNT treatment also prevents hemorrhage, edema, and decrease in GSH levels. Studies on the effect of MPSS, DNT sodium, and their combination on experimental SCI have indicated that these drugs do not reduce neuronal and glial loss, intrinsic pathway apoptosis, or promote functional recovery (Rosado et al., 2014).

OMEGA-3 FATTY ACIDS AND SCI

It is becoming increasingly evident that ω-3 polyunsaturated fatty acids (n-3 PUFAs) because of their antioxidant, antiinflammatory, and membrane stabilizing properties produce beneficial effects in neurotraumatic and neurodegenerative diseases (Farooqui, 2010). Thus, injections of α-linolenic acid (ALA) and DHA 30 minutes after SCI not only produce significant improvement in locomotor performance and neuroprotection but also reduce lesion size, inhibit apoptosis, and increase neuronal and oligodendrocyte survival (Lang-Lazdunski et al., 2003; King et al., 2006; Michael-Titus, 2007). The molecular mechanism associated with neuroprotective effects of DHA (Fig. 5.9) not only involves the modulation of neurotransmission and ion channel activities but also generation of resolvins and neuroprotectins. These DHA-derived lipid mediators protect neuronal cells from apoptotic cell death (King et al., 2006; Michael-Titus, 2007; Huang et al., 2009). DHA and its metabolites may also act by downregulating NF-κB, decreasing the expression of proinflammatory cytokines and enzymes (TNF-α, IL-1β, IL-6, iNOS, and COX-2), inhibiting proapoptotic protein, Bax immunoreactivity. Induction of these processes may also prevent apoptotic and necrotic neuronal death (Lang-Lazdunski et al., 2003). As stated in Chapter 4, SCI is accompanied by autonomic bladder dysfunction, consumption of DHA enriched diet not only results in amelioration of autonomic bladder function but also accelerates its complete recovery, suggesting reduced damage and/or activation of repair responses (Figueroa et al., 2013a, 2013b). The beneficial effects of DHA in SCI are long lasting, because behavioral function scores continued to improve in relation to controls for at least 8 weeks. These rapid and prolonged beneficial effects suggest that dietary ω-3 PUFA prophylaxis may be attributable to a combination of early (i.e., neuroprotection, plasticity, and remyelination) and late (i.e., sprouting and regeneration) protective/repair mechanisms (Figueroa et al., 2013a). Furthermore, diet enriched in ω-3 fatty acids may provide antinociceptive benefits in rats experiencing SCI-induced pain. Functional neurometabolomic profiling displays a distinctive deregulation in the metabolism of endocannabinoids (eCBs) and related N-acylethanolamines (NAEs) at 8weeks post-SCI. The tissue levels of these endocannabinoids are significantly correlated with the antihyperalgesic effects. In addition, rats consuming the ω-3 fatty acid enriched diet show reduction in sprouting of nociceptive fibers containing CGRP and dorsal horn neuron p38 MAPK expression, the well-established biomarkers of pain. Collectively, these results demonstrate the prophylactic value of dietary ω-3 fatty acid enriched diet against chronic pain in SCI supporting the view that ω-3 fatty acids may serve as promising therapeutic agents for the management of SCI (Figueroa et al., 2013b).

POLYETHYLENE GLYCOL AND SCI

Polyethylene glycol (PEG) (Fig. 5.9) is a nontoxic water-soluble fusogen, which is approved by the FDA. It is used as a vehicle or a base not only in food, cosmetics, and pharmaceuticals, but also in adjuvants for ameliorating drug pharmacokinetics. Some PEGs are also currently used as additives in organ preservation solutions before transplantation to limit the damage associated with cold ischemia reperfusion.

As stated earlier, the regeneration of injured neurons following SCI is not only retarded by glial scar formation but also due to the onset of Wallerian degeneration. However, the development of PEG-fusion technology along with concepts of biochemical engineering, cell biology, and clinical microsurgery has allowed PEG-mediated fusion of injured axons across the lesion site. After PEG-fusion repair, cut- or crush-severed or ablated peripheral nerve axons (PNAs) or crush-severed severing spinal tract axons (STAs) rapidly (within days to weeks), more completely, and permanently restore PNA- or STA-mediated behaviors compared to non-treated or conventionally treated animals. PEG-mediated fusion success is enhanced or decreased by the inclusion of antioxidants or oxidants, trimming cut ends or stretching axons, exposure to Ca^{2+}-free or -containing solutions, respectively (Bittner et al., 2015, 2016). PEG-mediated repair leads to spontaneous reassembly of cell membranes made possible by the action of targeted hydrophilic polymers, which first seal the compromised portion of the plasmalemma, and secondarily allow the lipidic core of the compromised membranes to resolve into each other (Koob et al., 2008; Bittner et al., 2016). Although, the molecular mechanism of PEG-mediated membrane fusion and neuroprotection after SCI remains unknown, but it is proposed that PEG reduces apoptotic cell death following SCI (Baptiste et al., 2009). PEG has been used to protect neurons in the rat models of SCI. In clip compression model of SCI at C8, intravenous injections of PEG not only reduce 200-kd neurofilament degradation but also promote spinal cord tissue sparing. This suggestion is based on retrograde axonal Fluoro-Gold tracing and morphometric histological assessment. PEGs also promote significant neurobehavioral recovery after SCI. In addition, intravenous injections of PEGs improve locomotor recovery and reduce pain but do not provide additional benefit compared with either treatment alone. Neither treatment, nor their combination, attenuate mean arterial pressure increases during autonomic dysreflexia (Ditor et al., 2007). The molecular mechanism of PEG-mediated neuroprotection in SCI is not fully understood. However, it is proposed that PEG may act by significantly declining the caspase-3 activity and increasing the generation of ROS. These processes may lead to the upregulation of prosurvival signaling including Akt, ERK, and GSK-3β phosphorylation. Furthermore, PEG may also preserve and stabilize sarcolemmal membrane lipid-raft architecture (Valuckaite et al., 2009). Because PEG does not scavenge superoxide anion or inhibit xanthine oxidase (Rubio-Gayosso et al., 2006), it is also suggested that PEG may also inhibit or reduce oxidative stress through preservation or restoration of membrane integrity. PEG treatments produce significant increases in dorsal myelin sparing, and the latter results in significant reductions in lesion volume, compared with saline-treated controls. Furthermore, mean lesion volumes correlate negatively with the corresponding mean locomotion BBB scores and positively with the corresponding mean pain scores (Ditor et al., 2007; Kwon et al., 2009). Collective evidence suggests that PEG protects key axonal cytoskeletal proteins after SCI, and that the protection is associated with axonal preservation. The modest extent of locomotor recovery after treatment with PEG suggests that this compound may not confer sufficient neuroprotection to be used clinically as a single treatment (Baptiste et al., 2009; Kwon et al., 2009). Derivatization of protein with PEG (pegylation) not only improves pharmacokinetic and pharmacodynamic properties of the proteins but improves efficacy and minimize the dose. Attachment of PEG with brain-derived neurotrophic factor (BDNF) and its intrathecal administration results in enhanced delivery of PEG-bound BDNF to the spinal cord. The biological activity of BDNF-PEG conjugate mixture has assessed with the goal of identifying a relationship between the number of PEG molecules attached to BDNF and biological activity. These preparations have been used to study their effects on SCI (Soderquist et al., 2009).

RESVERATROL AND SCI

Resveratrol (3, 4′, 5-trihydroxy stilbene), a polyphenolic compound, which exhibits neuroprotective effects in neurotraumatic and neurodegenerative diseases (Farooqui, 2012). The molecular mechanism of resveratrol action in animal models of SCI is unclear. It is proposed that the effect of resveratrol in SCI is associated with modulation of SIRT1/AMPK signaling pathway, autophagy, and apoptosis (Fig. 5.10). Nissl and HE staining reveals that resveratrol treatment significantly reduces the loss of motor neurons and lesion size in the spinal cord of injured rats when compared to vehicle-treated animals (Zhao et al., 2017). Western blotting reverse transcription-polymerase chain reaction and immunohistochemical analyses 7 days after SCI indicates that resveratrol-treated animals show increased expression of SIRT1, p-AMPK, Beclin-1, LC3-B, and Bcl-2, whereas expression of p62, Cleaved Caspase-3, Caspase-9, and Bcl-2 associated X protein (Bax) is inhibited (Zhao et al., 2017). Immunofluorescence analysis of primary neurons treated with resveratrol alone or in combination with Compound C (AMPK inhibitor) or EX527 (SIRT1 inhibitor) shows that treatment with the inhibitors blocks not only increases LC3-B expression but also increases the portion of TUNEL-positive cells. In addition, resveratrol also induces antioxidant effects in a variety of in vitro and in vivo models of neural injury. The antioxidant

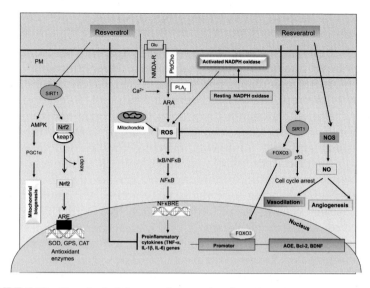

FIGURE 5.10 Hypothetical diagram showing the effect of resveratrol in animal models of SCI. Glu, glutamate; NMDA-R, N-Methyl-D-aspartate receptor; PtdCho, phosphatidyl-choline; lyso-PtdCho, lyso-phosphatidylcholine; PtdIns, phosphatidylinositol; InsP$_3$, inositol 1,4,5-trisphosphate; DAG, diacylglycerol; PKC, protein kinase C; ER, endoplasmic reticulum; Nrf2, nuclear factor E2-related factor 2; Keap1, kelch-like erythroid Cap'n'Collar homologue–associated protein 1; Akt, serine/threonine protein kinase; CREB, cAMP Response Element Binding; CBP/300, CREB binding protein; FOXO3, Forkhead box O3; SIRT1, sirtuin1; ROS, reactive oxygen species; NF-κB-RE, nuclear factor-κB-response element; I-κB, inhibitory subunit of NF-κB; Nrf2, NF-E2 related factor 2; ARE, antioxidant response element; CAT, catalase; GPS, glutathione peroxidase.

effects of resveratrol have assessed by measuring superoxide dismutase (SOD) activity and MDA level after SCI. Resveratrol treatment reverses the decrease of SOD activity and increase of MDA level caused by SCI, suggesting its antioxidant role of resveratrol in response to the injury. In addition, resveratrol treatment suppresses immunoreactivity and expression of inflammatory cytokines including IL-1β, IL-10, TNF-α, and myeloperoxidase after SCI, suggesting an antiinflammatory effect of resveratrol (Liu et al., 2011). In ischemic injury, resveratrol upregulates the expression of heme oxygenase-1 (HO-1) via the antioxidant response element (ARE)-mediated transcriptional activation of nuclear factor erythroid 2-related factor 2 (Nrf2) in a dose- and time-dependent manner (Farooqui, 2012). Resveratrol pretreatment protected mice subjected to an optimized ischemic–reperfusion (I/R) stroke model, which was absent in HO-1 knockout mice indicating the neuroprotective role of upregulated HO-1(Sakata et al., 2010; Bastianetto and Quirion, 2010). Taken together, these results suggest that resveratrol exerts neuroprotective effects in animal models of SCI by regulating autophagy and apoptosis mediated by the SIRT1-AMPK signaling pathway (Liu et al., 2011; Zhao et al., 2017).

NEUROTROPHINS AND SCI

It is well established that SCI permanently disrupts neuroanatomical circuitry leading to severe functional deficits. These functional deficits, however, are not immutable, and spontaneous recovery occurs in some patients. It is proposed this recovery depends not only upon spared tissue but also on endogenous neuroplasticity in brain and spinal cord. Neurotrophic factors are mediators of neuroplasticity throughout development and into adulthood, affecting proliferation of neuronal precursors, neuronal survival, axonal growth, dendritic arborization, and synapse formation. Neurotrophic factors are therefore excellent candidates for enhancing axonal plasticity and regeneration after SCI. Neurotrophins include nerve growth factor (NGF), BDNF, glial cell line-derived neurotrophic factor (GDNF), and neurotrophin-3 (NT-3). These molecules interact with neurons that express the appropriate tropomyosin-related kinase (Trk) receptors—TrkA (NGF), TrkB (BDNF), and TrkC (NT-3), as well as the p75 receptor common to all Trk-expressing neurons (Reichardt, 2006; Boyce and Mendell, 2014). The receptor biology and intracellular signaling associated with Trk receptors is reviewed elsewhere (Reichardt, 2006; Boyce and Mendell, 2014). Genes controlling growth-associated protein-43 (GAP-43), BDNF, and GDNF show significant changes in mRNA accumulation in spinal cord from 48 hours to 12 weeks after SCI (Boyce et al., 2012; Boyce and Mendell, 2014). Similarly, inhibitory genes, such as RhoA, LINGO-1, and others, are upregulated as late as 4–14 days after SCI suggesting that gene-specific regulatory changes, corresponding to repair and regenerative changes are naturally orchestrated over time after the injury. These delayed changes after SCI give ample time for therapeutic gene modulation through upregulation or silencing of specific genes responsible for the synthesis of the corresponding biogenic proteins. Neurotrophins promote recovery after SCI by multiple mechanisms. The main effects and mechanisms are (1) inhibition of c-fos and c-jun expressions in the spinal cord, thereby reducing apoptosis of spinal cord nerve cells; (2) decreasing TNF-α, IL-1β, and IL-8 expressions in the spinal cord, inhibiting the inflammatory response; and (3) reduction of inflammation and spinal cord I/R injury by inhibiting NF-κB and VCAM-1.

Among neurotrophins, BDNF is important in modulating neuro-plasticity and promoting recovery after SCI. Intrathecal delivery of BDNF enhances functional recovery following unilateral spinal cord hemisection (SH) at C2, a well-established model of incomplete cervical SCI. It is becoming increasingly evident that BDNF treatment following SCI increases survival of neurons and axonal sprouting when delivered by intrathecal infusion (Novikova et al., 2000, 2002), intraspinal viral transduction (Boyce et al., 2012), or stem cell transplantation (Lu et al., 2005, Lynskey et al., 2006). Although, the role of BDNF/TrkB signaling on motor pools below the level of injury is not well understood, it is proposed that increase in BDNF/TrkB signaling at the level of the phrenic motoneuron pool by intrathecal BDNF delivery not only enhances neuroplasticity and functional recovery of rhythmic diaphragm activity after cervical spinal cord hemisection but also quenches endogenous neurotrophins with the soluble fusion protein TrkB-Fc or by knocking down TrkB receptor expression in phrenic motoneurons using intrapleurally delivered siRNA impairs functional recovery after cervical spinal cord hemisection suggesting that BDNF/TrkB signaling in phrenic motoneuron pool plays a critical role in functional recovery after cervical SCI (Mantilla et al., 2013).

GDNF is another member of neurotrophin family. It is widely expressed in the brain and spinal cord. Human GDNF gene, which is located in the 5P13.1—P13.3 of the chromosome, has been successfully cloned (Bermingham et al., 1995). GDNF plays an important role in in the maintenance of viability of a number of cell different populations in the spinal cord, including the motor neurons (Cheng et al., 2002; Islamov et al., 2004). It not only reduces apoptosis and tissue degeneration (Mills et al., 2007) but also supports expression of neurofilament protein, CGRP, and growth associated protein 43 (GAP-43) (Cheng et al., 2002). GDNF not only protects spinal cord neurons but also promotes the recovery of peripheral nerve (Santos et al., 2016) in vivo. It is also revealed that GDNF transcription in the spinal cord began to increase within 30 minutes after injury and peaked within 3 hours. Immunohistochemical analysis indicates that GDNF immunoreactivity is present mainly in microglia and macrophages 1 day after injury but not in neurons or astrocytes. This immediate upregulation of GDNF gene expression may be a component of an inflammatory process and probably exerts a protective effect on neurons following SCI (Satake et al., 2000). Like BDNF, the infusion of GDNF promotes the SCI recovery following its infusion.

HYPOTHERMIA AND SCI

Moderate hypothermia (33°C) by intravascular cooling has gained significant attention as a potential therapy in neurotraumatic diseases such as SCI (Levi et al., 2009, 2010; Dietrich et al., 2011). In experimental models of SCI, moderate hypothermia has been shown to improve functional recovery and reduce overall structural damage. At the molecular level, hypothermia induces functional recovery and reduce overall structural damage by reducing cerebral metabolism and therefore provide energy required for maintaining ionic gradients and other mechanisms important in the normal regulation of neural cell function (Dietrich et al., 2009). Hypothermia also lowers metabolic and energy demands and has been shown to have beneficial effects in regards to adenosine-5' triphosphate (ATP) depletion following ischemia. In addition to metabolic changes, hypothermic therapy may not only have significant effects on cerebral blood flow alterations but also decreases the expression of proinflammatory cytokine (IL-1β, IL-18, and TNF-α) following both brain and SCI (Westergren et al., 2001; Kinoshita et al., 2002). In a recent Phase I clinical trial, systemic hypothermia has been shown to be safe and provide some encouraging results in terms of functional recovery. However, progress in the translation of preclinical treatments aimed at promoting regenerative growth has been slow (Thuret et al., 2006).

REGENERATION IN SCI

The majority of current spinal cord repair and regeneration therapies are at the experimental stage in vitro or animal models. Slow regeneration and reconstruction of spinal cord after SCI is not only caused by glial scar formation and cavitation but also by secondary axonal demyelination cause by oligodendrocytes apoptosis. Recovery from SCI is a very big challenge. It not only requires the rescue of degenerating neurons by neuroprotective agents, survival of transplanted cells, and induction of axonal regeneration and elongation, but also physiological targeting by growing axons to reconnect with their target neurons for establishing corrects to reconstitute original circuitry (or the equivalent), which will ultimately lead to functional restoration. There is a therapeutic window of opportunity within which the devastating consequences of the secondary injury can be slowed by preventing glial scar formation, retarding oligodendrocyte apoptosis, inducing neural regeneration. Cellular replacement (neural transplantation) and axon guidance are both necessary for the repair of injured spinal cord in animal model of SCI (Bartolomei and Greer, 2000). Two types of stem cells namely stem/progenitor cells and human umbilical cord blood stem cells (hUCBs) have been used for the treatment of SCI in animal models.

STEM/PROGENITOR CELL TRANSPLANTS IN SCI

Stem/progenitor cells provide a valuable cellular source for promoting repair following SCI. Stem/progenitor cells are multipotent and dynamic cells that have the capacity to expand in vitro. They not only can self-renew and differentiate into CNS cell lineages but are also capable of long-term survival following transplantation (Webber et al., 2007). Thus, they can be directed to differentiate into neurons or glia in vitro, which can be used for the replacement of neural cells lost, after SCI. Therapeutic transplantation of different types of stem cells and their derivatives, alone or in combination with other treatments, has been demonstrated to improve functional outcome in animal models of SCI, probably through cell replacement, trophic support, facilitation of axonal growth, remyelination, or modulation of neuroinflammation (Kim et al., 2007; Barnabé-Heider and Frisén, 2008; Sahni and Kessler, 2010). Although the field of stem cell therapy is in its infancy, some stem cell or cell-based transplantation using bone marrow-derived cells, umbilical cord blood cells, OECs, SCs, activated macrophages, or T cells have already been used in patients with SCI (Hernández et al., 2011; Saberi et al., 2008; Moviglia et al., 2006). To date, the existing results from clinical trials have shown some stem cell or cell transplants to be safe but with very limited or no therapeutic efficacy. Thus, stem cell therapies are not yet approved for SCI (Sahni and Kessler, 2010; Lindvall and Kokaia, 2010).

Four types of embryonic cells and other neural cells have been used for neural cell therapy in animal models of SCI: stem/progenitor cells, bone marrow mesenchymal stem cells, SCs, and olfactory ensheathing glia (Lu and Ashwell, 2002; Kim et al., 2007). These cells are preferred because they have clear capacity to become neurons or glial cells after transplantation into the injured spinal cord. Directed differentiation of stem/progenitor cells to oligodendrocyte lineage prior to transplantation may promote oligodendroglial differentiation. It is stated that this may be an effective strategy to increase the extent of remyelination. Transplanted stem/progenitor cells can also contribute to axonal regeneration by functioning as cellular scaffolds for growing axons. The combinatorial approaches using polymer scaffolds to fill the lesion cavity or introducing regeneration-promoting genes can greatly increase the efficacy of cellular transplantation strategies for SCI (Kim et al., 2007; Webber et al., 2007).

The use of OECs is another procedure for neural transplantation. OEGs are a specialized type of glial cells that guide primary olfactory axons from the neuroepithelium in the nasal cavity to the brain (Franssen et al., 2007). The ability of olfactory neurons to grow axons in the mature brain milieu has been attributed to the presence of OECs. It has been shown that transplanted OECs have ability to transform and migrate through glial scars facilitating axonal regrowth through an injury barrier. It is suggested that co-transplantation of stem/progenitor cells and OECs into an injured spinal cord may have a synergistic effect, promoting neural regeneration and functional reconstruction. The lost neurocytes can be replaced by stem/progenitor cells, while the OECs can promote the formation of "bridges" crossing the glial scaring that conduct axon elongation and promote myelinization simultaneously (Bartolomei and Greer, 2000). It is suggested that two types of cells may first be seeded into a bioactive scaffold, and then the cell seeded construct can be implanted into the injury site. This may facilitate treatment that may lead to improved neural regeneration and functional reconstruction after SCI (Ao et al., 2007). Therapeutic approaches using stem/progenitor cells transplants in animal models of SCI have provided mixed results. Some studies have provided positive results on behavioral recovery, whereas other investigators have reported that stem/progenitor cell transplants fail to promote significant functional recovery, with a small improvement observed in only one of the four tasks employed, primarily related to improvements in sensory function. Tracing of the corticospinal tract and ascending dorsal column pathway reveals no regeneration of the axons beyond the lesion site (Webber et al., 2007). In spite of this challenge, stem/progenitor cell therapy is likely to remain within the experimental arena for the foreseeable future.

HUMAN UMBILICAL CORD BLOOD CELLS TRANSPLANTATION IN SCI

Human umbilical cord blood cells (hUCBCs) provide great promise for therapeutic repair after SCI. Ultrastructural analysis of axons has revealed that hUCB can be transformed into morphologically normal appearing myelin sheaths around axons in the injured areas of spinal cord. It is becoming increasingly evident that hUCBCs have many of the properties that allow them to overcome major hurdles of SCI regeneration (Table 5.1). The transplantation of hUCBCs in SCI not only depresses neuroinflammatory response but also provides a neurotrophic influence and stimulates neovascularization (Chen et al., 2008). Injection of hUCBCs into the bloodstream after SCI decreases the expression of proapoptotic genes and promotes neuronal survival (Dasari et al., 2007, 2009). At 6 weeks after local transplantation of hUCBCs into the area of SCI results in significant improvement in behavioral recovery with elevation in levels of cytokines and growth factors with neuroprotective, angiogenic, and antiinflammatory actions (Chua et al., 2010). In dog model of SCI, hUCBCs enhance remyelination by promoting the formation of peripheral type myelin sheaths and functional recovery 3 years after the cell transplantation. (Mukhamedshina et al., 2016). Furthermore, transplantation of human umbilical cord blood

TABLE 5.1   Properties of Human Umbilical Cord Blood Cells that Promote Regeneration

Properties	Reference
Ability to induce antiinflammatory effects	Mukhamedshina et al. (2016)
Ability to induce antiapoptotic effects	Mukhamedshina et al. (2016)
Ability to induce neural cell migration	Mukhamedshina et al. (2016)
Ability to induce immunomodulatory effects	Mukhamedshina et al. (2016)
Ability to differentiate into endothelial cells, microglia, and astrocytes	Mukhamedshina et al. (2016)
Ability to reduce cavity volume and tissue retention at lesion site	Mukhamedshina et al. (2016)
Ability to increase neovascularization	Mukhamedshina et al. (2016)
Ability to enhance remyelination	Mukhamedshina et al. (2016)
Ability to secrete neurotrophic factors, cytokines, and chemokines	Mukhamedshina et al. (2016)
Ability to improve blood flow	Mukhamedshina et al., 2016
Ability to promote angiogenesis	Mukhamedshina et al., 2016

mononuclear cells (hUCB-MCs) also reduces cavity volume and tissue retention at the lesion site (both white and gray matter) (Mukhamedshina et al., 2016). It is reported that hUCB-MCs transduced with adenoviral vectors have ability to express VEGF and GDNF at the site of SCI. These growth factors induce behavioral recovery that correlated with tissue sparing. In humans, transplantation of umbilical cord mesenchymal stem cells (UCMSCs) into a 37-year-old female with SCI improves both functional recovery and sensory perception (Kang et al., 2005). Moreover, transplantation UCMSCs in combination with $CD34^+$ hUCBCs into a 29-year-old male patient with an L1 SCI results in recovery of muscle, bowel, and sexual function along with a decrease in ASIA score from "A" to "D" (Ichim et al., 2010). Collectively, these studies strongly suggest that the transplantation of hUCB-MCs transduced with adenoviral vectors expressing VEGF and GDNF genes after SCI may support functional tissue plasticity and its ability to regenerate. This approach for treating SCI may not only permit the delivery of growth and angiogenic factors into the damaged area of spinal cord but also reduces the severity of retrograde axonal degeneration, supports tissue reconstruction including remyelination, and elongation and collateral branching of axons to form synapses.

Patients with SCI also show deficits in volitional motor control and sensation limiting, not only the performance of daily tasks but also the overall activity level of these individuals. These patients have extremely sedentary lifestyle with an increased incidence of secondary complications including diabetes mellitus, hypertension, and atherogenic lipid profiles (Jacobs and Nash, 2004). To decrease secondary complications, physicians recommend daily exercise to SCI patients. Thus, physical rehabilitation following SCI traditionally focuses on teaching compensatory techniques that enable patients to achieve day-to-day function despite significant neurological and behavioral deficits (Sadowsky and McDonald, 2009). Rehabilitation SCI patients require a comprehensive, highly integrated, and intensive program that not only facilitates arm movement but also supports the conditioning of lower limbs after SCI. Furthermore, rehabilitation plans also include the use of braces, assistive devices, and multisensor activity for wheelchairs to achieve upright and seated mobility, orthopedic, and adjustment issues after SCI (Behrman et al., 2006; Mitcho and Kanko, 1999; Murphy, 1999). Teams of highly trained orthopedic surgeon, neurosurgeon, therapists, nurses, and psychosocial support are required for the treatment of SCI patient (Mitcho and Kanko, 1999)

CONCLUSION

SCI is accompanied by a primary insult (compression, contusion, or laceration) followed by a secondary injury cascade that propagates in disrupting motor, sensory, and/or autonomic functions. Depending on the location and severity of the SCI, deficits can range from weakness of limb movement to total paralysis and ventilator-assisted respiration. Spontaneous functional recovery is limited but can and often does occur in patients with initial sparing of sensorimotor function. This recovery, which plateaus between 12 and 18 months, is very likely due to sparing and sprouting of axons within the zone of partial preservation, an area where some motor function remains intact, immediately adjacent to the lesion site. Limited advances have been made in treatment of SCI in animal models and none in human SCI. Many therapeutic agents including MPSS, GM1 ganglioside, thyrotropin-releasing hormone, riluzole, glyburide, nimodipine, and minocycline have been used in animal models of SCI. Although, some beneficial effects are observed, but the primary outcome of these trials has been largely negative. A number of strategies have also been developed to facilitate regeneration (axonal growth) across the lesion with a variety of cellular substrates. These include fetal tissue transplants, stem/progenitor cells, OECs, and hUCBs.

Promising results have been obtained in experimental models of SCI with stem cells, which can differentiate into neurons or glia and used for the replacement of neural cells lost after SCI. Neuroprotective and axon regeneration-promoting effects have also been credited to transplanted stem cells. Human SCI is a heterogeneous condition, which requires specialized treatments based on the neurological and imaging assessment procedures. Many laboratories are concentrating on testing treatment strategies that can be given in the early injury setting to limit secondary injury mechanisms known to be active in acutely injured human patients. Cell transplantation approaches along with novel strategies to promote axonal regeneration in humans are needed to treat human SCI. A successful treatment of human SCI will require complete information on cell-signaling cascades, genetic factors, and the involvement of specific transcriptional factors have been reported to be important for successful neurite growth and axonal regeneration in various experimental settings.

References

Aggarwal, B.B., Deb, L., Prasad, S., 2014. Curcumin differs from tetrahydrocurcumin for molecular targets, signaling pathways and cellular responses. Molecules 20, 185–205.

Ahuja, C.S., Martin, A.R., Fehlings, M., 2016. Recent advances in managing a spinal cord injury secondary to trauma. F1000Res. 5, pii: F1000.

Anand, P., Thomas, S.G., Kunnumakkara, A.B., Sundaram, C., Harikumar, K.B., et al., 2008. Biological activities of curcumin and its analogues (Congeners) made by man and mother nature. Biochem. Pharmacol. 76, 1590–1611.

Ao, Q., Wang, A.J., Chen, G.O., Wang, S.T., Zuo, H.C., et al., 2007. Combined transplantation of neural stem cells and olfactory ensheathing cells for the repair of spinal cord injuries. Med. Hypotheses 69, 1234–1237.

Asher, R.A., Morgenstern, D.A., Properzi, F., Nishiyama, A., Levine, J.M., et al., 2005. Two separate metalloproteinase activities are responsible for the shedding and processing of the NG2 proteoglycan in vitro. Mol. Cell Neurosci. 29, 82–96.

Aslan, A., Cemek, M., Buyukokuroglu, M.E., Altunbas, K., Bas, O., Yurumez, Y., et al., 2009. Dantrolene can reduce secondary damage after spinal cord injury. Eur. Spine J. 18 (10), 1442–1451.

Bains, M., Hall, E.D., 2012. Antioxidant therapies in traumatic brain and spinal cord injury. Biochim. Biophys. Acta. 1822, 675–684.

Baptiste, D.C., Austin, J.W., Zhao, W., Nahirny, A., Sugita, S., et al., 2009. Systemic polyethylene glycol promotes neurological recovery and tissue sparing in rats after cervical spinal cord injury. J. Neuropathol. Exp. Neurol. 68, 661–676.

Barnabé-Heider, F., Frisén, J., 2008. Stem cells for spinal cord repair. Cell Stem Cell 3, 16–24.

Barres, B.A., Burne, J.F., Holtmann, B., Thoenen, H., Sendtner, M., et al., 1996. Ciliary neurotrophic factor enhances the rate of oligodendrocyte generation. Mol. Cell Neurosci. 8, 146–156.

Bartolomei, J.C., Greer, C.A., 2000. Olfactory ensheathing cells: bridging the gap in spinal cord injury. Neurosurgery 47, 1057–1069.

Bartus, K., James, N.D., Bosch, K.D., Bradbury, E.J., 2011. Chondroitin sulphate proteoglycans: key modulators of spinal cord and brain plasticity. Exp. Neurol. 235, 5–17.

Bastianetto, S., Quirion, R., 2010. Heme oxygenase 1: another possible target to explain the neuroprotective action of resveratrol, a multifaceted nutrient-based molecule. Exp. Neurol. 225, 237–239.

Becker, T., Becker, C.G., 2014. Axonal regeneration in zebrafish. Current Opinion in Neurobiology. 27, 186–191.

Behrman, A.L., Bowden, M.G., Nair, P.M., 2006. Neuroplasticity after spinal cord injury and training: an emerging paradigm shift in rehabilitation and walking recovery. Phys. Ther. 86, 1406–1425.

Bermingham, N., Hillermann, R., Gilmour, F., Martin, J.E., Fisher, E.M., 1995. Human glial cell line-derived neurotrophic factor (GDNF) maps to chromosome 5. Hum. Genet. 96, 671–673.

Bittner, G.D., Rokkappanavar, K.K., Peduzzi, J.D., 2015. Application and implications of polyethylene glycol-fusion as a novel technology to repair injured spinal cords. Neural Regen. Res. 10, 1406–1408.

Bittner, G.D., Sengelaub, D.R., Trevino, R.C., Peduzzi, J.D., Mikesh, M., et al., 2016. The curious ability of polyethylene glycol fusion technologies to restore lost behaviors after nerve severance. J. Neurosci. Res. 94, 207–230.

Boyce, V.S., Mendell, L.M., 2014. Neurotrophins and spinal circuit function. Front. Neural Circuits 8, 59.

Boyce, V.S., Park, J., Gage, F.H., Mendell, L.M., 2012. Differential effects of brain-derived neurotrophic factor and neurotrophin-3 on hindlimb function in paraplegic rats. Eur. J. Neurosci. 35, 221–232.

Bracken, M.B., Shepard, M.J., Collins, W.F., Holford, T.R., Young, W., et al., 1990. A randomized, controlled trial of methylprednisolone or naloxone in the treatment of acute spinal-cord injury. Results of the Second National Acute Spinal Cord Injury Study. N. Engl. J. Med. 322, 1405–1411.

Bracken, M.B., 2012. Steroids for acute spinal cord injury. Cochrane Database Syst Rev. 1, CD001046.

Bracken, M.B., Shepard, M.J., Collins, W.F., Holford, T.R., Baskin, D.S., et al., 1992. Methylprednisolone or naloxone treatment after acute spinal cord injury: 1-year follow-up data. Results of the second National Acute Spinal Cord Injury Study. J. Neurosurg. 76, 23–31.

Budh, C.N., Osteraker, A.L., 2007. Life satisfaction in individuals with a spinal cord injury and pain. Clin. Rehabil. 21, 89–96.

Buki, A., Farkas, O., Doczi, T., Povlishock, J.T., 2003. Preinjury administration of the calpain inhibitor MDL-28170 attenuates traumatically induced axonal injury. J. Neurotrauma. 20, 261–268.

Bunge, M.B., 2008. Novel combination strategies to repair the injured mammalian spinal cord. J. Spinal Cord Med. 31, 262–269.

Carvalho, M.O., Barros Filho, T.E., Tebet, M.A., 2008. Effects of methylprednisolone and ganglioside GM-1 on a spinal lesion: a functional analysis. Clinics (Sao Paulo). 63, 375–380.

Catala, A., 2012. Lipid peroxidation modifies the picture of membranes from the "Fluid Mosaic Model" to the "Lipid Whisker Model". Biochimie. 94, 101–109.

Cemil, B., Topuz, K., Demircan, M.N., Kurt, G., Tun, K., et al., 2010. Curcumin improves early functional results after experimental spinal cord injury. Acta Neurochir (Wien). 152, 1583–1590.

Chappell, E.T., 2002. Pharmacological therapy after acute cervical spinal cord injury. Neurosurgery 51, 855–856. author reply 856.

Chen, C.T., Foo, N.H., Liu, W.S., Chen, S.H., 2008. Infusion of human umbilical cord blood cells ameliorates hind limb dysfunction in experimental spinal cord injury through anti–inflammatory, vasculogenic and neurotrophic mechanisms. Pediatr. Neonatol. 49, 77–83.

Cheng, H., Wu, J.P., Tzeng, S.F., 2002. Neuroprotection of glial cell line–derived neurotrophic factor in damaged spinal cords following contusive injury. Neurosci. Res. 69, 397–405.

Chua, S.J., Bielecki, R., Yamanaka, N., Fehlings, M.G., Rogers, I.M., et al., 2010. The effect of umbilical cord blood cells on outcomes after experimental traumatic spinal cord injury. Spine 35, 1520–1526.

Coderre, T.J., Kumar, N., Lefebrvre, C.D., Yu, J.S., 2007. A comparison of the glutamate release inhibition and anti-allodynic effects of gabapentin, lamotrigine, and riluzole in a model of neuropathic pain. J. Neurochem. 100, 1289–1299.

Cooke, M.S., Evans, M.D., Dizdaroglu, M., Lunec, J., 2003. Oxidative DNA damage: mechanisms, mutation, and disease. FASEB J. 17, 1195–1214.

Cornago, P., Claramunt, R.M., Bouissane, L., Alkorta, I., Elguero, J., 2008. A study of the tautomerism of beta-dicarbonyl compounds with special emphasis on curcuminoids. Tetrahedron 64, 8089–8094.

Dasari, V.R., Spomar, D.G., Gondi, C.S., Sloffer, C.A., Saving, K.L., Gujrati, M., et al., 2007. Axonal remyelination by cord blood stem cells after spinal cord injury. J. Neurotrauma 24, 391–410.

Dasari, V.R., Veeravalli, K.K., Tsung, A.J., Gondi, C.S., Gujrati, M., et al., 2009. Neuronal apoptosis is inhibited by cord blood stem cells after spinal cord injury. J. Neurotrauma 26, 2057–2069.

David, S., Kroner, A., 2011. Repertoire of microglial and macrophage responses after spinal cord injury. Nat. Rev. Neurosci. 12, 388–399.

Dietrich, W.D., Atkins, C.M., Bramlett, H.M., 2009. Protection in animal models of brain and spinal cord injury with mild to moderate hypothermia. J. Neurotrauma 26, 301–312.

Dietrich, W.D., Cappuccino, A., Cappuccino, H., 2011. Systemic hypothermia for the treatment of acute cervical spinal cord injury in sports. Curr. Sports Med. Rep. 10, 50–54.

Ding, Y., Kastin, A.J., Pan, W., 2005. Neural plasticity after spinal cord injury. Curr. Pharm. Des. 11, 1441–1450.

Ditor, D.S., John, S.M., Roy, J., Marx, J.C., Kittmer, C., Weaver, L.C., 2007. Effects of polyethylene glycol and magnesium sulfate administration on clinically relevant neurological outcomes after spinal cord injury in the rat. J. Neurosci. Res. 85, 1458–1467.

Eftekharpour, E., Karimi-Abdolrezaee, S., Fehlings, M.G., 2008. Current status of experimental cell replacement approaches to spinal cord injury. Neurofocus 24, E19.

Farooqui, A.A., Ong, W.Y., Horrocks, L.A., 2004. Biochemical aspects of neurodegeneration in human brain: involvement of neural membrane phospholipids and phospholipases A_2. Neurochem. Res. 29, 1961–1977.

Farooqui, A.A., Ong, W.Y., Horrocks, L.A., 2006. Inhibitors of brain phospholipase A_2 activity: their neuropharmacological effects and therapeutic importance for the treatment of neurologic disorders. Pharmacol. Rev. 58, 591–620.

Farooqui, A.A., 2010. Neurochemical Aspects of Neurotraumatic and Neurodegenerative Diseases. Springer, New York.

Farooqui, A.A., 2012. Phytochemicals, Signal Transduction, and Neurological Disorders. Springer, New York.

Farooqui, A.A., 2014. Inflammation and Oxidative Stress in Neurological Disorders. Springer International Publishing Switzerland, New York.

Farooqui, A.A., 2016. Therapeutic Potentials of Curcumin for Alzheimer Disease. Springer, New York.

Farooqui, A.A., Horrocks, L.A., 2007. Glycerophospholipids in Brain. Springer, New York.

Farooqui, A.A., Horrocks, L.A., 2009. Glutamate and cytokines-mediated alterations of phospholipid in head injury and spinal cord trauma. In: Banik, N., Ray, S.K. (Eds.), Handbook of Neurochemistry and Molecular Neurobiology. Springer Science-Business LLC, New York.

Fehlings, M.G., Wilson, J.R., Cho, N., 2014. Methylprednisolone for the treatment of acute spinal cord injury: counterpoint. Neurosurgery 1 (61 Suppl), 36−42.

Festoff, B.W., Ameenuddin, S., Arnold, P.M., Wong, A., Santacruz, K.S., et al., 2006. Minocycline neuroprotects, reduces microgliosis, and inhibits caspase protease expression early after spinal cord injury. J. Neurochem. 97, 1314−1326.

Figueroa, J.D., Cordero, K., Llán, M.S., De Leon, M., 2013a. Dietary omega-3 polyunsaturated fatty acids improve the neurolipidome and restore the DHA status while promoting functional recovery after experimental spinal cord injury. J. Neurotrauma. 30, 853−868.

Figueroa, J.D., Cordero, K., Serrano-Illan, M., Almeyda, A., Baldeosingh, K., et al., 2013b. Metabolomics uncovers dietary omega-3 fatty acid-derived metabolites implicated in anti-nociceptive responses after experimental spinal cord injury. Neuroscience 255, 1−18.

Filbin, M.T., 2003. Myelin-associated inhibitors of axonal regeneration in the adult mammalian CNS. Nat. Rev. Neurosci. 4, 703−713.

Forgione, N., Fehlings, M.G., 2014. Rho-ROCK inhibition in the treatment of spinal cord injury. World Neurosurg. 82, e535−e539.

Fouad, K., Tse, A., 2008. Adaptive changes in the injured spinal cord and their role in promoting functional recovery. Neurol. Res. 30, 17−27.

Franssen, E.H., de Bree, F.M., Verhaagen, J., 2007. Olfactory ensheathing glia: their contribution to primary olfactory nervous system regeneration and their regenerative potential following transplantation into the injured spinal cord. Brain Res. Rev. 56, 236−258.

Fujimura, M., Usuki, F., Kawamura, M., Izumo, S., 2011. Inhibition of the Rho/ROCK pathway prevents neuronal degeneration in vitro and in vivo following methylmercury exposure. Toxicol. Appl. Pharmacol. 250, 1−9.

Gao, W., Chen, S.R., Wu, M.Y., Gao, K., Li, Y.L., et al., 2016. Methylprednisolone exerts neuroprotective effects by regulating autophagy and apoptosis. Neural Regen. Res. 11, 823−828.

Garrido-Mesa, N., Zarzuelo, A., Gálvez, J., 2013. Minocycline: far beyond an antibiotic. Br. J. Pharmacol. 169, 337−352.

Geisler, F.H., Dorsey, F.C., Coleman, W.P., 1991. Recovery of motor function after spinal-cord injury—a randomized, placebo-controlled trial with GM-1 ganglioside. N. Engl. J. Med. 324, 1829−1838.

Geisler, F.H., Coleman, W.P., Grieco, G., Poonian, D., 2001a. Measurements and recovery patterns in a multicenter study of acute spinal cord injury. Spine 26 (Suppl 24), 68−86 [PubMed].

Geisler, F.H., Coleman, W.P., Grieco, G., Poonian, D., 2001b. Recruitment and early treatment in a multicenter study of acute spinal cord injury. Spine 26 (Suppl 24), 58−67.

Guest, J., Benavides, F., Padgett, K., Mendez, E., Tovar, D., 2011. Technical aspects of spinal cord injections for cell transplantation. Clinical and translational considerations. Brain Res. Bull. 84, 267−279.

Hawryluk, G.W., Rowland, J., Kwon, B.K., Fehlings, M.G., 2008. Protection and repair of the injured spinal cord: a review of completed, ongoing, and planned clinical trials for acute spinal cord injury. Nurosurg. Focus 25, E14.

Herrmann, J.E., Imura, T., Song, B., Qi, J., Ao, Y., et al., 2008. STAT3 is a critical regulator of astrogliosis and scar formation after spinal cord injury. J. Neurosci. 28, 7231−7243.

Hernández, J., Torres-Espín, A., Navarro, X., 2011. Adult stem cell transplants for spinal cord injury repair: current state in preclinical research. Curr. Stem Cell Res. Ther. 6, 273−287.

Hesp, Z.C., Goldstein, E.A., Miranda, C.J., Kaspar, B.K., McTigue, D.M., 2015. Chronic oligodendrogenesis and remyelination after spinal cord injury in mice and rats. J. Neurosci. 35, 1274−1290.

Höke, A., Silver, J., 1996. Proteoglycans and other repulsive molecules in glial boundaries during development and regeneration of the nervous system. Prog. Brain Res. 108, 149–163.

Hsu, J.Y., Bourguignon, L.Y., Adams, C.M., Peyrollier, K., Zhang, H., Fandel, T., et al., 2008. Matrix metalloproteinase-9 facilitates glial scar formation in the injured spinal cord. J. Neurosci. 28, 13467–13477.

Huang, W., Bhavsar, A., Ward, R.E., Hall, J.C., Priestley, J.V., Michael-Titus, A.T., 2009. Arachidonyl trifluoromethyl ketone is neuroprotective after spinal cord injury. J. Neurotrauma 2009 (26), 1429–1434.

Hurlbert, R.J., 2014. Methylprednisolone for the treatment of acute spinal cord injury: point. Neurosurgery 61 (Suppl 1), 32–35. 1.

Ichim, T.E., Solano, F., Lara, F., Paris, E., Ugalde, F., et al., 2010. Feasibility of combination allogeneic stem cell therapy for spinal cord injury: a case report. Int. Arch. Med. 3, 30.

Ishibashi, T., Lee, P.R., Baba, H., Fields, R.D., 2009. Leukemia inhibitory factor regulates the timing of oligodendrocyte development and myelination in the postnatal optic nerve. J. Neurosci. Res. 87, 3343–3355.

Islamov, R.R., Chintalgattu, V., Pak, E.S., 2004. Induction of VEGF and its Flt-1 receptor after sciatic nerve crush injury. NeuroReport 15, 2117–2121.

Jacobs, P.L., Nash, M.S., 2004. Exercise recommendations for individuals with spinal cord injury. Sports Med. 34, 727–751.

Jones, L.L., Margolis, R.U., Tuszynski, M.H., 2003. The chondroitin sulfate proteoglycans neurocan, brevican, phosphacan, and versican are differentially regulated following spinal cord injury. Exp. Neurol. 182, 399–411.

Kang, K.S., Kim, S.W., Ohet, Y.H., Yu, J.W., Kim, K.Y., et al., 2005. A37-year-old spinal cord injured female patient, transplanted of multipotent stem cells from human UC blood, with improved sensory perception and mobility, both functionally and morphologically: a case study. Cytotherapy 7, 368–373.

Keightley, M.-C., Wang, C.-H., Pazhakh, V., Lieschke, G.J., 2014. Delineating the roles of neutrophils and macrophages in zebrafish regeneration models. Int. J. Biochem. Cell Biol. 56, 92–106.

Kim, H.M., Hwang, D.H., Lee, J.E., Kim, S.U., Kim, B.G., 2007. Stem cell-based cell therapy for spinal cord injury. Cell Transpl. 16, 355–364.

King, V.R., Huang, W.L., Dyall, S.C., Curran, O.E., Priestley, J.V., et al., 2006. Omega-3 fatty acids improve recovery, whereas omega-6 fatty acids worsen outcome, after spinal cord injury in the adult rat. J. Neurosci. 26, 4672–4680.

Kinoshita, K., Chatzipanteli, K., Vitarbo, E., Truettner, J.S., Alonzo, O.F., et al., 2002. Interleukin-1 b messenger ribonucleic acid and protein levels after fluid-percussion brain injury in rats; importance of injury severity and brain temperature. Neurosurgery 51, 195–203.

Koob, A.O., Colby, J.M., Borgens, R.B., 2008. Behavioral recovery from traumatic brain injury after membrane reconstruction using polyethylene glycol. J. Biol. Eng. 2, 9.

Kwok, J.C., Afshari, F., Garcia-Alias, G., Fawcett, J.W., 2008. Proteoglycans in the central nervous system: plasticity, regeneration and their stimulation with chondroitinase ABC. Restor. Neurol. Neurosci. 26, 131–145.

Kwon, B.K., Okon, E., Hillyer, J., Mann, C., Baptiste, D., Weaver, L.C., et al., 2011. A systematic review of non-invasive pharmacologicneuroprotective treatments for acute spinal cord injury. J. Neurotrauma. 28, 1545–1588.

Kwon, B.K., Roy, J., Lee, J.H., Okon, E.B., Zhang, H., Marx, J.C., et al., 2009. Magnesium chloride in a polyethylene glycol formulation as a neuroprotective therapy for acute spinal cord injury: preclinical refinement and optimization. J. Neurotrauma 26, 1379–1393.

Kyritsis, N., Kizil, C., Brand, M., 2014. Neuroinflammation and central nervous system regeneration in vertebrates. Trends Cell Biol. 24, 128–135.

Lang-Lazdunski, L., Biondeau, N., Jarretou, G., Heurteaux, C., 2003. Linolenic acid prevents neuronal cell death and paraplegia after transient spinal cord ischemia in rats. J. Vasc. Surg. 38, 564–575.

Lee, S.M., Yune, T.Y., Kim, S.J., Park, D.W., Lee, Y.K., et al., 2003. Minocycline reduces cell death and improves functional recovery after traumatic spinal cord injury in the rat. J. Neurotrauma 20, 1017–1027.

Lee, M.Y., Chen, L., Toborek, M., 2009. Nicotine attenuates iNOS expression and contributes to neuroprotection in a compressive model of spinal cord injury. J. Neurosci. Res. 87, 937–947.

Levi, A.D., Green, B.A., Wang, M.Y., et al., 2009. Clinical application of modest hypothermia after spinal cord injury. J. Neurotrauma 26, 407–415.

Levi, A.D., Casella, G., Green, B.A., et al., 2010. Clinical outcomes using modest intravascular hypothermia after acute cervical spinal cord injury. Neurosurgery 66, 670–677.

Li, G., Cao, Y., Shen, F., Wang, Y., Bai, L., et al., 2016. Mdivi-1 inhibits astrocyte activation and astroglial scar formation and enhances axonal regeneration after spinal cord injury in rats. Front. Cell Neurosci. 10, 241.

Lin, M.S., Lee, Y.H., Chiu, W.T., Hung, K.S., 2011a. Curcumin provides neuroprotection after spinal cord injury. J. Surg. Res. 166, 280–289.

Lin, M.S., Sun, Y.Y., Chiu, W.T., Chang, C.Y., Hung, C.C., et al., 2011b. Curcumin attenuates the expression and secretion of RANTES following spinal cord injury in vivo and lipopolysaccharide-induced astrocyte reactivation in vitro. J. Neurotrauma 28, 1259–1269.

Lindvall, O., Kokaia, Z., 2010. Stem cells in human neurodegenerative disorders—time for clinical translation? J. Clin. Investig. 120, 29–40.

Liu, N.K., Zhang, Y.P., Titsworth, W.L., Jiang, X., Han, S., et al., 2006. A novel role of phospholipase A_2 in mediating spinal cord secondary injury. Ann. Neurol. 59, 606–619.

Liu, N.K., Deng, L.X., Zhang, Y.P., Lu, Q.B., Wang, X.F., et al., 2014. Cytosolic phospholipase A_2 protein as a novel therapeutic target for spinal cord injury. Ann. Neurol. 75, 644–658.

Liu, N.K., Xu, X.M., 2010. Phospholipase A_2 and its molecular mechanism after spinal cord injury. Mol. Neurobiol. 41, 197–205.

Liu, C., Shi, Z., Fan, L., Zhang, C., Wang, K., Wang, B., 2011. Resveratrol improves neuron protection and functional recovery in rat model of spinal cord injury. Brain Res. 1374, 100–109.

Liu, Y., 2012. Rho-ROCK signal pathway. Zhongguo Ertong Baojian Za Zhi. 20, 822–825.

Lu, J., Ashwell, K., 2002. Olfactory ensheathing cells: their potential use for repairing the injured spinal cord. Spine (Phila Pa 1978) 27, 887–892.

Lu, P., Jones, L.L., Tuszynski, M.H., 2005. BDNF-expressing marrow stromal cells support extensive axonal growth at sites of spinal cord injury. Exp. Neurol. 191, 344–360.

Lu, G.B., Niu, F.W., Zhang, Y.C., Du, L., Liang, Z.Y., et al., 2016. Methylprednisolone promotes recovery of neurological function after spinal cord injury: association with Wnt/β-catenin signaling pathway activation. Neural Regen. Res. 11, 1816–1823.

Lynskey, J.V., Sandhu, F.A., Dai, H.N., McAtee, M., Slotkin, J.R., et al., 2006. Delayed intervention with transplants and neurotrophic factors supports recovery of forelimb function after cervical spinal cord injury in adult rats. J. Neurotrauma 23, 617–634.

Lynskey, J.V., Belanger, A., Jung, R., 2008. Activity-dependent plasticity in spinal cord injury. J. Rehabil. Res. Dev. 45, 229–240.

Mantilla, C.B., Gransee, H.M., Zhan, W.Z., Sieck, G.C., 2013. Motoneuron BDNF/TrkB signaling enhances functional recovery after cervical spinal cord injury. Exp. Neurol. 247, 101–109.

Marchand, F., Tsantoulas, C., Singh, D., Grist, J., Clark, A.K., et al., 2009. Effects of etanercept and minocycline in a rat model of spinal cord injury. Eur. J. Pain. 13, 673−681.

Marsala, J., Orendacova, J., Lukacova, N., Vanicky, I., 2007. Traumatic injury of the spinal cord and nitric oxide. Prog. Brain Res. 161, 171−183.

McKerracher, L., Rosen, K., 2015. MAG, myelin and overcoming growth inhibition in the CNS. Front. Mol. Neurosci 8, 1−6.

Michael-Titus, A.T., 2007. Omega-3 fatty acids and neurological injury. Prost. Leukot. Essent. Fatty Acids 2007 (77), 295−300.

Mills, C.D., Allchorne, A.J., Griffin, R.S., Woolf, C.J., Costigan, M., 2007. GDNF selectively promotes regeneration of injury−primed sensory neurons in the lesioned spinal cord. Mol. Cell Neurosci. 36, 185−194.

Miller, R.G., Mitchell, J.D., Lyon, M., Moore, D.H., 2007. Riluzole for amyotrophic lateral sclerosis (ALS)/motor neuron disease (MND). Cochrane Database Syst. Rev. CD001447.

Mitcho, K., Kanko, J.R., 1999. Acute care management of spinal cord injuries. Crit. Care Nurse 22, 60−79.

Moini-Zanjani, T., Ostad, S.N., Labibi, F., Ameli, H., Mosaffa, N., et al., 2016. Minocycline effects on IL-6 concentration in macrophage and microglial cells in a rat model of neuropathic pain Iran. Biomed J. 20, 273−279.

Moriwaki, A., Nishida, K., Matsushita, M., Ozaki, T., Kunisada, T., et al., 2005. Calpain inhibitors prevent neuronal cell death and ameliorate motor disturbances after compression-induced spinal cord injury in rats. J. Neurotrauma 22, 398−406.

Moviglia, G.A., Fernandez Viña, R., Brizuela, J.A., et al., 2006. Combined protocol of cell therapy for chronic spinal cord injury. Report on the electrical and functional recovery of two patients. Cytotherapy. 8, 202−209.

Mu, X., Azbill, R.D., Springer, J.E., 2000. Riluzole improves measure of oxidative stress following traumatic spinal cord injury. Brain Res. 870, 66−72.

Mukhamedshina, Y.O., Garanina, E.E., Masgutova, G.A., Galieva, L.R., Sanatova, E.R., et al., 2016. Assessment of glial scar, tissue sparing, behavioral recovery and axonal regeneration following acute transplantation of genetically modified human umbilical cord blood cells in a rat model of spinal cord contusion. PLoS One. 11, e0151745.

Murphy, M., 1999. Traumatic spinal cord injury: an acute care rehabilitation perspective. Crit. Care Nurs. Quar 22, 51−59.

Noble, L.J., Donovan, F., Igarashi, T., Gousseo, S., Werb, Z., 2002. Matrix metalloproteinases limit functional recovery after spinal cord injury by modulation of early vascular events. J. Neurosci. 22, 7526−7535.

Novikova, L.N., Novikov, L.N., Kellerth, J.O., 2000. BDNF abolishes the survival effect of NT-3 in axotomized Clarke neurons of adult rats. J Comp Neurol. 428, 671−680.

Novikova, L.N., Novikov, L.N., Kellerth, J.O., 2002. Differential effects of neurotrophins on neuronal survival and axonal regeneration after spinal cord injury in adult rats. J. Comp. Neurol. 452, 255−263.

Ohmi, Y., Ohkawa, Y., Yamauchi, Y., Tajima, O., Furukawa, K., et al., 2012. Essential roles of gangliosides in the formation and maintenance of membrane microdomains in brain tissues. Neurochem. Res. 37, 1185−1191.

Olivas, A.D., Noble-Haeusslein, L.J., 2006. Phospholipase A_2 and spinal cord injury: a novel target for therapeutic intervention. Ann. Neurol. 59, 577−579.

Parks, W.C., Wilson, C.L., López-Boado, Y.S., 2004. Matrix metalloproteinases as modulators of inflammation and innate immunity. Nat. Rev. Immunol. 4, 617−629.

Pizzi, M.A., Crowe, M.J., 2007. Matrix metalloproteinases and proteoglycans in axonal regeneration. Exp. Neurol. 204, 496−511.

Popovich, P.G., Guan, Z., Wei, P., Huitinga, I., van Rooijen, N., et al., 1999. Depletion of hematogenous macrophages promotes partial hindlimb recovery and neuroanatomical repair after experimental spinal cord injury. Exp. Neurol. 158, 351−365.

Ray, S.K., Hogan, E.L., Banik, N.L., 2003. Calpain in the pathophysiology of spinal cord injury: neuroprotection with calpain inhibitors. Brain Res. Rev. 42, 169–185.

Reichardt, L.F., 2006. Neurotrophin-regulated signalling pathways. Philos. Trans. R. Soc. Lond. B. Biol. Sci. 361, 1545–1564.

Rosado, I.R., Lavor, M.S., Alves, E.G., Fukushima, F.B., Oliveira, K.M., et al., 2014. Effects of methylprednisolone, dantrolene, and their combination on experimental spinal cord injury. Int. J. Clin. Exp. Pathol. 7, 4617–4626.

Rubio-Gayosso, I., Platts, S.H., Duling, B.R., 2006. Reactive oxygen species mediate modification of glycocalyx during ischemia-reperfusion injury. Am. J. Physiol. Heart Circ. Physiol. 290, 2247–2256.

Saberi, H., Moshayedi, P., Aghayan, H.-R., et al., 2008. Treatment of chronic thoracic spinal cord injury patients with autologous Schwann cell transplantation: an interim report on safety considerations and possible outcomes. Neurosci. Lett. 443, 46–50.

Sadowsky, C.L., McDonald, J.W., 2009. Activity-based restorative therapies: concepts and applications in spinal cord injury-related neurorehabilitation. Dev. Disabil. Res. Rev. 15, 112–126.

Sahni, V., Kessler, J.A., 2010. Stem cell therapies for spinal cord injury. Nat. Rev. Neurol. 6, 363–372.

Sakata, Y., Zhuang, H., Kwansa, H., Koehler, R.C., Doré, S., 2010. Resveratrol protects against experimental stroke: putative neuroprotective role of heme oxygenase 1. Exp. Neurol. 224, 325–329.

Sanivarapu, R., Vallabhaneni, V., Verma, V., 2016. The potential of curcumin in treatment of spinal cord injury. Neurol. Res. Int. 2016, 9468193.

Santos, D., Giudetti, G., Micera, S., Navarro, X., Del Valle, J., 2016. Focal release of neurotrophic factors by biodegradable microspheres enhance motor and sensory axonal regeneration in vitro and in vivo. Brain Res. 1636, 93–106.

Sapirstein, A., Bonventre, J.V., 2000. Phospholipases A_2 in ischemic and toxic brain injury. Neurochem. Res. 25, 745–753.

Satake, K., Matsuyama, Y., Kamiya, M., Kawakami, H., Iwata, H., et al., 2000. Up-regulation of glial cell line-derived neurotrophic factor (GDNF) following traumatic spinal cord injury. NeuroReport 11, 3877–3881.

Schmandke, A., Schmandke, A., Strittmatter, S.M., 2007. ROCK and Rho: biochemistry and neuronal functions of Rho-associated protein kinases. Neuroscientist 13, 454–469.

Schumacher, P.A., Siman, R.G., Fehlings, M.G., 2000. Pretreatment with calpain inhibitor CEP-4143 inhibits calpain I activation and cytoskeletal degradation, improves neurological function, and enhances axonal survival after traumatic spinal cord injury. J. Neurochem. 74, 1646–1655.

Schwab, J.M., Brechtel, K., Mueller, C.A., Failli, V., Kaps, H.P., et al., 2006. Experimental strategies to promote spinal cord regeneration--an integrative perspective. Prog. Neurobiol. 78, 91–116.

Shechter, R., London, A., Varol, C., Raposo, C., Cusimano, M., et al., 2009. Infiltrating blood-derived macrophages are vital cells playing an antiinflammatory role in recovery from spinal cord injury in mice. PLoS Med. 6, e1000113.

Silva, N.A., Sousa, N., Reis, R.L., Salgado, A.J., 2014. From basics to clinical: A comprehensive review on spinal cord injury. Prog. Neurobiol. 114, 25–57.

Smith, J.A., Park, S., Krause, J.S., Banik, N.L., 2013. Oxidative stress, DNA damage, and the telomeric complex as therapeutic targets in acute neurodegeneration. Neurochem. Int. 62, 764–775.

Snow, D.M., Lemmon, V., Carrino, D.A., et al., 1990. Sulfated proteoglycans in astroglial barriers inhibit neurite outgrowth in vitro. Exp. Neurol. 109, 111–130.

Soderquist, R.G., Milligan, E.D., Sloane, E.M., Harrison, J.A., Douvas, K.K., Potter, J.M., et al., 2009. PEGylation of brain-derived neurotrophic factor for preserved biological activity and enhanced spinal cord distribution. J. Biomed. Mater. Res. A 91 (3), 719–729.

Springer, J.E., Azbill, R.D., Kennedy, S.E., George, J., Geddes, J.W., 1997. Rapid calpain I activation and cytoskeletal protein degradation following traumatic spinal cord injury: attenuation with riluzole pretreatment. J. Neurochem. 69, 1592–1600.

Stirling, D.P., Koochesfahani, K.M., Steeves, J.D., Tetzlaff, W., 2005. Minocycline as a neuroprotective agent. Neuroscientist 11, 308–322.

Sun, D., Xu, J., 2013. Effect of curcumin on calcitonin gene related peptide expression after spinal cord injury in rats. Zhongguo Xiu Fu Chong Jian Wai Ke Za Zhi. 27, 1225–1229.

Tan, A.M., Zhao, P., Waxman, S.G., Hains, B.C., 2009. Early microglial inhibition preemptively mitigates chronic pain development after experimental spinal cord injury. J. Rehabi. Res. Dev. 46, 123–133.

Tator, C.H., Hashimoto, R., Raich, A., Norvell, D., Fehlings, M.G., et al., 2012. Translational potential of preclinical trials of neuroprotection through pharmacotherapy for spinal cord injury. J. Neurosurg. Spine 17 (Suppl), 157–229.

Teng, Y.D., Choi, H., Onario, R.C., Zhu, S., Desilets, F.C., Lan, S., et al., 2004. Minocycline inhibits contusion-triggered mitochondrial cytochrome c release and mitigates functional deficits after spinal cord injury. Proc. Natl. Acad. Sci. U.S.A. 101, 3071–3076.

Teramura, T., Takehara, T., Onodera, Y., Nakagawa, K., Hamanishi, C., et al., 2012. Mechanical stimulation of cyclic tensile strain induces reduction of pluripotent related gene expressions via activation of Rho/ROCK and subsequent decreasing of AKT phosphorylation in human induced pluripotent stem cells. Biochem. Biophys. Res. Commun. 417, 836–841.

Thorell, W.E., Leibrock, L.G., Agrawal, S.K., 2002. Role of RyRs and IP_3 receptors after traumatic injury to spinal cord white matter. J. Neurotrauma 19, 335–342.

Thuret, S., Moon, L.D.F., Gage, F.H., 2006. Therapeutic interventions after spinal cord injury. Nat. Rev. Neurosci. 7, 628–643.

Tripathi, R.B., McTigue, D.M., 2008. Chronically increased ciliary neurotrophic factor and fibroblast growth factor-2 expression after spinal contusion in rats. J. Comp. Neurol. 510, 129–144.

Tsintou, M., Dalamagkas, K., Seifalian, A.M., 2015. Advances in regenerative therapies for spinal cord injury: a biomaterials approach. Neural. Regen. Res. 10, 726–742.

Valuckaite, V., Zaborina, O., Long, J., Hauer-Jensen, M., Wang, J., et al., 2009. Oral PEG 15–20 protects the intestine against radiation: role of lipid rafts. Am. J. Physiol. Gastrointest. Liver Physiol. 297, G1041–G1052.

Varma, A.K., Das, A., Wallace 4th, G., Barry, J., Vertegel, A.A., et al., 2013. Spinal cord injury: a review of current therapy, future treatments, and basic science frontiers. Neurochem. Res. 38, 895–905.

Walker, J.B., Harris, M., 1993. GM-1 ganglioside administration combined with physical therapy restores ambulation in humans with chronic spinal cord injury. Neurosci. Lett. 161, 174–178.

Wang, Y.F., Zu, J.N., Li, J., Chen, C., Xi, C.Y., Yan, J.L., 2014. Curcumin promotes the spinal cord repair via inhibition of glial scar formation and inflammation. Neurosci. Lett. 560, 51–56.

Wanner, I.B., Anderson, M.A., Song, B., Levine, J., Fernandez, A., et al., 2013. Glial scar borders are formed by newly proliferated, elongated astrocytes that interact to corral inflammatory and fibrotic cells via STAT3-dependent mechanisms after spinal cord injury. J. Neurosci. 33, 12870–12886.

Webber, D.J., Bradbury, E.J., McMohan, S.B., Minger, S.L., 2007. Transplanted neural progenitor cells survive and differentiate but achieve limited functional recovery in the lesioned adult rat spinal cord. Regen. Med. 2, 929–945.

Wells, J.E., Rice, T.K., Nuttall, R.K., Edwards, D.R., Zekki, H., et al., 2002. An adverse role for matrix metalloproteinase 12 after spinal cord injury in mice. J. Neurosci. 23, 10107–10115.

Westergren, H., Farooque, M., Olsson, Y., et al., 2001. Spinal cord blood flow charges following systemic hypothermia and spinal cord compression injury: an experimental study in the rat using laser-Doppler flowmetry. Spinal Cord 39, 74–84.

Wilson, J.R., Forgione, N., Fehlings, M.G., 2013. Emerging therapies for acute traumatic spinal cord injury. CMAJ. 185, 485–492.

Wu, W., Chandler, L., Lu, Q., Wu, W., Eddelman, D.B., Parish, J.M., et al., 2017. RhoA/Rho kinase mediates neuronal death through regulating cPLA$_2$ activation. Mol. Neurobiol. 54, 6885–6895.

Yiu, G., He, Z., 2006. Glial inhibition of CNS axon regeneration. Nat. Rev. Neurosci. 7, 617–627.

Yong, V.W., 2005. Metalloproteinases: mediators of pathology and regeneration in the CNS. Nat. Rev. Neurosci. 6, 931–944.

Yong, V.W., Rivest, S., 2009. Taking advantage of the systemic immune system to cure brain diseases. Neuron. 64, 55–60.

Yuan, Y.M., He, C., 2013. The glial scar in spinal cord injury and repair. Neurosci. Bull. 29, 421–435.

Zai, L.J., Yoo, S., Wrathall, J.R., 2005. Increased growth factor expression and cell proliferation after contusive spinal cord injury. Brain Res. 1052, 147–155.

Zhao, H., Chen, S., Gao, K., Zhou, Z., Wang, C., et al., 2017. Resveratrol protects against spinal cord injury by activating autophagy and inhibiting apoptosis mediated by the SIRT1/AMPK signaling pathway. Neuroscience 348, 241–251.

Neurochemical Aspects of Traumatic Brain Injury

INTRODUCTION

Traumatic brain injury (TBI) is caused by a blow to the head by an external physical force or a sudden acceleration/deceleration movement of the head. TBI is one of the major causes of death and disability worldwide. It is estimated that in the United States 1.7 million people sustain TBI of whi ch 275,000 require hospitalization and 52,000 die (Faul et al., 2010). Rates of TBI-related deaths are even higher in developing countries (Thurman et al., 1999, 2007). TBI is the leading cause of death and disability for persons between the ages of 1 and 44 years, and an estimated 5.3 million Americans, almost 2% of the population, live with long-term disabilities due to a prior TBI (Thurman et al., 1999). In young children and elderly individuals, falls are the primary cause of TBI hospitalizations and deaths, whereas traffic crashes are the primary cause in adolescents and young adults (Faul et al., 2010). Symptoms of a TBI are unconsciousness, inability to remember the cause of the injury or when TBI has occurred immediately before or up to 24 hours after, confusion and disorientation, difficulty remembering new information, headache, dizziness, blurry vision, nausea and vomiting, ringing in the ears, trouble speaking coherently, and changes in emotions or sleep patterns. The severity of TBI is determined by the Glasgow Coma Scale (GCS) at the time of injury. A diagnosis of moderate TBI is made in patients with between 30 minutes and 6 hours of unconsciousness and a GCS score of 13–15, whereas severe TBI (GCS score of >9) refers to a longer period of unconsciousness and likely >24 hours of memory loss and has a 40% mortality rate and more extensive damage (Harmon et al., 2013; Shekhar et al., 2015). TBI is classified into (1) focal damage, which occurs in localized area and causes damage to the underlying brain tissues and vessels and (2) diffuse damage, which is not restricted but widespread throughout the brain. Diffuse type mainly involves

239

axonal injury also called diffuse axonal injury (DAI), brain swelling, and hypoxia (Farkas and Povlishock, 2007; Farooqui, 2010; Li et al., 2013). Axonal injury is a powerful predictor of morbidity and mortality (Czeiter et al., 2009). In axons, it causes an accumulation of proteins, including amyloid precursor protein (APP), which is carried by fast antero-grade axonal transport and serves as a sensitive marker of axonal damage. This may result in axonal disconnection leading to loss of axonal function and structure (Chen et al., 2004). Severe TBI is often life-threatening and requires immediate care. TBI usually affect the brain function such as cognitive status, executive function, memory, data processing, language skills, and attention (Yan et al., 2015). The disruption of normal functioning can lead to loss of homeostasis having devastating implication on the whole body. TBI not only disrupts blood—brain barrier (BBB) but also promote changes in brain vasculature depending upon the injury location and form of brain injury. As stated above, in human subjects, TBI is commonly caused by motor vehicle collisions, falls, sport-associated injuries, blast exposure, and shaken baby syndrome in infants (Table 6.1). In addition to the severity of the TBI, the time after the injury (i.e., acute vs chronic) dictates the observed symptoms to some extent. Favorable recovery has been observed in

TABLE 6.1   Common Causes of Traumatic Brain Injury

	Forms of TBI	Description	Reference
	Blast TBI	Blast energy-mediated injury	Turner et al., 2013
	Closed head injury	Blunt object-mediated injury	Turner et al., 2013
	Concussion	Violent blow-mediated injury	Angoa-Perez et al., 2014
TBI	Contusion	Contusion-mediated injury	Greer et al., 2013
	Fall-induced TBI	Rapid impact-mediated injury	Asl et al., 2013
	Penetrating TBI	Blunt object-mediated injury	Begum et al., 2014
	Shaken baby syndrome	Abusive head trauma-mediated injury	Foster et al., 2014
	Spinal cord injury	SCI-mediated injury	Xiong et al., 2013

80%−90% of TBI cases within the first 3 months of injury, and the remaining cases are termed as the "miserable minority" (Ruff, 2005). Besides characterizing the injury based on a specific inciting event, the TBI can be described as open or closed head injury, focal or global injury, and impact or blast-mediated injury (Covey and Born, 2010; Alford et al., 2011; Turner et al., 2013).

Like spinal cord injury, the pathophysiology of TBI is biphasic condition. The primary TBI occurs rapidly whereas secondary TBI is activated at later time points and may be more eventful involving may biochemical processes. Primary injury results in increase in intracranial pressure, rupturing of microvessels and neural cells, diffuse axonal shearing, disruption of BBB permeability, and necrosis of neural cells. In contrast, secondary injury involves Ca^{2+} influx, activation of microglial cells and astrocytes, cellular stress, neuroinflammation, and apoptotic cell death (Raghupathi, 2004) (Fig. 6.1). Cerebral edema is another process, which is induced by water imbalance, substance P (SP) release, and the development of functional deficits in response to TBI (Corrigan et al., 2016). Specifically, an elevation in cerebral perivascular SP is observed

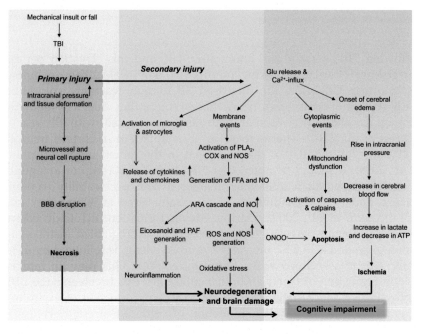

FIGURE 6.1 Hypothetical diagram showing mechanism of neurodegeneration and cognitive impairment following traumatic brain injury (TBI). BBB, blood−brain barrier; PLA₂, phospholipase A_2; COX, cyclooxygenase; NOS, nitric oxide synthase; NO, nitric oxide; PAF, platelet activating factor; ARA, arachidonic acid; ROS, reactive oxygen species; ONOO⁻, peroxynitrite.

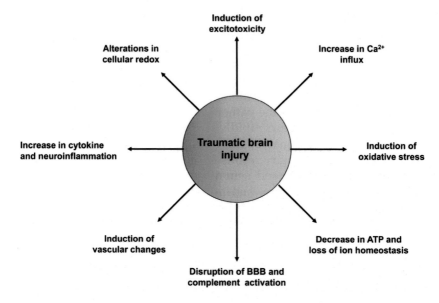

FIGURE 6.2 Traumatic brain injury (TBI)–induced alterations in neurochemical processes. BBB, blood–brain barrier.

following TBI as early as 5 hours after TBI, and this elevation persists for at least 24 hours following trauma (Donkin et al., 2009). In human postmortem TBI brain, the increased SP immunoreactivity colocalizes with APP in perivascular nerve fibers suggesting that TBI-mediated damage to these perivascular neurons is associated with SP release (Zacest et al., 2010). The increase in SP is apparent in cortical neurons and astrocytes, similar to that observed in the rodent models (Donkin et al., 2009). It should be noted that NK1 tachykinin receptor antagonist N-acetyl-L-tryptophan attenuates increased BBB permeability, cerebral edema, and functional deficits when administered at 30 minutes after TBI (Donkin et al., 2009). During edema formation, cytotoxic edema develops in acute stages of TBI as a result of dysregulated metabolism. Often in response to TBI, the early cytotoxic edema is followed by vasogenic edema associated with compromised BBB. Glia play an integral role in regulation of water and other molecules that transverse the BBB. Collective evidence suggests that TBI results in induction of excitotoxicity, increase in Ca^{2+}-influx, induction of oxidative stress, decrease in ATP, disruption of BBB, induction of vascular changes, increase in proinflammatory cytokines and chemokines, and changes in cellular redox (Fig. 6.2). Clinical symptoms of secondary injury appear slowly (days/week/months) after TBI (Table 6.2). After brain injury, microglia, monocytes, macrophages, and neutrophils invade areas along with

TABLE 6.2   Time-Dependence, Neurochemical Events, and Mode of Cell
Death Following TBI

Time Post-TBI	Pathological Events	Mode of Cell Death
1−3 hours	Disruption of the BBB, deformation of brain tissue, swelling, and ischemia	Alterations in ion homeostasis
6 hours	Rupture of neural cells, cell/axon stretching	Start of necrotic cell death
12 hours	Rupture of neural cells, cell/axon stretching	Maximum necrosis
1 week	Edema, vasospasm, inflammation, and oxidative stress	Start of apoptotic cell death
2 weeks	Edema, vasospasm, inflammation, and oxidative stress	Maximum apoptosis
1 month	Edema, inflammation, and oxidative stress	Some apoptotic cell death
3 months	Start of neurogenesis	Development of neurites
6−12 months		Neuropsychiatric symptoms

TBI rapidly initiates a series of secondary events that induce long-term neurological consequences, such as cognitive dysfunction due to neural injury (Agoston et al., 2009).

extensive upregulation of not only neutrophil adhesion factors (Corps et al., 2015) but also activation of integrin receptors and immunoglobulin superfamily members (Albelda et al., 1994; Kochanek and Hallenbeck, 1992) This process is carried out through innate signaling pathways and, in the case of TBI, through release of damage-associated molecular pattern molecules (DAMPs), called as danger signals (Bianchi, 2007). This response results not only in restoration of normal cellular homeostasis but also in the induction of maladaptive immune responses. This inflammatory response can persist for years and eventually contributes to neurodegeneration. Cerebral ischemia also contributes to the pathogenesis of secondary TBI. It is caused by a decrease in cerebral blood flow within the first hours after TBI (van Santbrink et al., 2003). As mentioned in Chapter 2, Molecular Aspects of Ischemic Injury, decrease in cerebral blood flow not only results mitochondrial damage but also induces alterations in ion homeostasis, edema, and greater reduction in cerebral blood flow. The disruption of mitochondrial function in neurons and glial cells is a characteristic feature of acute stages of TBI (Cheng et al., 2012; McGinn and Povlishock, 2016). An increase in mitochondrial membrane permeability in neurons involves the mitochondrial membrane permeability transition. This

Ca^{2+}-dependent process leads to the loss of mitochondrial membrane potential (Delta Psi), induction of mitochondrial swelling, and the rupture of outer mitochondrial membrane. These processes are not only intensified by activated glial cells but also result in the generation of reactive oxygen species (ROS). Neurons are limited in their antioxidant capacity and thus they rely on astrocytes to buffer ROS (Hamby and Sofroniew, 2010). Otherwise, neurons may become susceptible to irreversible damage. Importantly, a pro-oxidative environment also promotes ROS-mediated damage to lipid, protein, and nucleic acid resulting in further membrane disruption (Miller et al., 2015) and induction of neuroinflammation (Hsieh and Yang, 2013).

In humans, TBI can also be produced by blast exposure, motor vehicle collisions, falls, sport-associated injuries (American football, boxing), and in infants TBI can be by shaken baby syndrome. TBI-induced by above procedures promote axonal injury, the most important pathological features of TBI. There are several ways TBI can be introduced in experimental animals. Thus, onset of blast produces TBI by rotational and acceleration/deceleration components. Blast-mediated injury leads to a robust gliosis response and axonal degeneration (Creed et al., 2011; Turner et al., 2013). Axonal swelling and bulb formation are common morphological hallmarks of blast-mediated TBI (DiLeonardi et al., 2009). Closed head injuries are caused by blunt object strike without fracturing the bone (Angoa-Perez et al., 2014). Concision is produced by a violent blow to the head (Angoa-Perez et al., 2014). Contusion results in rupture of blood capillaries (Creed et al., 2011). During fall-induced injury, hit by the ground produces TBI (Asl et al., 2013). Injury by blunt object produces penetrating injury (Peek-Asa et al., 2001; Kuhajda et al., 2014). Abusive head trauma due to rapid acceleration and deceleration of skull when shaken results in Shaken baby syndrome (Foster et al., 2014) (Table 6.1). White matter tracts are particularly vulnerable to damage from impact-acceleration forces following TBI. Axonal injury not only includes demyelination, swelling, and disconnection of the proximal axon bulb from its distal segment but also Wallerian degeneration along with induction of demyelination and neuroinflammation. Axonal injury also involves the proliferation of activated microglia and the presence of myelin-containing macrophages at the injury site following TBI (Povlishock et al., 1983; Browne et al., 2011). In TBI, white matter tracts show thinning of white matter tracts (e.g., corpus callosum) and denervation and re-innervation along with activated microglia in some individuals up to 18 years postinjury (Johnson et al., 2013). These findings suggest ongoing axonal damage and resultant impaired integrity of white matter tracts as important components of the clinical deficits after TBI (Bigler, 2013) leading to the disruption of functional neural networks (Bigler, 2013). The use of advanced magnetic resonance imaging

(MRI) techniques allows the detection of white matter damage in patients with mild to moderate TBI. Diffusion tensor imaging (DTI) generates additional information from MRI sequences that detect changes in anisotropy, which is particularly advantageous for analysis of highly anisotropic myelinated nerve fibers that align within white matter tracts. DTI can be used to interpolate the pathways of fiber bundles, so that abnormal findings may indicate disrupted pathways. However, the inherent limitations of DTI tractography measures for anatomical accuracy must be recognized to appropriately interrogate white matter pathways for comparative changes in microstructure (Thomas et al., 2014; Armstrong et al., 2016).

CELLULAR AND NEUROCHEMICAL CHANGES IN TBI

Glutamate is a major transmitter in the nervous system. It plays a major role in rapid synaptic transmission. Thus, it is not only required for neuron-to-neuron communication, but it also plays an important roles in neuronal growth and axon guidance, brain development and maturation, and synaptic plasticity. Under normal physiologic conditions, the presence of glutamate in the synapse is regulated by active ATP-dependent transporters in neurons and glia. However, if these uptake mechanisms are impaired by metabolic disturbances brought about by TBI, glutamate excessively accumulates, stimulating sodium (Na^+) and calcium (Ca^{2+}) fluxes into the cell through glutamate receptors, thereby injuring or killing the cell. In humans and animals, TBI is accompanied by an acute increase in tissue glutamate concentrations that remain high for several days (Sundström and Mo, 2002; Faden et al., 1989). This sustained increase in extracellular glutamate levels leads to the overstimulation of the N-methyl-D-aspartate (NMDA) type of glutamate receptors and the subsequent overloading of neurons with Ca^{2+} and Na^+, resulting in the activation of phospholipases, endonucleases, nitric oxide synthases, protein phosphatases, and various protein kinases, matrix metalloproteinases (MMPs), and proteases such as calpain and caspases leading to eventually apoptotic and/or necrotic cell death (Fig. 6.3) (Raghupathi, 2004; Ray and Banik, 2003; Ellis et al., 2004; Ahn et al., 2004; Arundine and Tymianski, 2004; Arundine et al., 2004; Atkins et al., 2007, 2009). As stated above, TBI also results in reduction in ATP, disruption of BBB, alterations in cellular redox, vascular changes, and induction of neuroinflammation and oxidative stress (Fig. 6.2). Glutamate-mediated neuronal cell death has also been linked to autophagy (Bigford et al., 2009). It is shown that NR2B (NMDA receptor subunit) interacts with autophagic protein, Beclin-1 in membrane rafts of the normal rat cerebral cortex. Moderate TBI induces rapid recruitment and association of NR2B

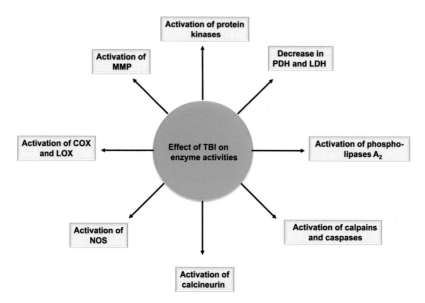

FIGURE 6.3   Stimulation of enzymes by traumatic brain injury (TBI). COX, cyclooxygenase; LOX, lipoxygenase; MMP, metalloproteinase; NOS, nitric oxide synthase; LDH, lactate dehydrogenase; PDH, pyruvate dehydrogenase.

and Ca^{2+}/calmodulin-dependent protein kinase II (CaMKII) to membrane rafts, and translocation of Beclin-1 out of membrane microdomains. Furthermore, TBI produces significant increases in the expression of key autophagic proteins. Morphological hallmarks of autophagy that are significantly attenuated by the treatment with the NR2B antagonist Ro 25-6981, suggesting that stimulation of autophagy by NR2B signaling may be regulated by redistribution of Beclin-1 in membrane rafts after TBI (Bigford et al., 2009). It is also suggested that the presence of high levels of glutamate produces glial cell demise by inhibiting cystine uptake leading to a decrease in glutathione and making glial cells vulnerable to oxidative stress (Matute et al., 2006; Pereire and Resende de Oliveira, 2000). It is recently shown that glutamate-mediated delayed posttraumatic white matter degeneration also involves the reversal of Na^+-dependent glutamate transport with subsequent activation of AMPA receptors and oligodendrocyte death (Park et al., 2004). Collective clinical and experimental evidence suggests that glutamate-mediated excitotoxicity is a significant contributor to acute posttraumatic neurodegenerative diseases (see below) (Yi and Hazell, 2006). The termination of glutamate-mediated toxicity and neurotransmission is achieved by rapid uptake of the released glutamate by presynaptic and/or astrocytic transporters (Szatkowski and Attwell, 1994) in a process that is driven by and coupled to ion gradients (Gegelashvili et al., 2000). The glutamate transporter EAAT2/GLT-1 (human/rat homolog) (Pines et al., 1992) is expressed predominantly in glia throughout the brain and spinal cord, and accounts for approximately 95% of glutamate uptake in the central nervous system (CNS) (Suchak et al., 2003), implicating this isoform in the maintenance of extracellular glutamate homeostasis in normal and pathological conditions (Sheldon and Robinson, 2007; Lauriat and McInnes, 2007).

Other mechanisms that contribute to TBI-mediated hypometabolic response include the overproduction of reactive oxygen and nitrogen species which can lead to poly(ADP) ribose polymerases (PARP) activation (Arundine et al., 2004; Kauppinen, 2007; Besson, 2009) and related reductions of nicotinamide adenine dinucleotide (NAD^+) and nicotinamide adenine dinucleotide phosphate ($NADP^+$) (Clark et al., 2007; Signoretti et al., 2010). This process may result in reduction in glucose metabolism through downregulation of glyceraldehyde-3-phosphate dehydrogenase (GAPDH) and pyruvate dehydrogenase. This process may inhibit glycolysis and the entry of pyruvate into the TCA cycle resulting in energy depletion and cell death. Reduced GAPDH activity has also been shown to act as a "molecular switch" resulting in increased flux of glucose into the PPP (Ralser et al., 2007; Grant, 2008). Here it should be recalled that many studies have indicated that PARP inhibitors can attenuate NAD^+ reductions, decrease neuronal damage, and improve behavioral outcome following experimental TBI (Clark et al., 2007; Besson, 2009).

In traumatized brain interactions among microvascular endothelia, astrocytes, microglial cells, and peripheral immune cells result in the initiation, maintenance, and prolongation of not only oxidative stress but also in induction of neuroinflammation through the generation of inflammatory mediators (da Silva Meirelles et al., 2017). Under physiological conditions, activity is suppressed by peptide signaling from healthy neurons (Wolf et al., 2013). TBI results in activation of microglial cells within minutes resulting not only in morphological changes and increase in cell motility but also in neural cell proliferation and upregulation of surface receptors (Nimmerjahn et al., 2005), along with the release of inflammatory mediators such as complement factors, cytokines, chemokines, proteolytic enzymes, and ROS and reactive nitrogen species (RNS) (Loane and Byrnes, 2010). Thus, the inflammatory response of the brain to TBI is multifactorial, encompassing the activation of resident CNS immune cells and the cerebral infiltration of peripheral immune cells (through a disrupted BBB), both of which mediate inflammatory processes through variety inflammatory cytokines, chemokines, adhesion molecules, ROS, and complement factors, among others (Rock and Kono, 2008). In response to perturbations in tissue homeostasis, local activation of microglia occurs (Nimmerjahn et al., 2005) mediating inflammation through the production of various cytokines, proteases, and ROS (Toklu and Tumer, 2015).

Thus, morphological and functional changes in astrocytes, microglia, and oligodendrocytes are associated with so called "glial reaction." Activated glial cells (microglia) are not only involved in eliminating and engulfing particles expelled from the site of injury but also in extending projections to fill in cavities from glial scars and produce MMPs to reconstruct damaged extracellular matrices after the progression of TBI. Glia cells also express insulin-like growth factor-1, epithelial growth factor, and other neurotrophic growth factors to decrease the rate of neuronal death and neural injury after the progression of TBI (Maegele et al., 2005; Park et al., 2007). Activation of glial cells following TBI also promotes neuron–glia and glia–glia interactions. Thus, chemokine CXCL-12, which is released from astrocytes, promotes the release of glutamate, which further promotes the release of large amounts of tumor necrosis factor alpha (TNF-α) from microglia. High concentrations of TNF-α impair the ability of microglia to eliminate glutamate, and this causes excitatory toxicity and injures neurons (Merali et al., 2015). Astrocytes also release the antiinflammatory factor interleukin 10 (IL-10), which inhibits the release of TGF-β from microglia and promotes the maturation of oligodendrocytes (Back et al., 2002; Schwab, 2010).

In post-TBI, there is a marked increase in neutrophilic and macrophages/monocytes infiltration, astrocytosis, edema, and increase in expression of both pro- and antiinflammatory cytokines from microglial cells (Ziebell and Morganti-Kossmann, 2010). Thus, there are marked alterations in regional, intrathecal, and systemic concentrations of several inflammatory cytokines including IL-1, IL-1β, IL-6, IL-8, IL-10, and IL-12, and TNF-α following human and experimental TBI (Morganti-Kossmann et al., 2002; Frugier et al., 2010). Depending on their concentrations and the timing/conditions of their expression following TBI, the members of interleukin family produce beneficial effects in the injured brain, possibly setting the stage for and promoting regenerative and reparative processes (McGinn and Povlishock, 2016). It is proposed that the dual role of the interleukin family shows a proinflammatory phase in the first hours and days after TBI followed by a reparative phase lasting for days to months (Schmidt et al., 2005). Importantly, IL-1β acts uniquely on astrocytes that when damaged stimulate the release of MMPs (Ralay Ranaivo et al., 2011). MMPs hydrolyze extracellular matrix and further facilitates BBB breakdown promoting and prolonging neuroinflammation (Roberts et al., 2013). Overall, in the acute stage of TBI, neuroinflammation mobilizes immune cells, astrocytes, cytokines, and chemokines toward the "traumatic penumbra" to promote an antiinflammatory response against neural injury progression, whereas, latter, excessive activation of inflammation leads to an "inflamed" brain (Krishnamurthy and Laskowitz, 2016). Additionally, peripheral injuries of the multi-injured patient may further increase circulating levels of many of the inflammatory cytokines worsening TBI outcomes (McDonald et al., 2016).

Parenchymal microglial activation has also been reported to occur through contact with components of CNS injury or through interaction with perivascular microglia or with peripheral immune cells that infiltrate via the impairment of BBB following TBI (Ziebell and Morganti-Kossmann, 2010). ATP, which is released by injured neural cells acts as an important activator of microglial cells (Davalos et al., 2005). Activated microglia are known to promote pro- or antiinflammatory effects depending on stimuli in the local microenvironment (Olah et al., 2011). Following TBI, proinflammatory processes facilitate the release of degradative, toxic, and activating autocrine and paracrine compounds. Activated microglia contribute to the removal of cell debris and harmful substances (Loane and Byrnes, 2010). Antiinflammatory processes mediated by microglial cells are associated with neuronal survival. Imbalanced or prolonged proinflammatory activation of microglial cells along with continuous release of cytotoxic proinflammatory cytokines and chemokines are injurious to neurons. This process may perpetuate microglial activation (Block et al., 2007), contributing to progressive CNS symptoms (Gao and Hong, 2008). Converging evidence suggests that TBI is accompanied by depolarization, excitotoxicity, disruption of calcium homeostasis, activation of calcium-dependent enzymes, free-radical generation, BBB disruption, induction of edema formation, development of intracranial hypertension, and induction of neuroinflammation and oxidative stress. Among these processes, oxidative stress and neuroinflammation are caused by distinct biochemical processes, which are closely intertwined and generally function in parallel, particularly in the brain, an organ especially prone to oxidative stress. The complex interplay between inflammatory mediators and markers for oxidative stress are closely associated with the pathogenesis of TBI (Farooqui, 2010). However, placing these pathways in the proper relationship to the onset, time course, and progress of neurodegeneration and its relationship to cytoskeletal pathology of TBI are challenging issues that are not fully understood (Farooqui, 2010). TBI-mediated damage to brain microvessels also promote the release of cytotoxic levels of iron into the brain parenchyma (Liu et al., 2013; Nisenbaum et al., 2014). Iron has been reported to promote and contribute to Ca^{2+}-dependent mechanisms, which either stimulate neuronal cell survival or trigger cell death depending on severity and duration of iron exposure (Munoz et al., 2011).

Ca^{2+}-dependent mechanisms associated with TBI not only promote the unfolded protein response (Ron and Walter, 2007; Farook et al., 2013), proteasomal degradation (Sano and Reed, 2013), and autophagy (Bernales et al., 2006) but also contribute to apoptotic cell death

(Clark et al., 2000) and neurodegeneration (Salminen et al., 2009). TBI-induced intracellular Ca^{2+} increase also prompts generation and accumulation of ROS (Cho et al., 2013) through the involvement of iron. Ferric iron (Fe^{3+}) is reduced to ferrous iron (Fe^{2+}) by the superoxide radical ($O_2^{\bullet-}$) ($Fe^{3+} + O_2^{\bullet-} \rightarrow Fe^{2+} + O_2$). Fe^{2+} reacts with H_2O_2 generating the highly reactive hydroxyl-free radical ($^{\bullet}OH$) ($Fe^{2+} + H_2O_2 \rightarrow Fe^{3+} + {}^{\bullet}OH + OH^{-}$, Fenton reaction) (Jomova and Valko, 2011). The combination of these reactions results in the so-called Haber–Weiss reaction ($O_2^{\bullet-} + H_2O_2 \rightarrow O_2 + {}^{\bullet}OH + OH^{-}$).

When the generation of ROS exceeds the capacity of cellular antioxidant mechanisms, a cell is said to be in a state of oxidative stress in which ROS are free to react with and damage proteins, lipids, and DNA, leading to cellular dysfunction and death. In addition, glutamate-mediated induction of neuroinflammatory cascades is initiated and promoted through the activation of NF-κB following TBI (Szmydynger-Chodobska et al., 2010; Shohami and Biegon, 2014). This transcription factor is present in the cytoplasm in an inactive form. TBI promotes the translocation of NF-κB to the nucleus, where it promotes the expression of proinflammatory cytokines and chemokines. Increased expression of cytokines and chemokines contribute to neuroinflammation in TBI. In the past, research on TBI had focused on neurons without any regard for glial cells and the cerebrovasculature. However, in recent years, studies are focused on the vasculature and the neurovascular unit following TBI. A paradigm shift in the importance of the vascular response to injury has opened new avenues of drug-treatment strategies for TBI. However, a connection between the vascular response to TBI and the development of chronic disease has yet to be elucidated (Rostami et al., 2017; Logsdon et al., 2015). Long-term cognitive deficits are common among those sustaining severe or multiple mild TBIs as well as severe TBIs. Collective evidence suggests that the immediate effects of TBI are complex. These effects include neural cell injury or death; neurovascular and BBB disruption; disturbances of ionic and neurotransmitter homeostasis; and electrical, chemical, and energetic dysfunction (Hall et al., 2004).

TBI-MEDIATED ALTERATIONS IN TRANSCRIPTION FACTORS

Transcription factors are key cellular components, which interact with specific DNA sequences and thereby control the transfer of genetic information from DNA to mRNA. Transcription factors perform their function alone or with other proteins in a complex by activating (activator) or inhibiting (repressor) the recruitment of RNA polymerase to specific genes. TBI influences activities of many transcription factors such as AP-1, NF-κB, CREB, p53, signal transducers and activators of transcription (STATs), and CCAAT/enhancer. Among these transcription factors activator protein-1 (AP-1) consists of a variety of dimers composed of members of the Jun and Fos families of proteins (Raivich and Behrens, 2006). However, it is the upregulation of c-jun that is a particularly common event in the adult as well as in injured nervous system that serves as a model of transcriptional control of brain function. It regulates genes expression in response to cytokines, neurotrophins, and oxidative stress. Depending on the AP-1 dimer combination, neuronal genes related to either apoptosis or survival is transcribed. A 35 kDa Fos-related antigen:JunD dimer is present in neurons that survive injury. Jun and JunD exists in neurons before undergoing apoptosis (Raivich and Behrens, 2006). During excitotoxicity, apoptotic cell death involves the activation of c-Jun, which affects hippocampal, nigral, and primary cultured neurons. The inhibition of JNKs exerts neuroprotective effects in neurons. Besides endogenous neuronal functions, the c-Jun/ AP-1 proteins can damage the nervous system by upregulation of harmful programs in non-neuronal cells (e.g., microglia) with release of neurodegenerative molecules. In contrast, the differentiation with neurite extension and maturation of neural cells in vitro indicate physiological and potentially neuroprotective functions of c-Jun and JNKs, including sensoring for alterations in the cytoskeleton (Raivich and Behrens, 2006).

NF-κB, an inducible transcription factor, acts as a master regulator of immune functions, inflammatory responses, secondary injury processes, and cell survival. NF-κB is rapidly activated in response to various stimuli, including trauma, infectious agents, and radiation-induced DNA double-strand breaks. Neuronal NF-κB is a mediator of trauma-triggered neuronal death, whereas astrocytic NF-κB is thought to be neuroprotective. Studies on the expression of NF-κB in human TBI indicate that a progressive upregulation of NF-κB activity occurs in the area surrounding the injured brain with the time from brain trauma to operation (Hang et al., 2006). In the brain, NF-κB regulates the expression of a large number of genes associated with immune responses, inflammation, cell survival, and apoptosis. STAT regulates infiltration of leukocytes into lesion-reactive hippocampus after axonal injury (Khorooshi et al., 2008).

CCAAT/enhancer binding proteins (C/EBPs) are a family of transcription factors that contain a basic-leucine zipper domain at the C-terminus that is involved in the dimerization and DNA binding. These transcription factors regulate gene expression to control cellular proliferation, differentiation, inflammation, and metabolism. Upregulation of C/EBPβ is observed 1 day following injury in both the adult and aged brain, but there were no major age-related differences in mRNA levels (Sandhir and Berman, 2009). C/EBP-β induces a variety of cytokines and thus may play a role in the induction of neuroinflammation. Differential expression of C/EBPβ, δ, and CCAAT/EBP homologous protein CHOP contributes to the hyperinflammatory response.

Involvement of nuclear factor E2-related factor 2 (Nrf2), a basic leucine zipper redox-sensitive transcription factor in TBI has also been reported (Yan et al., 2009). Nrf2 induces expression and upregulation of cytoprotective and antioxidant/detoxifying genes that attenuate tissue injury (Lee and Johnson, 2004). Nrf2 protein levels are significant increased following TBI (Yan et al., 2009). Studies on wild-type $Nrf2^{+/+}$ and $Nrf2^{-/-}$-deficient mice indicate that $Nrf2^{-/-}$ mice have more NF-κB activation, inflammatory cytokines TNF-α, IL-1β, and IL-6 production, and ICAM-1 expression in brain after TBI compared with their wild-type $Nrf2^{+/+}$ counterparts. These results suggest that Nrf2 plays an important protective role in limiting the cerebral upregulation of NF-κB activity, proinflammatory cytokine, and ICAM-1 after TBI. It is proposed that Nrf2 may play a protective role in the brain after TBI, possibly by reducing inflammation, oxidative stress, and brain edema (Jin et al., 2008). Collective evidence suggests that transcription factors play crucial roles in both cell death signaling pathways and DNA repair, respectively. Alterations in regulation of transcription factors may constitute one of the earliest events in TBI and may offer a therapeutic window of opportunity for intervention across a narrow time period prior to irreversible neuronal death (Kane, 2009). There has been considerable interest in the modulation of these cell death factors to prevent or mitigate damage to neurons with the goal of improving the lives of TBI patients. Following TBI, injured neurons degenerate while surviving neurons undergo neuritogenesis and synaptogenesis to establish neuronal connectivity disturbed and destroyed by the TBI.

TBI-MEDIATED ALTERATIONS IN COMPLEMENT SYSTEM

It is well known that under normal conditions, complement system plays a neuroprotective role and is a powerful and vital component of the innate immune system, but under pathological conditions, such as TBI marked changes have been observed. The immune response brain tissue after TBI is highly complex and involves both local and systemic events at the cellular and molecular level. It not only involves a dramatic overactivation of enzyme systems but also associated with increased expression of proinflammatory genes and the activation/recruitment of immune cells (Wagner and Frank, 2010; Wagner et al., 2012). Thus, the complement system represents a powerful component of the innate immunity and is highly involved in the inflammatory response. Complement components are synthesized predominantly by the liver and circulate in the bloodstream primed for activation. Moreover, neural cells can produce complement proteins and receptors. After acute TBI, the rapid and uncontrolled activation of the complement leads to massive release of inflammatory anaphylatoxins, recruitment of cells to the injury site, phagocytosis, and induction of BBB damage. Brain endothelial cells are particularly susceptible to complement-mediated effects, because they are exposed to both circulating and locally synthesized complement proteins (Wagner and Frank, 2010). The complement system consists of more than 30 fluid-phase and cell-associated proteins (Wagner and Frank, 2010), each with different functions including, but not limited to, initiator molecules, substrates, regulators, inhibitors, and receptors for complement proteins. The activation of the complement system can be triggered by exogenous and/or endogenous danger signals (pathogen-associated molecular patterns—PAMPs and/or DAMPs, respectively) through the classical, lectin, or alternative pathway (AP). These pathways are each activated by different types of danger signals but share the same cascade-like activation system consisting of a number of proteolytic reactions, during which an inactivated protein is cleaved into smaller and active peptide fragments. Activation of classical complement pathway involves the attachment of C1q to a target causing C1 dissociation. Amplification is facilitated through a cascade of proteases (C1r, C1s, C4, C2, and C3), and the hydrolyzed products C4b and C3b attach to the exposed sites close to the C1q binding site, opsonizing the target for phagocytosis. Following TBI, aggregated polypeptides can be potentially present their different charge patterns to C1q, which is a vital charge pattern of recognition molecule of the complement system. Consequently activation of complement leads to microglial activation, which in turn leads to defective clearance of the aggregated polypeptides by macrophages leading to chronic inflammation, especially in traumatized brain. As stated above, TBI is characterized, in part, by activation of the innate immune response, including the complement system. It is shown that mice devoid of a functional AP of complement activation (Factor $B^{-/-}$ mice) are protected from complement-mediated neuroinflammation and neuropathology after TBI (Leinhase et al., 2006). In addition, inhibition of the alternative complement pathway by posttraumatic administration of a neutralizing anti-factor B antibody may represent a new promising avenue for pharmacological attenuation of the complement-mediated neuroinflammatory response after TBI (Leinhase et al., 2007).

DIAGNOSIS OF TBI

The diagnosis of TBI can be performed by a neurological examination of the patient by a doctor. Currently, better diagnosis of TBI can be made using imaging radiology techniques such as computed tomography (CT) or MRI. The GCS assesses the severity of TBI on the basis of cognitive behavior (Teasdale et al., 2014). A total score of 13–15 refers to mTBI, 9–12 to moderate TBI, and 3–8 to severe TBI (Faul and Coronado, 2015). It is also reported that CT and MRI do not provide definitive means for the diagnostics of TBI because they fail to find alterations in a large proportion of patients who have a mild to moderate TBI (Hughes et al., 2004; Belanger et al., 2007). However, recently developed MRI technique called DTI provides better diagnosis. This procedure traces the direction of water molecules' diffusion and uses computed parameters of diffusivity as measures of axonal integrity (Delouche et al., 2016). This procedure allows for accurate 3D modeling of neural tracts (tractography) by means of computerized image analysis. DTI is considered a promising tool for diagnosing TBI because of the ability of this technique to focus on axonal structures, but the literature regarding the detection of acute mTBI is somewhat inconsistent. Another type of MRI is called as functional MRI (fMRI). This technique is used to study the activation of various brain regions using different stimuli or tasks. The fMRI detects changes in cerebral blood flow and oxygen consumption based on different magnetic properties between oxyhemoglobin and deoxyhemoglobin. In the diagnostics of mTBI, fMRI may be a promising technology. It is reported that functional alterations in the brain of concussed athletes who show no symptoms in clinical assessment and neuropsychological testing (Slobounov et al., 2011) can be diagnosed by fMRI even after 1 year of TBI (McAllister et al., 2008; McAllister et al., 2006). Furthermore, fMRI can also be used to evaluate the response of TBI patient to behavioral or pharmacological challenges and interventions targeting cognitive and behavioral sequelae of mTBI. There have been few fMRI studies examining mTBI. More studies with large and well-characterized samples are clearly needed (McDonald et al., 2012).

BIOMARKERS OF TBI

Biomarkers are of enormous importance for the diagnosis, prognosis, and therapeutic evaluation of TBI-mediated acute brain damage. Biomarkers for TBI can be detected in the cerebrospinal fluid (CSF) and in the blood directly after TBI (Zetterberg and Blennow, 2015). It is well known that BBB is almost impermeable to many proteins and neuroprotective drugs. TBI disrupts the integrity of BBB and allows the permeation of molecules (metabolites) from brain into the CSF and blood (Başkaya et al., 1997). Alternatively, they may be transported to the blood via the glymphatic system (Plog et al., 2015). Urine can be a good and noninvasive source of biomarkers. However, urine is indirect and may contain potential barriers and dilutive interfaces, yet markers of brain injury have been found in urine (Ottens et al., 2014; Oliver et al., 2015). As stated in Chapter 1, Classification and Molecular Aspects of Neurotraumatic Diseases: Similarities and Differences With Neurodegenerative and Neuropsychiatric Diseases, Putative biomarkers for TBI are CSF levels of total Tau protein, neuron-specific enolase, S100β (a Ca-binding protein), glial fibrillary acidic protein, ubiquitin C-terminal hydrolase-L1, myelin basic protein, microtubule-associated protein 2 (MAP2), α-spectrin and spectrin breakdown products, IL-6, and IL-10, and NMDA-R fragments (Fig. 6.4). These biomarkers are assessed via various immunoassays, such as Western blotting or enzyme-linked immunosorbent assay.

Furthermore, Tau proteins have been associated with elevated intracranial pressure, a characteristic feature of TBI (Zemlan et al., 2002), and phosphorylated Tau has been identified in serum up to several months after severe TBI (Rubenstein et al., 2015). Nevertheless, despite the identification of these biomarkers via targeted approaches, many of them suffer from lack of TBI specificity and may not indicate TBI chronic temporal changes. In addition, it is also reported that circulating levels of SP, soluble CD40 ligand (sCD40L), tissue inhibitor of matrix metalloproteinases (TIMP)-1, malondialdehyde (MDA), and cytokeratin (CK)-18 fragmented are associated with mortality in TBI patients (Lorente, 2015). Among above biomarkers, SP is a neuropeptide that belongs to the tachykinin family. It is mainly synthesized in the central and peripheral nervous system. It produces proinflammatory effects by binding with neurokinin-1 receptor (NK1R). Soluble CD40 ligand, a member of the TNF family that is released into circulation from activated platelets, exhibit proinflammatory, and procoagulant effects on binding to their cell surface receptor CD40. MMPs are a family of zinc-containing endoproteinases. It is involved neuroinflammation and TIMP-1 is the inhibitor of some of them. Malondialdehyde is an end-product formed during lipid peroxidation due to degradation of cellular membrane phospholipids, which is released into extracellular space and finally into the blood. CK-18 is cleaved by the action of caspases during apoptosis, and CK-18 fragmented is released into the blood (Lorente, 2015). Some biomarkers are related to neuroinflammation and coagulation, whereas others are linked with oxidation and apoptosis. Some of these biomarkers are associated with mortality in patients with TBI. These

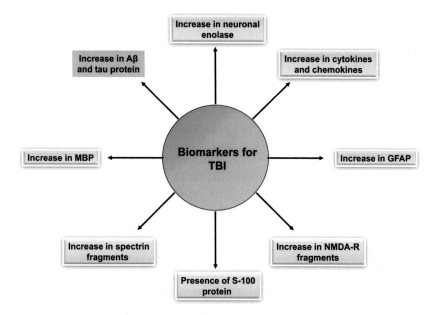

FIGURE 6.4   Biomarkers of traumatic brain injury (TBI). Aβ, amyloid beta; GFAP, glial fibrillary acidic protein; NMDA-R, N-methyl-D-aspartate receptor; MBP, myelin basic protein.

biomarkers may help in the prognostic classification of the patients and open new research lines in the treatment of patients with TBI. Among above biomarkers, some biomarkers are derived from neurons, while others are of glial origin. Recent years, neuroproteomic studies have proven to be a contemporary and convenient tool in biomarker discovery for many human diseases including CNS injury (Guingab-Cagmat et al., 2010). Neuroproteomic has been used to study biomarkers in rat TBI models. It is reported that out of 59 differential protein components of which 21 decreased and 38 increased in abundance after TBI. Proteins, which are decreased include collapsin response mediator protein 2 (CRMP-2), GAPDH, microtubule-associated proteins MAP2A/2B, and hexokinase. In contrast, C-reactive protein, transferrin, and breakdown products of CRMP-2, synaptotagmin, and alpha II-spectrin are markedly elevated after TBI. Differential changes in the above proteins have been confirmed by quantitative immunoblotting. These data may provide insight into molecular mechanisms of TBI and yield putative biochemical markers to potentially facilitate patient management by monitoring the severity, progression, and treatment of injury (Kobeissy et al., 2006).

Determination of temporal profiles of above-mentioned biomarkers is essential not only for evaluating diagnostic time window but also for determining the severity of TBI (Brophy et al. (2011). Many of the above-mentioned biomarkers are released during the first burst upon cellular injury and the concomitantly triggered catabolic processes. These markers peak early, within a few hours, and then decline after the molecule-specific half-life in the blood. The release of proinflammatory cytokines and chemokines (peaking at <48 hours after TBI) is a slow process. This results in induction of neuroinflammation. The induction of autoantibodies against brain proteins is a slow process. However, levels of autoantibodies remain elevated for a fairly long time. The severity of TBI affects the peak heights and durations. Delayed elevations in levels of some of these biomarkers are also observed in the blood after following TBI (Zetterberg et al., 2013; Adrian et al., 2016). Despite the above-mentioned information about biomarkers, FDA has not approved a specific biomarker for clinical use in TBI patients.

GENETIC INFLUENCES IN TBI

Many genes modulate TBI. These genes are categorized into three groups: (1) genes influencing the extent of the injury (e.g., pro- and anti-inflammatory cytokines), (2) genes contributing to repair and neuroplasticity (e.g., neurotrophic genes), and (3) genes modulating pre-and postinjury cognitive and neurobehavioral capacity (e.g., catecholamine genes) (McAllister, 2010). Based on the expression of above genes, the interindividual variability has been observed in terms of predicting functional and cognitive outcome following TBI (McAllister, 2010; Weaver et al., 2014). These variations in functional and cognitive outcome are due to alterations in the DNA sequence within a given gene and are referred to as genetic polymorphisms. Polymorphisms can arise from insertions or deletions of short lengths of DNA within a particular gene, interfering with the normal function of the gene or at a single nucleotide (G, A, T, or C). DNA modification caused by a single nucleotide is referred as a single nucleotide polymorphism or SNP. It is stated that SNPs are the most common type of genetic variation, occurring once every 100−300 nucleotides, amounting to approximately 10 million in the human genome (Bennett et al., 2016). A SNP can reside within the coding sequence of a gene where it may alter the amino acid composition of a protein or within a noncoding region of a gene, such as a promoter or intron, where it may influence expression of the gene and protein production (Bennett et al., 2016). To date, many genes have been implicated in the pathophysiology and outcome following moderate to severe TBI. These genes are associated with regulation of the brain's response to TBI and not only include both anti-and proinflammatory cytokines, DNA repair enzymes, signaling molecules, and mitochondrial genes but also several neurotrophins. How these diverse genes interact with one another following TBI remains to be elucidated and requires extensive investigations. Furthermore, very little is known about the influence of epigenetic factors and mechanisms (DNA methylation, histone modifications, nucleosome remodeling, and RNA editing) on TBI. Although inheriting a single "good" or "bad" allele of a specific gene may predispose an individual to better or worse outcome of TBI, it is becoming increasingly apparent that recovery from TBI is polygenic in nature, involving the interaction of numerous genes from multiple pathways (Bennett et al., 2016). Moreover, TBI is also modulated by epigenetic mechanisms (Graves and Munro, 2013; Qureshi and Mehler, 2010; Liyanage et al., 2014) and signal transduction processes that can modulate gene expression without altering the DNA sequence (e.g., DNA methylation, chromatin modifications) (Bennett et al., 2016). The majority of TBI-genetic association studies reported in the literature have been conducted in adult populations, despite the observation that the vast majority of TBIs occur in children and young adults. Clearly, additional genetic association studies are essential to facilitate both the prediction of outcome and clinical management in the pediatric TBI population (Bennett et al., 2016).

APOPTOTIC CELL DEATH IN TBI

TBI has been reported to induce apoptotic cell death in neuronal and glial cells in both animals and humans (Raghupathi et al., 2000). In traumatized human brain and injured experimental animal brain, apoptotic cells have been observed alongside of cells undergoing necrosis. Apoptotic cell death is also observed in oligodendrocytes and astrocytes within injured white matter tracts. In TBI, apoptotic cell death is triggered by interactions between excitotoxicity and oxidative stress. Apoptosis not only involves enhancement of glycerophospholipid, sphingolipid, and cholesterol metabolism due to changes in activities of phospholipases, sphingomyelinases, and cytochrome P450 oxygenases but also by alterations in levels of glycerophospholipid, sphingolipid, and cholesterol-derived lipid mediators. These processes along with abnormalities in signal transduction processes bring about neural cell demise through apoptosis (Farooqui, 2010). Neurochemical changes in apoptotic cell death occur in an orderly fashion due to sufficient levels of ATP that maintains normal ion homeostasis. The dead cells undergo phagocytosis without spilling cellular contents.

The clearance of debris after TBI is a critical step for restoration of the injured neural network. Although, microglia contribute to the elimination of degenerating neurons and axons and facilitate the restoration of favorable environment after TBI, the mechanism underlying debris clearance remains elusive. However, it is proposed that activation of p38 mitogen-activated protein kinase (MAPK) in microglia facilitates the engulfment of cellular debris. This engulfment of axon debris can be blocked by the p38 MAPK inhibitor SB203580, indicating that p38 MAPK is required for phagocytic activity (Tanaka et al., 2009). In contrast, in necrosis rapid permeabilization of plasma membrane, rapid decrease in ATP, sudden loss of ion homeostasis, and activation of lysosomal enzymes result in a passive cell death through lysis (Farooqui and Horrocks, 2007). During necrosis release of cellular contents is accompanied by neuroinflammation and oxidative stress (Farooqui, 2014). In TBI, neurons die rapidly (hours to days) at the injury core by necrotic cell death, whereas in the surrounding area neurons undergo apoptotic cell death (several days to months) (Farooqui, 2014).

TBI AND NEUROLOGICAL DISORDERS

Neurodegenerative diseases are a debilitating group of diseases associated with site-specific premature and slow death of specific neuronal populations and synapses in brain and spinal cord that modulate thinking, skilled movements, decision-making, cognition, and memory (Soto and Estrada, 2008). The molecular mechanisms associated with pathogenesis of neurodegenerative diseases remain elusive. However, it is becoming increasingly evident that the accumulation of misfolded protein aggregates, induction of chronic oxidative stress, onset of chronic neuroinflammation may contribute to synaptic dysfunction, neuronal apoptosis, and brain damage in neurodegenerative diseases (Amor et al., 2014). The burden of above biologic mechanisms on degenerative pathophysiology is influenced not only by environmental factors and behavioral determinants including diet and exercise (Gomez-Pinilla, 2011; Farooqui, 2015) but also by enhanced rate (upregulation) of interplay among excitotoxity, oxidative stress, and neuroinflammation (Farooqui and Horrocks, 2007; Deleidi et al., 2015). Most neurodegenerative diseases are also accompanied by elevations in levels of lipid mediators (Farooqui, 2011). Converging evidence suggests that diet, genetic, exercise, and environmental factors may also contribute to the increase in the vulnerability of neurons in neurodegenerative diseases (Kidd, 2005; Farooqui, 2015).

Given that 1.3 million Americans seek emergency care for TBI each year, any potential long-term effects of such injuries are likely to be substantial. TBI is not only linked with an increased risk for such as Alzheimer's disease (AD) and Parkinson's disease (PD) but also for epilepsy, depression, and posttraumatic dementia (Fig. 6.5). Of note, both AD and PD are characterized by the accumulation of misfolded protein aggregates composed of amyloid-beta (Aβ), hyperphosphorylated Tau protein (p-τ protein), α-synuclein (α-Syn), and transactive response DNA-binding protein 43 kDa (TDP-43) accumulates in frontotemporal dementia and amyotrophic lateral sclerosis (ALS) (Neumann et al., 2006) in neurons, respectively. While the role of these proteins in the initiation of neurodegenerative diseases is still under debate, it is clear that this abnormal accumulation is indicative of abnormal cellular processes and cerebral dysfunction. A unifying feature of acute and chronic pathology after severe TBI or repeat mild TBIs is the abnormal accumulation of pathological proteins related to neurodegenerative disease. Acutely TBI brains can present with Aβ, p-tau, and α-synuclein pathology (Uryu et al., 2007). Chronically TBI brains can present with Aβ, p-tau, TDP-43, and α-synuclein pathology (Johnson et al., 2012; McKee et al., 2013). These proteins have been reported to play an important role in the induction of neurodegeneration. Hyperphosphorylation of Tau leads to destabilization of microtubules, interrupting axonal transport, while Tau aggregates are associated with synaptic dysfunction (Khanna et al., 2016). Similarly, beta amyloid oligomers (AβOs) cause impaired synaptic plasticity, loss of memory function, synapse elimination, induction of oxidative and endoplasmic reticulum stress, inflammatory microglial activation, and neurodegeneration (Viola and Klein, 2015; Farooqui, 2017). The exact mechanisms through which TBI

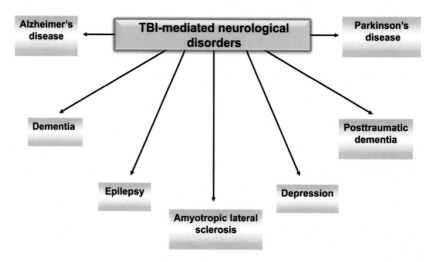

FIGURE 6.5   Neurological disorders promoted by traumatic brain injury (TBI).

contributes to tauopathy later and its role in the later induction of dementia are yet to be fully determined. TBI-mediated axonal injury may provide the initial perturbation of Tau, by promoting its dissociation from microtubules, facilitating its phosphorylation and aggregation. Changes in Tau and AβO dynamics may then be exacerbated by the chronic persistent inflammatory response that has been shown to persist for decades following the initial impact of TBI. Importantly, immune responses have also been reported to play a role in accelerating disease progression in other neurodegenerative diseases, with high levels of proinflammatory cytokines (TNF-α, IL-1β, and IL-6). These cytokines have also been shown to activate kinases that promote Tau hyperphosphorylation (Farooqui, 2017).

LINK BETWEEN TBI AND AD

AD is a progressive, irreversible, and multifactorial neurodegenerative disease, which is characterized by the accumulation of extracellular β-amyloid (Aβ) plaques (senile plaques) and intracellular neurofibrillary tangles composed of hyperphosphorylated Tau amyloid fibrils (Farooqui, 2017) leading to the loss of synapses and degeneration of neurons in multiple brain regions (cortical and subcortical areas and hippocampus), causing a loss of cognitive brain functions, along with progressive impairment of activities of daily living and often behavioral and physiological changes like apathy and depression (Fig. 6.6) (Farooqui, 2017). Among seniors AD has reached epidemic proportions, with no slowdown in sight. On the contrary, evidence suggests the trend is worsening. At present, AD affects an estimated 5.4 million Americans (Alzheimer's-Association, 2013). Projections suggest the disease will affect one in four Americans within the next two decades, and by 2050, Alzheimer's diagnoses are projected to triple (Mapstone et al., 2014). The primary mechanism of Aβ peptide production is thought to be via transmembrane cleavage of APP by β- and γ-secretases (Nunan and Small, 2000). Besides acute primary damage, TBI also promotes secondary neurodegeneration, which elevates the risk for developing AD by ~3- to 5-fold (Guo et al., 2000; Fleminger et al., 2003). The question of whether a single moderate-to-severe TBI triggers the development of late-onset dementia remains somewhat controversial. AD accounts for 60%−80% of all dementias, and most studies on TBI and dementia risk have focused specifically on the development of AD after injury. Following TBI in humans and several experimental animal models, a marked accumulation of APP has been observed in damaged axons, suggesting that there may be ample substrate for Aβ production

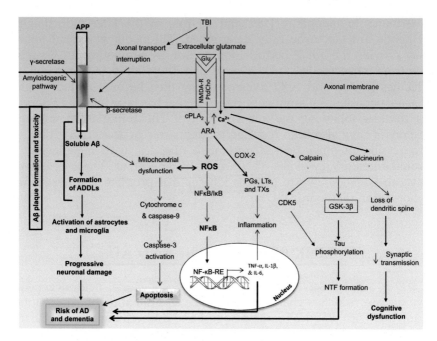

FIGURE 6.6　Hypothetical mechanism showing the contribution of traumatic brain injury (TBI) in the pathogenesis of Alzheimer's disease (AD). APP, amyloid precursor protein; PM, Plasma membrane; NMDA-R, N-methyl-D-aspartate receptor; Glu, Glutamate; Aβ, amyloid beta; ADDLs, Aβ-derived diffusible ligands; PtdCho, phosphatidylcholine; ARA, arachidonic acid; ROS, reactive oxygen species; cPLA$_2$, cytosolic phospholipase A$_2$; lyso-PtdCho, lyso-phosphatidylcholine; PGs, prostaglandins; LTs, leukotrienes; TXs, thromboxanes; IκB/NF-κB, nuclear factor κB inhibited form; NFκB-RE, nuclear factor κB-response element; IκB, inhibitory subunit of NF-κB; TNF-α, tumor necrosis factor-α; IL-1β, interleukin 1β; GSK3β, glycogen synthase kinase 3 beta; CDK5, cyclin-dependent kinase 5; NTF, neurofibrillary tangle.

(Smith et al., 1999, 2003; Xiong et al., 2013). These observations suggest that damaged axons serve as a key source of Aβ following TBI (Ikonomovic et al., 2004; Uryu et al., 2007). Although intra-axonal proteolysis of APP to Aβ is not a typical process proposed for the pathogenesis of AD, a recent study has demonstrated Aβ production within the axon membrane compartment of peripheral nerves (Kamal et al., 2000; Kamal et al., 2001). This process is mediated by β-site APP-cleaving enzyme (BACE1) (Esler and Wolfe, 2001). BACE1 levels are markedly increased following experimental TBI, and this increase coincides with increase in Aβ production (Loane et al., 2009; Walker et al., 2012). It should be noted that BACE1 activity is regulated at many levels within the neural cell including, at the transcriptional, translational, and posttranslational levels (Walker et al., 2012). The posttranslational regulation of BACE1 facilitated by the adaptor protein called GGA3. This adaptor protein plays a key role in trafficking BACE1 from the endosomes to the lysosomes for degradation (Kang et al., 2010). GGA3 regulates BACE1 levels both in vitro and in vivo and that it impairs the degradation of BACE1 due to caspase-3-mediated cleavage of GGA3 resulting in dramatically increased Aβ levels in vitro (Walker et al., 2012). GGA3 levels are reduced by 50% in the temporal cortex of AD patients concurrently with caspase-3 activation, supporting the view that reduced levels of GGA3 may play an important role in regulating BACE1 levels in the brains of AD patients (Tesco et al., 2007). It is also demonstrated that caspase-3 mediated cleavage of GGA3 and its closely related homolog GGA1 synergistically regulate BACE1 levels and Aβ production in the acute phase (48 hours) following experimental TBI in rodents. Importantly, using GGA3$^{+/-}$ mice, it is shown that a 50% reduction in GGA3 is sufficient to cause a sustained elevation of BACE1 levels and activity and Aβ production in subacute phase (7 days) of TBI when GGA1 levels have returned to normal. Collectively, these results indicate that GGA3 plays a key role in regulating BACE1 levels in vivo, impaired degradation of BACE1 due to reduced levels of GGA3 represents an attractive molecular mechanism linking acute TBI to chronic Aβ production and neurodegeneration. Postmortem histological analysis shows that deposition of amyloid ß-protein in the brain occurs in approximately one-third of individuals who die shortly after a severe head injury (Roberts et al., 1994). Levels of Aβ are also altered in cerebrospinal and interstitial cerebral fluid in patients with TBI (Magnoni and Brody, 2010; Tsitsopoulos and Marklund, 2013) and correlate with clinical outcome (Magnoni and Brody, 2010). A history of TBI prior to the onset of dementia correlates with greater amyloid burden in patients with mild cognitive deficits (Milman et al., 2005; Mielke et al., 2014) and is associated with faster rates of cognitive dysfunction in AD patients (Moretti et al., 2012; Gilbert et al., 2014). In TBI patients, APP transcription is upregulated and its axonal transport is interrupted due to DAI, which results in deposition of APP and its products in axonal "bulbs" (Hayashi et al., 2015). These results from human studies are in line with a large body of evidence from various models of TBI in mice and rats, where APP overexpression following TBI has been extensively studied (Stone et al., 2002; Iwata et al., 2002; Chen et al., 2004; Farooqui, 2016). The association between TBI and AD is further strengthened by commonality of genetic factors such as apolipoprotein E (APOE), the lipid transport protein APOE. This protein influences the amyloid pathology and outcome following TBI (Smith et al., 2006). Thus, changes in APOE ε4 seem to worsen the prognosis following TBI and predispose individuals to the formation of Aβ plaques in AD (Kim et al., 2009). These reports argue that TBI may be a risk factor for the long-term development of AD (Fleminger et al., 2003; Johnson et al., 2010, 2012; Magnoni and Brody, 2010). Collective evidence suggests that the pathology of TBI-induced AD is complex and dependent not only on injury severity and age-at-injury but also on the length of time between injury and neuropathological evaluation. In addition, processes and mechanisms modulating pathology and recovery after TBI may involve genetic/epigenetic factors, which may be related to aging as well as vascular health. In this regard, dysfunction of the aging neurovascular system can be an important link between TBI and chronic neurodegenerative diseases, either as a precipitating event or related to accumulation of AD-like pathology which is amplified in the context of aging. Thus, with advanced age and vascular dysfunction, TBI can trigger self-propagating cycles of neuronal injury, pathological protein aggregation, and synaptic loss resulting in chronic neurodegenerative disease (Ikonomovic et al., 2017).

LINK BETWEEN TBI AND PD

PD is a chronic and progressive neurodegenerative disorder characterized by the selective loss of pigmented dopaminergic neurons of the substantia nigra pars compacta. Clinical features of PD include rigidity, dyskinesia, gait imbalance, and tremor at rest (Jankovic, 2008). The pathogenesis of PD remains unknown. However, experimental studies have indicated the involvement of oxidative stress, mitochondria dysfunction, apoptosis, and inflammation either separately or cooperatively to induce neurodegeneration in PD (Dauer and Przedborski, 2003). The degeneration of dopaminergic neurons in the substantia nigra pars compacta may be due to monoamine oxidase—mediated abnormal dopamine (DA) metabolism, generation of hydrogen peroxide, and oxygen radical superoxide (O_2^-). Excessive production of O_2^- and H_2O_2 can result in brain damage (Fig. 6.7), which often involves generation of highly reactive hydroxyl radical ($\cdot OH$) and other oxidants in the presence of "catalytic" iron ions. A major form of antioxidant defense is the storage and transport of iron ions in forms that will not catalyze formation of reactive radicals. Oxidative stress in the brain can produce damage by several interacting mechanisms, including rises in intracellular free Ca^{2-} and, possibly, release of excitatory amino acids. PD is also characterized by the presence of α-synuclein aggregates as Lewy body (LB) inclusions in specific regions of the brain such as substantia nigra, thalamus, and neocortex (Uversky and Eliezer, 2009). α-Synuclein is primarily localized at the presynaptic terminals of neurons (Iwai et al., 1995). LBs consist of a heterogeneous mixture of more than 90 molecules, including PD-linked gene products (α-synuclein, DJ-1, LRRK2, parkin, and PINK-1), mitochondria-related proteins, and molecules implicated in the ubiquitin-proteasome system, autophagy, and aggresome formation. Among these components and gene products,

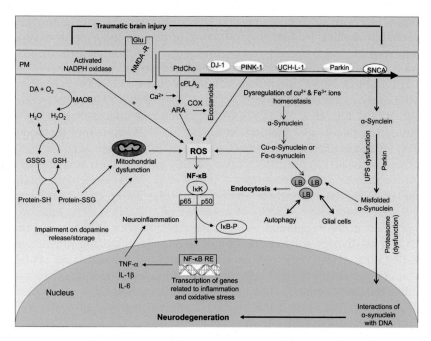

FIGURE 6.7 Hypothetical mechanism showing the contribution of traumatic brain injury (TBI) in the pathogenesis of Parkinson's disease (PD). PM, Plasma membrane; NADPH, Nicotinamide adenine dinucleotide phosphate; Glu, Glutamate; ROS, reactive oxygen species; PtdCho, phosphatidylcholine; cPLA$_2$, cytosolic phospholipase A$_2$; IκB/NF-κB, nuclear factor κB inhibited form; NFκB-RE, nuclear factor κB-response element; IκB, inhibitory subunit of NF-κB; NOS, nitric oxide synthase; NO, nitric oxide; TNF-α, tumor necrosis factor-α; IL-1β, interleukin 1β; MAOB, monoamine oxidase B.

α-synuclein (α-Synuclein, a 140 amino acid, soluble protein) plays an important role in the regulation of synaptic vesicle release and trafficking, maintenance of synaptic vesicle pools, fatty acid binding, neurotransmitter release, synaptic plasticity, and neuronal survival (Uversky and Eliezer, 2009). Similar to Aβ in AD, α-synuclein undergoes rapid self-aggregation in vivo with an accelerated rate in the presence of transition metal ions, DA, proteins, and lipids. Oxidative stress upregulates the expression of α-synuclein and promotes its fibrillization and aggregation (Vila et al., 2000). Conversely, a high degree of fibrillization and aggregation of α-synuclein results in an increase of ROS and neurotoxicity (Hsu et al., 2000; McAllister et al., 2005). This vicious cycle between α-synuclein and oxidative stress may contribute to the progression of loss of substantia nigra pars compacta dopaminergic neurons in PD. In addition, multiple neurochemical processes, which have been negatively impacted in the pathogenesis of PD. In addition, oligomeric α-synuclein is released from neurons, allowing α-synuclein to propagate to neighboring neurons and glia (Lee et al., 2010). Oligomeric α-synuclein is a potent activator of microglia and macrophages via engagement of Toll-like receptors, leading to production of proinflammatory mediators (Fellner et al., 2013; Daniele et al., 2015) suggesting that neuroinflammation is a common mechanism, which is involved in the neuronal injury in TBI and PD. Neuroinflammation is supported by high levels of proinflammatory cytokines such as IL-1β, IL-6, IL-8, IL-33, TNF-α, chemokine (C-C motif) ligand 2 (CCL2), CCL5, granulocyte macrophage colony-stimulating factor, glia maturation factor, SP, ROS, and RNS (Farooqui, 2011; Farooqui, 2017). Other mechanisms of α-Synuclein involve in the pathogenesis of PD are interactions of this protein with mitochondria and the membranes of lysosomes (Cuervo et al., 2004) along with inhibition of lysosomal function (Stefanis et al., 2001) and chaperone-mediated autophagy (CMA) (Cuervo et al., 2004). CMA has been implicated in the regulation of the transcription factor MEF2D, and that this can be disrupted by expression of α-synuclein, leading to neuronal death (Yang et al., 2009). As another example of misregulated protein turnover, α-synuclein (and specifically α-synuclein oligomers) can also inhibit the proteasome (Tanaka et al., 2001; Emmanouilidou et al., 2008), although it is not clear if the predicted altered turnover of proteasome substrates occurs in vivo (Chen et al., 2006).

Investigating a causal relation between TBI and PD is complicated by the fact that PD is a disorder of mobility and cognition that predisposes one to falls and other types of physical injury. Furthermore, PD is a slowly progressive disorder with insidious onset; thus, the diagnosis by a physician can postdate the onset of symptoms by years. Therefore, it is important to consider the timing of TBI in light of this latency between onset of Parkinsonism and diagnosis of PD to be alert to the possibility of reverse causation. Functional imaging studies have indicated that there is bilateral impairment of DA function in the nigrostriatal terminals, raising the possibility that the TBI may cause more substantial damage than is evident on anatomical imaging. Bilateral reduction in tracer uptake also raises the possibility that symptoms of patients may be consistent with idiopathic PD, or that unilateral structural damage can cause bilateral striatal dopaminergic dysfunction with retrograde degeneration of nigrostriatal terminals. For example, bilateral striatal DA depletion induced by unilateral lesion dorsal to substantia nigra was described in monkeys (Lawler et al., 1995). The nigral DA was severely reduced on both sides in the chronic experiments weeks after a unilateral caudate lesion in cats (Cheramy et al., 1981).

Several studies have indicated that there is a link between TBI and increased risk of PD (Bower et al., 2003; Goldman et al., 2006). Many mechanisms contribute to the PD pathology. Thus, accumulation of α-synuclein is coupled with TBI appears to synergistically impact on PD symptoms (Shahaduzzaman et al., 2013; Ulusoy and Di Monte, 2013). Furthermore, in animal models 30 days after TBI, levels of PD-like markers (α-synuclein) are significantly upregulated. In addition, midbrain tissue of chronic TBI mice displayed a remarkable decrease in the immune-histochemical expression of dopaminergic markers, along with an evident accumulation of α-synuclein in neurons. Based on the above studies, it has been hypothesized that TBI exacerbates nigrostriatal dopaminergic degeneration by modulating PD-associated genes including α-synuclein, DJ-1, LRRK2, among others. Furthermore, the chronic consequences of TBI may result not only in the development of chronic neuroinflammation and sensory motor problems but also in cognitive dysfunction in the form of PD years after the initial insult (Ettenhofer and Abeles, 2009; Ozen and Fernandes, 2012; Acosta et al., 2013). Thus, there may be a pathological overlap among genetic components of TBI and PD.

LINK BETWEEN TBI AND DEMENTIA

Dementia is a progressive cognitive syndrome, which is not only characterized by memory deficits and cognitive impairment (speech, comprehension, execution, orientation) but also by disturbances of higher cortical functions. Dementia is accompanied by deterioration in emotional control and social behavior (Xu et al., 2004; Qaseem et al., 2008). The deterioration of cognitive function is more than what is typically experienced in normal aging and results from damage caused by the disease, such as AD, PD, ALS, and TBI (Sonnen et al., 2009). Dementia syndrome can be classified into vascular dementia, progressive dementia, LB dementia, Alzheimer type of dementia, PD linked dementia, and dementia as a result of diseases such as stroke, AIDS, and multiple sclerosis, and posttraumatic dementia (Ritchie and Lovestone, 2002). Major risk factors for dementia include advancing age, physical and cognitive inactivity, and environmental factors (Fig. 6.8). Other risk factors such as (1) cardiovascular and cerebrovascular problems; (2) excessive alcohol consumption; (3) social isolation; (4) head injury; and (5) having one or two copies of the APOE-ε4 genetic variant also contribute to the pathogenesis of dementia (Xu et al., 2004; Sonnen et al., 2009; Qaseem et al., 2008). The presence APOE-ε4 may contribute to a poor outcome in cognitive dysfunction and functionality following brain injury rehabilitation (Koponen et al., 2004; Crawford et al., 2002). APOE-ε4 is also associated with a rapid cognitive decline in AD (Wilson and Montgomery, 2007). A combination of all these factors is known to contribute to the pathogenesis and development of the dementia, but information on underlying molecular mechanisms contributing to dementia still remains speculative. Clinical and preclinical studies have indicated that symptoms of dementia may be linked with alterations in neuroplasticity in corticolimbic brain regions. In particular, divergent responses such as neuronal

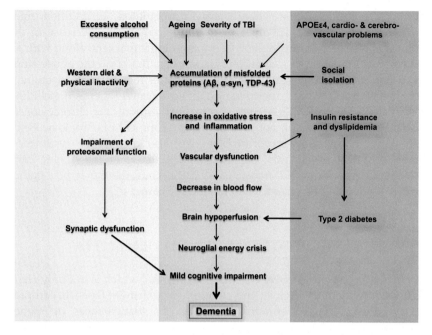

FIGURE 6.8   Risk factors contributing to the pathogenesis of dementia. TBI, traumatic brain injury; TDP-43, TAR DNA-binding protein 43; APOE-ε4, apolipoprotein E4 allele; Aβ, amyloid beta.

atrophy and synapse loss in the prefrontal cortex and hippocampus, and neuronal hypertrophy and increased synaptic density in the amygdala and nucleus accumbens are reported (Christoffel et al., 2011).

Very little is known about molecular mechanisms linking TBI with dementia. However, it is proposed that accumulation of misfolded proteins (Aβ and Tau) in AD, α-synuclein in PD, and TDP-43 in ALS may be common mechanisms that may contribute to TBI-mediated decline in cognitive function, vascular dysfunction, decrease in blood causing brain hypofunction leading to neuroglial crisis that may promote changes in emotion or behavior (Farooqui, 2017) (Fig. 6.8). All these processes may contribute to the pathogenesis of dementia (Farooqui, 2010). In addition, induction of chronic neuroinflammation in TBI and dementia may be another common mechanism to both these conditions (Cederberg and Siesjo, 2010). It is well known that the inflammatory response from TBI persists over time demonstrating that the initial effects of TBI may be more long lasting than previously believed (Das et al., 2012). Thus, in animal models of TBI persistent inflammation in the brain occurs for at least a year (Nagamoto-Combs et al., 2007) and in postmortem human studies for many years after TBI (Gentleman et al., 2004). A recent study using positron emission tomography to examine in vivo the inflammatory response after brain injury demonstrates increase in microglial activation up to 17 years after injury, with activation in the thalamus being associated with more severe cognitive impairment (Ramlackhansingh et al., 2011). Collective evidence suggests that TBI may trigger an inflammatory response, particularly in subcortical regions, which may persist and further evolve over time. This persistent inflammation may be an initial trigger of a larger cascade ultimately leading to TBI-related dementia, neurodegenerative, or cerebrovascular disease.

LINK BETWEEN TBI AND EPILEPSY

Epilepsy is a neurological disorder characterized by an enduring predisposition to generate epileptic seizures, and by the neurobiological, cognitive, psychological, and social consequences of this condition. The definition of epilepsy requires the occurrence of at least one unprovoked seizure (Fisher et al., 2005). Depending on the time delay from the TBI to the occurrence of the first seizure, post-TBI seizures have been categorized into immediate (<24 hours), early (1−7 days), or late seizures (>1week after TBI) (Annegers et al., 1998). Thus, when TBI is associated with one unprovoked late seizure, it qualifies for diagnosis of posttraumatic epilepsy (PTE). The molecular mechanisms associated with TBI-mediated seizures are not fully understood. However, it is well known that immediately after TBI, the brain undergoes distinct electrophysiological changes, which can be detected with electroencephalography (Schmitt and Dichter, 2015). At the molecular level, both NMDA and non-NMDA type of glutamate receptors contribute to seizures after TBI. In addition, it is well known that TLRs trigger the innate immune system and regulate non-NMDA type of glutamate channels (Maroso et al., 2010). Following TBI, the activation of TLRs intensifies glutamate excitotoxicity for several weeks (Li et al., 2015). Among TLRs, specifically, TLR 4 is associated with temporal lobe seizures following trauma (Liang et al., 2014). TLRs on glia trigger a robust gliosis response postinjury (Atmaca et al., 2014). Following TBI, the overstimulation of NMDA type of glutamate receptors is called as excitotoxicity, which results in the calcium influx and stimulation of cytosolic PLA_2, cyclooxygenase-2 (COX-2) and lipoxygenases (Fig. 6.9) (Farooqui and Horrocks, 2007). These processes initiate and support the generation of eicosanoids (prostaglandins, leukotrienes, and thromboxanes), which contribute to neuroinflammation. In addition, at high levels arachidonic acid (ARA) undergoes uncontrolled ARA cascade resulting in generation of high levels of ROS, which are responsible for the induction of

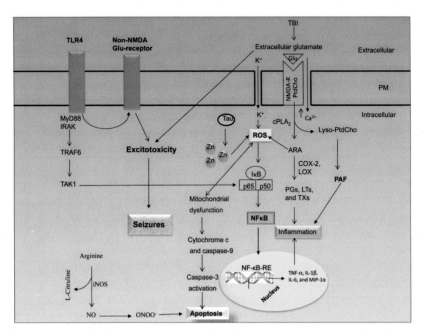

FIGURE 6.9 Hypothetical mechanism showing the contribution of traumatic brain injury (TBI) in the pathogenesis of epilepsy. PM, Plasma membrane; Glu, Glutamate; TLR, Toll-like receptor 4; NMDA-R, N-methyl-D-aspartate receptor; Glu, Glutamate; iNOS, inducible nitric oxide synthase; NO, nitric oxide; PtdCho, phosphatidylcholine; $cPLA_2$, cytosolic phospholipase A_2; ARA, arachidonic acid; COX-2, cyclooxygenase 2; LOX, lipoxygenase; ROS, reactive oxygen species; lyso-PtdCho, lyso-phosphatidylcholine; PGs, prostaglandins; LTs, leukotrienes; TXs, thromboxanes; IκB/NF-κB, nuclear factor κB inhibited form; IκB, inhibitory subunit of NF-κB; PAF, platelet activating factor; NF-κB-RE, nuclear factor κB-response element; MYD88, myeloid differentiation primary response gene 88; IRAK, Interleukin-1 receptor–associated kinase; TRAF, TNF receptor–associated factor; TAK1, Transforming growth factor b-activated kinase 1; NOS, nitric oxide synthase; NO, nitric oxide; ONOO−, peroxynitrite; TNF-α, tumor necrosis factor-α; IL-1β, interleukin 1β.

oxidative stress. High ROS also promote the migration of NF-κB from cytosol to the nucleus, where it binds with NF-κB response element and upregulates the expression of cytokines (TNF-α, IL-1β, and IL-6) and chemokine (MIP-1α), which may be responsible for the induction of neuroinflammation. Thus, oxidative stress and neuroinflammation are caused by distinct biochemical cascades that are closely intertwined and generally function in parallel, particularly in the brain, an organ especially prone to oxidative stress. Both these processes regulate the progression of TBI (Farooqui, 2010). Induction of excitotoxicity and high oxidative stress is known to promote epileptic seizures (Fig. 6.9) following TBI (Farooqui, 2014). Reducing excitotoxicity, oxidative stress, and neuroinflammation through selective brain cooling proves promising in preventing late onset seizures in a rodent model (Atkins et al., 2010). Recent evidence implicates IL-1β as a CSF marker predictive of persistent neuroinflammation seen with PTE (Diamond et al., 2014). Severe seizure activity not only accounts for heightened morbidity and mortality in the early stages following TBI but also remains the leading cause of death several years following TBI (Rao and Parko, 2015). It is also reported that unprovoked seizures develop in patients with AD at a higher rate than what is observed in the general population, raising questions about some inherent link between AD and epilepsy (Amatniek et al., 2006). It is suggested that in AD patients, neuronal hyperexcitability increases synaptic release of Aβ, which causes an accelerated cycle of cell death and cognitive decline in patients with AD (Noebels, 2011). There have been suggestions that a similar process involving Aβ dysfunction or related mechanisms may contribute to the progression of cognitive deficits and other behavioral features observed in patients with epilepsy (Chin and Scharfman, 2013).

LINK BETWEEN TBI AND DEPRESSION

In addition to above conditions, TBI may also contribute to high incidence of posttraumatic depression and other neuropsychiatric disorders such as anxiety and substance misuse are common in patients with TBI (Deb et al., 1999). Based on modern neuroimaging techniques DTI may help in recognizing degrees of DAI on the basis of measurement of the integrity of white matter (Maller et al., 2010). It is also reported that posttraumatic depression and other neuropsychiatric disorders persist at a 30-year follow-up of TBI. It is reported that these TBI patients were particularly susceptible to depressive episodes, delusional disorder, and persistent changes in personality (Koponen et al., 2004). Who develops these neuropsychiatric problems and why are poorly understood? Furthermore, the molecular mechanisms contributing to link between TBI and posttraumatic depression are not fully understood. However, there are several neurochemical mechanisms that may contribute to the link between TBI and posttraumatic depression (Fig. 6.10) (Zgaljardic et al., 2015). Inflammatory mediators, including proinflammatory cytokines are markedly elevated in the brain of TBI patients (Uzan et al., 2006). These markers are linked with the depression not only in intact adults (Raison et al., 2006; Schiepers et al., 2005) and older adults (Dimopoulos et al., 2006) but also in individuals with chronic conditions associated with inflammation, including TBI (Juengst et al., 2015; Devoto et al., 2017). Thus, high levels of inflammatory markers such as sVCAM-1, sICAM-1, and sFAS are associated with a significant increase

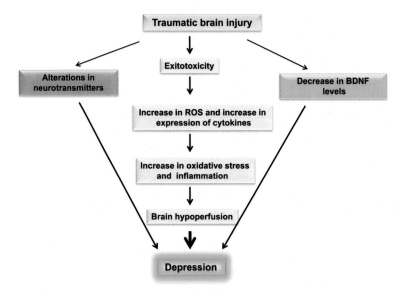

FIGURE 6.10   Hypothetical molecular mechanism linking traumatic brain injury (TBI) with posttraumatic depression. ROS, reactive oxygen species; BDNF, brain-derived neurotrophic factor.

in risk for depression 6 months post-TBI. Similarly, elevated CSF levels of IL-12 are also associated with PTD at 12 months (Juengst et al., 2015). In addition, to inflammatory cytokines both TBI and posttraumatic depression are also accompanied by low levels of brain-derived neurotrophic factor. It is also reported that the incidences of anxiety and depression are more strongly associated with unhealthy lifestyle style of patients than with severity of TBI (Curran et al., 2000).

CONCLUSION

Like spinal cord injury, the pathophysiology of TBI is biphasic with the initial presence of contusions, hematomas, and diffuse cell injury followed by secondary injury, which involves the release of glutamate from intracellular stores. The secondary brain injury is caused by a dynamic interplay between ischemic, inflammatory, and cytotoxic processes. Early symptoms of TBI include blood flow irregularities leading to metabolic imbalance, ischemia, hypoxia, and excitotoxicity. These processes not only contribute to the disruption of the BBB and alterations in signaling cascades but also result in complex interactions between pathological processes within the neurovascular unit. These interactions also cause brain edema, induce local inflammatory response, and increase neuronal excitability. These early events may promote and initiate acute complications, such as increased intracranial pressure, ischemic cell damage, seizures, and necrotic and apoptotic cell death. In parallel, slower pathophysiological mechanisms, such as neovascularization, transformation and dysfunction of astrocytes, and changes in synaptic wiring, may be associated with cognitive disabilities. At present, the severity of TBI is judged by the GCS, in which patients are scored on the basis of clinical symptoms, and the resulting overall score classifies their injury as mild (score: 13−15), moderate (score: 9−12), or severe (score: <9). Symptoms of mild to moderate TBI can include headaches, dizziness, nausea, and amnesia; these TBIs usually resolve within days to weeks of the insult. However, occasionally these injuries can result in long-term cognitive and behavioral deficits. Furthermore, there is evidence to suggest that moderate to severe TBI, and even repeat mild TBI may result in the onset of several neurological disorders including AD, PD, dementia, and epilepsy through many possible mechanisms including the accumulation of misfolded proteins (Aβ and α-synuclein), induction of oxidative stress and neuroinflammation. Collective evidence suggests that TBI is accompanied by depolarization, excitotoxicity, disruption of calcium homeostasis, mitochondrial dysfunction, activation of calcium-dependent enzymes, free-radical generation, BBB disruption, edema formation, induction of neuroinflammation, intracranial hypertension, and apoptotic cell death.

References

Acosta, S.A., Tajiri, N., Shinozuka, K., Ishikawa, H., Grimmig, B., et al., 2013. Long-term upregulation of inflammation and suppression of cell proliferation in the brain of adult rats exposed to traumatic brain injury using the controlled cortical impact model. PLoS One. 8, e53376.

Adrian, H., Mårten, K., Salla, N., Lasse, V., 2016. Biomarkers of traumatic brain injury: temporal changes in body fluids. eNeuro. 3.

Agoston, D.V., Gyorgy, A., Eidelman, O., Pollard, H.B., 2009. Proteomic biomarkers for blast neurotrauma: targeting cerebral edema, inflammation, and neuronal death cascades. J. Neurotrauma 26, 901−911.

Ahn, M.J., Sherwood, E.R., Prough, D.S., Lin, C.Y., DeWitt, D.S., 2004. The effects of traumatic brain injury on cerebral blood flow and brain tissue nitric oxide levels and cytokine expression. J. Neurotrauma 21, 1431−1442.

Albelda, S.M., Smith, C.W., Ward, P.A., 1994. Adhesion molecules and inflammatory injury. FASEB J. 8, 504−512.

Alford, P.W., Dabiri, B.E., Goss, J.A., Hemphill, M.A., Brigham, M.D., et al., 2011. Blast-induced phenotypic switching in cerebral vasospasm. Proc. Natl. Acad. Sci. USA 108, 12705−12710.

Alzheimer's-Association, 2013. Alzheimer's disease facts and figures. Alzheimer Dement. 9, 208−245.

Amatniek, J.C., Hauser, W.A., DelCastillo-Castenada, C., Jacobs, D.M., Marder, K., et al., 2006. Incidence and predictors of seizures in patients with Alzheimer's disease. Epilepsia 47, 867−872.

Amor, S., Peferoen, L.A., Vogel, D.Y., Breur, M., van der Valk, P., et al., 2014. Inflammation in neurodegenerative diseases—an update. Immunology 142, 151−166.

Angoa-Perez, M., Kane, M.J., Briggs, D.I., Herrera-Mundo, N., Viano, D.C., et al., 2014. Animal models of sports-related head injury: bridging the gap between pre-clinical research and clinical reality. J. Neurochem. 129, 916−931.

Annegers, J.F., Hauser, A., Coan, S.P., Rocca, W.A., 1998. A population-based study of seizures after traumatic brain injuries. N. Engl. J. Med. 338, 20−24.

Armstrong, R.C., Mierzwa, A.J., Marion, C.M., Sullivan, G.M., 2016. White matter involvement after TBI: clues to axon and myelin repair capacity. Exp. Neurol. 275 (Pt 3), 328−333.

Arundine, M., Tymianski, M., 2004. Molecular mechanisms of glutamate-dependent neurodegeneration in ischemia and traumatic brain injury. Cell Mol. Life Sci. 61, 657−668.

Arundine, M., Aarts, M., Lau, A., Tymianski, M., 2004. Vulnerability of central neurons to secondary insults after in vitro mechanical stretch. J. Neurosci. 24, 8106−8123.

Asl, S.Z., Khaksari, M., Khachki, A.S., Shahrokhi, N., Nourizade, S., 2013. Contribution of estrogen receptors alpha and beta in the brain response to traumatic brain injury. J. Neurosurg. 119, 353−361.

Atkins, C.M., Oliva Jr, A.A., Alonso, O.F., Pearse, D.D., Bramlett, H.M., et al., 2007. Modulation of the cAMP signaling pathway after traumatic brain injury. Exp. Neurol. 208, 145−158.

Atkins, C.M., Chen, S., Alonso, O.F., Dietrich, W.D., Hu, B.R., 2009. Activation of calcium/calmodulin-dependent protein kinases after traumatic brain injury. J. Cereb. Blood Flow Metab. 26, 1507−1518.

Atkins, C.M., Truettner, J.S., Lotocki, G., Sanchez-Molano, J., Kang, Y., et al., 2010. Posttraumatic seizure susceptibility is attenuated by hypothermia therapy. Eur. J. Neurosci. 32, 1912−1920.

Atmaca, H.T., Kul, O., Karakus, E., Terzi, O.S., Canpolat, S., et al., 2014. Astrocytes, microglia/macrophages, and neurons expressing Toll-like receptor 11 contribute to innate immunity against encephalitic Toxoplasma gondii infection. Neuroscience 269, 184−191.

Back, S.A., Han, B.H., Luo, N.L., et al., 2002. Selective vulnerability of late oligodendrocyte progenitors to hypoxia-ischemia. J. Neurosci. 22, 455−463.

Başkaya, M.K., Rao, A.M., Doğan, A., Donaldson, D., Dempsey, R.J., 1997. The biphasic opening of the blood-brain barrier in the cortex and hippocampus after traumatic brain injury in rats. Neurosci. Lett. 226, 33−36.

Belanger, H.G., Vanderploeg, R.D., Curtiss, G., Warden, D.L., 2007. Recent neuroimaging techniques in mild traumatic brain injury. J. Neuropsychiatr. Clin. Neurosci. 19, 5−20.

Bennett, E.R., Reuter-Rice, K., Laskowitz, D.T., 2016. Genetic influences in traumatic brain injurychapter 9 In: Laskowitz, D., Grant, G. (Eds.), Translational Research in Traumatic Brain Injury. CRC Press/Taylor and Francis Group, Boca Raton (FL), pp. 34−44.

Bernales, S., McDonald, K.L., Walter, P., 2006. Autophagy counterbalances endoplasmic reticulum expansion during the unfolded protein response. PLoS Biol. 4, e423.

Besson, V.C., 2009. Drug targets for traumatic brain injury from poly(ADP-ribose)polymerase pathway modulation. Br. J. Pharmacol. 157, 695−704.

Bianchi, M.E., 2007. DAMPs, PAMPs and alarmins: all we need to know about danger. J. Leukoc. Biol. 81, 1−5.

Bigford, G.E., Alonso, O.F., Dietrich, D., Keane, R.W., 2009. A novel protein complex in membrane rafts linking the NR2B glutamate receptor and autophagy is disrupted following traumatic brain injury. J. Neurotrauma 26, 703−720.

Bigler, E.D., 2013. Neuroinflammation and the dynamic lesion in traumatic brain injury. Brain 136, 9−11.

Block, M.L., Zecca, L., Hong, J.S., 2007. Microglia-mediated neurotoxicity: uncovering the molecular mechanisms. Nat. Rev. Neurosci. 8, 57–69.

Bower, J.H., Maraganore, D.M., Peterson, B.J., McDonnell, S.K., Ahlskog, J.E., et al., 2003. Head trauma preceding PD: a case-control study. Neurology 60, 1610–1615.

Brophy, G.M., Mondello, S., Papa, L., Robicsek, S.A., Gabrielli, A., et al., 2011. Biokinetic analysis of ubiquitin C-terminal hydrolase-L1 (UCH-L1) in severe traumatic brain injury patient biofluids. J. Neurotrauma 28, 861–870.

Browne, K.D., Chen, X.H., Meaney, D.F., Smith, D.H., 2011. Mild traumatic brain injury and diffuse axonal injury in swine. J. Neurotrauma 28, 1747–1755.

Cederberg, D., Siesjo, P., 2010. What has inflammation to do with traumatic brain injury? Child Nerv. Syst. 26, 221–226.

Chen, X.H., Siman, R., Iwata, A., Meaney, D.F., Trojanowski, J.Q., et al., 2004. Long-term accumulation of amyloid-β, β-secretase, presenilin-1, and caspase-3 in damaged axons following brain trauma. Am. J. Pathol. 165, 357–371.

Chen, L., Thiruchelvam, M.J., Madura, K., Richfield, E.K., 2006. Proteasome dysfunction in aged human alpha-synuclein transgenic mice. Neurobiol. Dis. 23, 120–126.

Cheng, G., Kong, R.-H., Zhang, L.-M., Zhang, J.N., 2012. Mitochondria in traumatic brain injury and mitochondrial-targeted multipotential therapeutic strategies. Br. J. Pharmacol. 167, 699–719.

Cheramy, A., Leviel, V., Daudet, F., Guibert, B., Chesselet, M.F., et al., 1981. Involvement of the thalamus on the reciprocal regulation of the two nigrostriatal dopaminergic pathways. Neuroscience 6, 2657–2668.

Chin, J., Scharfman, H.E., 2013. Shared cognitive and behavioral impairments in epilepsy and Alzheimer's disease and potential underlying mechanisms. Epilepsy Behav. 26, 343–351.

Cho, H.J., Sajja, V.S., Vandevord, P.J., Lee, Y.W., 2013. Blast induces oxidative stress, inflammation, neuronal loss and subsequent short-term memory impairment in rats. Neuroscience. 253, 9–20.

Christoffel, D.J., Golden, S.A., Russo, S.J., 2011. Structural and synaptic plasticity in stress-related disorders. Rev. Neurosci. 22, 535–549.

Clark, R.S., Kochanek, P.M., Watkins, S.C., Chen, M., Dixon, C.E., et al., 2000. Caspase-3 mediated neuronal death after traumatic brain injury in rats. J. Neurochem. 74, 740–753.

Clark, R.S., Vagni, V.A., Nathaniel, P.D., Jenkins, L.W., Dixon, C.E., et al., 2007. Local administration of the poly(ADP-ribose) polymerase inhibitor INO-1001 prevents NAD$^+$ depletion and improves water maze performance after traumatic brain injury in mice. J. Neurotrauma 24, 1399–1405.

Corps, K.N., Roth, T.L., McGavern, D.B., 2015. Inflammation and neuroprotection in traumatic brain injury. JAMA Neurol. 72, 355–362.

Corrigan, F., Vink, R., Turner, R.J., 2016. Inflammation in acute CNS injury: a focus on the role of substance P. Br. J. Pharmacol. 173, 703–715.

Covey, D.C., Born, C.T., 2010. Blast injuries: mechanics and wounding patterns. J. Surg. Orthop. Adv. 19, 8–12.

Crawford, F.C., Vanderploeg, R.D., Freeman, M.J., Singh, S., Waisman, M., et al., 2002. APOE genotype influences acquisition and recall following traumatic brain injury. Neurology. 58, 1115–1118.

Creed, J.A., DiLeonardi, A.M., Fox, D.P., Tessler, A.R., Raghupathi, R., 2011. Concussive brain trauma in the mouse results in acute cognitive deficits and sustained impairment of axonal function. J. Neurotrauma 28, 547–563.

Cuervo, A.M., Stefanis, L., Fredenburg, R., Lansbury, P.T., Sulzer, D., 2004. Impaired degradation of mutant α-synuclein by chaperone-mediated autophagy. Science 305, 1292–1295.

Curran, C.A., Ponsford, J.L., Crowe, S., 2000. Coping strategies and emotional outcome following traumatic brain injury: a comparison with orthopedic patients. J. Head Trauma Rehabil. 15, 1256–1274.

Czeiter, E., Buki, A., Bukovics, P., Farkas, O., Pal, J., et al., 2009. Calpain inhibition reduces axolemmal leakage in traumatic axonal injury. Molecules 14, 5115–5123.

Daniele, S.G., Béraud, D., Davenport, C., Cheng, K., Yin, H., Maguire-Zeiss, K.A., 2015. Activation of MyD88-dependent TLR1/2 signaling by misfolded alpha-synuclein, a protein linked to neurodegenerative disorders. Sci Signal l 8:ra45.

da Silva Meirelles, L., Simon, D., Regner, A., 2017. Neurotrauma: the crosstalk between neurotrophins and inflammation in the acutely injured brain. Int. J. Mol. Sci. 18, pii: E1082.

Das, M., Mohapatra, S., Mohapatra, S.S., 2012. New perspectives on central and peripheral immune responses to acute traumatic brain injury. J. Neuroinflammation. 9, 236.

Dauer, W., Przedborski, S., 2003. Parkinson's disease: mechanisms and models. Neuron 39, 889–909.

Davalos, D., Grutzendler, J., Yang, G., et al., 2005. ATP mediates rapid microglial response to local brain injury in vivo. Nat. Neurosci. 8, 752–758.

Deb, S., Lyons, I., Koutzoukis, C., 1999. Neurobehavioural symptoms one year after a head injury. Br. J. Psychiatry 174, 360–365.

Deleidi, M., Jäggle, M., Rubino, G., 2015. Immune aging, dysmetabolism, and inflammation in neurological diseases. Front. Neurosci. 9, 172.

Delouche, A., Attyé, A., Heck, O., Grand, S., Kastler, A., et al., 2016. Diffusion MRI: pitfalls, literature review and future directions of research in mild traumatic brain injury. Eur. J. Radiol. 85, 25–30.

Devoto, C., Arcurio, L., Fetta, J., et al., 2017. Inflammation relates to chronic behavioral and neurological symptoms in military with traumatic brain injuries. Cell Transplant. 26, 1169–1177.

Diamond, M.L., Ritter, A.C., Failla, M.D., Boles, J.A., Conley, Y.P., et al., 2014. IL-1beta associations with posttraumatic epilepsy development: a genetics and biomarker cohort study. Epilepsia. 55, 1109–1119.

DiLeonardi, A.M., Huh, J.W., Raghupathi, R., 2009. Impaired axonal transport and neurofilament compaction occur in separate populations of injured axons following diffuse brain injury in the immature rat. Brain Res. 1263, 174–182.

Dimopoulos, N., Piperi, C., Salonicioti, A., et al., 2006. Elevation of plasma concentration of adhesion molecules in late-life depression. Int. J. Geriatr. Psychiatry. 21, 965–971.

Donkin, J.J., Nimmo, A.J., Cernak, I., Blumbergs, P.C., Vink, R., 2009. Substance P is associated with the development of brain edema and functional deficits after traumatic brain injury. J. Cereb. Blood Flow Metab. 29, 1388–1398.

Ellis, R.C., Earnhardt, J.N., Hayes, R.L., Wang, K.K., Anderson, D.K., 2004. Cathepsin B mRNA and protein expression following contusion spinal cord injury in rats. J. Neurochem. 88, 689–697.

Emmanouilidou, E., Stefanis, L., Vekrellis, K., 2008. Cell-produced alpha-synuclein oligomers are targeted to, and impair, the 26S proteasome. Neurobiol. Aging. 31, 953–968.

Esler, W.P., Wolfe, M.S., 2001. A portrait of Alzheimer secretases: new features and familiar faces. Science. 293, 1449–1454.

Ettenhofer, K.S., Abeles, N., 2009. The significant of mild traumatic brain injury to cognition and self-reported sympons in long term recovery from injury. J. Clin. Exp. Neuropsychol. 31, 363–372.

Faden, A.I., Demediuk, P., Panter, S.S., Vink, R., 1989. The role of excitatory amino acids and NMDA receptors in traumatic brain injury. Science 244, 798–800.

Farkas, O., Povlishock, J.T., 2007. Cellular and subcellular change evoked by diffuse traumatic brain injury: a complex web of change extending far beyond focal damage. Prog. Brain Res. 161, 43–59.

Farook, J.M., Shields, J., Tawfik, A., Markand, S., Sen, T., Smith, S.B., et al., 2013. GADD34 induces cell death through inactivation of Akt following traumatic brain injury. Cell Death Dis. 4, e754.

Farooqui, A.A., 2010. Neurochemical Aspects of Neurotraumatic and Neurodegenerative Diseases. Springer, New York.

Farooqui, A.A., 2011. Lipid Mediators and Their Metabolism in the Brain. Springer, New York.

Farooqui, A.A., 2014. Inflammation and Oxidative Stress in Neurological Disorders. Springer International Publishing Switzerland.

Farooqui, A.A., 2015. High Calorie Diet and the Human Brain: Metabolic Consequences of Long-Term Consumption. Springer International Publishing Switzerland.

Farooqui, A.A., 2016. Therapeutic Potentials of Curcumin for Alzheimer Disease. Springer International Publishing Switzerland.

Farooqui, A.A., 2017. Neurochemical Aspects of Alzheimer's Disease: Risk Factors, Pathogenesis, Biomarkers, and Potential Treatment Strategies. Academic Press, London, UK.

Farooqui, A.A., Horrocks, L.A., 2007. Glycerophospholipids in the Brain: Phospholipases A_2 in Neurological Disorders. Springer, New York.

Faul, M., Xu, L., Wald, M.W., Coronado, V.G., 2010. Traumatic Brain Injury in the United States: Emergency Department Visits, Hospitalizations, and Deaths 2002—2006. Centers for Disease Control and Prevention, National Center for Injury Prevention and Control, Atlanta, GA.

Faul, M., Coronado, V., 2015. Epidemiology of traumatic brain injury. Handb. Clin. Neurol. 127, 3—13.

Fellner, L., Irschick, R., Schanda, K., Reindl, M., Klimaschewski, L., et al., 2013. Toll-like receptor 4 is required for alpha-synuclein dependent activation of microglia and astroglia. Glia. 61, 349—360.

Fisher, R.S., van Emde Boas, W., Blume, W., Elger, C., Genton, P., et al., 2005. Epileptic seizures and epilepsy: definitions proposed by the International League Against Epilepsy (ILAE) and the International Bureau for Epilepsy (IBE). Epilepsia. 46, 470—472.

Fleminger, S., Oliver, D.L., Lovestone, S., Rabe-Hesketh, S., Giora, A., 2003. Head injury as a risk factor for Alzheimer's disease: the evidence 10 years on; a partial replication. J. Neurol. Neurosurg. Psychiatry 74, 857—862.

Foster, K.A., Recker, M.J., Lee, P.S., Bell, M.J., Tyler-Kabara, E.C., 2014. Factors associated with hemispheric hypodensity after subdural hematoma following abusive head trauma in children. J. Neurotrauma 31, 1625—1631.

Frugier, T., Morganti-Kossmann, M.C., O'Reilly, D., McLean, C.A., 2010. In situ detection of inflammatory mediators in post mortem human brain tissue after traumatic injury. J. Neurotrauma 27, 497—507.

Gao, H.M., Hong, J.S., 2008. Why neurodegenerative diseases are progressive: uncontrolled inflammation drives disease progression. Trends Immunol. 29, 357—365.

Gegelashvili, G., Dehnes, Y., Danbolt, N.C., Schousboe, A., 2000. The high-affinity glutamate transporters GLT1, GLAST, and EAAT4 are regulated via different signalling mechanisms. Neurochem. Int. 37, 163—170.

Gentleman, S.M., Leclercq, P.D., Moyes, L., Graham, D.I., Smith, C., et al., 2004. Long-term intracerebral inflammatory response after traumatic brain injury. Forensic Sci. Int. 146, 97—104.

Gilbert, M., Snyder, C., Corcoran, C., Norton, M.C., Lyketsos, C.G., et al., 2014. The association of traumatic brain injury with rate of progression of cognitive and functional impairment in a population-based cohort of Alzheimer's disease: the Cache County dementia progression study. Int. Psychogeriatr. 26, 1593—1601.

Goldman, S.M., Tanner, C.M., Oakes, D., Bhudhikanok, G.S., Gupta, A., et al., 2006. Head injury and Parkinson's disease risk in twins. Ann. Neurol. 60, 65–72.

Gomez-Pinilla, F., 2011. The combined effects of exercise and foods in preventing neurological and cognitive disorders. Prev. Med. 52 (Suppl 1), S75–S80.

Grant, C.M., 2008. Metabolic reconfiguration is a regulated response to oxidative stress. J. Biol. 7, 1.

Graves, B.T., Munro, C.L., 2013. Epigenetics in critical illness: a new frontier. Nurs. Res. Pract. 2013, 503686.

Guingab-Cagmat, J.D., Kobeissy, F., Ratliff, M.V., Shi, P., Zhang, Z., Wang, K.W., 2010. Neurogenomics and neuroproteomics approaches of studying neural injury. In: Fehlings, M., et al., (Eds.), Essentials of Spinal Cord Injury. Thieme, Toronto, pp. 605–618.

Guo, Z., Cupples, L.A., Kurz, A., Auerbach, S.H., Volicer, L., et al., 2000. Head injury and the risk of AD in the MIRAGE study. Neurology 54, 1316–1323.

Hall, E.D., Detloff, M.R., Johnson, K., Kupina, N.C., 2004. Peroxynitritemediated protein nitration and lipid peroxidation in a mouse model of traumatic brain injury. J. Neurotrauma 21, 9–20.

Hamby, M.E., Sofroniew, M.V., 2010. Reactive astrocytes as therapeutic targets for CNS disorders. Neurotherapeutics 7, 494–506.

Hang, C.H., Chen, G., Shi, J.X., Zhang, X., Li, J.S., 2006. Cortical expression of nuclear factor kappaB after human brain contusion. Brain Res. 1109, 14–21.

Harmon, K.G., Drezner, J., Gammons, M., Guskiewicz, K., Halstead, M., et al., 2013. American Medical Society for Sports Medicine position statement: concussion in sport. Clin. J. Sport. Med 23, 1–18.

Hayashi, T., Ago, K., Nakamae, T., Higo, E., Ogata, M., 2015. Two different immunostaining patterns of beta-amyloid precursor protein (APP) may distinguish traumatic from nontraumatic axonal injury. Int. J. Legal Med. 129, 1085–1090.

Hsieh, H.-L., Yang, C.-M., 2013. Role of redox signaling in neuroinflammation and neurodegenerative diseases. Biomed. Res. Int. 2013, 18.

Hsu, L.J., Sagara, Y., Arroyo, A., Rockenstein, E., Sisk, A., et al., 2000. Alpha-synuclein promotes mitochondrial deficit and oxidative stress. Am. J. Pathol 157, 401–410.

Hughes, D.G., Jackson, A., Mason, D.L., Berry, E., Hollis, S., et al., 2004. Abnormalities on magnetic resonance imaging seen acutely following mild traumatic brain injury: correlation with neuropsychological tests and delayed recovery. Neuroradiology 46, 550–558.

Ikonomovic, M.D., Uryu, K., Abrahamson, E.E., Ciallella, J.R., Trojanowski, J.Q., Lee, V.M., et al., 2004. Alzheimer's pathology in human temporal cortex surgically excised after severe brain injury. Exp. Neurol. 190, 192–203.

Ikonomovic, M.D., Mi, Z., Abrahamson, E.E., 2017. Disordered APP metabolism and neurovasculature in trauma and aging: combined risks for chronic neurodegenerative disorders. Ageing Res. Rev. 34, 51–63.

Iwata, A., Chen, X.H., McIntosh, T.K., Browne, K.D., Smith, D.H., 2002. Long-term accumulation of amyloid-β in axons following brain trauma without persistent upregulation of amyloid precursor protein genes. J. Neuropathol. Exp. Neurol. 61, 1056–1068.

Iwai, A., Masliah, E., Yoshimoto, M., Ge, N.F., Flanagan, L., et al., 1995. The precursor protein of non-a-beta component of Alzheimers-disease amyloid Is a presynaptic protein of the central-nervous-system. Neuron. 14, 467–475.

Jankovic, J., 2008. Parkinson's disease: clinical features and diagnosis. J. Neurol. Neurosurg. Psychiatr. 79, 368–376.

Jin, W., Wang, H., Yan, W., Xu, L., Wang, X., et al., 2008. Disruption of Nrf2 enhances upregulation of nuclear factor-kappaB activity, proinflammatory cytokines, and intercellular adhesion molecule-1 in the brain after traumatic brain injury. Mediators Inflamm. 2008, 725174.

Johnson, V.E., Stewart, W., Smith, D.H., 2010. Traumatic brain injury and amyloid-beta pathology: a link to Alzheimer's disease?. Nat. Rev. Neurosci. 11, 361−370.

Johnson, V.E., Stewart, W., Smith, D.H., 2012. Widespread tau and amyloid-beta pathology many years after a single traumatic brain injury in humans. Brain Pathol. 22, 142−149.

Johnson, V.E., Stewart, J.E., Begbie, F.D., Trojanowski, J.Q., Smith, D.H., Stewart, W., 2013. Inflammation and white matter degeneration persist for years after a single traumatic brain injury. Brain. 136, 28−42.

Jomova, K., Valko, M., 2011. Advances in metal-induced oxidative stress and human disease. Toxicology. 283, 65−87.

Juengst, S.B., Kumar, R.G., Failla, M.D., Goyal, A., Wagner, A.K., 2015. Acute inflammatory biomarker profiles predict depression risk following moderate to severe traumatic brain injury. J. Head Trauma Rehabil. 30, 207−218.

Kamal, A., Stokin, G.B., Yang, Z., Xia, C.H., Goldstein, L.S., 2000. Axonal transport of amyloid precursor protein is mediated by direct binding to the kinesin light chain subunit of kinesin-I. Neuron. 28, 449−459.

Kamal, A., Almenar-Queralt, A., LeBlanc, J.F., Roberts, E.A., Goldstein, L.S., 2001. Kinesin-mediated axonal transport of a membrane compartment containing beta-secretase and presenilin-1 requires APP. Nature. 414, 643−648.

Kane, M.J., Citron, B.A., 2009. Transcription factors as therapeutic targets in CNS disorders. Recent Pat. Nanotechnol. 4, 190−199.

Kang, E.L., Cameron, A.N., Piazza, F., Walker, K.R., Tesco, G., 2010. Ubiquitin regulates GGA3-mediated degradation of BACE1. J. Biol. Chem. 285, 24108−24119.

Kauppinen, T.M., 2007. Multiple roles for poly(ADP-ribose)polymerase-1 in neurological disease. Neurochem. Int. 50, 954−958.

Khanna, M.R., Kovalevich, J., Lee, V.M., Trojanowski, J.Q., Brunden, K.R., 2016. Therapeutic strategies for the treatment of tauopathies: hopes and challenges. Alzheimers Dement. 12, 1051−1065.

Khorooshi, R., Babcock, A.A., Owens, T., 2008. NF-kappaB-driven STAT2 and CCL2 expression in astrocytes in response to brain injury. J. Immunol. 181, 7284−7291.

Kidd, P.M., 2005. Neurodegeneration from mitochondrial insufficiency: nutrients, stem cells, growth factors, and prospects for brain rebuilding using integrative management. Altern. Med. Rev. 10, 268−293.

Kim, J., Basak, J.M., Holtzman, D.M., 2009. The role of apolipoprotein E in Alzheimer's disease. Neuron. 63, 287−303.

Kobeissy, F.H., Ottens, A.K., Zhang, Z., Liu, M.C., Denslow, N.D., et al., 2006. Novel differential neuroproteomics analysis of traumatic brain injury in rats. Mol. Cell Proteomics. 5, 1887−1898.

Kochanek, P.M., Hallenbeck, J.M., 1992. Polymorphonuclear leukocytes and monocytes/macrophages in the pathogenesis of cerebral ischemia and stroke. Stroke. 23, 1367−1379.

Koponen, S., Taiminen, T., Kairisto, V., Portin, R., Isoniemi, H., et al., 2004. APOE-epsilon4 predicts dementia but not other psychiatric disorders after traumatic brain injury. Neurology 63, 749−750.

Krishnamurthy, K., Laskowitz, D.T., 2016. Cellular and molecular mechanisms of secondary neuronal injury. In: Laskowitz, D., Grant, G. (Eds.), Translational Research in Traumatic Brain Injury. CRC Press/Taylor and Francis Group, Boca Raton, FL.

Kuhajda, I., Zarogoulidis, K., Kougioumtzi, I., Huang, H., Li, Q., et al., 2014. Penetrating trauma. J. Thorac. Dis. 6 (Suppl 4), S461−S465.

Lauriat, T., McInnes, L.A., 2007. EAAT2 regulation and splicing: relevance to psychiatric and neurological disorders. Mol. Psychiatry 12, 1065−1078.

Lawler, C.P., Gilmore, J.H., Watts, V.J., Walker, Q.D., Southerland, S.B., et al., 1995. Interhemispheric modulation of dopamine receptor interactions in unilateral 6-OHDA rodent model. Synapse 21, 299−311.

Lee, J.M., Johnson, J.A., 2004. An important role of Nrf2-ARE pathway in the cellular defense mechanism. J. Biochem. Mol. Biol. 37, 139—143.

Lee, H.J., Suk, J.E., Patrick, C., Bae, E.J., Cho, J.H., et al., 2010. Direct transfer of α-synuclein from neuron to astroglia causes inflammatory responses in synucleinopathies. J. Biol. Chem. 285, 9262—9272.

Leinhase, I., Schmidt, O.I., Thurman, J.M., Hossini, A.M., Rozanski, M., et al., 2006. Pharmacological complement inhibition at the C3 convertase level promotes neuronal survival, neuroprotective intracerebral gene expression, and neurological outcome after traumatic brain injury. Exp. Neurol. 199, 454—464.

Leinhase, I., Rozanski, M., Harhausen, D., Thurman, J.M., Schmidt, O.I., et al., 2007. Inhibition of the alternative complement activation pathway in traumatic brain injury by a monoclonal anti-factor B antibody: a randomized placebo-controlled study in mice. J. Neuroinflammation. 4, 13.

Li, S., Sun, Y., Shan, D., Feng, B., Xing, J., et al., 2013. Temporal profiles of axonal injury following impact acceleration traumatic brain injury in rats—a comparative study with diffusion tensor imaging and morphological analysis. Int. J. Legal Med. 127, 159—167.

Li, Y., Korgaonkar, A.A., Swietek, B., Wang, J., Elgammal, F.S., Elkabes, S., et al., 2015. Toll-like receptor 4 enhancement of non-NMDA synaptic currents increases dentate excitability after brain injury. Neurobiol. Dis. 74, 240—253.

Liang, Y., Lei, Z., Zhang, H., Xu, Z., Cui, Q., et al., 2014. Toll-like receptor 4 is associated with seizures following ischemia with hyperglycemia. Brain Res. 1590, 75—84.

Liu, H.D., Li, W., Chen, Z.R., Zhou, M.L., Zhuang, Z., Zhang, D.D., et al., 2013. Increased expression of ferritin in cerebral cortex after human traumatic brain injury. Neurol. Sci. 34, 1173—1180.

Liyanage, V.R., Jarmasz, J.S., Murugeshan, N., Del Bigio, M.R., Rastegar, M., et al., 2014. DNA modifications: function and applications in normal and disease States. Biology (Basel) 3, 670—723.

Loane, D.J., Pocivavsek, A., Moussa, C.E., Thompson, R., Matsuoka, Y., et al., 2009. Amyloid precursor protein secretases as therapeutic targets for traumatic brain injury. Nat. Med. 15, 377—379.

Loane, D.J., Byrnes, K.R., 2010. Role of microglia in neurotrauma. Neurotherapeutics. 7, 366—377.

Logsdon, A.F., Lucke-Wold, B.P., Turner, R.C., Huber, J.D., Rosen, C.L., et al., 2015. Role of microvascular disruption in brain damage from traumatic brain injury. Compr. Physiol. 5, 1147—1160.

Lorente, L., 2015. New prognostic biomarkers in patients with traumatic brain injury. Arch. Trauma Res. 4, e301165.

Maegele, M., Riess, P., Sauerland, S., et al., 2005. Characterization of a new rat model of experimental combined neurotrauma. Shock 23, 476—481.

Magnoni, S., Brody, D., 2010. New perspectives on amyloid-β dynamics after acute brain injury: moving between experimental approaches and studies in the human brain. Arch. Neurol. 67, 1068—1073.

Maller, J.J., Thomson, R.H., Lewis, P.M., Rose, S.E., Pannek, K., et al., 2010. Traumatic brain injury, major depression, and diffusion tensor imaging: making connections. Brain Res. Rev. 64, 213—240.

Mapstone, M., Cheema, A.K., Fiandaca, M.S., Zhong, X., Mhyre, T.R., et al., 2014. Plasma phospholipids identify antecedent memory impairment in older adults. Nat. Med. 20, 415—418.

Maroso, M., Balosso, S., Ravizza, T., Liu, J., Aronica, E., et al., 2010. Toll-like receptor 4 and high-mobility group box-1 are involved in ictogenesis and can be targeted to reduce seizures. Nat. Med. 16, 413—419.

Matute, C., Domercq, M., Sánchez-Gómez, M.V., 2006. Glutamate-mediated glial injury: mechanisms and clinical importance. Glia 53, 212–224.

McAllister, T.W., Rhodes, C.H., Flashman, L.A., McDonald, B.C., Belloni, D., et al., 2005. Effect of the dopamine D2 receptor T allele on response latency after mild traumatic brain injury. Am. J. Psychiatry 162, 1749–1751.

McAllister, T.W., Flashman, L.A., McDonald, B.C., Saykin, A.J., 2006. Mechanisms of working memory dysfunction after mild and moderate TBI: evidence from functional MRI and neurogenetics. J. Neurotrauma 23, 1450–1467.

McAllister, T.W., Flashman, L.A., Harker Rhodes, C., Tyler, A.L., Moore, J.H., et al., 2008. Single nucleotide polymorphisms in ANKK1 and the dopamine D2 receptor gene affect cognitive outcome shortly after traumatic brain injury: a replication and extension study. Brain Inj. 22, 705–714.

McAllister, T.W., 2010. Genetic factors modulating outcome after neurotrauma. PM R. 2 (Suppl 2), S241–S252.

McDonald, B.C., Saykin, A.J., McAllister, T.W., 2012. Functional MRI of mild traumatic brain injury (mTBI): progress and perspectives from the first decade of studies. Brain Imaging Behav. 6, 193–207.

McDonald, S.J., Sun, M., Agoston, D.V., Shultz, S.R., 2016. The effect of concomitant peripheral injury on traumatic brain injury pathobiology and outcome. J. Neuroinflamm. 13, 90.

McGinn, M.J., Povlishock, J.T., 2016. Pathophysiology of traumatic brain injury. Neurosurg. Clin. N. Am. 27, 397–407.

McKee, A.C., Stern, R.A., Nowinski, C.J., Stein, T.D., Alvarez, V.E., et al., 2013. The spectrum of disease in chronic traumatic encephalopathy. Brain. 136, 43–64.

Merali, Z., Leung, J., Mikulis, D., Silver, F., Kassner, A., 2015. Longitudinal assessment of imatinib's effect on the blood-brain barrier after ischemia/reperfusion injury with permeability MRI. Transl. Stroke Res 6, 39–49.

Mielke, M.M., Savica, R., Wiste, H.J., Weigand, S.D., Vemuri, P., et al., 2014. Head trauma and in vivo measures of amyloid and neurodegeneration in a population-based study. Neurology 2014 (82), 70–76.

Miller, D.M., Singh, I.N., Wang, J.A., Hall, E.D., 2015. Nrf2-ARE activator carnosic acid decreases mitochondrial dysfunction, oxidative damage and neuronal cytoskeletal degradation following traumatic brain injury in mice. Exp. Neurol. 264, 103–110.

Milman, A., Rosenberg, A., Weizman, R., Pick, C.G., 2005. Mild traumatic brain injury induces persistent cognitive deficits and behavioral disturbances in mice. J. Neurotrauma 22, 1003–1010.

Moretti, L., Cristofori, I., Weaver, S.M., Chau, A., Portelli, J.N., et al., 2012. Cognitive decline in older adults with a history of traumatic brain injury. Lancet Neurol. 11, 1103–1112.

Morganti-Kossmann, M.C., Rancan, M., Stahel, P.F., Kossmann, T., 2002. Inflammatory response in acute traumatic brain injury: a double-edged sword. Curr. Opin. Crit. Care. 8, 101–105.

Munoz, P., Humeres, A., Elgueta, C., Kirkwood, A., Hidalgo, C., Nunez, M.T., 2011. Iron mediates N-methyl-D-aspartate receptor-dependent stimulation of calcium-induced pathways and hippocampal synaptic plasticity. J. Biol. Chem. 286, 13382–13392.

Nagamoto-Combs, K., McNeal, D.W., Morecraft, R.J., Combs, C.K., 2007. Prolonged microgliosis in the rhesus monkey central nervous system after traumatic brain injury. J. Neurotrauma 24, 1719–1742.

Neumann, M., Sampathu, D.M., Kwong, L.K., Truax, A.C., Micsenyi, M.C., et al., 2006. Ubiquitinated TDP-43 in frontotemporal lobar degeneration and amyotrophic lateral sclerosis. Science. 314, 130–133.

Nimmerjahn, A., Kirchhoff, F., Helmchen, F., 2005. Resting microglial cells are highly dynamic surveillants of brain parenchyma in vivo. Science. 308, 1314–1318.

Nisenbaum, E.J., Novikov, D.S., Lui, Y.W., 2014. The presence and role of iron in mild traumatic brain injury: an imaging perspective. J. Neurotrauma 31, 301–307.

Noebels, J., 2011. A perfect storm: converging paths of epilepsy and Alzheimer's dementia intersect in the hippocampal formation. Epilepsia 52 (suppl 1), 39–46.

Nunan, J., Small, D.H., 2000. Regulation of APP cleavage by α-, β-, and γ-secretases. FEBS Lett. 483, 6–10.

Olah, M., Biber, K., Vinet, J., Boddeke, H.W., 2011. Microglia phenotype diversity. CNS Neurol. Disord. Drug Targets. 10, 108–118.

Oliver, J., Abbas, K., Lightfoot, J.T., Baskin, K., Collins, B., et al., 2015. Comparison of neurocognitive testing and the measurement of marinobufagenin in mild traumatic brain injury: a preliminary report. J. Exp. Neurosci. 9, 67–72.

Ottens, A.K., Stafflinger, J.E., Griffin, H.E., Kunz, R.D., Cifu, D.X., et al., 2014. Post-acute brain injury urinary signature: a new resource for molecular diagnostics. J. Neurotrauma 31, 782–788.

Ozen, L.J., Fernandes, M.A., 2012. Slowing down after a mild traumatic brain injury: a strategy to improve cognitive task performance. Arch. Clin. Neuropsychol. 27, 85–100.

Park, E., Velumian, A.A., Fehlings, M.G., 2004. The role of excitotoxicity in secondary mechanisms of spinal cord injury: a review with an emphasis on the implications for white matter degeneration. J. Neurotrauma 21, 754–774.

Park, E., Liu, E., Shek, M., Park, A., Baker, A.J., 2007. Heavy neurofilament accumulation and α-spectrin degradation accompany cerebellar white matter functional deficits following forebrain fluid percussion injury. Exp. Neurol. 204, 49–57.

Peek-Asa, C., McArthur, D., Hovda, D., Kraus, J., 2001. Early predictors of mortality in penetrating compared with closed brain injury. Brain Inj. 15, 801–810.

Pereire, C.F.M., Resende, de Oliveira, C., 2000. Oxidative glutamate toxicity involves mitochondrial dysfunction and perturbation of intracellular Ca^{2+} homeostasis. Neurosci. Res. 83, 2758–2762.

Pines, G., Danbolt, N.C., Bjoras, M., Zhang, Y., Bendahan, A., et al., 1992. Cloning and expression of a rat brain L-glutamate transporter. Nature 360, 464–467.

Plog, B.A., Dashnaw, M.L., Hitomi, E., Peng, W., Liao, Y., et al., 2015. Biomarkers of traumatic injury are transported from brain to blood via the glymphatic system. J. Neurosci. 35, 518–526.

Povlishock, J.T., Becker, D.P., Cheng, C.L., Vaughan, G.W., 1983. Axonal change in minor head injury. J. Neuropathol. Exp. Neurol. 42, 225–242.

Qaseem, A., Snow, V., Cross Jr, J., Forciea, M.A., Hopkins Jr, R., et al., 2008. Current pharmacologic treatment of dementia: a clinical practice guideline from the American College of Physicians and the American Academy of Family Physicians. Ann. Intern. Med. 148, 370–378.

Qureshi, I.A., Mehler, M.F., 2010. Emerging role of epigenetics in stroke: part 1: DNA methylation and chromatin modifications. Arch. Neurol. 67, 1316–1322.

Raghupathi, R., 2004. Cell death mechanisms following traumatic brain injury. Brain Path. 14, 215–222.

Raghupathi, R., Graham, D.I., McIntosh, T.K., 2000. Apoptosis after traumatic brain injury. J. Neurotrauma 17, 927–938.

Raison, C.L., Capuron, L., Miller, A.H., 2006. Cytokines sing the blues: inflammation and the pathogenesis of depression. Trends Immunol. 27, 24–31.

Raivich, G., Behrens, A., 2006. Role of the AP-1 transcription factor c-Jun in developing, adult and injured brain. Prog. Neurobiol. 78, 347–363.

Ralay Ranaivo, H., Zunich, S.M., Choi, N., Hodge, J.N., Wainwright, M.S., 2011. Mild stretch-induced injury increases susceptibility to interleukin-1β-induced release of matrix metalloproteinase-9 from astrocytes. J. Neurotrauma 28, 1757–1766.

Ralser, M., Wamelink, M.M., Kowald, A., Gerisch, B., Heeren, G., et al., 2007. Dynamic rerouting of the carbohydrate flux is key to counteracting oxidative stress. J. Biol. 6, 10.

Ramlackhansingh, A.F., Brooks, D.J., Greenwood, R.J., Bose, S.K., Turkheimer, F.E., et al., 2011. Inflammation after trauma: microglial activation and traumatic brain injury. Ann. Neurol 70, 374–383.

Rao, V.R., Parko, K.L., 2015. Clinical approach to posttraumatic epilepsy. Semin. Neurol. 35, 57–63.

Ray, S.K., Banik, N.L., 2003. Calpain and its involvement in the pathophysiology of CNS injuries and diseases: therapeutic potential of calpain inhibitors for prevention of neurodegeneration. Curr. Drug Targets CNS Neurol. Disord. 2, 173–189.

Ritchie, K., Lovestone, S., 2002. The dementias. Lancet. 360, 1759–1766.

Roberts, G.W., Gentleman, S.M., Lynch, A., Murray, L., Landon, M., et al., 1994. Beta amyloid protein deposition in the brain after severe head injury: implications for the pathogenesis of Alzheimer's disease. J. Neurol. Neurosurg. Psychiatr. 57, 419–425.

Roberts, D.J., Jenne, C.N., Leger, C., Kramer, A.H., Gallagher, C.N., et al., 2013. Association between the cerebral inflammatory and matrix metalloproteinase responses after severe traumatic brain injury in humans. J. Neurotrauma 30, 1727–1736.

Rock, K.L., Kono, H., 2008. The inflammatory response to cell death. Annu. Rev. Pathol. 3, 99–126.

Ron, D., Walter, P., 2007. Signal integration in the endoplasmic reticulum unfolded protein response. Nat. Rev. Mol. Cell Biol. 8, 519–529.

Rostami, R., Salamati, P., Yarandi, K.K., Khoshnevisan, A., Saadat, S., et al., 2017. Effects of neurofeedback on the short-term memory and continuous attention of patients with moderate traumatic brain injury: a preliminary randomized controlled clinical trial. Chin. J. Traumatol. pii: S1008-1275.

Rubenstein, R., Chang, B., Davies, P., Wagner, A.K., Robertson, C.S., Wang, K.K., 2015. A novel, ultrasensitive assay for tau: potential for assessing traumatic brain injury in tissues and biofluids. J. Neurotrauma 32, 342–352.

Ruff, R., 2005. Two decades of advances in understanding of mild traumatic brain injury. J. Head Trauma Rehabil. 20, 5–18.

Salminen, A., Kauppinen, A., Suuronen, T., Kaarniranta, K., Ojala, J.E.R., 2009. Stress in Alzheimer's disease: a novel neuronal trigger for inflammation and Alzheimer's pathology. J. Neuroinflamm 6, 41.

Sandhir, R., Berman, N.E., 2009. Age-dependent response of CCAAT/enhancer binding proteins following traumatic brain injury in mice. Neurochem. Int. 56, 188–193.

Sano, R., Reed, J.C., 2013. ER stress-induced cell death mechanisms. Biochim. Biophys. Acta. 1833, 3460–3470.

Schiepers, O.J.G., Wichers, M.C., Maes, M., 2005. Cytokines and major depression. Prog. Neuropsychopharmacol. Biol. Psychiatry 29, 201–217.

Schmidt, O.I., Heyde, C.E., Ertel, W., Stahel, P.F., 2005. Closed head injury—an inflammatory disease? Brain Res. Rev. 48, 388–399.

Schmitt, S., Dichter, M.A., 2015. Electrophysiologic recordings in traumatic brain injury. Handb. Clin. Neurol. 127, 319–339.

Schwab, M.E., 2010. Functions of Nogo proteins and their receptors in the nervous system. Nat. Rev. Neurosci. 11, 799–811.

Shahaduzzaman, M., Acosta, S., Bickford, P.C., Borlongan, C.V., 2013. Alpha-Synuclein is a pathological link and therapeutic target for Parkinson's disease and traumatic brain injury. Med. Hypotheses 81, 675–680.

Shekhar, C., Gupta, L.N., Premsagar, I.C., et al., 2015. An epidemiological study of traumatic brain injury cases in a trauma centre of New Delhi (India). J. Emerg. Trauma Shock. 8, 131–139.

Sheldon, A.L., Robinson, M.B., 2007. The role of glutamate transporters in neurodegenerative diseases and potential opportunities for intervention. Neurochem. Int. 51, 333–355. 2007.

Shohami, E., Biegon, A., 2014. Novel approach to the role of NMDA receptors in traumatic brain injury. CNS Neurol. Disord. Drug Targets 13, 567–573.

Signoretti, S., Vagnozzi, R., Tavazzi, B., Lazzarino, G., 2010. Biochemical and neurochemical sequelae following mild traumatic brain injury: summary of experimental data and clinical implications. Neurosurg. Focus 29, E1.

Slobounov, S.M., Gay, M., Zhang, K., Johnson, B., Pennell, D., et al., 2011. Alteration of brain functional network at rest and in response to YMCA physical stress test in concussed athletes: RsFMRI study. NeuroImage 55, 1716–1727.

Smith, D.H., Chen, X.H., Nonaka, M., Trojanowski, J.Q., Lee, V.M., et al., 1999. Accumulation of amyloid beta and tau and the formation of neurofilament inclusions following diffuse brain injury in the pig. J. Neuropathol. Exp. Neurol. 58, 982–992.

Smith, D.H., Chen, X.H., Iwata, A., Graham, D.I., 2003. Amyloid-β accumulation in axons after traumatic brain injury in humans. J. Neurosurg. 98, 1072–1077.

Smith, C., Graham, D.I., Murray, L.S., Stewart, J., Nicoll, J.A., 2006. Association of APOE ε4 and cerebrovascular pathology in traumatic brain injury. J. Neurol. Neurosurg. Psychiatry. 77, 363–366.

Sonnen, J.A., Larson, E.B., Haneuse, S., Woltjer, R., Li, G., et al., 2009. Neuropathology in the adult changes in thought study: a review. J. Alzheimers Dis. 18, 703–711.

Soto, C., Estrada, L.D., 2008. Protein misfolding and neurodegeneration. Arch. Neurol. 65, 184–189.

Stefanis, L., Larsen, K.E., Rideout, H.J., Sulzer, D., Greene, L.A., 2001. Expression of A53T mutant but not wild-type alpha-synuclein in PC12 cells induces alterations of the ubiquitin-dependent degradation system, loss of dopamine release, and autophagic cell death. J. Neurosci. 21, 9549–9560.

Stone, J.R., Okonkwo, D.O., Singleton, R.H., Mutlu, L.K., Helm, G.A., et al., 2002. Caspase-3-mediated cleavage of amyloid precursor protein and formation of amyloid β peptide in traumatic axonal injury. J. Neurotrauma 19, 601–614.

Suchak, S.K., Baloyianni, N.V., Perkinton, M.S., Williams, R.J., Meldrum, B.S., et al., 2003. The 'glial' glutamate transporter, EAAT2 (Glt-1) accounts for high affinity glutamate uptake into adult rodent nerve endings. J. Neurochem 84, 522–532. 2003.

Sundström, E., Mo, L.L., 2002. Mechanisms of glutamate release in the rat spinal cord slices during metabolic inhibition. J. Neurotrauma 19, 257–266.

Szatkowski, M., Attwell, D., 1994. Triggering and execution of neuronal death in brain ischaemia: two phases of glutamate release by different mechanisms. Trends Neurosci. 17, 359–365.

Szmydynger-Chodobska, J., Fox, L.M., Lynch, K.M., Zink, B.J., Chodobski, A., 2010. Vasopressin amplifies the production of proinflammatory mediators in traumatic brain injury. J. Neurotrauma 27, 1449–1461.

Tanaka, Y., Engelender, S., Igarashi, S., Rao, R.K., Wanner, T., et al., 2001. Inducible expression of mutant alpha-synuclein decreases proteasome activity and increases sensitivity to mitochondria-dependent apoptosis. Hum. Mol. Genet. 10, 919–926.

Tanaka, T., Ueno, M., Yamashita, T., 2009. Engulfment of axon debris by microglia requires p38 MAPK activity. J. Biol. Chem. 284, 21626–21636.

Teasdale, G., Maas, A., Lecky, F., Manley, G., Stocchetti, N., et al., 2014. The Glasgow Coma Scale at 40 years: standing the test of time. Lancet Neurol. 13, 844–854.

Tesco, G., Koh, Y.H., Kang, E.L., Cameron, A.N., Das, S., et al., 2007. Depletion of GGA3 stabilizes BACE and enhances beta-secretase activity. Neuron 54, 721–737.

Thomas, C., Ye, F.Q., Irfanoglu, M.O., Modi, P., Saleem, P.K., et al., 2014. Anatomical accuracy of brain connections derived from diffusion MRI tractography is inherently limited. Proc. Natl. Acad. Sci. USA 111, 16574–16579.

Thurman, D.J., Coronado, V., Selassie, A., 2007. The epidemiology of TBI: implications for public health. In: Zasler, N.D., Katz, D.I., Zafonte, R.D. (Eds.), Brain Injury Medicine: Principles and Practice. Demos, New York, NY, pp. 45–55.

Thurman, D.J., Alverson, C., Dunn, K.A., Guerrero, J., Sniezek, J.E., 1999. Traumatic brain injury in the United States: a public health perspective. J. Head Trauma Rehabil. 14, 602–615.

Toklu, H.Z., Tumer, N., 2015. Oxidative stress, brain edema, blood-brain barrier permeability, and autonomic dysfunction from traumatic brain injury. In: Kobeissy, F.H. (Ed.), Brain Neurotrauma: Molecular, Neuropsychological, and Rehabilitation Aspects. CRC Press/Taylor and Francis Group, Boca Raton, FL.

Tsitsopoulos, P.P., Marklund, N., 2013. Amyloid-β peptides and tau protein as biomarkers in cerebrospinal and interstitial fluid following traumatic brain injury: a review of experimental and clinical studies. Front. Neurol. 4, 79.

Turner, R.C., Dodson, S.C., Rosen, C.L., Huber, J.D., 2013. The science of cerebral ischemia and the quest for neuroprotection: navigating past failure to future success. J. Neurosurgery. 118, 1072–1085.

Ulusoy, A., Di Monte, D.A., 2013. Alpha-Synuclein elevation in human neurodegenerative diseases: experimental, pathogenetic, and therapeutic implications. Mol. Neurobiol. 47, 484–494.

Uryu, K., Chen, X.H., Martinez, D., Browne, K.D., Johnson, V.E., et al., 2007. Multiple proteins implicated in neurodegenerative diseases accumulate in axons after brain trauma in humans. Exp. Neurol. 208, 185–192.

Uversky, V.N., Eliezer, D., 2009. Biophysics of Parkinson's disease: structure and aggregation of alpha-synuclein. Curr. Protein Pept. Sci. 10, 483–499.

Uzan, M., Erman, H., Tanriverdi, T., Sanus, G.Z., Kafadar, A., et al., 2006. Evaluation of apoptosis in cerebrospinal fluid of patients with severe head injury. Acta Neurochir. (Wien) 148, 1157–1164.

van Santbrink, H., Vd Brink, W.A., Steyerberg, E.W., Carmona Suazo, J.A., Avezaat, C.J., et al., 2003. Brain tissue oxygen response in severe traumatic brain injury. Acta Neurochir. 145, 429–438.

Vila, M., Vukosavic, S., Jackson-Lewis, V., Neystat, M., Jakowec, M., et al., 2000. α-Synuclein up-regulation in substantia nigra dopaminergic neurons following administration of the parkinsonian toxin MPTP. J. Neurochem. 74, 721–729.

Viola, K.L., Klein, W.L., 2015. Amyloid β oligomers in Alzheimer's disease pathogenesis, treatment, and diagnosis. Acta Neuropathol. 129, 183–206.

Wagner, A.K., Hatz, L.E., Scanlon, J.M., Niyonkuru, C., Miller, M.A., et al., 2012. Association of KIBRA rs17070145 polymorphism and episodic memory in individuals with severe TBI. Brain Inj. 26, 1658–1669.

Wagner, E., Frank, M.M., 2010. Therapeutic potential of complement modulation. Nat. Rev. Drug Discov. 9, 43–56.

Walker, K.R., Kang, E.L., Whalen, M.J., Shen, Y., Tesco, G., 2012. Depletion of GGA1 and GGA3 mediates postinjury elevation of BACE1. J. Neurosci. 32, 10423–10437.

Weaver, S.M., Portelli, J.N., Chau, A., Cristofori, I., et al., 2014. Genetic polymorphisms and traumatic brain injury: the contribution of individual differences to recovery. Brain Imaging Behav. 8, 420–434.

Wilson, M., Montgomery, H., 2007. Impact of genetic factors on outcome from brain injury. Br. J. Anaesth. 99, 43–48.

Wolf, Y., Yona, S., Kim, K.W., Jung, S., 2013. Microglia, seen from the CX3CR1 angle. Front. Cell Neurosci. 7, 26.

Xiong, Y., Mahmood, A., Chopp, M., 2013. Animal models of traumatic brain injury. Nat. Rev. Neurosci. 14, 128–142.

Xu, W.L., Qiu, C.X., Wahlin, A., Winblad, B., Fratiglioni, L., 2004. Diabetes mellitus and risk of dementia in the Kungsholmen project: a 6-year follow-up study. Neurology 63, 1181−1186.

Yi, J.H., Hazell, A.S., 2006. Excitotoxic mechanisms and the role of astrocytic glutamate transporters in traumatic brain injury. Neurochem. Int. 48, 394−403.

Yan, W., Wang, H.D., Feng, X.M., Ding, Y.S., Jin, W., Tang, K., et al., 2009. The expression of NF-E2-related factor 2 in the rat brain after traumatic brain injury. J. Trauma. 66, 1431−1435.

Yan, H.Q., Osier, N.D., Korpon, J., et al., 2015. Persistent cognitive deficits: implications of altered dopamine in traumatic brain injury. In: Kobeissy, F.H. (Ed.), Brain Neurotrauma: Molecular, Neuropsychological, and Rehabilitation Aspects. CRC Press/ Taylor & Francis, Boca Raton, FL, p. 33.

Yang, Q., She, H., Gearing, M., Colla, E., Lee, M., et al., 2009. Regulation of neuronal survival factor MEF2D by chaperone-mediated autophagy. Science. 323, 124−127.

Zacest, A.C., Vink, R., Manavis, J., Sarvestani, G.T., Blumbergs, P.C., 2010. Substance P immunoreactivity increases following human traumatic brain injury. Acta Neurochir Suppl. 106, 211−6.10.

Zemlan, F.P., Jauch, E.C., Mulchahey, J.J., Gabbita, S.P., Rosenberg, W.S., et al., 2002. C-tau biomarker of neuronal damage in severe brain injured patients: association with elevated intracranial pressure and clinical outcome. Brain Res. 947, 131−139.

Zetterberg, H., Blennow, K., 2015. Fluid markers of traumatic brain injury. Mol. Cell Neurosci. 66, 99−102.

Zetterberg, H., Smith, D.H., Blennow, K., 2013. Biomarkers of mild traumatic brain injury in cerebrospinal fluid and blood. Nat. Rev. Neurol. 9, 201−210.

Ziebell, J.M., Morganti-Kossmann, M.C., 2010. Involvement of pro- and anti-inflammatory cytokines and chemokines in the pathophysiology of traumatic brain injury. Neurotherapeutics. 7, 22−30.

Zgaljardic, D.J., Seale, G.S., Schaefer, L.S., Temple, R.O., Foreman, J., et al., 2015. Psychiatric disease and post-acute traumatic brain injury. J. Neurotrauma 32, 1911−1925.

Potential Neuroprotective Strategies for Traumatic Brain Injury

INTRODUCTION

Traumatic brain injury (TBI) is a heterogeneous disease that involves multiple mechanisms. TBI not only produces alterations in the brain function, but also is a risk factor for other neurological disorders such as Alzheimer's disease (AD), Parkinson's disease (PD), and dementia. Many psychiatric pathological conditions, such as major depression, generalized anxiety disorder, and posttraumatic stress disorder, are also escalated after TBI (Warren et al., 2015; Alway et al., 2016). TBI and above-mentioned neurological disorders are major causes of mortality and morbidity worldwide (Gardner and Zafonte, 2016; Taylor et al., 2017). An estimated 1.6–3 million TBIs occur in the United States each year resulting over 1 million emergency department visits, 290,000 hospitalizations, and 51,000 deaths. As stated in Chapter 6, Neurochemical Aspects of Traumatic Brain Injury, TBI is classified as mild, moderate, or severe using the Glasgow Coma Scale (mild = 13–15; moderate = 9–12; severe = less than or equal to 8 out of 15). TBI can result in significant motor, sensory, cognitive, and emotional impairments. Even mild TBI can be associated with headache, dizziness, nausea/vomiting, impaired balance and coordination, vision changes, tinnitus, mood and memory changes, difficulty with memory and attention, and fatigue and/or sleep disturbances (Gardner and Zafonte, 2016; Taylor et al., 2017). Some TBI symptoms appear immediately, while others do not appear until several days or weeks. Mild TBI symptoms include headache, confusion, lightheadedness, dizziness, blurred vision, fatigue, and trouble with memory (Bahraini et al., 2009). Moderate TBI produces a headache that gets worse with time, seizures, inability to awaken from

Ischemic and Traumatic Brain and Spinal Cord Injuries
DOI: https://doi.org/10.1016/B978-0-12-813596-9.00007-9

287

sleep, dilation of one or both pupils of the eyes, slurred speech, loss of coordination, increased confusion. Severe TBI not only produces very severe seizures, but loss of consciousness, coma, and death. *Diagnosis is suspected clinically and confirmed by neuroimaging (primarily CT).* CT can rapidly detect intracranial hematoma, intraparenchymal contusion, skull fracture, and cerebral edema, as well as transependymal flow and obliteration of the basal cisterns, which are concerns for increased intracranial pressure (Chun et al., 2009). It should be noted that commonly used methods such as behavioral assessment and structural neuroimaging do not allow for precise monitoring of the evolution of TBI-mediated changes in neuronal functionality in the damaged brain. Only electrophysiological studies can provide the high-precision information needed monitoring and understand the temporal evolution of neuronal functionality in normal and injured brain.

As stated in Chapter 6, Neurochemical Aspects of Traumatic Brain Injury, TBI is accompanied by primary and secondary injuries. Primary injury is irreversible and caused by the direct mechanical damage to neurons, axons, glial cells, and blood vessels. Secondary injury involves glutamate-mediated excitotoxicity, a key initiator of cell death following TBI. Excessive glutamate-mediated activation of extra-synaptic NMDA receptors results in a dramatic increase in intracellular calcium levels. Impaired calcium homeostasis in turn initiates a number of crucial downstream cellular injury processes including mitochondrial oxidative stress as well as the activation of the calcium-sensitive enzymes such as phospholipase A2, nitric oxide synthases, protein kinases, and proteases (caspases and calpains). Activation of these enzymes has been demonstrated to induce neural cell death in vitro (and hence loss of neurons and synapses) via caspase-3 activation and the cleavage of tau into a 17 kDa toxic tau fragment. TBI also produces activation of microglial cells and astrocytes leading to increase in expression of cytokine and chemokine and induction of neuroinflammation. These processes play an important role in neural cell death following TBI. Inflammation may amplify excitotoxic cell death by reducing glial glutamate transporters leading to increased glutamate at the synapse exacerbating calcium dysregulation. Experimental evidence also suggests calcium-mediated activation of calpain and calcineurin induces dendritic spine remodeling and loss and hence impairs synaptic transmission. Additionally, calpain and calcineurin have both been implicated in the induction of neurofibrillary tangle (NFT) formation via cleavage induced activation of GSK-3β leading to hyperphosphorylation of Tau. As stated in Chapter 6, Neurochemical Aspects of Traumatic Brain Injury, TBI also results in formation of elevated levels of soluble Aβ which is capable of inducing synaptic dysfunction. Many studies have also indicated that soluble Aβ is capable of directly mediating many of the cellular injury processes characteristic of the secondary phase of TBI and hence elevated Aβ levels may be key initiating events in the development of a "feed forward" toxic cascade that links TBI to chronic neurodegeneration (Farooqui, 2017). Collectively above studies indicate that the cascade of secondary injury culminates in neuronal, endothelial, and glial cell death and white matter degeneration. The consequences of TBI can be far-reaching and vary depending on the type and location of the injuries. In comparison to strokes, which result in local damage to the brain due to circulation disruptions, TBI is often mediated by diffuse to high-acceleration traumatic forces. In addition, TBIs are frequently associated with other injuries to internal organs or the locomotor system. This leads to a high degree of heterogeneity in the manifestation of clinical symptoms and makes the treatment of the accident victims particularly challenging. Based on above-mentioned information, the *initial treatment of severe TBI patients in the United States consists of ensuring a reliable airway and maintaining adequate ventilation, oxygenation, and blood pressure.* The second event of treatment of TBI involves inhibition of endogenous cascade of cellular and neurochemical events in the brain that occurs within minutes and continues for months after the primary brain injury, leading to ongoing traumatic axonal injury and neuronal cell damage (delayed brain injury), and ultimately, neuronal cell death (Lenzlinger et al., 2001). In Switzerland, TBI is mostly treated in the surgical intensive care units of university hospitals and specific regional hospitals in a nonstandardized interdisciplinary way. In Germany the "Bundesarbeitsgemeinschaft für Rehabilitation," a federal institution to define standards in rehabilitation, has published recommendations for early rehabilitation of neurological patients including TBI patients in 1995. These recommendations have influenced the OPS 8-552 in the German DRG-system. The German DRG-system defines a "minimum standard" to treat neurological/neurosurgical early rehabilitation patients (e.g., minimum of 300-minute therapy/day consisting of physiotherapy, and occupational therapy) (Rollnik et al., 2010). However, while these standards define the duration of therapy, they do not specify its methods.

AXONAL GROWTH AFTER TRAUMATIC BRAIN INJURY

Functional recovery in TBI victims is very limited because injured axons in the mammalian central nervous system (CNS) have a limited capacity for regeneration after injury (Farooqui, 2010). Lesions in the CNS cause a complex sequence of pathological responses (Farooqui,

2010). Immediately after TBI, there is extravasation of blood into the lesion site due to the disruption of blood vessels. This results in local ischemia, hypoxemia, and hypoglycemia, which help cause secondary damage to the CNS tissue surrounding the lesion site. Several weeks after the injury, microglia and macrophages clear the tissue debris at the lesion site, resulting in cyst formation and cavitation (Greitz, 2006). Astrocytes close to the lesion become reactive and undergo hyperplasia and hypertrophy. Under these conditions astrocytes have been shown to upregulate molecules such as tenascin, semaphorin 3, slit proteins, and chondroitin sulfate proteoglycans (CSPGs) (Apostolova et al., 2006; Brodkey et al., 1995). It is reported that a transmembrane protein tyrosine phosphatase (PTPσ) transduces CSPG-mediated inhibition of axon growth (Shen et al., 2009) (Fig. 7.1). CSPGs also interact with leukocyte common antigen-related phosphatase (LAR), and NgR1/3 receptors (Fisher et al., 2011). After TBI, deletion of LAR reverses CSPG-induced neurite growth inhibition. Blocking LAR with a peptide enhances axonal growth of serotonergic fibers. Furthermore, CSPGs

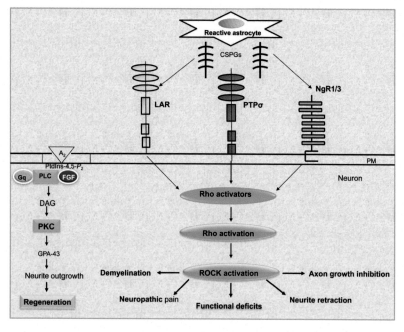

FIGURE 7.1   Inhibition of axonal growth by CSPGs and its receptors. *CSPGs*, chondroitin sulfate proteoglycans; *DAG*, diacylglycerol; *FGF*, fibroblast growth factor; *GAP-43*, growth associated protein-43; *LAR*, leukocyte common antigen-related phosphatase; *NgR1/3*, Nogo receptor1/3; *PKC*, protein kinase C; *PLC*, phospholipase C; *PM*, plasma membrane; *PtdIns-4,5-P$_2$*, phosphatidylinositol 4,5-bisphosphate; *PTPσ*, transmembrane protein tyrosine phosphatase; *ROCK*, Rho kinase; small GTPase RhoA.

inhibit neurite outgrowth through the activation of the RhoA/ROCK pathway since inhibition of RhoA/ROCK signaling blocks the inhibitory effects of CSPGs on neurite outgrowth (Borisoff et al., 2003; Monnier et al., 2003; Hou et al., 2008). The RhoA/ROCK pathway not only mediates the effects of myelin-associated axon growth inhibitors and Nogo, myelin-associated glycoprotein (MAG), but also oligodendrocyte-myelin glycoprotein (OMgp), and repulsive guidance molecule. Blocking RhoA/ROCK signaling can reverse the inhibitory effects of these molecules on axon outgrowth, and promotes axonal sprouting and functional recovery in animal models of CNS injury (Fujita and Yamashita, 2014). Following TBI, the growth cone collapsing and alterations in cytoskeletal proteins (Hou et al., 2008) are supported by the induction of semaphorins, ephrins, slits, netrins, Wnts, and myelin-secreted inhibitory glycoproteins (MAG and Nogo). Collective evidence suggests that brain tissue contains multiple axon growth inhibitors that contribute to inability of the injured axons to regenerate. However, some regeneration in adult injured brain (neurogenesis) does occur in limited areas where synaptic plasticity is prevalent. In the absence of axonal regeneration, there is not only an inevitable loss of functional connections, but also a loss of neurons. It is stated that a detailed understanding of the molecular mechanisms that limit neuronal growth in the injured brain will be an important step toward the development of specific strategies aimed at restoring functional connectivity lost as a consequence of injury (Skaper et al., 2001; Yamashita, 2007; Hou et al., 2008).

POTENTIAL NEUROPROTECTIVE STRATEGIES FOR TRAUMATIC BRAIN INJURY

As stated in Chapter 6, Neurochemical Aspects of Traumatic Brain Injury, TBI is a devastating and complex clinical condition caused by both primary and secondary injury mechanisms (Farooqui, 2010; Loane and Faden, 2010). Primary injury mechanisms result from the mechanical damage that occurs at the time of trauma to neurons, axons, glia, and blood vessels as a result of shearing, tearing, or stretching. In contrast, secondary injury involves induction of excitotoxicity, generation of reactive oxygen species (ROS), release of proinflammatory cytokines and chemokines (neuroinflammation), and production of nitric oxide. These processes result in a progressive injury entailing neuronal loss, axonal destruction, disruption of blood−brain barrier (BBB), demyelination not only at the site of impact, but also in the surrounding area. Secondary injury is also accompanied by the development of edema and neuronal apoptosis (Farooqui, 2010; Loane and Faden, 2010; Loane

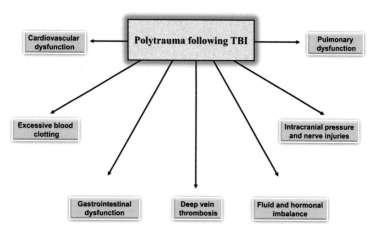

FIGURE 7.2   Polytrauma caused by TBI. *TBI*, traumatic brain injury.

et al., 2015). These processes result in short-term complications of TBIs, which include cognitive deficits, difficulties with sensory processing and communication, immediate seizures, hydrocephalus, cerebrospinal fluid (CSF) leakage, vascular or cranial nerve injuries, tinnitus, organ failure, and polytrauma (Fig. 7.2) (Center for Disease Control and Prevention, 2016). Polytrauma may include pulmonary, cardiovascular, gastrointestinal dysfunction, fluid and hormonal imbalances, deep vein thrombosis, excessive blood clotting, and nerve injuries (Ahmed et al., 2017). In addition, TBI also results in an increase in metabolic rate, which leads to an excessive amount of heat generation within the body. Long-term complications of TBI include AD, PD, dementia pugilistica, and posttraumatic epilepsy (Ahmed et al., 2017). The delayed nature and onset of above processes and complications suggest that there may be a window for therapeutic intervention (pharmacologic or other) to prevent progressive tissue damage and improve functional recovery after TBI. There are two strategic approaches to treat TBI (Xiong et al., 2015): (1) a neuroprotective approach, which not only targets the injured brain with a focus on reducing/preventing secondary injury and neural cell death, but also promotes reduction in the lesion size and (2) a neurorestorative approach, which is designed to improve neurological recovery by treating the entire CNS to promote neurovascular remodeling including angiogenesis, neurogenesis, oligodendrogenesis, and dendrite/axon outgrowth. Many studies have indicated that many neuroprotective agents (Table 7.1) limit brain damage and/or improve behavioral outcome in animal models of TBI. However, translation of such neuroprotective strategies to human injury has been disappointing,

TABLE 7.1 Neuroprotective Agents Used for the Treatment of TBI in Animal Models

Neuroprotective Agents	Reference
Progesterone	Stein (2013); Skolnick et al. (2014)
Erythropoietin	Peng et al. (2014); Robertson et al. (2014)
Cyclosporin	Sullivan et al. (2000); Aminmansour et al. (2014)
Glibenclamide	Kurland et al. (2013); Khanna et al. (2014)
Minocycline	Homsi et al. (2010)
NNZ-2566	Wei et al. (2009)
Nerve growth factor	Lv et al. (2014); Tian et al. (2012)
Propranolol	Ley et al. (2010); Patel et al. (2012)
Statins	Li et al. (2009); Wible and Laskowitz (2010)
Stem cell therapy	Lu et al. (2001); Mahmood et al. (2005)
Tranexamic acid	Zehtabchi et al. (2014); Roberts et al. (2013)
Thymosin β4	Morris et al. (2010); Sun and Kim (2007); Xiong et al. (2011)
Exosomes	Stoorvogel et al. (2002)
IL-1 receptor antagonists	Clark et al. (2008); Helmy et al. (2014)
microRNAs	Sandhir et al. (2014); Ge et al. (2014)

with the failure of more than 30 controlled clinical trials. Both conceptual issues and methodological differences between preclinical and clinical injury have undoubtedly contributed to these translational difficulties (Farooqui, 2010; Loane and Faden, 2010; Loane et al., 2015). In addition, pharmacokinetics-related factors, such as the rate of drug penetration in animal and human brains and therapeutic window limitations, may be very different in animal models and human patients. Safety and tolerability of the drug may also contribute to differences between human and experimental models of TBI. Moreover, it should also be recognized that there are substantial anatomical differences between animal and human brains, particularly that the rodent brain has a higher gray to white matter ratio. Also, it has become very clear in recent years that TBI is a very heterogeneous clinical condition with highly variable pathologies and functional consequences. All these differences in TBI animal models and human subjects may account for the failure of controlled clinical trials in human subjects.

PROGESTERONE AND TRAUMATIC BRAIN INJURY

Progesterone is a female reproductive steroid hormone, which can also be synthesized and actively metabolized in the central and peripheral nervous system (Fig. 7.3) (Melcangi et al., 2014). Progesterone not only contributes to the development of neurons, but is also associated with the regulation of cognition, mood, inflammation, mitochondrial function, neurogenesis, regeneration, and myelination (Brinton et al., 2008). The action of progesterone is mediated by a progesterone receptor (PR), which is widely expressed in the developing and adult brain, so various brain regions are the normal targets of progesterone PR (Kato et al., 1994). Indeed, there is 10-fold increase in progesterone synthesis during fetal growth to protect the fetus during gestation. Because many processes contribute to CNS repair after TBI, it is proposed that progesterone may actively contribute to recovery from TBI. The molecular mechanisms of actions of progesterone are not fully understood. However, it is becoming increasingly evident that progesterone not only attenuates glutamate excitotoxicity (Smith, 1991) and modulates apoptotic pathways (Djebaili et al., 2005), but also reduces membrane lipid peroxidation (Roof et al., 1997), and limits inflammation after TBI (Fig. 7.4) (Pan et al., 2007). Progesterone also elicits its neuroprotective effects via nongenomic mechanisms such as through the activation of signal

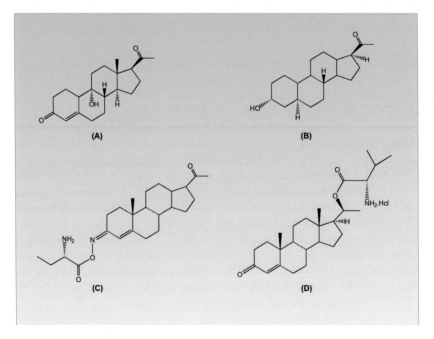

FIGURE 7.3   Chemical structures of (A) progesterone, (B) allopregnanolone, (C) oxime derivative of progesterone, and (D) valine tethered progesterone analogs.

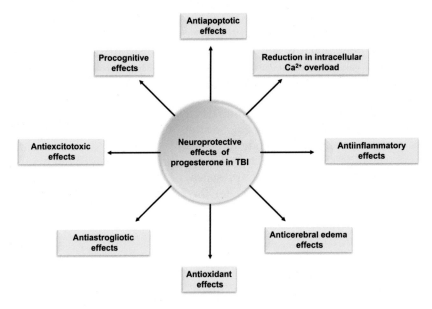

FIGURE 7.4 Neuroprotective effects of progesterone in TBI. *TBI*, traumatic brain injury.

transduction pathways. Signal transduction systems, which are activated by progesterone include cAMP/PKA (Collado et al., 1985), MAPK (ERK1/2) (Singh, 2001; Migliaccio et al., 1998), TLRs/NF-κB (Chen et al., 2008), and the PtdIns 3K/Akt signaling pathway (Baulieu and Robel, 1990). It is also speculated that in TBI, progesterone acts through the pleiotropic effects involving Nrf2/ARE signal pathway (Zhang et al., 2017). In addition, progesterone may also act by not only increasing the brain-derived neurotrophic factor (BDNF)-mediated survival of neurons, rebuilding of BBB, improving vascular tone, but also by upregulating GABA signaling and by promoting the formation of new myelin sheaths (Chen et al., 2008). Collectively, these studies indicate that progesterone acts by inhibiting neuroinflammation, lipid peroxidation, and apoptotic cell death in TBI and these processes influence on the cognitive outcome (Sayeed and Stein, 2009; Si et al., 2013).

ERYTHROPOIETIN AND TRAUMATIC BRAIN INJURY

Erythropoietin (EPO) is a 30-kDa glycoprotein (165-amino-acid protein) that regulates red cell production by binding to an erythroid progenitor cell surface receptor (Patel et al., 2011). EPO acts through a specific erythropoietin receptor (EPOR) on the surface of red cell precursors in the bone marrow and facilitates their transformation into mature red blood cells. EPO and its receptor (EPOR) are weakly expressed in the human brain. However, their local production is rapidly induced in response to acute hypoxia, as evidenced by the increased expression of EPO in CSF or postmortem brain tissue in humans with stroke and hypoxia (Siren et al., 2001; Springborg et al., 2003). EPO contains four glycosylated chains that include three N-linked and one O-linked acidic oligosaccharide side chains. The production and secretion of the mature EPO is dependent upon the presence of N- and O-linked chains. The carbohydrates are important for the clearance of EPO. In addition, the oligosaccharides may offer protection from free radical activity, the carbohydrate chains stabilize the EPO protein, and the glycosylated chains prevent EPO degradation during free radical oxygen exposure (Maiese et al., 2008, 2012).

The first evidence that EPO is able to protect tissues/organs comes from several models of ischemic injury in the brain. Based on these studies it is concluded that EPO is also a multifunctional tissue-protecting agent that exerts antiapoptotic, antiinflammatory, antioxidative, angiogenic, and neurotrophic effects (Fig. 7.5) (Ehrenreich et al., 2004; Peng et al., 2014). In the brain, the major sites of EPO production and secretion are the hippocampus, internal capsule, cortex, midbrain, cerebral endothelial cells, and astrocytes (Genc et al., 2003; Marti, 2004). At the molecular level, the action of EPO involves PtdIns 3K and Akt. Akt is downstream target of phosphatidylinositol 3-kinase (PtdIns 3K). The PtdIns 3K/Akt cascade has been reported not only to inhibit apoptosis (Maiese et al., 2012), but also promote cell survival through insulin and growth factors (Maiese et al., 2012). After phosphoinositide-dependent protein kinase (PDK) phosphorylating Akt-1, glycogen synthase kinase (GSK-3β, a serine/threonine kinase), is inhibited (Maiese et al., 2012). It is demonstrated that GSK-3β plays an important role in fundamental functions of cell, such as cell cycle, cytoskeletal integrity, apoptosis, transcription factors expression, and formation of NFTs (Maiese et al., 2012). For example, GSK-3β regulates neurogenesis, neuronal polarization, and axon growth in the developing brain (Hur and Zhou, 2010). These findings implied that PtdIns 3K kinase/Akt signaling pathway is related to the survival of neural cells in TBI. When EPO was first discovered, it was thought that such a large protein could not cross the BBB. However, recent report indicates that EPO does indeed have the capacity to cross the BBB, which protects against a variety of potential brain injuries, including transient ischemia and reperfusion (Brines et al., 2000). EPO acts a neuroprotective agent in animal models of TBI (Peng et al., 2014). Delayed posttraumatic

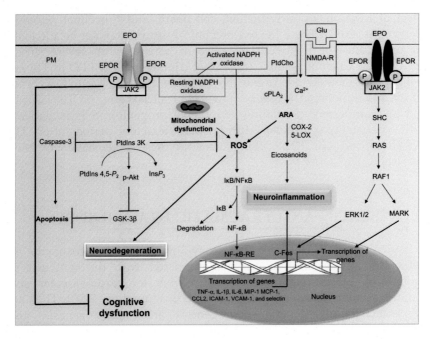

FIGURE 7.5 Hypothetical diagram showing neuroprotective mechanisms associated with beneficial effects of erythropoietin. *Akt*, serine/threonine kinase; *ARA*, arachidonic acid; *COX-2*, cyclooxygenase-2; *cPLA₂*, cytosolic phospholipase A$_2$; *EPO*, erythropoietin; *EPOR*, erythropoietin receptor; *Glu*, glutamate; *GSK-3β*, glycogen synthase kinase 3 beta; *I-κB*, inhibitory subunit of NF-κB; *I-κB/NF-κB*, inhibitory form of nuclear factor kappa B; *IL-1β*, interleukin-1β; *IL-6*, interleukin-6; *InsP₃*, inositol 1,4,5-trisphosphate; *JAK1*, Janus kinase 1; *JAK2*, Janus kinase 2; *5-LOX*, 5-lipoxygenase; *NF-κB*, nuclear factor-kappa B; *NF-κB-RE*, nuclear factor κB-response element; *NMDA-R*, N-methyl-D-aspartate receptor; *PM*, plasma membrane; *PtdCho*, phosphatidylcholine; *PtdIns-4,5-P₂*, phosphatidylinositol 4,5-bisphosphate; *ROS*, reactive oxygen species; *TNF-α*, tumor necrosis factor-α.

administration of EPO significantly improves histological and long-term functional outcomes compared with saline treatment in rats after TBI. The triple doses of delayed EPO treatment induce better histological and functional outcomes in rats, although a single dose provided substantial benefits (Xiong et al., 2009). Studies on the treatment of injured rat with recombinant EPO, carbamylated erythropoietin (CEPO) and asialoerythropoietin (ASEPO) indicate that EPO and CEPO are equally effective in enhancing spatial learning and promoting neural plasticity after TBI (Mahmood et al., 2009b). A recent randomized clinical trial of 200 patients (EPO, $n = 102$; placebo, $n = 98$) with severe closed head TBI has indicated that the administration of EPO does not improve the outcomes of TBI at 6 months (Robertson et al., 2014). It should be noted that most preclinical studies have been performed with the moderate controlled cortical impact (CCI) injury model of TBI to investigate the effect of EPO on lesion reduction, cell death, and functional recovery (Peng et al., 2014). These limited preclinical results may not be adequate for predicting the treatment response in patients with severe closed head injury. Currently, there are several clinical trials of EPO in TBI are being performed to determine the effect of EPO on secondary brain injury and functional recovery (www.clinicaltrials.gov, NCT00987454), and on numbers of circulating endothelial progenitor cells in patients with persistent symptoms during the subacute period after TBI (NCT02148367, NCT02226848). Results of these trials have not been published.

STATIN AND TRAUMATIC BRAIN INJURY

Statins inhibit HMG-CoA (3-hydroxy-3-methylglutaryl coenzyme A) reductase, a rate limiting enzyme associated with the synthesis of cholesterol. Statins significantly reduce risk for cardiovascular and cerebrovascular diseases (Endres, 2005, 2006; Vaughan, 2003). They act by inducing angiogenesis, neurogenesis and synaptogenesis, and enhancing functional recovery following TBI in rats (Lu et al., 2004, 2007a,b). Commercially available statins include lovastatin and pravastatin (naturally occurring statins), simvastatin (semisynthetic statins), and atorvastatin, fluvastatin, cerivastatin, rosuvastatin, and pitavastatin (synthetic statins). Structural differences among statins (Fig. 7.6) determine their lipophilicity, half-lives, and potency in mammalian tissues. Because of their lipophilicity, simvastatin, lovastatin, and cerivastatin pass the BBB. In contrast, pravastatin, fluvastatin, and atorvastatin do not pass the BBB (Vuletic et al., 2006).

Beneficial effects of statins in TBI are due to their antiexcitotoxic, antioxidant, and antiinflammatory properties. Treatment of rats with atorvastatin and simvastatin 1 day after TBI and daily for 14 days not only improves spatial learning on days 31–35 after onset of TBI, but also reduces the neuronal loss in hippocampal CA3 region, lowers microglial activation, and decreases TBI-mediated increases in beta amyloid (Aβ) (Lu et al., 2007a,b; Abrahamson et al., 2009). At the molecular level simvastatin not only stimulates phosphorylation of Akt, glycogen synthase kinase-3beta (GSK-3β), and cAMP response element-binding proteins (CREBs), but also upregulates the expression of BDNF and vascular endothelial growth factor (VEGF) in the dentate gyrus, increases in the cell proliferation and differentiation in the dentate gyrus, and enhances the recovery of spatial learning (Wu et al., 2008a). In addition, statin may also affect microvasculature by increasing nitric oxide bioavailability, which regulates cerebral perfusion and improves

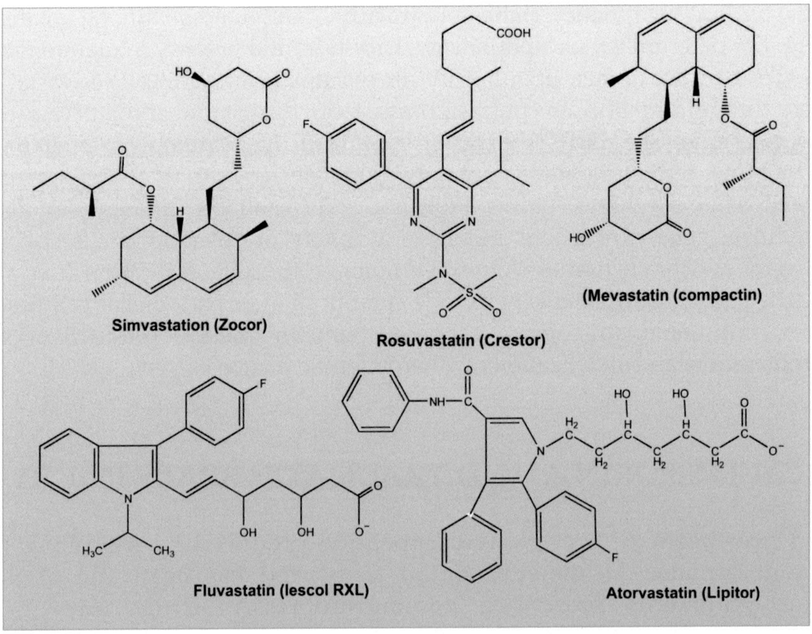

FIGURE 7.6 Chemical structures of statins.

endothelial function. These processes may lead to restoration of cognitive function and improved outcome after TBI in rats (Nakazawa et al., 2007; Wu et al., 2008b; Mahmood et al., 2009a). Furthermore, simvastatin also suppresses the activation of caspase-3 and apoptotic cell death leading to neuronal function recovery after TBI (Wu et al., 2008a,b). Given the wide use, favorable safety profile and positive clinical data for statins, the rare occurrence of serious adverse events, and the extensive available preclinical data demonstrating neuroprotection and neurorestoration (Wible and Laskowitz, 2010), clinical trials are warranted to determine the neuroprotective and neurorestorative properties of statins following TBI. The effect of rosuvastatin on TBI-induced cytokine change is ongoing in a Phase I/II trial (NCT00990028).

Statins are drugs that inhibit HMG-CoA (3-hydroxy-3-methylglutarylcoenzyme A) reductase and significantly reduce risk for cardiovascular and cerebrovascular diseases (Endres, 2005, 2006; Vaughan, 2003). Beneficial effects of statins in cardiovascular and cerebrovascular systems are due to their antiexcitotoxic, antioxidant, and anti-inflammatory properties. Statins are commercially available and include lovastatin and pravastatin (naturally occurring statins), simvastatin (semisynthetic statins), and atorvastatin, fluvastatin, cerivastatin, rosuvastatin, and pitavastatin (synthetic statins). Structural differences among statins (Fig. 7.6) determine their lipophilicity, half-lives, and potency in mammalian tissues. Because of their lipophilicity simvastatin, lovastatin, and cerivastatin pass through the BBB. In contrast, pravastatin, fluvastatin, and atorvastatin do not cross the BBB (Vuletic et al., 2006). In addition to inhibiting HMG-CoA reductase, statins not only modulate activities of other enzymes (nitric oxide synthases, PtdIns 3-kinases, and metalloproteinases), but also modulate gene expression, and have a variety of "pleiotropic effects" in visceral and brain tissues (Johnson-Anuna et al., 2005, 2007; Kirsch et al., 2003). The pleiotropic effects include modification of endothelial cell function, immunoinflammatory responses, smooth muscle cell activation, proliferation, and stabilization of atherosclerotic plaques.

CYCLOSPORIN A AND TRAUMATIC BRAIN INJURY

Cyclosporin A, a cyclic undecapeptide produced by a number of fungi, contains 11 unusual amino acids, and has been one of the most commonly prescribed immunosuppressive drugs (Fig. 7.7).

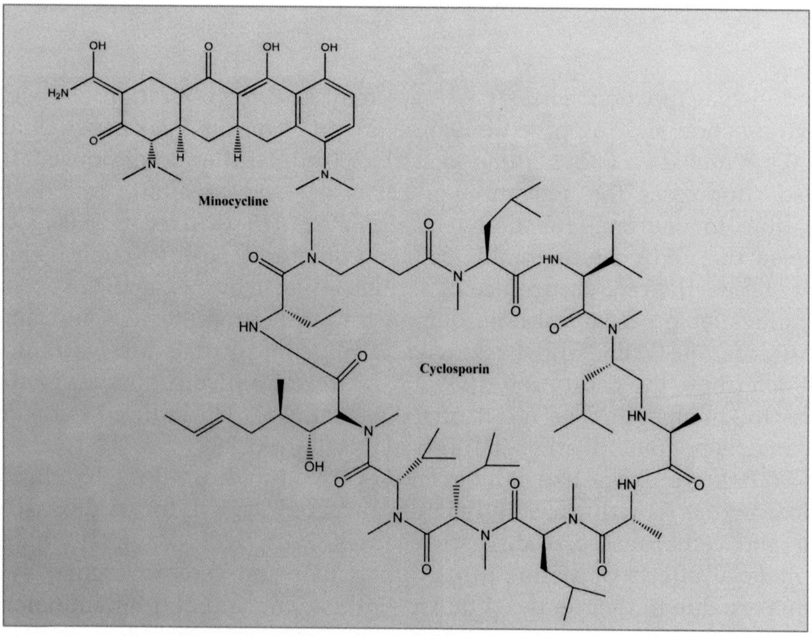

FIGURE 7.7   Chemical structures of minocycline and cyclosporin.

Cyclosporin interacts with cytosolic protein cyclophilin in T cells, and the cyclosporin–cyclophilin complex inhibits calcineurin (Liu et al., 1991; Laupacis et al., 1982). Cyclosporin A not only inhibits the Ca^{2+}-mediated mitochondrial membrane permeability transition (MPT) but may also reduce unrelated increase in posttraumatic Ca^{2+} accumulation (Mirzayan et al., 2008). Alterations in MPT may be responsible for the loss of $\Delta\psi$, mitochondrial swelling, and rupture of the outer mitochondrial membrane leading to the opening of a channel known as permeability transition pore (PTP). PTP consists of the voltage-dependent anion channel, the adenine nucleotide translocator, cyclophilin-D, and other molecule(s) (Tsujimoto and Shimizu, 2007). In mouse model of TBI, treatment with cyclosporin A significantly reduces mitochondrial dysfunction marker (alpha-spectrin degradation) (Mbye et al., 2009). In rat model of TBI, cyclosporin A interacts with N-acetylaspartate and promotes the restoration of ATP loss (Signoretti et al., 2004). Cyclosporin A treatment also results in a significant reduction in amyloid precursor protein (APP) mRNA, and neuronal perikaryal APP antigen expression in a large animal model using sheep (Van Den Heuvel et al., 2004). Also, in animal experiments, intravenous cyclosporin A achieves therapeutic levels in brain parenchyma, and 10 mg/kg is the most effective dose in attenuating axonal damage after TBI (Okonkwo et al., 2003). Based on this useful information in animal models, prospective, randomized, placebo-controlled Phase I/II trials have been performed (Mazzeo et al., 2009) to evaluate the safety, tolerability, and pharmacokinetics of a single intravenous infusion of cyclosporin in patients with severe TBI (Mazzeo et al., 2009). Fifty adult patients with severe TBI were enrolled over a 22-month period and received treatment within 12 hours of the injury. Although cyclosporin A did not produce significant adverse effects compared to placebo, there was no significant difference in neurological outcomes. Furthermore, a clinical study of 50 adults with severe TBI demonstrated the beneficial effect of cyclosporin A treatment on brain extracellular metabolites using in vivo microdialysis. Results indicate that levels of glutamate concentration and lactate/pyruvate ratio are significantly higher in the placebo group than in cyclosporin A treated patients, 1–2 days, and 2–3 days after the end of the 24-hour drug infusion (NCT01825044). The administration of cyclosporin A also contributes to a significant increase in mean arterial pressure and cerebral perfusion pressure (Mazzeo et al., 2008).

GLUTATHIONE, N-ACETYLCYSTEINE, TRAUMATIC BRAIN INJURY

Studies in animal models of mild cortical injury, transcranial administration of the reduced glutathione at 15 minutes or 3 hours after injury significantly reduces inflammation, glial limitans breakdown, and parenchymal (but not meningeal) cell death by up to approximately 70% (Roth et al., 2014). Pretreatment with glutathione reduces meningeal cell death by approximately 50%. These observations indicate that ROS are a primary inducer of cell death and inflammation after focal brain injury and that an antioxidant (glutathione) can have a major effect on lesion expansion if given early. The advantage of passing a neuroprotective compound directly through the skull bone (transcranial delivery) is that a high local drug concentration can be achieved in the CNS with a limited off-target effect on the periphery. N-Acetylcysteine, an active agent in Mucomyst, an FDA-approved medication with a 40-year safety history also reduces brain damage and improves recovery after TBI. N-Acetylcysteine is the cellular precursor to glutathione. A randomized, double-blind, placebo-controlled clinical trial performed on blast TBI patient to assess efficacy this agent indicates that patients who received N-acetylcysteine within 24 hours show significantly improved recovery during a 7-day period when compared with a placebo control group (Hoffer et al., 2013; Eakin et al., 2014). These findings have been corroborated in two different rodent models of TBI (weight drop and fluid percussion), which revealed that N-acetylcysteine reversed the behavioral deficits associated with mTBI and moderate TBI (Eakin et al., 2014). Further studies are needed to determine whether this promising neuroprotective intervention will be efficacious in patients with diverse types of brain injury.

MINOCYCLINE AND TRAUMATIC BRAIN INJURY

As stated in Chapter 5, Potential Neuroprotective Strategies for Experimental Spinal Cord Injury, minocycline is a lipophilic second-generation tetracycline analog that crosses BBB and produces neuroprotective effects in animal models of acute neural trauma and neurodegenerative diseases (Fig. 7.7). The molecular mechanisms contributing to beneficial effects of minocycline in neurotraumatic and neurodegenerative diseases are not fully understood. However, it is reported that minocycline may not only act by blocking mitochondrial permeability transition mediated cytochrome c release from mitochondria, inhibiting caspase-1 and 3 expressions, but also by upregulating iNOS, inhibiting

NADH-cytochrome c reductase and cytochrome c oxidase activities, and suppressing microglial activation (Garcia-Martinez et al., 2010). In addition, minocycline also downregulates the expression and inhibiting activities of phospholipase A_2 (PLA_2), cyclooxygenase-2 (COX-2), 5-lipoxygenase (LOX), MMP-2, MMP-9, p38 mitogen-activated protein kinase (MAPK), and decreasing the expression of c-Fos in brain (Hua et al., 2005; Machado et al., 2006; Marchand et al., 2009). These enzymes are associated with nociception, neuroinflammation, and apoptotic cell death. Minocycline reduces the number of reactive astrocytes and augment survival of oligodendrocytes in the spared white matter. Thus minocycline is a multifaceted therapeutic agent that has proven clinical safety and efficacy during a clinically relevant therapeutic window. It can be effective in treating acute SCI. Because of the high tolerance and the excellent penetration through BBB, minocycline has been used for the treatment of many neurological disorders, including stroke, multiple sclerosis, TBI, SCI, amyotrophic lateral sclerosis, Huntington's disease, and PD (Kim and Suh, 2009).

Cerebral edema, microglial activation, and thrombin formation are important complications of TBI. They contribute to brain injury after intracerebral hemorrhage and should be treated to prevent further brain damage. Minocycline administration not only reduces cerebral edema, but also downregulates inflammatory markers at 6 hours post-TBI without effecting TBI-induced oxidized glutathione increases. The antiedematous effect of minocycline persists up to 24 hours and is accompanied by a neurological recovery (Homsi et al., 2010). Minocycline decreases thrombin-mediated increase in TNF-α and IL-1β levels. In vivo, minocycline reduces neurological deficits and brain atrophy (Wu et al., 2009). Studies on gene expression patterns of sham TBI and minocycline-treated brain TBI indicate that many genes are modulated by minocycline treatment and significant differences are observed in genes modulating chemokines, proinflammatory cytokines, and genes involved in cell surface receptor-linked signal transduction. Expression levels of some key genes are validated by real-time quantitative PCR and it is suggested that multiple regulatory pathways are affected following brain injury and these genes are affected by minocycline following brain injury (Crack et al., 2009). Collective evidence suggests that minocycline is safe and effectively penetrates of the BBB and provides neuroprotection in TBI through its antiinflammatory and antiapoptotic effects, and protease inhibition properties. Studies on the effect of minocycline in TBI in a mouse model of closed head injury indicate that a single dose of minocycline decreases lesion volume and improves short-term (1-day) neurological outcome, which is associated with reduced microglial activation and interleukin-1beta expression (Bye et al., 2007). A triple (5 minutes, 3 hours, and 9 hours postinjury) minocycline administration reduces cerebral edema up to 24 hours, and improves long-term (12-weeks) neurological recovery (Homsi et al., 2009, 2010). A Phase I/II clinical trial is ongoing to assess the safety and efficacy of minocycline administration after TBI as a therapeutic agent for severe human TBI (NCT01058395).

OMEGA-3 FATTY ACIDS AND TRAUMATIC BRAIN INJURY

Cognitive impairment in animal models of TBI can be prevented by decreasing inflammation and oxidative damage. Docosahexaenoic acid (DHA) and DHA-derived lipid mediators (neuroprotectins and resolvins) decrease cognitive impairment, oxidative stress, and white matter injury in adult rats after TBI (Schober et al., 2016). It is hypothesized that DHA not only decreases early inflammatory markers (proinflammatory eicosanoids and cytokines and chemokines) and oxidative stress, but also improves cognitive outcome. It is well known that the silent information regulator 2 (Sir2) is closely associated with maintenance of genomic stability and cellular homeostasis under challenging situation. Mild TBI reduces the expression of Sir2α in the hippocampus and increases levels of protein oxidation. The dietary supplementation of ω-3 fatty acids not only ameliorates protein oxidation, but also reverses the reduction of Sir2α level in injured rats (Wu et al., 2007). TBI also reduces levels of phosphorylated AMPK (p-AMPK), which is an indicator of the energy status of neural cells. Hippocampal levels of total and phosphorylated AMPK can be normalized by supplementation of ω-3 fatty acts. Furthermore, TBI also reduces ubiquitous mitochondrial creatine kinase (uMtCK), an enzyme implicated in the energetic regulation of Ca^{2+}-pumps and in the maintenance of Ca^{2+}-homeostasis. Omega-3 fatty acids supplements normalized the levels of uMtCK after lesion. Collective evidence suggests that DHA attenuates the release of proinflammatory cytokines, decreases COX activity, inhibits formation of proinflammatory eicosanoids and cytokines, and promotes levels of antiinflammatory lipid mediators (neuroprotectins and resolvins). In addition, DHA also promotes neuronal survival, neurogenesis, neurite development, neuronal cell migration, synaptogenesis, and modulation of inflammatory cascade (Kawakita et al., 2006; Bailes and Mills, 2010; Farooqui, 2010; Lewis et al., 2013).

FAILURE OF CLINICAL TRIALS USING SOME ANTIOXIDANT AND ANTIINFLAMMATORY AGENTS IN TBI

Attempts to treat TBI using promising preclinical antioxidative and antiinflammatory agents in phase III human trials have failed (Kabadi and Faden, 2014; Helmy et al., 2011). Reasons for the failure in human TBI patients have not been fully understood. However, it is proposed that inadequate dosing, inappropriate delivery route, inadequate therapy duration, and timing of drug delivery in relation to the onset of the TBI may contribute to the failure (Kabadi and Faden, 2014; Helmy et al., 2011). In addition, complexity and permeability of BBB and adequate drug penetration not only in the brain, but also at the injury site may also contribute to the failure. In fact, large Phase III studies, including corticosteroids (CRASH trial) (Roberts et al., 2004), progesterone (Wright et al., 2014; Skolnick et al., 2014), and erythropoietin (Nichol et al., 2015), have failed to detect the presence of the antioxidant and antiinflammatory agents in the brain. The presence of agents can be determined by microdialysis (Thelin et al., 2017). Moreover, due to poor penetration of pharmacological compounds across the BBB, lower concentrations of the drug may have reached the brain explaining the lack of expected neuroprotection (Shannon et al., 2013). Before deciding to embark on large Phase III ventures, which are costly and consume much time and resources, adequate Phase II clinical studies with informative surrogate endpoints should be performed, including microdialysis, to ascertain the degree to which the drug can cross the BBB and exert changes on relevant biomarkers, including immune response-related molecules such as proinflammatory cytokines and chemokines.

GLIBENCLAMIDE AND TRAUMATIC BRAIN INJURY

Glibenclamide is an adopted name for glyburide, a member of the sulfonylurea class of drugs, which are clinically used as an oral hypoglycemic agent for the treatment of diabetes (Fig. 7.8). These drugs act by inhibiting K_{ATP} sulfonylurea receptor 1 channels (Sur1-Kir6.2) in pancreatic β islet cells leading to increase in insulin release (Panten et al., 1996). In the brain, glibenclamide exerts its effects primarily via inhibition of the Sur1-Trpm4 channel (Woo et al., 2013) (formerly, the Sur1-regulated nonselective cation (NC_{Ca-ATP}) channel). Inhibition of Sur1 with glibenclamide has been found to be an effective treatment in

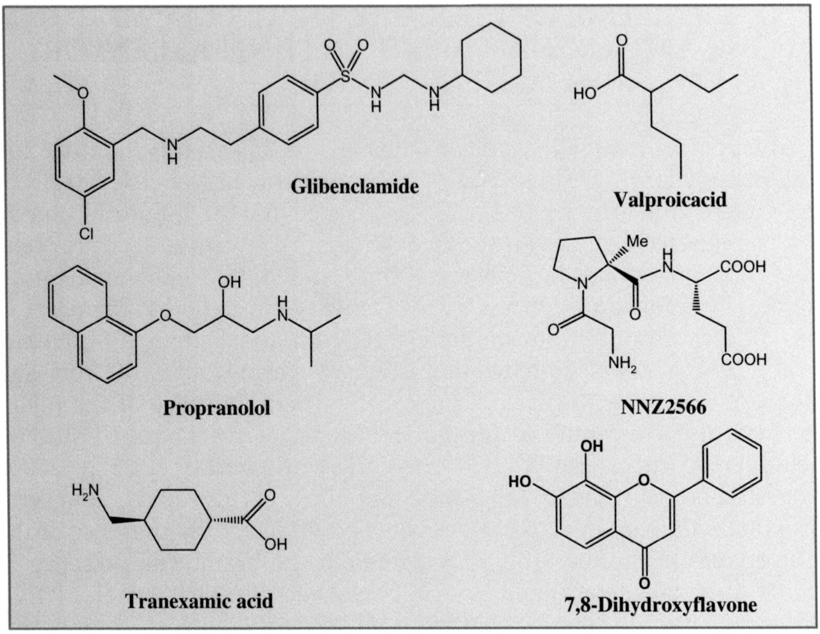

FIGURE 7.8 Chemical structures of glibenclamide, valproic acid, propranolol, NNZ2566, tranexamic acid, and 7,8-dihydroxyflavone.

rodent models of various neurological pathologies such as ischemic (Simard et al., 2006; Wali et al., 2012) and hemorrhagic stroke (Simard et al., 2009; Tosun et al., 2013a,b), spinal cord injury (Simard et al., 2012) neonatal encephalopathy of prematurity (Tosun et al., 2013a,b; Zhou et al., 2009). In addition, glibenclamide not only reduces edema formation and secondary hemorrhage, inhibits necrotic cell death, but also exerts potent antiinflammatory effects and promotes neurogenesis (Kurland et al., 2013). Treatment with low-dose glibenclamide reduces posttraumatic brain edema and contusion volume following an open head injury in rats (Zweckberger et al., 2014). Glibenclamide has long-term protective effects on the hippocampus in rats after mild-to-moderate TBI (Patel et al., 2010). Collective evidence suggests that in TBI glibenclamide produces beneficial effects by regulating NCCa-ATP (SUR1/TRPM4) channels in ischemic astrocytes, neurons, and capillaries. Furthermore, the depletion of ATP results in depolarization and opening of the channel leading to cytotoxic edema. A recent Phase IIa clinical stroke trial (NCT01268683) indicates that glibenclamide significantly reduces cerebral edema and lowers the rate of hemorrhagic conversion following ischemic stroke (Sheth et al., 2014), suggesting the potential use of glibenclamide to improve outcomes in humans after brain injury (Khanna et al., 2014). A Phase II clinical trial is underway to assess whether patients with severe, moderate, or complicated mild TBI administered glibenclamide will show a decrease in edema and/or hemorrhage, compared to patients administered placebo (NCT01454154).

NNZ-2566 AND TRAUMATIC BRAIN INJURY

NNZ-2566 is a synthetic analogue of the endogenous N-terminus tripeptide, Glycine-Proline-Glutamate (GPE, Neuren Pharmaceuticals) (Fig. 7.8), which is proteolytically cleaved from insulin-like growth factor-1 (IGF-1) (Sara et al., 1989). GPE does not bind to IGF-1 receptors. However, in vitro studies have demonstrated its ability to stimulate acetylcholine and dopamine release, as well as to protect neurons from a variety of brain injuries. GPE has been reported to cross the BBB and produces neuroprotective effects against TBI. However, it is rapidly metabolized (Batchelor et al., 2003). Its half-life is >70 minutes (Wei et al., 2009). In penetrating ballistic-like brain injury (PBBI), NNZ-2566 significantly decreases PBBI-mediated upregulation of inflammatory cytokines including TNF-α, IFN-γ, and IL-6. The mechanism of action of NNZ-2566 is not known. However, it is reported that activating transcription factor-3 (ATF3) act by repressing the expression of TNF-α, IFN-γ, and IL-6 (Cartagena et al., 2013). It is also reported that NNZ-2566 treatment alters ATF3 expression 12 hours following PBBI. It is known that PBBI alone significantly increases ATF3 mRNA levels by 13-fold at 12 hours and these levels are increased by an additional 4-fold with NNZ-2566 treatment (Cartagena et al., 2013). To confirm that changes in mRNA translated to changes in protein expression, ATF3 expression levels are determined in vivo in microglia/macrophages, T cells, natural killer cells (NKCs), astrocytes, and neurons. It is reported that PBBI significantly increases ATF3 in microglia/macrophages (820%), NKCs (58%), and astrocytes (51%), but decreased levels in T cells (48%). Finally, PBBI increases ATF3 levels by 55% in neurons and NNZ-2566 treatment further increases these levels an additional 33%. Since increased ATF3 may be an innate protective mechanism to limit inflammation following injury, these results support the view that the antiinflammatory and neuroprotective drug NNZ-2566 increases both mRNA and protein levels of ATF3 in multiple cell types, provide a cellular mechanism for NNZ-2566 modulation of neuroinflammation following PBBI (Cartagena et al., 2013). At present, two clinical trials are ongoing to investigate the dosing of NNZ-2566 for safety and tolerability with efficacy in nonpenetrating TBI (NCT00805818 and NCT01366820). Interestingly, these clinical trials will include nonpenetrating TBI, while NNZ-2566 efficacy has not been investigated in the animal models of nonpenetrating TBI.

PROPRANOLOL AND TRAUMATIC BRAIN INJURY

It is well known that TBI is associated with a systemic hyperadrenergic state, which results in an immediate and profound sympathetic nervous system activation with massive release of both central and peripheral catecholamines. The elevated catecholamine levels may be associated with unfavorable outcome after TBI (Loftus et al., 2016). The administration of β-adrenergic receptor blockers (BBs) contributes to the improvement of outcome following TBI. Propranolol (Fig. 7.8) may be an ideal BB because it not only nonselective inhibits elevated levels of catecholamines, reduces sympathetic activation, modifies glucose homeostasis and cytokine expression, but also has ability to cross the BBB. In TBI, early administration of propranolol after TBI is associated with lower mortality. In preclinical mouse model of TBI, propranolol reduces brain edema, increases cerebral perfusion, decreases cerebral hypoxia, and improves neurologic outcomes (Ley et al., 2010). Also, propranolol can reduce the maximum intensity of agitated episodes, and even reduces aggressive behavior months after TBI (Fleminger et al., 2006). The DASH (Decreasing adrenergic or sympathetic hyperactivity after TBI, NCT01322048) study is the first randomized, double-blinded, placebo-controlled trial powered to determine safety and outcomes associated with adrenergic blockade in patients with severe TBI (Patel et al., 2012). If the study results in positive trends, this can provide pilot data for a larger multicenter randomized clinical trial.

TRANEXAMIC ACID AND TRAUMATIC BRAIN INJURY

Tranexamic acid (TXA) is an antifibrinolytic agent (Fig. 7.8), which has an ability to reduce blood loss in patients undergoing surgery and the risk of death in patients with TBI, with no apparent increase in vascular occlusive events (Henry et al., 2007). These findings raise the possibility that it may be effective in other situations in which bleeding can be life threatening or disabling. Posttraumatic coagulopathy occurs in one-third of TBI patients and is associated with an increased risk of death (Harhangi et al., 2008). One of the most important and devastating parts of the TBI is the progression of intracranial hemorrhage (ICH), which often occurs within the first 24 hours. The intensity of ICH varies with severity of TBI. Thus severe, moderate, and mild TBI produce 25%−45%, 3%−12%, and 0.2% ICH among most patients, respectively (Bullock et al., 2006). TXA reduces ICH growth after TBI. It is demonstrated that the release of thromboplastin after TBI is followed by the activation of the coagulation and fibrinolytic pathways. Recently, TXA has been used to reduce mortality compared with placebo in severely bleeding trauma patients in the CRASH-2 (Clinical Randomization of an Antifibrinolytic in Significant Hemorrhage) trial, which enrolled 20,211 patients in 40 countries (Shakur et al., 2010). Based on several TBI treatment studies, it is suggested that TXA significantly reduces intracerebral hemorrhage progression but produce no significant improvement in clinical outcomes of TBI patients (Zehtabchi et al., 2014; Yutthakasemsunt et al., 2013). Thus more studies are needed to determine the routine use of TXA in patients with TBI. An ongoing, international, multicenter, Phase III trial (NCT01402882, CRASH-3) evaluating the use of TXA on death and disability in TBI patients, with a planned enrollment of 10,000 patients, will certainly shed light on this particular question (Dewan et al., 2012).

VALPROIC ACID AND TRAUMATIC BRAIN INJURY

Valproate (2-propylpentanoic acid; VPA) is one of the most commonly prescribed antiepileptic drug that has been shown to reduce the neuronal damage induced by epileptic activity (Fig. 7.8). For example, in a model of rodent status epilepticus, VPA not only decreases neuronal damage in the hippocampal formation, but also improves neurological and memory functions (Brandt et al., 2006). It is reported that the antiepileptic activity of VPA is due to its influence on a number of targets in the brain including inhibition of GABA transamination, reduction of NMDA-mediated neuronal excitation, inhibition of histone deacetylases and glycogen synthase kinase-3beta (GSK-3β), and blockade of voltage-gated sodium and T-type calcium channels (Rosenberg, 2007). In a rat model of TBI, postinjury systemic administration of VPA at a high dose (400 mg/kg) decreases cortical contusion volume, disrupts BBB permeability, and, of most importance, improves motor function and spatial memory following TBI (Dash et al., 2010). It is proposed that VPA at low dose (30 mg/kg) improves motor function in adult rats through increased histone acetylation, p-ERK, and p-CREB expression in the brain (Tai et al., 2014). In a 2-year randomized double-blind trial for prevention of posttraumatic seizures, VPA treatment initiated within 24 hours after TBI substantially reduces the rate of early seizure, but this benefit was not significant, compared with short-term (1 week) treatment with an antiepileptic drug phenytoin; neither drug prevented late seizures (Temkin et al., 1999). Of note, there was a trend toward increased mortality in the VPA groups, although it was not statistically significant compared to phenytoin. In addition, no significant adverse or beneficial effects are associated with VPA treatment in another clinical study, as assessed by a battery of neuropsychological measurements administered 1, 6, and 12 months after TBI (Dikmen et al., 2000). Accumulating evidence suggests that VPA produces robust benefits in preclinical TBI models (Dash et al., 2010; Tai et al., 2014). A clinical trial is underway to evaluate whether VPA at 400 mg/kg can provide neuroprotection and recovery of brain function after severe TBI (primary outcome) and to explore whether VPA can block or slow the onset of late epilepsy after severe nonpenetrating TBI (secondary outcome, NCT02027987).

The lack of translational success of above therapies has prompted researchers and clinicians to reconsider the use of single drug (monotherapeutic) for the treatment of TBI. It is proposed that combination drugs (polytherapies), which affect multiple targets and complementary mechanisms should be evaluated for the efficient treatment and recovery from TBI. It has been suggested those therapies that produce beneficial effects on their own may provide additive benefit when combined, or that have modest effects on their own but act synergistically to exert positive outcomes should be pursued (Kline et al., 2016). This form of therapy is called as polytherapy. Fortunately, a small number of early studies given positive results (Menkü et al., 2003; Barbre and Hoane, 2006), supporting the view that the correct combination of drugs for the treatment of TBI during the appropriate therapeutic window can be efficacious and thus may serve as the impetus for further investigation for the treatment of a complex and heterogenous condition like TBI.

BDNF AND BDNF MIMICS AND TRAUMATIC BRAIN INJURY

It is well known that TBI reduces in the expression of BDNF, a growth factor which is synthesized by neurons in an activity-dependent manner (Stranahan et al., 2008). This growth factor plays an important role in the survival, maintenance, growth and is essential for learning and memory. BDNF mediates its action by interacting and activating transmembrane receptors linked with tropomyosin-related kinase B (TrkB), a high-affinity receptor tyrosine kinase found in the brain. This receptor is located in the plasma membrane, dendrites, and presynaptic terminals. The binding to the TrkB receptor with BDNF results in dimerization and autophosphorylation of this receptor, which causes internalization of the TrkB receptor and initiates intracellular signaling cascades (Levine et al., 1996) (Fig. 7.9) involving phosphatidylinositol 3-kinase (PtdIns 3K) pathway, the PLCγ pathway, and the MAPK pathway. The PtdIns 3K pathway activates protein kinase B (Akt), which ultimately promotes cell survival by inhibiting Bad and consequently allowing the expression of antiapoptotic proteins, such as BcL2 (Yoshii and Constantine-Paton, 2010). Phosphorylation of Akt at the proper site also results in the suppression of proapoptotic proteins, procaspase-9 and Forkhead (Kaplan and Miller, 2007). Upregulated BcL2 levels are correlated with positive outcomes, such as attenuated cell death and a better prognosis (Nathoo et al., 2004). The PLCγ pathway leads to the release of intracellular calcium stores via activation of the inositol

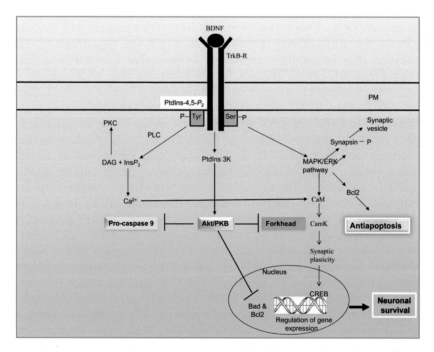

FIGURE 7.9 Hypothetical diagram showing BDNF-mediated signaling. *Akt/PKB*, protein kinase B; *CaM*, calmodulin; *CamK*, calmodulin kinase; *CREB*, cyclic AMP response element-binding protein; *CREM*, cAMP responsive element modulator; *DAG*, diacylglycerol; *InsP₃*, inositol 1,4,5-trisphosphate; *PKC*, protein kinase C; *PLC*, phospholipase C; *PtdIns 3K*, phosphatidylinositol 3-kinases; *PtdIns-4,5-P₂*, phosphatidylinositol 4,5-bisphosphate; *TrkB*, tyrosine kinase B receptor.

triphosphate (InsP$_3$) receptor, and helps to increase calmodulin kinase (CamK) activity, and thus synaptic plasticity via the transcription factor CREB. The MAPK pathway, also referred to as extracellular related signal kinase (ERK) pathway, aids in cell growth and differentiation. PLCγ mediated response is probably responsible for quick, short-term actions, while MAPK and PtdIns 3K pathways involve long-term transcriptional effects (Yoshii and Constantine-Paton, 2010).

In response to TBI, the mRNA expression level of BDNF is transiently and significantly increased. Many studies have indicated that within hours post-TBI, the expression level of BDNF mRNA is significantly upregulated in the injured cortex and in the hippocampus (Yang et al., 1996). The level of BDNF declines at 24 hours postinjury, and is no longer significant at 36 hours postinjury (Oyesiku et al., 1999). Similarly following TBI, the mRNA expression level of TrkB receptor is also transiently upregulated in the hippocampus and dentate gyrus (Merlio et al., 1993). This transient surge of BDNF and its receptor following TBI suggests that BDNF acts as an endogenous neuroprotective response attempting to attenuate secondary cell damage following TBI (Mattson and Scheff, 1994). Due to its short half-life (<10 minutes) and inability to cross the BBB BDNF cannot be used for the treatment of TBI. However, it is becoming increasingly evident that 7,8-DHF is a TrkB receptor agonist, which mimics BDNF functions due to its ability to bind with extracellular domain of TrkB receptor (Chen et al., 2011; Zeng et al., 2012). Like BDNF, 7,8-DHF (Fig. 7.8) promotes dimerization and autophosphorylation of TrkB receptor (Jang et al., 2010), producing the activation of downstream signaling pathways (Fig. 7.9). Studies on therapeutic potential of 7,8-DHF in TBI have been performed in several experimental models of TBI. Thus, in in vitro stretch injury model, 7,8-DHF treatment attenuates stretch injury-mediated cytotoxicity and apoptosis in cultured primary neurons (Wu et al., 2014). In a mouse focal CCI model of TBI, intraperitoneal injection of 7,8-DHF at the dose of 20 mg/kg beginning at 10 minutes following moderate CCI injury, and subsequent single daily doses for 3 days produce significant beneficial effects including reducing brain edema, cortical contusion volume, neuronal cell death and apoptosis, as well as improving motor functions of injured animals (Wu et al., 2014). Similarly, in a fluid percussion injury (FPI) rat model of TBI, a single injection (daily dose of 5 mg/kg for 7 consecutive days) of 7,8-DHF not only stimulates learning and memory functions (Agrawal et al., 2015), but also enhances phosphorylation of TrkB receptor and activation of Akt and CREB pathways (Wu et al., 2014; Agrawal et al., 2015). Furthermore, CN2097, a peptidomimetic ligand which targets the synaptic scaffold protein, postsynaptic density protein 95, enhances downstream signaling of TrkB, improves neurological function after TBI (Marshall et al., 2017). Moderate to severe TBI elicits neuroinflammation and c-Jun-N-terminal kinase (JNK) activation, which is associated with memory deficits. It is also reported that CN2097 significantly reduces the posttraumatic synthesis of proinflammatory mediators and retards the posttraumatic activation of JNK in a rodent model of TBI (Marshall et al., 2017). Furthermore, CN2097 significantly improves the complex auditory processing deficits, which are impaired after injury supporting the view that the multi-functionality of CN2097 strongly suggests that CN2097 can be highly efficacious in targeting complex secondary injury processes resulting from TBI (Marshall et al., 2017).

MICRORNAs AND TRAUMATIC BRAIN INJURY

MicroRNAs (miRNA) are small, noncoding RNA fragments. miRNAs are approximately 22 nucleotides long and are associated with posttranscriptional regulation of gene expression (Guan et al., 2010; Cheng et al.,2013). In mammalian cells, miRNAs work through base pairing with complementary sequences within messenger RNA (mRNA) molecules, usually resulting in gene silencing via translational repression. After processing by endonucleases (Cheng et al., 2013), the resultant single-stranded miRNAs combine with other macromolecules to form RNA-induced silencing complexes (RISCs). These RISCs target complementary mRNA strands for degradation, altering cellular function (Cheng et al., 2013; Freischmidt et al., 2013). miRNAs are abundantly found in the brain, where they are key regulators of different biological functions including synaptic plasticity, neurogenesis, apoptosis, and differentiation. Also, they can indirectly influence neural cell proliferation and self-renewal of neural stem cells (Grasso et al., 2014).

Alterations in levels of miRNAs expression have been reported to occur in the brain of animal with TBI (Lei et al., 2009; Harrison et al., 2016) and in plasma of TBI patients (Redell et al., 2010). Microarray analysis has revealed several miRNAs are dysregulated following TBI (Lei et al., 2009). Of the miRNAs that are altered following TBI, miR-21 has been shown to be globally and consistently upregulated after TBI. Further, Redell et al. (2011) have also observed increased expression of miR-21 along with altered expression of its targets after TBI. miR-21 plays a key role in a plethora of biological functions that may influence outcome of TBI. More importantly, miRNAs have been used as potential therapeutic targets in TBI. For example, miR-21, a strong prosurvival miRNA, is upregulated in adult rat brains after TBI but downregulated in aged rat brains after TBI (Sandhir et al., 2014). A recent study manipulated the expression level of miR-21 in brain using intracerebroventricular infusion of miR-21 agomir or antagomir to evaluate the potential effect of miR-21 on neurological function in the FPI rat model of TBI (Ge et al., 2014). Upregulation of miR-21 level in brain conferred a better neurological outcome after TBI by alleviating brain edema and decreasing lesion volume. miR-21 inhibited apoptosis and promoted angiogenesis through regulating the expression of apoptosis- and angiogenesis-related molecules including VEGF, angiopoietin-1 (Ang-1) and Tie-2 (receptor of Ang-1) in brain. In addition, the expression of phosphatase and tensin homolog deleted on chromosome10, a miR-21 target gene, is inhibited and Akt signaling is activated in the brain (Ge et al., 2014). These data indicate that miRNAs including miR-21 can be a potential therapeutic target for interventions after TBI.

STEM CELL THERAPY AND TRAUMATIC BRAIN INJURY

Because the adult brain cells have a limited capacity to regenerate at sites of injury, stem cell transplantations may provide enormous potential to replace the lost cells following TBI. Several types of cell lines such as immortalized progenitors cells, embryonic rodent and human stem cells, bone marrow-derived cells, and neural stem/progenitor cells have been successfully transplanted in experimental models of TBI, resulting in reduced neurobehavioral deficits and attenuation of histological damage (Longhi et al., 2005).

Neural stem/progenitor cells provide great promise for therapeutic repair after TBI. Ultrastructural analysis of axons has revealed that neural stem/progenitor cells can be transformed into morphologically normal appearing myelin sheaths around axons in the injured areas of the brain. It is becoming increasingly evident that neural stem/progenitor cells have many of the properties that allow them to overcome major hurdles of TBI regeneration. The transplantation of neural stem/progenitor cells in TBI not only depresses neuroinflammatory response, but also provides a neurotrophic influence and stimulates neovascularization (Jain, 2009). However, the clinical use of fetal tissues or embryonic stem cells is limited not only due to ethical considerations, but also because of scientific problems. It is becoming increasingly evident that multipotent mesenchymal stromal cells (MSCs), which are derived from mesodermal cells, are primarily resident in adult bone marrow, adipose tissue, skin, umbilical cord blood, and peripheral blood (Ho et al., 2008). MSCs can transform themselves not only into neuronal cells, but also in many tissue-specific cell phenotypes (Kassem and Abdallah, 2008). Thus MSCs represent an important and alternative source of stem cells for cell replacement therapies.

Administration of MSCs 24 hours after TBI significantly improves functional outcome in animal models of TBI (Mahmood et al., 2005). Beneficial effects of MSCs in TBI are due to secretion and release of various growth factors including nerve growth factor, BDNF, and basic fibroblast growth factor (Mahmood et al., 2004). MSCs not only influence and support synaptogenesis (Mahmood et al., 2004), angiogenesis (Mahmood et al., 2004; Qu et al., 2008), neurogenesis (Chen and Chopp, 2006), but also promote axonal reorganization (Jiang et al., 2011). Collective evidence suggests that MSCs can be used to stimulate brain remodeling. Although MSCs alone do not reduce the lesion volume after TBI, a recent study indicates that collagen scaffolds populated with MSCs improve spatial learning and sensorimotor function, reduce the lesion volume, and foster the migration of MSCs into the lesion boundary zone after TBI in rats compared to MSCs without scaffolds (Lu et al., 2007a,b). Transplanting human MSCs with the scaffolds downregulates neurocan and Nogo-A transcription (major forms of growth-inhibitory molecule that suppresses axonal regeneration and neurite regrowth after neural injury) and protein expression (Mahmood et al., 2014a,b), which may partially contribute to the enhanced axonal regeneration after TBI.

The safety and feasibility of MSCs has been evaluated in TBI patients by directly applying to the injured area during the cranial operation followed by a second intravenous dose of MSCs. No immediate or delayed toxicity related to the cell administration was observed within the 6-month follow-up period. It is reported that neurologic function of TBI patient is significantly improved at 6 months after MSC therapy (Zhang et al., 2008). The safety and feasibility of MSC therapy has been confirmed by transplanting autologous MSCs into the subarachnoid space via lumbar puncture in another single center (Zhang et al., 2008; Tian et al., 2013). A recent Phase I clinical trial demonstrates that intravenous infusion of autologous bone marrow-derived mononuclear cell therapy within 48 hours after severe TBI in children is feasible and safe (Cox et al., 2011; Liao et al., 2015). Several Phase I/II clinical trials are ongoing to further study the safety of autologous bone marrow mononuclear cells and their effect on functional outcome in TBI patients of children and adults (NCT01851083, NCT01575470, and NCT02028104).

EXOSOMES THERAPY AND TRAUMATIC BRAIN INJURY

Exosomes are endosomal origin membrane-enclosed small vesicles (30–100 nm), which contain various molecular constituents including proteins, lipids, mRNAs, and miRNAs. Exosomes play a pivotal role in intercellular communication. It is reported that MSC-generated exosomes effectively improve functional recovery, at least in part, not only by promoting endogenous angiogenesis and neurogenesis, but also by reducing neuroinflammation in rats after TBI. Thus MSC-generated exosomes may provide a novel cell-free therapy for TBI and possibly for other neurological diseases (Xiong et al., 2017; Yang et al., 2017). A recent study indicates that the therapeutic efficacy of extracellular vesicles from MSCs is similar to efficacy of MSCs in a rodent stroke model (Doeppner et al., 2015). It is reported that exosomes transfer RNAs and proteins to other cells which then act epigenetically to alter the function of the recipient cells. The development of cell-free exosomes derived from MSCs for treatment of TBI is just in its infancy (Zhang et al., 2015, 2016; Kim et al., 2016). In a proof-of-principle study, an intravenous delivery of MSC-derived exosomes improves functional recovery and promotes neuroplasticity in young adult male rats subjected to TBI induced by CCI (Zhang et al., 2015).

HYPOTHERMIA AND TRAUMATIC BRAIN INJURY

It is well known that hypothermia decreases endogenous antioxidant consumption and decreases lipid peroxidation after TBI (Sahuguillo and Vilalta, 2009). However, hypothermic therapy in TBI patients has been very controversial and results have been inconsistent (Hutchison et al., 2008; Grände et al., 2009). Hypothermic therapy improves survival and the neurologic outcome in animal models of TBI (Sahuguillo and Vilalta, 2009). Hypothermic therapy reduces brain edema and intracranial pressure in TBI patients. It produces alterations in temperature-sensitive miRNAs (miR-34a, miR-874, and miR-451) in TBI and this process may be involved in the regulation of cellular apoptosis after TBI. miR-34a is associated with the regulation of the proliferation of neural stem cells in the hippocampus through crosstalk with Notch signaling (Wang et al., 2012), and miR-107 can influence the process of wound repair by regulating granulin expression after TBI (Wang et al., 2010). In addition, several studies have examined the miRNA profiles of CSF and blood samples from patients and TBI rats, and identified potential miRNAs biomarkers in TBI (Redell et al., 2010; Balakathiresan et al., 2012). The molecular mechanism by which hypothermic therapy provides neuroprotection is multifactorial and includes (1) reduction in brain metabolic rate, (2) modulation in cerebral blood flow, (3) reduction of the critical threshold for oxygen delivery, (4) blockade of excitotoxic mechanisms and inhibition of calcium influx, (5) preservation of protein synthesis, and (6) reduction of brain thermopooling (Sahuguillo and Vilalta, 2009). Hypothermic therapy decreases JNK activation, which is involved in the reduction of caspase-3 expression (Huang et al., 2009). In contrast, hyperthermic therapy activates both ERK and JNK and upregulates expression of cleaved caspase-3. These observations support the involvement of JNK activation in apoptosis after TBI. In addition, hypothermia protects against TNF-α-induced endothelial barrier dysfunction and apoptosis through a MAPK phosphatase-1 (MKP-1)-dependent mechanism (Yang et al., 2009). It should be noted that hypothermic therapy in TBI suffers from many problems. The main problem is the lack of a systematic methodology to induce and maintain hypothermic conditions. It is reported that rapid rewarming after TBI prevents the beneficial effects of hypothermic therapy on axonal injury and microvascular damage (Povlishock and Wei, 2009). While hypothermic therapy combined with a slow rewarming phase results in improved protection, rapid rewarming canceled the beneficial effects of cooling. Rewarming rates are now considered a critical factor when using therapeutic hypothermia in clinical studies. Thus, more studies are required on determination of optimal duration of hypothermic therapy and timing for bringing the body to the normal temperature. Collective evidence suggests that it is essential to establish velocity and other important parameters needed for rewarming the body (Sahuguillo and Vilalta, 2009).

ACUPUNCTURE AND TRAUMATIC BRAIN INJURY

Acupuncture is a traditional Chinese medicine method that has been used for both disease prevention and treatment for over 3000 years. It may be a promising treatment strategy for neurological disorders including TBI (Xu et al., 2015; Tian et al., 2016). Acupuncture involves the stimulation at the combined acupoint of Baihui, Renzhong, Hegu, and Zusanli with fine needles. Earlier studies have indicated that acupuncture can not only improve the ischemic and hypoxic changes after TBI, but also promote the regeneration of nerve in injured tissues (Jiang et al., 2016; Shi et al., 2015; Nam et al., 2013). The molecular mechanism associated with acupuncture therapy in neurotraumatic diseases has not been established. However, it is reported that acupuncture significantly increases levels of BDNF not only immediately after TBI, but also at 168 hours after TBI compared with TBI simple group, indicating that acupuncture can persistently enhance the expression of BDNF (Li et al., 2017). The placebo acupuncture group shows no obvious change in TBI simple group. It is also reported that BDNF interacts with the TrkB receptor to activate the downstream signaling pathways, modulating a series of pathological and physiological changes (Xu et al., 2015; Yama and Nabeshima, 2004). Besides BDNF, the levels of TrkB are subsequently increased after acupuncture compared with TBI group, suggesting that BDNF/TrkB may be activated indicate that both phosphorylated Akt and phosphorylated Erk1/2 are significantly increased showing the activation of BDNF/TrkB pathway (Numakawa et al., 2010). In addition to BDNF/TrkB signaling pathway in ischemia, acupuncture therapy markedly decreases the ischemic damaged areas in the cerebral cortex and hippocampus. Concomitantly, acupuncture therapy upregulates GABA immunoexpression in MCAO rats suggesting that acupuncture therapy on specific and established acupoints produces neuroprotective effects by upregulating GABA receptor expression (Xu et al., 2015; Yama and Nabeshima, 2004) that would have a neuroprotective effect.

EXERCISE AND TRAUMATIC BRAIN INJURY

Exercise produces beneficial effects in patient with TBI. The under-lying mechanisms associated with beneficial effects include changes in the brain structural integrity by enhancing neurogenesis and angiogenesis with more secretions of growth factors promoting synaptic plasticity (Fig. 7.10) (Gomez-Pinilla et al., 2008; Farooqui, 2014). These processes improve cognitive function through increase in gray matter volume (Hillman et al., 2008) and neurogenesis in the dentate gyrus. Neurogenesis is coupled with angiogenesis, which in turn related to cerebral blood volume (van Praag et al., 1999). It is hypothesized that measurement of cerebral blood volume may provide an in vivo correlation between neurogenesis and increased cerebral blood flow due to exercise. At the molecular level many molecules mediate exercise-induced neurogenesis, angiogenesis, and cerebral blood flow. These molecules include VEGF, BDNF, catechol-O-methyltransferase, endorphins, and nitric oxide (Neeper et al., 1996; Stroth et al., 2010; Camargo et al., 2013). In addition, exercise also modulates gene involved in insulin-like signaling, energy metabolism, neurogenesis, and synaptic plasticity along with learning and memory (Reagan, 2007; van Praag et al., 2005). Notably, aerobic exercises such as Tai chi and Yoga have been popularly promoted for its potential advantages in healthy and ill-attacked populations (Manko et al., 2013; Schmid et al., 2016); however, the frequency and burden of exercise after TBI differ from one to another and remain to be further elucidated (Kandola et al., 2016).

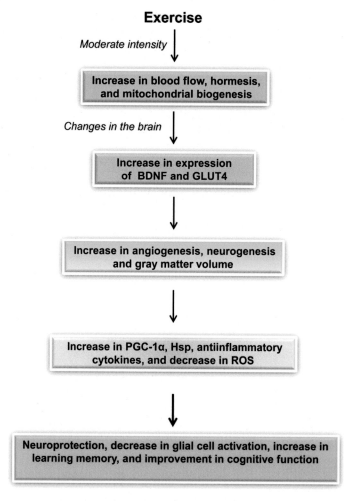

FIGURE 7.10   Effects of exercise on the brain. *BDNF*, brain-derived neurotrophic factor; *GLUT-4*, glucose transporter type 4; *PGC-1α*, peroxisome proliferator-activated receptor-gamma coactivator-1α; *ROS*, reactive oxygen species.

CONCLUSION

TBI survivors suffer from long-lasting disability, which is mainly related to cognitive deficits. Such deficits include slow information processing, deficits of learning and memory, of attention, of working memory, and of executive functions, associated with behavioral and personality modifications. Many clinical trials using glutamate receptor antagonists, progesterone, erythropoietin, statins, monocycline, cyclosporin, glibenclamide, propranolol, and NNZ2566, have been performed and achieved some success in animal model of TBI. However, these trials have failed in human patients. These observations suggest that it is time to leave single drug or monotherapeutic approaches to treat TBI and try to treat TBI with combined drug treatment (polytherapies) to target multiple and complementary mechanisms for the treatment of TBI.

Fortunately, a small number of early studies on polytherapies revealed positive benefits, indicating that the correct combination of treatments during the appropriate therapeutic window can be efficacious and thus served as the impetus for further investigation into this complex, but more realistic and potentially more successful strategy for the treatment and rehabilitation of TBI. These drugs may provide neuroprotection by facilitating and promoting angiogenesis, neurogenesis, and synaptogenesis. Large clinical trials with combined drugs therapy have been planned. It is expected that the next decade will witness an increasing number of clinical trials that seek to translate preclinical research discoveries to the clinic.

References

Abrahamson, E.E., Ikonomovic, M.D., Dixon, C.E., DeKosky, S.T., 2009. Simvastatin therapy prevents brain trauma-induced increases in beta-amyloid peptide levels. Ann. Neurol. 66, 407–414.

Agrawal, R., Noble, E., Tyagi, E., Zhuang, Y., Ying, Z., et al., 2015. Flavonoid derivative 7,8-DHF attenuates TBI pathology via TrkB activation. Biochim. Biophys. Acta 1852, 862–872.

Ahmed, S., Venigalla, H., Mekala, H.M., Dar, S., Hassan, M., et al., 2017. Traumatic brain injury and neuropsychiatric complications. Indian J. Psychol. Med. 39, 114–121.

Alway, Y., Gould, K.R., Johnston, L., McKenzie, D., Ponsford, J., 2016. A prospective examination of Axis I psychiatric disorders in the first 5 years following moderate to severe traumatic brain injury. Psychol. Med. 12, 1–11.

Aminmansour, B., Fard, S.A., Habibabadi, M.R., Moein, P., Norouzi, R., et al., 2014. The efficacy of cyclosporine-A on diffuse axonal injury after traumatic brain injury. Adv. Biomed. Res. 3, 35.

Apostolova, I., Irintchev, A., Schachner, M., 2006. Tenascin-R restricts posttraumatic remodeling of motoneuron innervation and functional recovery after spinal cord injury in adult mice. J. Neurosci. 26, 7849–7859.

Bahraini, N.H., Brenner, L.A., Harwood, J.E., Homaifar, B.Y., Ladley-O'Brien, S.E., et al., 2009. Utility of the trauma symptom inventory for the assessment of post-traumatic stress symptoms in veterans with a history of psychological trauma and/or brain injury. Mil. Med. 174, 1005–1009.

Bailes, J.E., Mills, J.D., 2010. Docosahexaenoic acid reduces traumatic axonal injury in a rodent head injury model. J. Neurotrauma 27, 1617–1624.

Balakathiresan, N., Bhomia, M., Chandran, R., Chavko, M., McCarron, R.M., et al., 2012. MicroRNA let-7i is a promising serum biomarker for blast-induced traumatic brain injury. J. Neurotrauma 29, 1379–1387.

Barbre, A.B., Hoane, M.R., 2006. Magnesium and riboflavin combination therapy following cortical contusion injury in the rat. Brain Res. Bull. 69, 639–646.

Batchelor, D.C., Lin, H., Wen, J.Y., Keven, C., Van Zijl, P.L., et al., 2003. Pharmacokinetics of glycine-proline-glutamate, the N-terminal tripeptide of insulin-like growth factor-1, in rats. Anal. Biochem. 323, 156−163.

Baulieu, E.E., Robel, P., 1990. Neurosteroids: a new brain function? J. Steroid Biochem. Mol. Biol. 37, 395−403.

Borisoff, J.F., Chan, C.C., Hiebert, G.W., Oschipok, L., Robertson, G.S., et al., 2003. Suppression of Rho-kinase activity promotes axonal growth on inhibitory CNS substrates. Mol. Cell. Neurosci. 22, 405−416.

Brandt, C., Gastens, A.M., Sun, M., Hausknecht, M., Loscher, W., 2006. Treatment with valproate after status epilepticus: effect on neuronal damage, epileptogenesis, and behavioral alterations in rats. Neuropharmacology 51, 789−804.

Brines, M.L., Ghezzi, P., Keenan, S., Agnello, D., De Lanerolle, N.C., et al., 2000. Erythropoietin crosses the blood−brain barrier to protect against experimental brain injury. Proc. Natl. Acad. Sci. USA. 97, 10526−10531.

Brinton, R.D., Thompson, R.F., Foy, M.R., Baudry, M., Wang, J., et al., 2008. Progesterone receptors: form and function in brain. Front. Neuroendocrinol. 29, 313−339.

Brodkey, J.A., Laywell, E.D., O'Brien, T.F., Faissner, A., Stefansson, K., et al., 1995. Focal brain injury and upregulation of a developmentally regulated extracellular matrix protein. J. Neurosurg. 82, 106−112.

Bullock, M.R., Chesnut, R., Ghajar, J., Gordon, D., Hartl, R., et al., 2006. Surgical management of traumatic parenchymal lesions. Neurosurgery 58 (3 Suppl.), S1−S3. Discussion Si−iv.

Bye, N., Habgood, M.D., Callaway, J.K., Malakooti, N., Potter, A., et al., 2007. Transient neuroprotection by minocycline following traumatic brain injury is associated with attenuated microglial activation but no changes in cell apoptosis or neutrophil infiltration. Exp. Neurol. 204, 220−233.

Camargo, L.H., Alves, F.H., Biojones, C., Correa, F.M., Resstel, L.B., et al., 2013. Involvement of N-methyl-d-aspartate glutamate receptor and nitric oxide in cardiovascular responses to dynamic exercise in rats. Eur. J. Pharmacol. 713, 16−24.

Cartagena, C.M., Phillips, K.L., Williams, G.L., Konopko, M., Tortella, F.C., et al., 2013. Mechanism of action for NNZ-2566 anti-inflammatory effects following PBBI involves upregulation of immunomodulator ATF3. Neuromol. Med. 15, 504−514.

Center for Disease Control and Prevention, 2016. Heads up: concussion in youth sports. Available from: <http://www.cdc.gov/headsup/basics/concussion_symptoms.html> (Last updated on 16.02.15. Last accessed on 16.10.16.).

Chen, G., Shi, J., Jin, W., Wang, L., Xie, W., et al., 2008. Progesterone administration modulates TLRs/NF-kappaB signaling pathway in rat brain after cortical contusion. Ann. Clin. Lab. Sci. 38, 65−74.

Chen, J., Chopp, M., 2006. Neurorestorative treatment of stroke: cell and pharmacological approaches. NeuroRx 3, 466−473.

Chen, J., Chua, K.W., Chua, C.C., Yu, H., Pei, A., et al., 2011. Antioxidant activity of 7,8-dihydroxyflavone provides neuroprotection against glutamate-induced toxicity. Neurosci. Lett. 499, 181−185.

Cheng, L., Quek, C.Y., Sun, X., Bellingham, S.A., Hill, A.F., 2013. The detection of microRNA associated with Alzheimer's disease in biological fluids using next-generation sequencing technologies. Front. Genet. 4, 150.

Chun, K.A., Manley, G.T., Stiver, S.I., Aiken, A.H., Phan, N., et al., 2009. Interobserver variability in the assessment of CT imaging features of traumatic brain injury. J. Neurotrauma 27, 325−330.

Clark, S.R., McMahon, C.J., Gueorguieva, I., Rowland, M., Scarth, S., et al., 2008. Interleukin-1 receptor antagonist penetrates human brain at experimentally therapeutic concentrations. J. Cereb. Blood Flow Metab. 28, 387–394.

Collado, M.L., Rodriguez-Manzo, G., Cruz, M.L., 1985. Effect of progesterone upon adenylate cyclase activity and cAMP levels on brain areas. Pharmacol. Biochem. Behav. 23, 501–504.

Cox Jr., C.S., Baumgartner, J.E., Harting, M.T., Worth, L.L., Walker, P.A., et al., 2011. Autologous bone marrow mononuclear cell therapy for severe traumatic brain injury in children. Neurosurgery 68, 588–600.

Crack, P.J., Gould, J., Bye, N., Ross, S., Ali, U., et al., 2009. The genomic profile of the cerebral cortex after closed head injury in mice: effects of minocycline. J. Neural Transm. 116, 1–12.

Dash, P.K., Orsi, S.A., Zhang, M., Grill, R.J., Pati, S., et al., 2010. Valproate administered after traumatic brain injury provides neuroprotection and improves cognitive function in rats. PLoS One 5, e11383.

Dewan, Y., Komolafe, E.O., Mejia-Mantilla, J.H., et al., 2012. CRASH-3-tranexamic acid for the treatment of significant traumatic brain injury: study protocol for an international randomized, double-blind, placebo-controlled trial. Trials 13, 87.

Djebaili, M., Guo, Q., Pettus, E.H., Hoffman, S.W., Stein, D.G., 2005. The neurosteroids progesterone and allopregnanolone reduce cell death, gliosis, and functional deficits after traumatic brain injury in rats. J. Neurotrauma 22, 106–118.

Dikmen, S.S., Machamer, J.E., Winn, H.R., Anderson, G.D., Temkin, N.R., et al., 2000. Neuropsychological effects of valproate in traumatic brain injury: a randomized trial. Neurology 54, 895–902.

Doeppner, T.R., Herz, J., Gorgens, A., Schlechter, J., Ludwig, A.K., et al., 2015. Extracellular vesicles improve post-stroke neuroregeneration and prevent postischemic immunosuppression. Stem Cells Transl. Med. 4, 1131–1143.

Eakin, K., Baratz-Goldstein, R., Pick, C.G., et al., 2014. Efficacy of N-acetyl cysteine in traumatic brain injury. PLoS One 9, e90617.

Ehrenreich, H., Aust, C., Krampe, H., et al., 2004. Erythropoietin: novel approaches to neuroprotection in human brain disease. Metab. Brain Dis. 19, 195–206.

Fleminger, S., Greenwood, R.J., Oliver, D.L., 2006. Pharmacological management for agitation and aggression in people with acquired brain injury. Cochrane Database Syst. Rev. 4, CD003299.

Endres, M., 2005. Statins and stroke. J. Cereb. Blood Flow Metab. 25, 1093–1110.

Endres, M., 2006. Statins: potential new indications in inflammatory conditions. Atheroscler. Suppl. 7, 31–35.

Farooqui, A.A., 2010. Neurochemical Aspects of Neurotraumatic and Neurodegenerative Diseases. Springer, New York, NY.

Farooqui, A.A., 2014. Inflammation and Oxidative Stress in Neurological Disorders. Springer International Publishing, Switzerland.

Farooqui, A.A., 2017. Neurochemical Aspects of Alzheimer's Disease. Academic Press, an Imprint of Elsevier, San Diego, CA, USA.

Fisher, D., Xing, B., Dill, J., Li, H., Hoang, H.H., et al., 2011. Leukocyte common antigen-related phosphatase is a functional receptor for chondroitin sulfate proteoglycan axon growth inhibitors. J. Neurosci. 31, 14051–14066.

Freischmidt, A., Müller, K., Ludolph, A.C., Weishaupt, J.H., 2013. Systemic dysregulation of TDP-43 binding microRNAs in amyotrophic lateral sclerosis. Acta Neuropathol. Commun. 1, 42.

Fujita, Y., Yamashita, T., 2014. Axon growth inhibition by RhoA/ROCK in the central nervous system. Front. Neurosci. 8, 338.

Garcia-Martinez, E.M., Sanz-Blasco, S., Karachitos, A., Bandez, M.J., Fernandez-Gomez, F.J., et al., 2010. Mitochondria and calcium flux as targets of neuroprotection caused by minocycline in cerebellar granule cells. Biochem. Pharmacol. 79, 239–2350.

Gardner, A.J., Zafonte, R., 2016. Neuroepidemiology of traumatic brain injury. Handb. Clin. Neurol. 138, 207–223.

Ge, X.T., Lei, P., Wang, H.C., Han, Z.L., Chen, X., et al., 2014. miR-21 improves the neurological outcome after traumatic brain injury in rats. Sci. Rep. 4, 6718.

Genc, S., Koroglu, T.F., Genc, K., 2003. Erythropoietin as a novel neuroprotectant. Restor. Neurol. Neurosci. 22, 105–119.

Gomez-Pinilla, F., Vaynman, S., Ying, Z., 2008. Brain-derived neurotrophic factor functions as a metabotrophin to mediate the effects of exercise on cognition. Eur. J. Neurosci. 28, 2278–2287.

Grände, P.O., Reinstrup, P., Romner, B., 2009. Active cooling in traumatic brain-injured patients: a questionable therapy?. Acta Anaesthesiol. Scand. 53, 1233–1238.

Grasso, M., Piscopo, P., Confaloni, A., Denti, M.A., 2014. Circulating miRNAs as biomarkers for neurodegenerative disorders. Molecules 19, 6891–6910.

Greitz, D., 2006. Unraveling the riddle of syringomyelia. Neurosurg. Rev. 29, 251–263. Discussion 264.

Guan, Y., Mizoguchi, M., Yoshimoto, K., Hata, N., Shono, T., et al., 2010. MiRNA-196 is upregulated in glioblastoma but not in anaplastic astrocytoma and has prognostic significance. Clin. Cancer Res. 16, 4289–4297.

Harhangi, B.S., Kompanje, E.J., Leebeek, F.W., Maas, A.I., 2008. Coagulation disorders after traumatic brain injury. Acta Neurochir. (Wien) 150, 165–175.

Harrison, E.B., Hochfelder, C.G., Lamberty, B.G., Meays, B.M., Morsey, B.M., et al., 2016. Traumatic brain injury increases levels of miR-21 in extracellular vesicles: implications for neuroinflammation. FEBS Open Bio. 6, 835–846.

Helmy, A., Carpenter, K.L., Menon, D.K., Pickard, J.D., Hutchinson, P.J., 2011. The cytokine response to human traumatic brain injury: temporal profiles and evidence for cerebral parenchymal production. J. Cereb. Blood Flow Metab. 31, 658–670.

Helmy, A., Guilfoyle, M.R., Carpenter, K.L., Pickard, J.D., Menon, D.K., et al., 2014. Recombinant human interleukin-1 receptor antagonist in severe traumatic brain injury: a phase II randomized control trial. J. Cereb. Blood Flow Metab. 34, 845–851.

Henry, D.A., Carless, P.A., Moxey, A.J., O'Connell, D., Stokes, B.J., et al., 2007. Anti-fibrinolytic use for minimising perioperative allogeneic blood transfusion. Cochrane Database Syst. Rev. 17. CD001886.

Hillman, C.H., Erickson, K.I., Kramer, A.F., 2008. Be smart, exercise your heart: exercise effects on brain and cognition. Nat. Rev. Neurosci. 9, 58–65.

Ho, A.D., Wagner, W., Franke, W., 2008. Heterogeneity of mesenchymal stromal cell preparations. Cytotherapy 10, 320–330.

Hoffer, M.E., Balaban, C., Slade, M.D., Tsao, J.W., Hoffer, B., 2013. Amelioration of acute sequelae of blast induced mild traumatic brain injury by N-acetyl cysteine: a double-blind, placebo controlled study. PLoS One 8, e54163.

Homsi, S., Federico, F., Croci, N., Palmier, B., Plotkine, M., et al., 2009. Minocycline effects on cerebral edema: relations with inflammatory and oxidative stress markers following traumatic brain injury in mice. Brain Res. 1291, 122–132.

Homsi, S., Piaggio, T., Croci, N., Noble, F., Plotkine, M., et al., 2010. Blockade of acute microglial activation by minocycline promotes neuroprotection and reduces locomotor hyperactivity after closed head injury in mice: a twelve-week follow-up study. J. Neurotrauma 27, 911−921.

Hou, S.T., Jiang, S.X., Smith, R.A., 2008. Permissive and repulsive cues and signalling pathways of axonal outgrowth and regeneration. Int. Rev. Cell Mol. Biol. 267, 125−181.

Hua, X.Y., Svensson, C.I., Matsui, T., Fitzsimmons, B., Yaksh, T.L., et al., 2005. Intrathecal minocycline attenuates peripheral inflammation-induced hyperalgesia by inhibiting p38 MAPK in spinal microglia. Eur. J. Neurosci. 22, 2431−2440.

Huang, T., Solano, J., He, D., Loutfi, M., Dietrich, W.D., et al., 2009. Traumatic injury activates MAP kinases in astrocytes: mechanisms of hypothermia and hyperthermia. J. Neurotrauma 26, 1535−1545.

Hur, E., Zhou, F., 2010. GSK3 signalling in neural development. Nat. Rev. Neurosci. 11, 539−551.

Hutchison, J.S., Ward, R.E., Lacroix, J., Hébert, P.C., Barnes, M.A., et al., 2008. Hypothermia therapy after traumatic brain injury in children. N. Engl. J. Med. 358, 2447−2456.

Jain, K.K., 2009. Cell therapy for CNS trauma. Mol. Biotechnol. 42, 367−376.

Jang, S.W., Liu, X., Yepes, M., Shepherd, K.R., Miller, G.W., et al., 2010. A selective TrkB agonist with potent neurotrophic activities by 7,8-dihydroxyflavone. Proc. Natl. Acad. Sci. USA. 107, 2687−2692.

Jiang, Q., Qu, C., Chopp, M., Ding, G.L., Davarani, S.P., et al., 2011. MRI evaluation of axonal reorganization after bone marrow stromal cell treatment of traumatic brain injury. NMR Biomed. 24, 1119−1128.

Jiang, S., Chen, W., Zhang, Y., Zhang, Y., Chen, A., et al., 2016. Acupuncture induces the proliferation and differentiation of endogenous neural stem cells in rats with traumatic brain injury. Evid. Based Complem. Alternat. Med. 8, 2047412.

Johnson-Anuna, L.N., Eckert, G.P., Keller, J.H., Igbavboa, U., Franke, C., et al., 2005. Chronic administration of statins alters multiple gene expression patterns in mouse cerebral cortex. J. Pharmacol. Exp. Ther. 312, 786−793.

Johnson-Anuna, L.N., Eckert, G.P., Franke, C., Igbavboa, U., Müller, W.E., et al., 2007. Simvastatin protects neurons from cytotoxicity by up-regulating Bcl-2 mRNA and protein. J. Neurochem. 101, 77−86.

Kabadi, S.V., Faden, A.I., 2014. Neuroprotective strategies for traumatic brain injury: improving clinical translation. Int. J. Mol. Sci. 15, 1216−1236.

Kandola, A., Hendrikse, J., Lucassen, P.J., Yücel, M., 2016. Aerobic exercise as a tool to improve hippocampal plasticity and function in humans: practical implications for mental health treatment. Front. Hum. Neurosci. 10, 373.

Kaplan, D.R., Miller, F.D., 2007. Developing with BDNF: a moving experience. Neuron 55, 1−2.

Kassem, M., Abdallah, B.M., 2008. Human bone-marrow-derived mesenchymal stem cells: biological characteristics and potential role in therapy of degenerative diseases. Cell Tissue Res. 331, 157−163.

Kato, J., Hirata, S., Nozawa, A., Yamada-Mouri, N., 1994. Gene expression of progesterone receptor isoforms in the rat brain. Horm. Behav. 28, 454−463.

Kawakita, E., Hashimoto, M., Shido, O., 2006. Docosahexaenoic acid promotes neurogenesis in vitro and in vivo. Neuroscience 139, 991−997.

Khanna, A., Walcott, B.P., Kahle, K.T., Simard, J.M., 2014. Effect of glibenclamide on the prevention of secondary brain injury following ischemic stroke in humans. Neurosurg. Focus 36, E11.

Kim, D.K., Nishida, H., An, S.Y., Shetty, A.K., Bartosh, T.J., et al., 2016. Chromatographically isolated CD63 + CD81 + extracellular vesicles from mesenchymal stromal cells rescue cognitive impairments after TBI. Proc. Natl. Acad. Sci. USA. 113, 170–175.

Kim, H.S., Suh, Y.H., 2009. Minocycline and neurodegenerative diseases. Behav. Brain Res. 196, 168–179.

Kirsch, C., Eckert, G.P., Müller, W.E., 2003. Statin effects on cholesterol microdomains in brain plasma membranes. Biochem. Pharmacol. 65, 843–856.

Kline, A.E., Leary, J.B., Radabaugh, H.L., Cheng, J.P., Bondi, C.O., 2016. Combination therapies for neurobehavioral and cognitive recovery after experimental traumatic brain injury: is more better? Prog. Neurobiol. 142, 45–67.

Kurland, D.B., Tosun, C., Pampori, A., et al., 2013. Glibenclamide for the treatment of acute CNS injury. Pharmaceuticals (Basel) 6, 1287–1303.

Laupacis, A., Keown, P.A., Ulan, R.A., McKenzie, N., Stiller, C.R., 1982. Cyclosporin A: a powerful immunosuppressant. Can. Med. Assoc. J. 126, 1041–1046.

Lei, P., Li, Y., Chen, X., Yang, S., Zhang, J., 2009. Microarray based analysis of microRNA expression in rat cerebral cortex after traumatic brain injury. Brain Res. 1284, 191–201.

Lenzlinger, P.M., Saatman, K., Raghupathi, R., 2001. Overview of basic mechanisms underlying neuropathological consequences of head trauma. In: Miller, G., Hayes, R. (Eds.), Head Trauma: Basic, Preclinical, and Clinical Directions. Wiley-Liss, New Jersey, pp. 3–36.

Levine, E.S., Dreyfus, C.F., Black, I.B., Plummer, M.R., 1996. Selective role for trkB neurotrophin receptors in rapid modulation of hippocampal synaptic transmission. Brain Res. Mol. Brain Res. 38, 300–303.

Ley, E.J., Park, R., Dagliyan, G., Palestrant, D., Miller, C.M., et al., 2010. In vivo effect of propranolol dose and timing on cerebral perfusion after traumatic brain injury. J. Trauma 68, 353–356.

Lewis, M., Ghassemi, P., Hibbeln, J., 2013. Therapeutic use of omega-3 fatty acids in severe head trauma. Am. J. Emerg. Med. 31 (273), e5–e8.

Li, B., Mahmood, A., Lu, D., Wu, H., Xiong, Y., et al., 2009. Simvastatin attenuates microglial cells and astrocyte activation and decreases interleukin-1beta level after traumatic brain injury. Neurosurgery 65, 179–185.

Li, X., Chen, C., Yang, X., Wang, J., Zhao, M.L., Sun, H., et al., 2017. Acupuncture improved neurological recovery after traumatic brain injury by activating BDNF/TrkB pathway. Evid. Based Complement. Alternat Med. 2017, 8460145.

Liao, G.P., Harting, M.T., Hetz, R.A., et al., 2015. Autologous bone marrow mononuclear cells reduce therapeutic intensity for severe traumatic brain injury in children. Pediatr. Crit. Care Med. 16, 245–255.

Liu, J., Farmer Jr, J.D., Lane, W.S., Friedman, J., Weissman, I., et al., 1991. Calcineurin is a common target of cyclophilin-cyclosporin A and FKBP-FK506 complexes. Cell 66, 807–815.

Loane, D.J., Faden, A.I., 2010. Neuroprotection for traumatic brain injury: translational challenges and emerging therapeutic strategies. Trends Pharmacol. Sci. 31, 596–604.

Loane, D.J., Stoica, B.A., Faden, A.I., 2015. Neuroprotection for traumatic brain injury. Handb. Clin. Neurol. 127, 343–366.

Loftus, T.J., Efron, P.A., Moldawer, L.L., Mohr, A.M., 2016. β-Blockade use for traumatic injuries and immunomodulation: a review of proposed mechanisms and clinical evidence. Shock 46, 341–351.

Longhi, L., Zanier, E.R., Royo, N., Stocchetti, N., McIntosh, T.K., 2005. Stem cell transplantation as a therapeutic strategy for traumatic brain injury. Transpl. Immunol. 15, 143–148.

Lu, D., Mahmood, A., Wang, L., Li, Y., Lu, M., et al., 2001. Adult bone marrow stromal cells administered intravenously to rats after traumatic brain injury migrate into brain and improve neurological outcome. Neuroreport 12, 559–563.

Lu, D., Goussev, A., Chen, J., Pannu, P., Li, Y., et al., 2004. Atorvastatin reduces neurological deficit and increases synaptogenesis, angiogenesis, and neuronal survival in rats subjected to traumatic brain injury. J. Neurotrauma 21, 21–32.

Lu, D., Qu, C., Goussev, A., Jiang, H., Lu, C., et al., 2007a. Statins increase neurogenesis in the dentate gyrus, reduce delayed neuronal death in the hippocampal CA3 region, and improve spatial learning in rat after traumatic brain injury. J. Neurotrauma 24, 1132–1146.

Lu, D., Mahmood, A., Qu, C., Hong, X., Kaplan, D., et al., 2007b. Collagen scaffolds populated with human marrow stromal cells reduce lesion volume and improve functional outcome after traumatic brain injury. Neurosurgery 61, 596–602.

Lv, Q., Lan, W., Sun, W., Ye, R., Fan, X., et al., 2014. Intranasal nerve growth factor attenuates tau phosphorylation in brain after traumatic brain injury in rats. J. Neurol. Sci. 345, 48–55.

Machado, L.S., Kozak, A., Erqul, A., Hess, D.C., Borlougan, C.V., et al., 2006. Delayed minocycline inhibits ischemia-activated matrix metalloproteinases 2 and 9 after experimental stroke. BMC 7, 56.

Mahmood, A., Lu, D., Chopp, M., 2004. Intravenous administration of marrow stromal cells (MSCs) increases the expression of growth factors in rat brain after traumatic brain injury. J. Neurotrauma 21, 33–39.

Mahmood, A., Lu, D., Qu, C., Goussev, A., Chopp, M., et al., 2005. Human marrow stromal cell treatment provides long-lasting benefit after traumatic brain injury in rats. Neurosurgery 57, 1026–1031. Discussion-31.

Mahmood, A., Lu, D., Qu, C., Goussev, A., Zhang, Y., et al., 2009a. Treatment of traumatic brain injury in rats with erythropoietin and carbamylated erythropoietin. J. Neurosurg. 107, 392–397.

Mahmood, A., Gousser, A., Kazmi, H., Qu, C., Lu, D., Chopp, M., et al., 2009b. Long-term benefits after treatment of traumatic brain injury with simvastatin in rats. Neurosurgery 65, 187–191.

Mahmood, A., Wu, H., Qu, C., Mahmood, S., Xiong, Y., et al., 2014a. Suppression of neurocan and enhancement of axonal density in rats after treatment of traumatic brain injury with scaffolds impregnated with bone marrow stromal cells. J. Neurosurg. 120, 1147–1155.

Mahmood, A., Wu, H., Qu, C., Mahmood, S., Xiong, Y., et al., 2014b. Down-regulation of Nogo-A by collagen scaffolds impregnated with bone marrow stromal cell treatment after traumatic brain injury promotes axonal regeneration in rats. Brain Res. 1542, 41–48.

Maiese, K., Chong, Z.Z., Hou, J., Shang, Y.C., 2008. Erythropoietin and oxidative stress. Curr. Neurovasc. Res. 5, 125–142.

Maiese, K., Chong, Z.Z., Shang, Y.C., Wang, S., 2012. Erythropoietin: new directions for the nervous system. Int. J. Mol. Sci. 13, 11102–11129.

Manko, G., Ziolkowski, A., Mirski, A., Kłosiński, M., 2013. The effectiveness of selected tai chi exercises in a program of strategic rehabilitation aimed at improving the self-care skills of patients aroused from prolonged coma after severe TBI. Med. Sci. Monit. 19, 767–772.

Marchand, F., Tsantoulas, C., Singh, D., Grist, J., Clark, A.K., et al., 2009. Effects of Etanercept and Minocycline in a rat model of spinal cord injury. Eur. J. Pain 13, 673–681.

Marti, H.H., 2004. Erythropoietin and the hypoxic brain. J. Exp. Biol. 207, 3233–3242.

Marshall, J., Szmydynger-Chodobska, J., Rioult-Pedotti, M.S., Lau, K., Chin, A.T., et al., 2017. TrkB-enhancer facilitates functional recovery after traumatic brain injury. Sci. Rep. 7, 10995.

Mattson, M.P., Scheff, S.W., 1994. Endogenous neuroprotection factors and traumatic brain injury: mechanisms of action and implications for therapy. J. Neurotrauma 11, 3–33.

Mazzeo, A.T., Alves, O.L., Gilman, C.B., Hayes, R.L., Tolias, C., et al., 2008. Brain metabolic and hemodynamic effects of cyclosporin A after human severe traumatic brain injury: a microdialysis study. Acta Neurochir. 150, 1019–1031.

Mazzeo, A.T., Beat, A., Singh, A., Bullock, M.R., 2009. The role of mitochondrial transition pore, and its modulation, in traumatic brain injury and delayed neurodegeneration after TBI. Exp. Neurol. 218, 363–370.

Mbye, L.H., Singh, I.N., Carrico, K.M., Saatman, K.E., Hall, E.D., 2009. Comparative neuroprotective effects of cyclosporin A and NIM811, a nonimmunosuppressive cyclosporin A analog, following traumatic brain injury. J. Cereb. Blood Flow Metab. 29, 87–97.

Melcangi, R.C., Giatti, S., Calabrese, D., Pesaresi, M., Cermenati, G., et al., 2014. Levels and actions of progesterone and its metabolites in the nervous system during physiological and pathological conditions. Prog. Neurobiol. 113, 56–69.

Menkü, A., Koç, R.K., Tayfur, V., Saraymen, R., Narin, F., Akdemir, H., 2003. Effects of mexiletine, ginkgo biloba extract (EGb 761), and their combination on experimental head injury. Neurosurg. Rev. 26, 288–291.

Merlio, J.P., Ernfors, P., Kokaia, Z., Middlemas, D.S., Bengzon, J., et al., 1993. Increased production of the TrkB protein tyrosine kinase receptor after brain insults. Neuron 10, 151–164.

Migliaccio, A., Piccolo, D., Castoria, G., Di Domenico, M., Bilancio, A., et al., 1998. Activation of the Src/p21ras/Erk pathway by progesterone receptor via cross-talk with estrogen receptor. EMBO J. 17, 2008–2018.

Mirzayan, M.J., Klinge, P.M., Ude, S., Hotop, A., Samii, M., et al., 2008. Modified calcium accumulation after controlled cortical impact under cyclosporin A treatment: a 45Ca autoradiographic study. Neurol. Res. 30, 476–479.

Monnier, P.P., Sierra, A., Schwab, J.M., Henke-Fahle, S., et al., 2003. The Rho/ROCK pathway mediates neurite growth-inhibitory activity associated with the chondroitin sulfate proteoglycans of the CNS glial scar. Mol. Cell. Neurosci. 22, 319–330.

Morris, D.C., Chopp, M., Zhang, L., Zhang, Z.G., 2010. Thymosinbeta4: a candidate for treatment of stroke? Ann. N. Y. Acad. Sci. 1194, 112–117.

Nakazawa, T., Takahashi, H., Nishijima, K., Shimura, Fuse, N., 2007. Pitavastatin prevents NMDA-induced retinal ganglion cell death by suppressing leukocyte recruitment. J. Neurochem. 100, 1018–1031.

Nam, M.-H., Ahn, K.S., Choi, S.-H., 2013. Acupuncture stimulation induces neurogenesis in adult brain. Int. Rev. Neurobiol. 111, 67–90.

Nathoo, N., Narotam, P.K., Agrawal, D.K., Connolly, C.A., van Dellen, J.R., Barnett, G.H., et al., 2004. Influence of apoptosis on neurological outcome following traumatic cerebral contusion. J. Neurosurg. 101, 233–240.

Neeper, S.A., Gomez-Pinilla, F., Choi, J., Cotman, C.W., 1996. Physical activity increases mRNA for brain-derived neurotrophic factor and nerve growth factor in rat brain. Brain Res. 726, 49–56.

Nichol, A., French, C., Little, L., Haddad, S., Presneill, J., Arabi, Y., et al., 2015. Erythropoietin in traumatic brain injury (EPO-TBI): a double-blind randomised controlled trial. Lancet 386, 2499–2506.

Numakawa, T., Suzuki, S., Kumamaru, E., Adachi, N., Richards, M., et al., 2010. BDNF function and intracellular signaling in neurons. Histol. Histopathol. 25, 237–258.

Okonkwo, D.O., Melon, D.E., Pellicane, A.J., Mutlu, L.K., Rubin, D.G., et al., 2003. Dose-response of cyclosporin A in attenuating traumatic axonal injury in rat. Neuroreport 14, 463–466.

Oyesiku, N.M., Evans, C.O., Houston, S., Darrell, R.S., Smith, J.S., et al., 1999. Regional changes in the expression of neurotrophic factors and their receptors following acute traumatic brain injury in the adult rat brain. Brain Res. 833, 161–172.

Pan, D.S., Liu, W.G., Yang, X.F., Cao, F., 2007. Inhibitory effect of progesterone on inflammatory factors after experimental traumatic brain injury. Biomed. Environ. Sci. 20, 432–438.

Panten, U., Schwanstecher, M., Schwanstecher, C., 1996. Sulfonylurea receptors and mechanism of sulfonylurea action. Exp. Clin. Endocrinol. Diabetes 104, 1–9.

Patel, A.D., Gerzanich, V., Geng, Z., Simard, J.M., 2010. Glibenclamide reduces hippocampal injury and preserves rapid spatial learning in a model of traumatic brain injury. J. Neuropathol. Exp. Neurol. 69, 1177–1190.

Patel, M.B., McKenna, J.W., Alvarez, J.M., Sugiura, A., Jenkins, J.M., et al., 2012. Decreasing adrenergic or sympathetic hyperactivity after severe traumatic brain injury using propranolol and clonidine (DASH After TBI Study): study protocol for a randomized controlled trial. Trials 13, 177.

Patel, N.S., Collino, M., Yaqoob, M.M., et al., 2011. Erythropoietin in the intensive care unit: beyond treatment of anemia. Ann. Intensive Care 1, 40.

Peng, W., Xing, Z., Yang, J., et al., 2014. The efficacy of erythropoietin in treating experimental traumatic brain injury: a systematic review of controlled trials in animal models. J. Neurosurg. 121, 653–664.

Povlishock, J.T., Wei, E.P., 2009. Posthypothermic rewarming considerations following traumatic brain injury. J. Neurotrauma 26, 333–340.

Qu, C., Mahmood, A., Lu, D., Goussev, A., Xiong, Y., et al., 2008. Treatment of traumatic brain injury in mice with marrow stromal cells. Brain Res. 1208, 234–239.

Reagan, L.P., 2007. Insulin signaling effects on memory and mood. Curr. Opin. Pharmacol. 7, 633–637.

Redell, J.B., Moore, A.N., Ward 3rd, N.H., Hergenroeder, G.W., Dash, P.K., 2010. Human traumatic brain injury alters plasma microRNA levels. J. Neurotrauma 27, 2147–2156.

Redell, J.B., Zhao, J., Dash, P.K., 2011. Altered expression of miRNA-21 and its targets in the hippocampus after traumatic brain injury. J. Neurosci. Res. 89, 212–221.

Roberts, I., Yates, D., Sandercock, P., Farrell, B., Wasserberg, J., et al., 2004. Effect of intravenous corticosteroids on death within 14 days in 10008 adults with clinically significant head injury (MRC CRASH trial): randomised placebo-controlled trial. Lancet 364, 1321–1328.

Roberts, I., Shakur, H., Coats, T., Hunt, B., Balogun, E., et al., 2013. The CRASH-2 trial: a randomised controlled trial and economic evaluation of the effects of tranexamic acid on death, vascular occlusive events and transfusion requirement in bleeding trauma patients. Health Technol. Assess. 17, 1–79.

Robertson, C.S., Hannay, H.J., Yamal, J.M., Yamal, J.M., Gopinath, S., et al., 2014. Effect of erythropoietin and transfusion threshold on neurological recovery after traumatic brain injury: a randomized clinical trial. JAMA 312, 36–47.

Rollnik, J.D., Berlinghof, K., Lenz, O., Bertomeu, A.M., 2010. Mechanical ventilation in neurological early rehabilitation. Akt Neurol. 37, 316–318.

Roof, R.L., Hoffman, S.W., Stein, D.G., 1997. Progesterone protects against lipid peroxidation following traumatic brain injury in rats. Mol. Chem. Neuropathol. 31, 1–11.

Rosenberg, G., 2007. The mechanisms of action of valproate in neuropsychiatric disorders: can we see the forest for the trees? Cell. Mol. Life Sci. 64, 2090–2103.

Roth, T.L., Nayak, D., Atanasijevic, T., Koretsky, A.P., Latour, L.L., et al., 2014. Transcranial amelioration of inflammation and cell death after brain injury. Nature 505, 223–228.

Sahuguillo, J., Vilalta, A., 2009. Cooling the injured brain: how does moderate hypothermia influence the pathophysiology of traumatic brain injury. Curr. Pharm. Des. 13, 2310–2322.

Sandhir, R., Gregory, E., Berman, N.E., 2014. Differential response of miRNA-21 and its targets after traumatic brain injury in aging mice. Neurochem. Int. 78, 117–121.

Sara, V.R., Carlsson-Skwirut, C., Bergman, T., Jörnvall, H., Roberts, P.J., et al., 1989. Identification of Gly-Pro-Glu (GPE), the aminoterminal tripeptide of insulin-like growth factor 1 which is truncated in brain, as a novel neuroactive peptide. Biochem. Biophys. Res. Commun. 165, 766–771.

Sayeed, I., Stein, D.G., 2009. Progesterone as a neuroprotective factor in traumatic and ischemic brain injury. Prog. Brain Res. 175, 219–237.

Schmid, A.A., Miller, K.K., Van Puymbroeck, M., Schalk, N., 2016. Feasibility and results of a case study of yoga to improve physical functioning in people with chronic traumatic brain injury. Disabil. Rehabil. 38, 914–920.

Schober, M.E., Requena, D.F., Abdullah, O.M., Casper, T.C., Beachy, J., et al., 2016. Dietary docosahexaenoic acid improves cognitive function, tissue sparing, and magnetic resonance imaging indices of edema and white matter injury in the immature rat after traumatic brain injury. J. Neurotrauma 33, 390–402.

Shakur, H., Roberts, I., Bautista, R., Caballero, J., Coats, T., Dewan, Y., et al., 2010. Effects of tranexamic acid on death, vascular occlusive events, and blood transfusion in trauma patients with significant haemorrhage (CRASH-2): a randomised, placebo-controlled trial. Lancet 376, 23–32.

Shannon, R.J., Carpenter, K.L., Guilfoyle, M.R., Helmy, A., Hutchinson, P.J., 2013. Cerebral microdialysis in clinical studies of drugs: pharmacokinetic applications. J. Pharmacokinet. Pharmacodyn. 40, 343–358.

Sheth, K.N., Kimberly, W.T., Elm, J.J., et al., 2014. Pilot study of intravenous glyburide in patients with a large ischemic stroke. Stroke 45, 281–283.

Shen, Y., Tenney, A.P., Busch, S.A., Horn, K.P., Cuascut, F.X., et al., 2009. PTPsigma is a receptor for chondroitin sulfate proteoglycan, an inhibitor of neural regeneration. Science 326, 592–596.

Shi, G.-X., Wang, X.-R., Yan, C.-Q., He, T., Yang, J.W., et al., 2015. Acupuncture elicits neuroprotective effect by inhibiting NAPDH oxidase-mediated reactive oxygen species production in cerebral ischaemia. Sci. Rep. 2015, 17981.

Si, D., Wang, H., Wang, Q., Zhang, C., Sun, J., et al., 2013. Progesterone treatment improves cognitive outcome following experimental traumatic brain injury in rats. Neurosci. Lett. 553, 18–23.

Signoretti, S., Marmarou, A., Tavazzi, B., Dunbar, J., Amorini, A.M., et al., 2004. The protective effect of cyclosporin A upon N-acetylaspartate and mitochondrial dysfunction following experimental diffuse traumatic brain injury. J. Neurotrauma 21, 1154–1167.

Simard, J.M., Chen, M., Tarasov, K.V., Bhatta, S., Ivanova, S., Melnitchenko, L., et al., 2006. Newly expressed SUR1-regulated NC(Ca-ATP) channel mediates cerebral edema after ischemic stroke. Nat. Med. 12, 433–440.

Simard, J.M., Yurovsky, V., Tsymbalyuk, N., Melnichenko, L., Ivanova, S., et al., 2009. Protective effect of delayed treatment with low-dose glibenclamide in three models of ischemic stroke. Stroke 40, 604–609.

Simard, J.M., Woo, S.K., Tsymbalyuk, N., Voloshyn, O., Yurovsky, V., et al., 2012. Glibenclamide-10-h treatment window in a clinically relevant model of stroke. Transl. Stroke Res. 3, 286–295.

Singh, M., 2001. Ovarian hormones elicit phosphorylation of Akt and extracellular signal regulated kinase in explants of the cerebral cortex. Endocrine 14, 407—415.

Siren, A.L., Knerlich, F., Poser, W., Gleiter, C.H., Bruck, W., 2001. Erythropoietin and erythropoietin receptor in human ischemic/hypoxic brain. Acta Neuropathol. 101, 271—276.

Skaper, S.D., Moore, S.E., Walsh, F.S., 2001. Cell signaling cascades regulating neuronal growth-promoting and inhibitory cues. Prog. Neurobiol. 65, 593—608.

Skolnick, B.E., Maas, A.I., Narayan, R.K., et al., 2014. A clinical trial of progesterone for severe traumatic brain injury. N. Engl. J. Med. 371, 2467—2476.

Smith, S.S., 1991. Progesterone administration attenuates excitatory amino acid responses of cerebellar Purkinje cells. Neuroscience 42, 309—320.

Springborg, J.B., Sonne, B., Frederiksen, H.J., Foldager, N., Poulsgaard, L., 2003. Erythropoietin in the cerebrospinal fluid of patients with aneurysmal subarachnoid haemorrhage originates from the brain. Brain Res. 984, 143—148.

Stein, D.G., 2013. A clinical/translational perspective: can a developmental hormone play a role in the treatment of traumatic brain injury? Horm. Behav. 63, 291—300.

Stoorvogel, W., Kleijmeer, M.J., Geuze, H.J., Raposo, G., 2002. The biogenesis and functions of exosomes. Traffic 3, 321—330.

Stranahan, A.M., Norman, E.D., Lee, K., Cutler, R.G., Telljohann, R.S., Egan, J.M., et al., 2008. Diet-induced insulin resistance impairs hippocampal synaptic plasticity and cognition in middle-aged rats. Hippocampus 18, 1085—1088.

Stroth, S., Reinhardt, R.K., Thöne, J., Hille, K., Schneider, M., et al., 2010. Impact of aerobic exercise training on cognitive functions and affect associated to the COMT polymorphism in young adults. Neurobiol. Learn. Mem. 94, 364—372.

Sullivan, P.G., Rabchevsky, A.G., Hicks, R.R., Gibson, T.R., Fletcher-Turner, A., et al., 2000. Dose-response curve and optimal dosing regimen of cyclosporin A after traumatic brain injury in rats. Neuroscience 101, 289—295.

Sun, W., Kim, H., 2007. Neurotrophic roles of the beta-thymosins in the development and regeneration of the nervous system. Ann. N. Y. Acad. Sci. 1112, 210—218.

Tai, Y.T., Lee, W.Y., Lee, F.P., Lin, T.J., Shih, C.L., et al., 2014. Low dose of valproate improves motor function after traumatic brain injury. Biomed. Res. Int. 2014, 980657.

Taylor, C.A., Bell, J.M., Breiding, M.J., Xu, L., 2017. Traumatic Brain Injury-Related Emergency Department Visits, Hospitalizations, and Deaths-United States, 2007 and 2013. MMWR Surveill. Summ. 66, 1—16.

Temkin, N.R., Dikmen, S.S., Anderson, G.D., Wilensky, A.J., Holmes, M.D., et al., 1999. Valproate therapy for prevention of posttraumatic seizures: a randomized trial. J. Neurosurg. 91, 593—600.

Thelin, E.P., Carpenter, K.L., Hutchinson, P.J., Helmy, A., 2017. Microdialysis monitoring in clinical traumatic brain injury and its role in neuroprotective drug development. AAPS J. 19, 367—376.

Tian, C., Wang, X., Wang, L., Wang, L., Wang, X., et al., 2013. Autologous bone marrow mesenchymal stem cell therapy in the subacute stage of traumatic brain injury by lumbar puncture. Exp. Clin. Transplant. 11, 176—181.

Tian, L., Guo, R., Yue, X., Lv, Q., Ye, X., et al., 2012. Intranasal administration of nerve growth factor ameliorate beta-amyloid deposition after traumatic brain injury in rats. Brain Res. 1440, 47—55.

Tian, T., Sun, Y., Wu, H., et al., 2016. Acupuncture promotes mTOR-independent autophagic clearance of aggregation-prone proteins in mouse brain. Sci. Rep. 6, 19714.

Tosun, C., Kurland, D.B., Mehta, R., Castellani, R.J., deJong, J.L., et al., 2013a. Inhibition of the Sur1-Trpm4 channel reduces neuroinflammation and cognitive impairment in subarachnoid hemorrhage. Stroke 44, 3522—3528.

Tosun, C., Koltz, M.T., Kurland, D.B., Ijaz, H., Gurakar, M., et al., 2013b. The protective effect of glibenclamide in a model of hemorrhagic encephalopathy of prematurity. Brain Sci. 3, 215−238.

Tsujimoto, Y., Shimizu, S., 2007. Role of the mitochondrial membrane permeability transition in cell death. Apoptosis 12, 835−840.

Van Den Heuvel, C., Donkin, J.J., Finnie, J.W., Blumbergs, P.C., Kuchel, T., et al., 2004. Downregulation of amyloid precursor protein (APP) expression following post-traumatic cyclosporin-A administration. J. Neurotrauma 21, 1562−1572.

van Praag, H., Kempermann, G., Gage, F.H., 1999. Running increases cell proliferation and neurogenesis in the adult mouse dentate gyrus. Nat. Neurosci. 2, 266−270.

van Praag, H., Shubert, T., Zhao, C., Gage, F.H., 2005. Exercise enhances learning and hippocampal neurogenesis in aged mice. J. Neurosci. 25, 8680−8685.

Vaughan, C.J., 2003. Prevention of stroke and dementia with statins: effects beyond lipid lowering. Am. J. Cardiol. 91, 23B−29B.

Vuletic, S., Riekse, R.G., Marcovina, S.M., Peskind, E.R., Hazzard, W.R., et al., 2006. Statins of different brain penetrability differentially affect CSFPLTP activity. Dement. Geriatr. Cogn. Disord. 22, 392−398.

Wali, B., Ishrat, T., Atif, F., Hua, F., Stein, D.G., et al., 2012. Glibenclamide administration attenuates infarct volume, hemispheric swelling, and functional impairments following permanent focal cerebral ischemia in rats. Stroke Res. Treat. 460909.

Wang, Y., Guo, F., Pan, C., Lou, Y., Zhang, P., et al., 2012. Effects of low temperatures on proliferation-related signaling pathways in the hippocampus after traumatic brain injury. Exp. Biol. Med. (Maywood) 237, 1424−1432.

Wang, W.X., Wilfred, B.R., Madathil, S.K., Tang, G., Hu, Y., et al., 2010. miR-107 regulates granulin/progranulin with implications for traumatic brain injury and neurodegenerative disease. Am. J. Pathol. 177, 334−345.

Warren, A.M., Boals, A., Elliott, T.R., Reynolds, M., Weddle, R.J., et al., 2015. Mild traumatic brain injury increases risk for the development of posttraumatic stress disorder. J. Trauma Acute Care Surg. 79, 1062−1066.

Wei, H.H., Lu, X.C., Shear, D.A., Waghray, A., Yao, C., et al., 2009. NNZ-2566 treatment inhibits neuroinflammation and pro-inflammatory cytokine expression induced by experimental penetrating ballistic-like brain injury in rats. J. Neuroinflammation 6, 19.

Wible, E.F., Laskowitz, D.T., 2010. Statins in traumatic brain injury. Neurotherapeutics 7, 62−73.

Woo, S.K., Kwon, M.S., Ivanov, A., Gerzanich, V., Simard, J.M., 2013. The sulfonylurea receptor 1 (Sur1)-transient receptor potential melastatin 4 (Trpm4) channel. J. Biol. Chem. 288, 3655−3667.

Wright, D.W., Yeatts, S.D., Silbergleit, R., Palesch, Y.Y., Hertzberg, V.S., Frankel, M., et al., 2014. Very early administration of progesterone for acute traumatic brain injury. N. Engl. J. Med. 371, 2457−2466.

Wu, A., Ying, Z., Gomez-Pinilla, F., 2007. Omega-3 fatty acids supplementation restores mechanisms that maintain brain homeostasis in traumatic brain injury. J. Neurotrauma 24, 1587−1595.

Wu, C.H., Hung, T.H., Chen, C.C., Ke, C.H., Lee, C.Y., et al., 2014. Post-injury treatment with 7,8-dihydroxyflavone, a TrkB receptor agonist, protects against experimental traumatic brain injury via PI3K/Akt signaling. PLoS One 9, e113397.

Wu, H., Lu, D., Jiang, H., Xiong, Y., Qu, C., et al., 2008a. Increase in phosphorylation of Akt and its downstream signaling targets and suppression of apoptosis by simvastatin after traumatic brain injury. J. Neurosurg. 109, 691−698.

Wu, H., Lu, D., Jiang, H., Xiong, Y., Qu, C., et al., 2008b. Simvastatin-mediated upregulation of VEGF and BDNF, activation of the PI3K/Akt pathway, and increase of neurogenesis are associated with therapeutic improvement after traumatic brain injury. J. Neurotrauma 25, 130–139.

Wu, J., Yang, S., Xi, G., Fu, G., Keep, R.F., et al., 2009. Minocycline reduces intracerebral hemorrhage-induced brain injury. Neurol. Res. 31, 183–188.

Xiong, Y., Mahmood, A., Meng, Y., Zhang, Y., Qu, C., et al., 2009. Delayed administration of erythropoietin reducing hippocampal cell loss, enhancing angiogenesis and neurogenesis, and improving functional outcome following traumatic brain injury in rats: comparison of treatment with single and triple dose. J. Neurosurg. 113, 598–608.

Xiong, Y., Mahmood, A., Meng, Y., et al., 2011. Treatment of traumatic brain injury with thymosin beta(4) in rats. J. Neurosurg. 114, 102–115.

Xiong, Y., Zhang, Y., Mahmood, A., Chopp, M., 2015. Investigational agents for treatment of traumatic brain injury. Expert Opin. Investig. Drugs 24, 743–760.

Xiong, Y., Mahmood, A., Chopp, M., 2017. Emerging potential of exosomes for treatment of traumatic brain injury. Neural Regen. Res. 12, 19–22.

Xu, Q., Yang, J.-W., Cao, Y., Zhang, L.W., Zeng, X.H., et al., 2015. Acupuncture improves locomotor function by enhancing GABA receptor expression in transient focal cerebral ischemia rats. Neurosci. Lett. 588, 88–94.

Yama, K., Nabeshima, T., 2004. Interaction of BDNF/TrkB signaling with NMDA receptors in learning and memory. Drug News Perspect. 17, 435–438.

Yamashita, T., 2007. Molecular mechanism and regulation of axon growth inhibition. Brain Nerve 59, 1347–1353.

Yang, D., Xie, P., Guo, S., Li, H., 2009. Induction of MAPK phosphatase-1 by hypothermia inhibits TNF-(alpha)-induced endothelial barrier dysfunction and apoptosis. Cardiovasc. Res. 85, 520–529.

Yang, K., Perez-Polo, J.R., Mu, X.S., Yan, H.Q., Xue, J.J., et al., 1996. Increased expression of brain-derived neurotrophic factor but not neurotrophin-3 mRNA in rat brain after cortical impact injury. J. Neurosci. Res. 44, 157–164.

Yang, Y., Ye, Y., Su, X., He, J., Bai, W., et al., 2017. MSCs-derived exosomes and neuroinflammation, neurogenesis and therapy of traumatic brain injury. Front. Cell Neurosci. 11, 55.

Yoshii, A., Constantine-Paton, M., 2010. Postsynaptic BDNF-TrkB signaling in synapse maturation, plasticity, and disease. Dev. Neurobiol. 70, 304–322.

Yutthakasemsunt, S., Kittiwatanagul, W., Piyavechvirat, P., et al., 2013. Tranexamic acid for patients with traumatic brain injury: a randomized, double-blinded, placebo-controlled trial. BMC Emerg. Med. 13, 20.

Zehtabchi, S., Abdel Baki, S.G., Falzon, L., Nishijima, D.K., 2014. Tranexamic acid for traumatic brain injury: a systematic review and meta-analysis. Am. J. Emerg. Med 32, 1503–1509.

Zeng, Y., Liu, Y., Wu, M., Liu, J., Hu, Q., 2012. Activation of TrkB by 7,8-dihydroxyflavone prevents fear memory defects and facilitates amygdalar synaptic plasticity in aging. J. Alzheimer's Dis. 31, 765–778.

Zhang, M., Wu, J., Ding, H., Wu, W., Xiao, G., et al., 2017. Progesterone provides the pleiotropic neuroprotective effect on traumatic brain injury through the Nrf2/ARE signaling pathway. Neurocrit. Care 26, 292–300.

Zhang, Y., Chopp, M., Meng, Y., Katakowski, M., Xin, H., et al., 2015. Effect of exosomes derived from multipluripotent mesenchymal stromal cells on functional recovery and neurovascular plasticity in rats after traumatic brain injury. J. Neurosurg. 122, 856–867.

Zhang, Y., Chopp, M., Zhang, Z.G., Katakowski, M., Xin, H., et al., 2016. Systemic administration of cell-free exosomes generated by human bone marrow derived mesenchymal stem cells cultured under 2D and 3D conditions improves functional recovery in rats after traumatic brain injury. Neurochem. Int. S0197-0186 (16), 30251–30260.

Zhang, Z.X., Guan, L.X., Zhang, K., Zhang, Q., Dai, L.J., 2008. A combined procedure to deliver autologous mesenchymal stromal cells to patients with traumatic brain injury. Cytotherapy 10, 134–139.

Zhou, Y., Fathali, N., Lekic, T., Tang, J., Zhang, J.H., 2009. Glibenclamide improves neurological function in neonatal hypoxia-ischemia in rats. Brain Res. 1270, 131–139.

Zweckberger, K., Hackenberg, K., Jung, C.S., Hertle, D.N., Kiening, K.L., et al., 2014. Glibenclamide reduces secondary brain damage after experimental traumatic brain injury. Neuroscience 272, 199–206.

Molecular Aspects of Concussion and Chronic Traumatic Encephalopathy

INTRODUCTION

Boxers and players of contact sports such as American football, wrestling, rugby, hockey, lacrosse, soccer, and skiing as well as military veterans expose themselves to repetitive concussions or mild traumatic injuries (mild traumatic brain injuries [mTBIs]) throughout their careers. According to the Centers for Disease Control (CDC), 1.4–3.8 million concussions occur annually in the United States (Laker, 2011). Attempts are underway to develop therapeutic treatments to deal with the effects of concussions as well as possible measures to prevent the secondary effects of concussion in military or sports related situations. These efforts are based on an understanding of what constitutes mild repeated traumatic brain injury (TBI), what conditions contribute to the severity of TBI, and what may be the treatment "window" for interventional therapeutics. It is becoming increasingly evident that concussion is a complex neurological syndrome induced by mild traumatic biomechanical acceleration and deceleration forces initiated by either a direct blow to the head, face, or neck or via excessive force elsewhere on the body transmitted to the head (Meaney et al., 1995; McCrory et al., 2009). When the brain is subjected to rapid acceleration, deceleration, and rotational forces, the brain elongates and deforms, stretching individual components such as neurons, glial cells, and blood vessels and altering membrane permeability. Concussion may also disrupt the blood—brain barrier (BBB) and result in multifaceted consequences. Secondary repercussions of postconcussion BBB dysfunction may manifest as neuronal loss, impaired consciousness, memory and motor impairment, cognitive decline, and even increased dementia risk (Omalu et al., 2005;

Ischemic and Traumatic Brain and Spinal Cord Injuries
DOI: https://doi.org/10.1016/B978-0-12-813596-9.00008-0

Guskiewicz et al., 2005). Importantly, the magnitude of postconcussion BBB dysfunction may influence the time course and extent of neuronal recovery. Some studies have indicated that forces that contribute to concussion can markedly effect and disrupt the neurons that run along the vestibulospinal tracts, control the vestibular−ocular reflex, and link central vestibular pathways (Fife and Giza, 2013; Nashner and Peters, 1990). In addition, peripheral vestibular receptors can also be injured during a concussion (Fife and Giza, 2013; Ouchterlony et al., 2016). Other studies indicate that traumatic stretch injuries not only affect neuronal cell bodies, axons, dendrites, blood vessels, and glial cells but also traumatized axons, which are often extend long distances from the neuronal cell bodies and may be injured even without the death of the neuron of origin (Povlishock, 1992). Concussions can vary from mild to severe. Symptoms of concussion include dizziness, nausea, confusion, disorientation, slow thinking, loss of balance, headaches, blurred or double vision, slurred speech, and amnesia (Fig. 8.1). Sport related concussion is the most common type of mTBI in youth and sports players account for over half of the concussions sustained by young players each year. The latest estimates from the CDC indicate that sport related concussions have increased to approximately 1.6−3.0 million per year

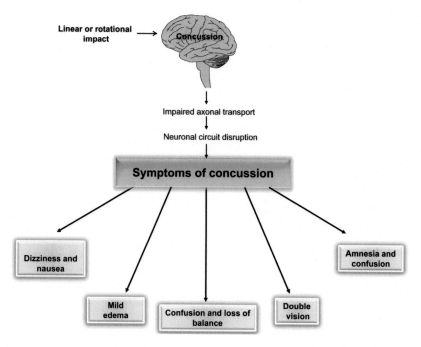

FIGURE 8.1   Symptoms concussion.

(Centers for Disease Control and Prevention, 2006). Moreover, recent studies report that the incidence of concussion at both the high school and collegiate level has been on the rise, as 8.9% of all high school and 5%—18% of all collegiate athletic injuries are concussions (Hootman et al., 2007; Bazarian et al., 2005, 2010; Langlois et al., 2006). In addition, concussion also occur in military personnel exposed to an explosive blast during their deployment in in Iraq and Afghanistan. Of the nearly 2 million military service members, 15%—25% of individuals have sustained at least one TBI during deployment (Hoge et al., 2008; Fortier et al., 2014). The vast majority of these injuries are identified as either mild or moderate (Defense and Veterans Brain Injury Center, 2016) and are often the direct result of either blunt force (direct blow to the head) or blast related (pressure wave from an explosive device) trauma. It has been hypothesized that concussions disrupt auditory processes (Kraus et al., 2016). Specifically, concussions disrupt the processing of the fundamental frequency, a key acoustic cue for identifying and tracking sounds and talkers, and, consequently, understanding speech in noise. Children, who sustained a concussion, exhibit a signature neural profile. They have worse representation of the fundamental frequency and smaller and more sluggish neural responses. Neurophysiological responses to the fundamental frequency partially recover to control levels as concussion symptoms abate, suggesting a gain in biological processing following partial recovery (Kraus et al., 2016). Neural processing of sound correctly identifies 90% of concussion cases and clears 95% of control cases, suggesting this approach has practical potential as a scalable biological marker for sports related concussion and other types of mTBIs. Collective evidence suggests that concussion is the mildest type of TBI, which typically results in altered brain function, in the absence of gross structural abnormalities. Symptoms of concussion (Fig. 8.1) can be resolved within 7—10 days in most adults (McCrory et al., 2009, 2013; Noble and Hesdorffer, 2013). Thus, most patients with concussion often recover spontaneously after a short period of time. However, long term consequences of concussion remain uncertain. Despite the transient nature of the clinical symptoms of concussion, neurochemical changes of concussion take over a month to return to baseline and neuropathological evaluation shows that concussion induced axonopathy may persist for years. The cumulative effects of multiple concussions or accumulation of subconcussive impacts remain poorly understood. Many studies have indicated that multiple concussions may cause greater functional impairments than mediated by only a single concussion (Longhi et al., 2005; Prins et al., 2013), indicating that long term structural changes may occur, possibly with each such incident (Giza and Kutcher, 2014). Furthermore, repeated concussions may cause long term cognitive, motor, and psychiatric deficits

(Riemann and Guskiewicz, 2000; Montenigro et al., 2016). Based on many animal and human studies, it is proposed that repeated concussions may cause gross and microscopic pathological changes in the brain leading into a condition called chronic traumatic encephalopathy (CTE) (see below) (McKee et al., 2009; Bennett and Brody, 2014). Thus, it is becoming increasingly evident that concussion is predominantly a functional or microstructural injury to neural tissue (axons). Functional axonal injury can refer to perturbations of cellular or physiological function including but not limited to ionic shifts, metabolic changes, or impaired neurotransmission. Microstructural injury refers to physical changes not readily evident on computed tomography (CT) scanning but can be detected by advanced neuroimaging techniques such as functional magnetic resonance imaging (MRI), resting state functional connectivity, diffusion tensor imaging (DTI), and magnetic resonance spectroscopy. DTI studies have indicated the presence of white matter (WM) injury indicating cortical network dysfunction in concussed individuals and using positron emission tomography (PET) ligands to the peripheral benzodiazepine receptor to confirm the presence of microglia and macrophage in TBI patients (Zhang et al., 2010; Cubon et al., 2011; Bazarian et al., 2012). Collectively, these techniques offer promising aid in research into understanding the complexities and nuances of concussion which may ultimately influence clinical management of the condition. It should be noted that in the American football game, specific positions may have a differential risk of concussion and exposure to subconcussive impacts leading to stroke and chronic neurodegenerative diseases (Lehman, 2013). It is proposed that "speed" players (quarterback, running back, wide receiver, defensive back, safety, linebacker, etc.) and "non speed" players (offensive and defensive lineman) may modulate the severity of concussion, due to the nature of their positions (Slobounov et al., 2017). "Speed" players often build up momentum prior to tackling or being tackled, whereas "non speed" players typically engage in hits immediately after the ball is snapped (Broglio et al., 2012; Pellman et al., 2004). However, there is still great debate regarding whether greater risk of concussion exists for players exposed to the higher magnitude impacts (i.e., speed players) or those exposed to the repetitive immediate head impacts (i.e., non speed players) (Slobounov et al., 2017). Of interest here, several studies have shown that linemen receive more cumulative impacts (especially at the front of the head) and develop more postimpact symptoms than other positions (Baugh et al., 2015; Crisco et al., 2010). Although the results of many football studies do not provide a cause−effect relationship between football related head injury and neurodegenerative disorders, a growing body of research supports the hypothesis that professional football players are at an increased risk of neurodegenerative diseases. Programs aimed to limit repeated concussion, particularly before recovery from an initial concussion, like return to play and return to work are all based on the provision of an accurate knowledge of the history of concussion symptoms by the patient to a doctor or another person such as a coach or an athletic trainer. As such, recognizing and understanding the symptoms of concussion is paramount for accurate patient management and for the prevention of future events. The clinical management of sports induced concussion has not changed much over the past decade.

NEUROCHEMICAL CHANGES IN CONCUSSION

The basic neurochemistry of concussion has been elucidated and perfected in animal models is increasingly corroborated in human studies. It is reported that a neurometabolic cascade of events that involves bioenergetic challenges produces oxidative stress, cytoskeletal and axonal alterations leading to abnormalities in signal transduction processes, impairments in neurotransmission resulting in decrease in neuroplasticity, memory loss, and behavioral changes and vulnerability to delayed cell death and chronic dysfunction leading to neuronal dysfunction (acidosis, membrane damage, altered BBB permeability, and cerebral edema promoting cognitive deficits) (Barkhoudarian et al., 2011; Giza and Hovda, 2014). Converging evidence suggests that pathophysiology of concussion involves a complex cascade of neurochemical changes, which include potassium efflux, and sodium and calcium influx, in discriminant release of excitatory neurotransmitter (glutamate) leading to neuronal membrane depolarization, acute hyperglycolysis, and subacute metabolic depression (MacFarlane and Glenn, 2015). Alterations in brain glucose metabolism vary with injury severity and age. Glucose metabolic depression can be maintained for 5, 10, or 14 days after mild, moderate, or severe fluid percussion injury in adults, respectively (Hovda et al., 1994). Duration of behavioral deficits in the Morris water maze also correlated with injury severity (Moore et al., 2000). Consequently, these metabolic changes not only induce impairment in neurotransmission and alterations in synaptic plasticity but also promote changes in protein expression (MacFarlane and Glenn, 2015). In order to restore ionic and cellular homeostasis, neuronal cell requires adenosine triphosphate (ATP) dependent membrane ionic pumps. Consequently, these pumps go into overdrive resulting in hyperglycolysis, causing a relative reduction in intracellular ATP, and elevation in adenosine diphosphate (ADP) (Yoshino et al., 1991). Thus, very early phase of concussion is accompanied by reduction in cerebral blood flow (CBF) and uncoupling or mismatch between energy supply and demand. This is followed by influx of calcium, which persists longer than other ionic disturbances. This leads into sequestration of calcium into mitochondria producing mitochondrial dysfunction and induction of oxidative stress along with neuroglial energy crisis in the injured brain. In addition to the acute neuroglial energy crisis, alterations in intracellular redox state are also observed following concussion This puts additional stress on the system through the generation of free radicals (superoxide anions, hydroxyl, alkoxyl, peroxyl radicals, and hydrogen peroxide) producing oxidative stress. This triggers not only long lasting impairments in neuronal function but also setting the stage for repeated neuronal injury, which is particularly relevant for the clinical setting of sports related concussion. In some cases, this type of injury may last for few days (3—7 days) causing behavioral impairments in spatial learning (Yoshino et al., 1991; Hovda, 1996). It is also reported that duration of this hypometabolic period may vary with age. Younger animals show shorter periods (3 days) of impairment, whereas older animals display longer periods (7—10 days) (Thomas et al., 2000). Posttraumatic changes in metabolism may cause alterations not only in gene expression (Li et al., 2004) but also in enzyme/transporter regulation (Tavazzi et al., 2007). The molecular mechanisms underlying the association between single or repetitive mTBI and progressive neurodegeneration are not fully understood. However, it is becoming increasingly evident that some biochemical tests of diffuse axonal, neuronal, and astroglial injury can be helpful in identifying a severe TBI from concussion. Based on many mTBI studies, it can be suggested that concussion is a complex brain injury, which is accompanied by diffuse axonal, microhemorrhage, microglial activation, and small vessel injury in the brain (McKee et al., 2014). Concussion may result in two primary complications namely postconcussion syndrome and second impact syndrome. The postconcussion syndrome is defined as persistence of concussion mediated symptomatology for greater than 3 months postinjury leading to both neurophysiological and neuropathological changes secondary to the initial concussion (Silverberg and Iverson, 2011). In contrast, second impact syndrome is defined as a condition in which a second head impact is sustained during a "vulnerable period" before the complete symptomatic resolution of the initial impact leading to profound engorgement, massive edema, and rapid elevation in intracranial pressure within minutes of the impact and resulting in brain herniation, edema, decrease in CBF followed by coma and death (Lam et al., 1997; Cantu, 1998). Second impact syndrome has a morbidity rate of 100% and a mortality rate of 50% (McCrory, 2001). In some subjects with concussion show somatic symptoms such as headache, dizziness/nausea, fatigue or lethargy, and changes in sleep pattern (Riggio and Wong, 2009). Neuropsychiatric sequelae after concussion include cognitive deficits and behavioral disorders, which are identified in almost all TBI patients for up to 3 months, with a small percentage exhibiting persistent (months–years) symptoms. Cognitive deficits are characterized not only by impaired attention, memory, and/or executive function but also irritability, anxiousness, and depression.

STANDARDIZED ASSESSMENT OF CONCUSSION

Although in recent years, many clinical tools have become available for the assessment of concussion (McCrea et al., 2003, 2005; Guskiewicz et al., 2003; Churchill et al., 2017), these tools are based on symptom scales, computerized neurocognitive tests, and balance assessment tools. However, there is no objective test that can confirm the concussion diagnosis. So, concussion remains a clinical diagnosis, which is based on the athlete's presenting signs and symptoms and the impression of the evaluating medical officer. Interestingly, the definition of concussion as a pathophysiological process is separate and distinct from the clinical presentation on which diagnosis is based. Without an objective test capable of confirming the presence or absence of cellular dysfunction, there is a degree of uncertainty about the diagnosis of concussion. The Standardized Assessment of Concussion (SAC) involves 6-minute administration, a test to assess four neurocognitive domains—orientation, immediate memory, concentration, and delayed recall—for use by nonphysicians on the sidelines of an athletic event. The SAC is likely to identify the presence of concussion in the early stages postinjury (sensitivity 80%–94%, specificity 76%–91%) (multiple Class III studies) (Barr and McCrea, 2001; McCrea et al., 2003, 2005). The SAC is based on neuropsychological testing, balance error scoring testing, and sensory organization testing (Giza et al., 2013). Collectively, these studies indicate that due to the subjective, complex, and, at times, ambiguous presentations of potentially concussed individuals, clinical outcomes research studying concussion must be interpreted with a potentially significant degree of diagnostic uncertainty and more studies are urgently needed on this important topic.

BIOCHEMICAL MARKERS OF CONCUSSION

As described in Chapter 6, Neurochemical Aspects of Traumatic Brain Injury, moderate and severe TBI can be easily identified because their signs and symptoms, but about 70%–90% of TBIs, which are mild are still difficult to recognize (Cassidy et al., 2004). Additionally, the World

Health Organization estimates that many mild injuries are not even seen by a health-care practitioner because this lack of obvious and urgent symptoms fails to motivate patients to seek care (Cassidy et al., 2004). Unfortunately, there are no currently accepted biomarkers for clinical diagnosis of concussions. Different organizations use schematic tools for diagnosis, but they are subjective and the organizations do not completely agree on what constitutes a concussion (Rutherford and Corrigan, 2009). At present, it must be admitted that there is insufficient information available on biomarkers of concussion. Potential biomarkers for distinguishing between focal injuries (skull fracture and brain contusion) and diffuse injuries [concussion, subdural hematoma, and diffuse axonal injury (DAI)] are astrocyte enriched proteins S100β and glial fibrillary acidic protein (GFAP), along with the neuron-enriched neuron specific enolase (NSE), ubiquitin (Ub) C terminal hydrolase L1 (UCH L1), and calpain cleaved αII spectrin N terminal fragment (SNTF) (Yokobori et al., 2013; Siman et al., 2013; Di Battista et al., 2015; Kawata et al., 2016; Papa, 2016). Among these biomarkers, increased plasma SNTF postconcussion is related not only to structural evidence for DAI but also functional evidence for long term cognitive impairment (Johnson et al., 2016).

It should be noted that most of abovementioned biomarkers are rapidly elevated after injury, and they serve as diagnostics tools for some times. Some biomarkers remain elevated for months after injury, although the literature on long term biomarkers is scarce. Unfortunately, none of these biomarkers has advanced for the use in the clinical setting. So presently, the diagnosis of concussion and various types of TBIs is made on the basis of a neurological examination and additionally using imaging radiology techniques such as CT or MRI or DTI (Delouche et al., 2016). The Glasgow Coma Scale assesses the severity of TBI on the basis of cognitive behavior (Teasdale et al., 2014). A total score of 13–15 refers to mTBI, 9–12 to moderate TBI, and 3–8 to severe TBI (Faul and Coronado, 2015).

In addition, cerebral microdialysis has also been used for monitoring damage to the brain tissue by determining biochemical metabolites such as glucose, lactate, pyruvate, glutamate, glycerol, interleukin-6 (IL-6), interleukin-1b (IL-1b), and monocyte chemoattractant protein (MCP)-1. Furthermore, small noncoding RNAs have also presented themselves as potential markers of concussions for future studies (Kulbe and Geddes, 2016).

SPINAL CORD CONCUSSION

Spinal cord concussion is a transient disturbance in spinal cord function, with or without vertebral damage. Clinically, spinal cord concussion is called as transient paraplegia or neurapraxia. There is motor and sensory weakness without demonstrable pathological changes. Spinal cord dysfunction is typically resolved within 24–72 hours without permanent deficits or damage (Del Bigio and Johnson, 1989; Zwimpfer and Bernstein, 1990; Torg et al., 1997). Spinal cord concussion is predominantly associated with sport related injury that occurs during contact sports (wrestling, hockey, gymnastics, American football, whiplash during minor car accidents, and falls) (Zwimpfer and Bernstein, 1990). In contact sports, the cervical spine is particularly susceptible to injury because of axial loading forces to the head with the neck in flexion or extension. According to Fischer et al., spinal cord concussion mediated injury may be caused by disc hernia- tion, buckling of the ligamentum flavum or the posterior longitudinal ligament, or by compression of the spinal cord between vertebral bodies (Fischer et al., 2016). There is a mechanistic difference in spinal cord concussion mediated injury between adults and children groups. In the adult, a stenotic spinal canal or a diminished spinal canal to vertebral body diameter predispose patients to cervical concussion at the level of stenosis after hyperextension, hyperflexion, or axial loading (Fischer et al., 2016). In contrast, in children, spines have increased mobility, pre- disposing the spinal cords to contact with bony elements even in absence of focal stenosis (Clark et al., 2011). Guidelines regarding return to play have been developed based upon the duration of neurological symptoms, neurapraxia, and MRI analysis, but they are based on a lim- ited number of small scale retrospective studies (Tempel et al., 2015). Unlike brain concussion, there have been no appropriate models to study the effects and risks of spinal cord concussion. So, the long term consequences of single and repeated spinal cord concussions are not known. Attempts are underway to study the histological and functional deficits in rats after repeated spinal cord concussions (Jin et al., 2015; Fischer et al., 2016). Attempts are underway to generate animal models for spinal cord concussions.

NEUROLOGICAL DISORDERS ASSOCIATED WITH CONCUSSION

Following concussion, at the molecular level, the damage to the brain tissue is caused by the rapid acceleration–deceleration force applied to the head. This process damages the brain by producing shear forces within nervous tissue resulting in DAI due to an impact with the cranial wall (Shaw, 2002). As stated above, these injuries can be ipsilateral or contralateral to the blow and have been described in literature as coup and counter coup, respectively (Ommaya et al., 1971). Concussion mediated brain damage is frequently mediated by the generation of free radicals and reactive oxygen species, induction of excitotoxicity, and onset of neuroinflammation (Farooqui, 2010; Cornelius et al., 2013). Initial concussion not only results in axonal damage from the shear forces of primary injury. Concussion also promotes changes in neural membrane permeability and alterations in ionic balance (Werner and Engelhard, 2007). In particular, uptake of calcium through either membrane disruption or through the activation of N-methyl-D-aspartate (NMDA) and α amino-3-hydroxy-5-methyl-4-isoxazolepropionic acid (AMPA) receptors by glutamate can result in mitochondrial dysfunction and overproduction of free radicals and activation of apoptotic caspase signaling (Zhang and Bhavnani, 2006; Farooqui, 2014). Subsequent inflammatory processes such as activation of native microglia may also contribute to oxidative stress via oxidative burst or through secondary effects of inflammatory cytokines (Farooqui, 2014). These reactive radicals can overwhelm endogenous antioxidant systems and inflict cellular damage via lipid peroxidation and protein modifications (Farooqui, 2014).

While most football players and veterans, who experience concussion, do not require immediate or emergency medical care at the time of injury, in the long run (postinjury), they undergo a host of troubling cognitive (executive dysfunction, attention, and memory deficits) (Combs et al., 2015), post concussive (headaches, dizziness, and fatigue) (King et al., 2012; Lippa et al., 2010), and psychiatric symptoms (anxiety and depression) (Brenner, 2011; Yurgil et al., 2014). Concussion induced neural injury may increase the risk of several neurological conditions such as headaches, stroke, dementia, posttraumatic stress, anxiety, and depression (Fig. 8.2).

CONCUSSION AND HEADACHES

Headache is the primary symptom reported after concussion. Posttraumatic headaches (PTHs) commonly fall into one of three categories: tension, migraine, or a combination of the two. The evaluation of PTH includes assessment for neurologic findings suggestive of serious intracranial abnormalities. Cumulative incidence and prevalence of PTH are higher following concussion compared with moderate to-severe TBI. Frequency is higher in those with more severe PTH. Migraine or probable migraine is the most common headache type after any severity TBI using primary headache disorder criteria. The molecular mechanisms of PTH are not fully understood. However, it is

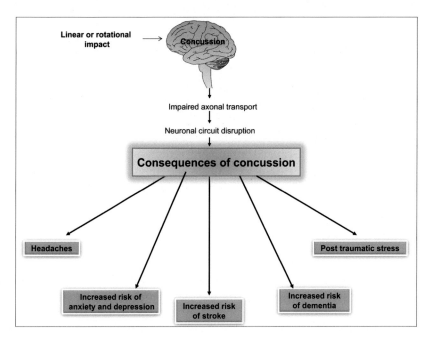

FIGURE 8.2   Increased risk of neurological disorders by concussion.

known that concussion increases the concentration of extracellular potassium, which will trigger neuronal depolarization and release of neurotransmitters (excitatory amino acids) along with alterations in serotonin, abnormalities in catecholamines, and endogenous opioids. In addition, PTH is also promoted by also decrease in magnesium levels and increase in intracellular calcium; impairment in glucose utilization; and induction of abnormalities in nitric oxide generation and alterations in neuropeptides. All these processes promote headaches (Ruff and Blake, 2016).

Concussion is accompanied by increase in extracellular potassium and intracellular sodium, calcium, and chloride; excessive release of excitatory amino acids; alterations in serotonin; abnormalities in catecholamines and endogenous opioids; decline in magnesium levels and increase in intracellular calcium along with impaired glucose utilization; abnormalities in nitric oxide formation; and alterations in neuropeptides (Ruff and Blake, 2016). In addition, concussion also promotes neuroinflammation. This process not only enhances neuronal death and impairs recovery of function but can also alter central nervous system (CNS) pain processing to induce migraine. Neuroinflammation is characterized by the activation of microglia; the release of proinflammatory chemicals, including chemokines, specific interleukins, and tumor necrosis factor alpha; and possibly the invasion of the CNS by inflammatory lymphocytes and phagocytic white cells coming through cerebral blood vessels (Farooqui, 2014).

CONCUSSION AND RISK OF STROKE

As stated in Chapter 2, Molecular Aspects of Ischemic Injury, stroke is a metabolic trauma caused by severe reduction or blockade in CBF due to the formation of a clot. This blockade not only decreases delivery of oxygen and glucose to the brain tissue but also results in the breakdown of BBB and buildup of potentially toxic products in brain (Farooqui, 2010). Two types of stroke have been reported to occur in humans: ischemic and hemorrhagic. Although concussion causes little structural damage to the brain, there is a growing concern that it increases the risk of stroke. Concussion's victims often recover spontaneously after a period of time; investigators have designed population based cohort studies to investigate the association between concussion and stroke. It is reported that concussion may be a potential unrecognized risk factor for stroke. During concussion, trauma to the head and neck may not only increase microvascular injury but also promote abnormal blood coagulation, which may contribute to stroke (Liu et al., 2017; Lu et al., 2004).

CONCUSSION AND DEMENTIA

Dementia is a progressive syndrome, which is associated with memory deficits, cognitive impairment, and deterioration in emotional control and social behavior (Xu et al., 2004; Qaseem et al., 2008). The loss in cognitive function is more than what is typically experienced in normal aging and results from brain damage produced by neurodegenerative processes (Sonnen et al., 2009). Several types of dementia have been described in human patients including vascular dementia, progressive dementia, Lewy body dementia, Alzheimer type of dementia, and dementia as a result of diseases such as stroke, AIDS, or multiple sclerosis (Ritchie and Lovestone, 2002). Major risk factors for dementia are age, physical and cognitive inactivity, cardiovascular and cerebrovascular diseases, and concussion (Xu et al., 2004; Povlishock and Katz, 2005; Qaseem et al., 2008). At present, very little is known about the temporal course and neuropathological consequences of concussion (Greve and Zink, 2009; Eierud et al., 2014; Niogi and Mukherjee, 2010; Clark et al., 2016). However, there is some evidence to suggest that concussion mediated changes in CBF and damage to WM tracts may be associated with the pathogenesis of dementia (Croall et al., 2014). PET has indicated that metabolic demands of brain are efficiently met when CBF is maintained to approximately 750 mL/minute or about 50 mL/ 100 mL of brain tissue per minute (Ito et al., 2005; Roher et al., 2012). CBF has been reported to be decreased in patients with diabetes and Alzheimer's disease (AD) (30%−40%) compared to age matched control subjects (Erol, 2008). Reduced CBF not only reduces oxygen and/or glucose supply to the brain but also decreases their utilization by the brain. This may cause an energy crisis in neurons and affect the function of ion pumps such as Na^+/K^+ ATPases that maintain the resting potential in neurons. This results in depolarization, excessive calcium entry into neurons and induces slow excitotoxicity in the aged brain (Farooqui, 2010). Reduction in CBF due to cerebrovascular diseases such as dementia may also promote cognitive problems induced by the accumulation of endogenous toxic products such as ammonia, lactic acid, nitric oxide, proinflammatory eicosanoids, cytokines, and chemokines. Accumulation of these toxic products may contribute to the pathogenesis of ischemic stroke, dementia, and AD. Reduced brain perfusion not only decreases glucose metabolism, decreases mitochondrial function, and induces neuroglial crisis leading to cognitive dysfunction and dementia (Fig. 8.3). These processes

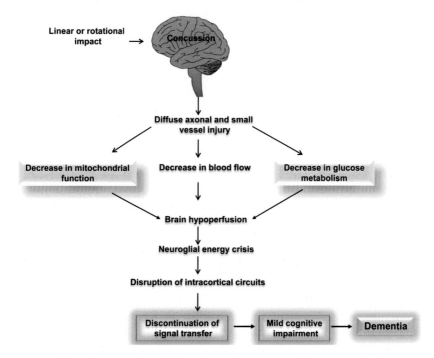

FIGURE 8.3 Hypothetical diagram showing processes associated with concussion mediated risk of dementia.

not only increase the risk of immune exhaustion (Brod, 2000), induce synaptic dysfunction (Farooqui, 2010, 2017), but may also inhibit neurogenesis and negatively affect the synthesis of proteins required for the formation of memory and learning (Dong et al., 2004; Jin et al., 2004; Li et al., 2008). Furthermore, changes in CBF along with induction of vascular inflammation and endothelial dysfunction may also contribute to the onset of clinical cognitive decline and dementia.

CONCUSSION AND POSTTRAUMATIC STRESS DISORDER

Posttraumatic stress disorder (PTSD) is a chronic and disabling, anxiety disorder induced by exposure to life threatening events such as a serious accident, abuse, or combat (Haber et al., 2016). PTSD is characterized by avoidance, negative alterations in cognitions and mood, and heightened arousal and reactivity. In addition, veterans with PTSD complaint dizziness, disorientation, and/or postural imbalance in environments such as grocery stores and shopping malls. The etiology of these symptoms in PTSD is poorly understood and some attribute them to anxiety or mTBI or concussion (Haber et al., 2016). It is proposed that an impaired vestibular system may contribute to abovementioned symptoms of PTSD. The molecular mechanisms contributing to the pathogenesis of PTSD are not fully understood. However, it is proposed that an altered fear response mechanism, behavioral sensitization, and failure of the extinction of fear play an important role in the pathophysiology of PTSD (Charney et al., 1993). Furthermore, it has been shown that patients with PTSD show significant deficits in memory (Bremner et al., 1995). Alterations in memory are correlated with specific brain structures and functional pathways that may be altered and are therefore possibly dysfunctional in patients with PTSD. It is also proposed that at the molecular level chronic stress induces structural and functional changes in the brain (Romeo, 2016). For example, brain derived neurotrophic factor (BDNF) expression in specific brain regions (i.e., mesocorticolimbic brain reward areas and the learning related circuit) (Holly et al., 2015) is altered by social defeat stress. Some studies have demonstrated that the brain may adapt through neural plasticity to cope with stressful situations. BDNF plays a key role in neural plasticity (Morrison and Ressler, 2014). Serotonin (5-HT) plays important roles in the brain and the dysregulation of 5-HT systems may be associated with a variety of stress disorders (Olivier, 2015). Selective 5-HT reuptake inhibitors clinically alleviate stress related disorders (Amos et al., 2014). These studies indicate that 5-HT may play a key role in the PTSD pathogenesis.

TRAUMATIC BRAIN INJURY

As stated in Chapter 6, Neurochemical Aspects of Traumatic Brain Injury, severe TBI is a neurological event marked by structural, cellular, molecular pathology, and/or functional disturbances in the CNS. It is triggered by severe head trauma. TBI frequently involves contusion, edema, and hemorrhage of the brain tissue and its patients show long term unconsciousness and repeated very severe seizures. Elevated troponin, posttraumatic cerebral infarction, and coagulopathy are frequently observed after severe TBI (Salim et al., 2008). Diagnosis of severe TBI is made by neuroimaging either through CT or by MRI, which can rapidly detect intracranial hematoma, skull fracture, and cerebral edema, as well as transependymal flow and obliteration of the basal cisterns (Chun et al., 2010).

NEUROCHEMICAL CHANGES IN TRAUMATIC BRAIN INJURY

As stated in Chapter 6, Neurochemical Aspects of Traumatic Brain Injury, TBI is caused by direct impact to the head or from acceleration–deceleration injury. TBI results in functional deficits due to both primary and secondary injury. Primary injury involves immediate mechanical damage to parenchyma (tissue, vessels), whereas secondary injury develops over a period of hours to days to even months after the primary insult to the brain tissue. These events result in neurochemical and physiological processes (excitotoxicity, mitochondrial dysfunction, free radical generation, induction of neuroinflammation, and onset of apoptosis), which ultimately lead to neuronal cell death (Farooqui, 2010). Molecular aspects of TBI have been described in Chapter 6, Neurochemical Aspects of Traumatic Brain Injury, and will not be discussed here.

BIOCHEMICAL MARKERS OF TRAUMATIC BRAIN INJURY

The diagnosis of TBI can be made after neurological examination by neuroimaging cranial CT scanning and MRI. Putative biomarkers for severe TBI are levels of total tau protein, changes in NSE, S100β (a Ca-binding protein), GFAP, UCH-L1, microtubule associated protein 2, IL-6, and IL-10. Information on biomarkers of TBI has been described in Chapter 6, Neurochemical Aspects of Traumatic Brain Injury.

NEUROLOGICAL DISORDERS ASSOCIATED WITH TRAUMATIC BRAIN INJURY

Most survivors of TBI develop cognitive deficits and motor dysfunctions. The most common cognitive impairment among severe TBI patients is memory loss. Maximal natural recovery among TBI patients occurs within the first 6 months and is more gradual after that, but outcome varies with different types of TBI. Depending on intensity, TBI patients develop AD, Parkinson's disease (PD), amyotrophic lateral sclerosis (ALS), depression, and dementia.

CHRONIC TRAUMATIC ENCEPHALOPATHY

CTE is a progressive neurodegenerative tauopathy associated with repetitive mild brain trauma (RMBT). Because millions of athletes and thousands of military veterans are exposed to RMBTs and subconcussive insults and TBI, CTE represents an important public health issue (Cassidy et al., 2004; Holm et al., 2005). However, the incidence rates and pathological mechanisms are still largely illusive, primarily due to the fact that there is no in vivo diagnostic tool. CTE was initially described in boxers but now has been found in a variety of contact sport athletes, military veterans, and civilians exposed to repetitive RMBT (Cassidy et al., 2004; Holm et al., 2005). Postmortem microscopic diagnosis of CTE is almost exclusively limited to the use of antibodies (Abs) directed against phosphorylated tau (p-tau) protein, with p-tau immunoreactivity observed in a perivascular pattern and at the depths of the sulci in addition to p-tau immune positive glial and neuronal profiles in subpial regions and astrocytic p-tau-positive plaques (Omalu et al. 2010). This perivascular pattern of p-tau accumulation is unique to CTE and from other tauopathies, including AD and frontotemporal lobar degeneration (FTLD). Based on immunoreactivity patterns of tight junction components claudin-5 and zonula occludens-1, it is hypothesized that the disruption in the BBB may be closely associated with the pathogenesis of CTE (Doherty et al., 2016). Thus, BBB dysfunction may represent a correlate of neural dysfunction in live subjects suspected of being at risk for development of CTE (Doherty et al., 2016). CTE is not only found in athletes, who have experienced repetitive head impacts, including epileptics, but also in developmentally disabled individuals who head bang, and victims of physical abuse (McKee et al., 2013). Two forms of p-tau have been reported to occur: *cis* p-tau and *trans* p-tau which are associated with CTE and neuronal survival, respectively.

The conversion of *trans* p-tau into *cis* p-tau is catalyzed by the peptidyl-prolyl isomerase Pin1, an enzyme whose expression inversely not only correlates with the predicted neuronal vulnerability in normally aged brain but also with actual neurofibrillary degeneration in AD brain (Fig. 8.4). Moreover, deletion of the gene encoding Pin1 in mice causes progressive age dependent neuropathy characterized by motor and behavioral deficits, tau hyperphosphorylation, tau filament formation, and neuronal degeneration (Lim and Lu, 2005). Collectively, these studies indicate that depletion of Pin1 may be associated with age dependent neurodegeneration and tau pathologies. Thus, Pin1 is pivotal in maintaining normal neuronal function and preventing age dependent neurodegeneration (Lim and Lu, 2005).

According to Albayram et al. (2016), p-tau and *trans* p-tau can be distinguished by a polyclonal and monoclonal Abs. Histological studies have shown that early stages of human mild cognitive impairment, AD, and CTE are accompanied by the appearance of robust *cis* p-tau in the brains not only in sport related TBI but also military veterans. The appearance of *cis* p-tau within hours after closed head injury and long before other known pathogenic p-tau conformations including

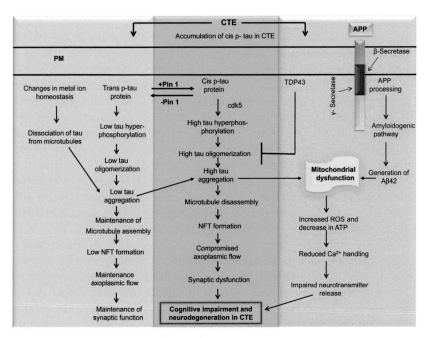

FIGURE 8.4 Hypothetical diagram showing existence two forms of p-tau in the brain and their role in neuronal survival and degradation.
PM, Plasma membrane; *ROS*, reactive oxygen species; *Cdk5*, cyclin dependent kinase 5; *NFT*, neurofibrillary tangles; *APP*, amyloid precursor protein; *Aβ*, beta-amyloid.

oligomers, prefibrillary tangles, and neurofibrillary tangles (NFTs) suggests that *cis* p-tau is an early driver of tau pathology in TBI and CTE. Importantly, *cis* p-tau monoclonal antibody treatment not only eliminates *cis* p-tau induction and tau pathology but also restores many neuropathological and functional outcome in TBI mouse models (Albayram et al., 2016). The detection of *cis* p-tau in human bodily fluids can potentially provide new diagnostic and prognostic tools. This information can be used to develop treatment for AD, TBI, and CTE (Albayram et al., 2016). The exact relationship between concussion and CTE is not clear. However, it is reported that number of concussions is not significantly correlated with CTE stage (McKee et al., 2013, 2015) and is less predictive than the cumulative head impact index of cognitive and neurobehavioral impairment (Montenigro et al., 2016). Furthermore, 16% of individuals diagnosed with CTE have no history of concussions supporting the view that subconcussive hits are sufficient for the development of CTE (Stein et al., 2015).

The clinical features of CTE are often progressive, leading to dramatic changes in mood, behavior, and cognition. At late stages, CTE is characterized by movement and speech disorders. CTE can be distinguished from other neurodegenerative diseases by a distinctive topographic location and cellular pattern of tau NFTs. In CTE, hyper-p-tau abnormalities begin focally, as perivascular NFTs and neurites at the depths of the cerebral sulci, and then spread to involve superficial layers of adjacent cortex before becoming a widespread degeneration affecting medial temporal lobe structures, diencephalon, and brainstem. The lack of development of full blown dementia in the majority of CTE sufferers can be attributed to the high suicide rates, which are a prominent feature of CTE (Gavett et al., 2011). Based on many studies on boxer and American football players, it is proposed that repetitive axonal injury initiates a series of metabolic, ionic, and cytoskeletal disturbances that trigger a pathological cascade leading to CTE in susceptible individuals. In most instances, the clinical symptoms of the disease begin after several decades of latency period. The diagnosis CTE can only be made at the postmortem (McKee et al., 2013, 2015).

Neuropsychological, mood, and neurobehavioral dysfunctions in CTE typically present in midlife after a latency period (usually years or decades) after exposure to the RMBTs. Early identification usually includes a history of direct trauma to the head and brief loss of consciousness. The mood related symptoms of CTE involve depression, apathy, irritability, and suicidality. Behavior symptoms are impulse control, disinhibition, and aggression as well as comorbid substance abuse (Baugh et al., 2012). As stated above, CTE is accompanied with the accumulation of p-tau in neurons and glial cells of perivascular areas of the cerebral cortex. Tau is a 45–65-kDa protein, which is encoded by a single gene located on chromosome 17 (17q21). Six tau isoforms are present in the brain containing either three (3R-tau) or four (4R-tau) repeat domains that together with the flanking regions mediate physiological tau—microtubule binding and stability. Tau is degraded by the ubiquitin—proteasome system (UPS) and the autophagy—lysosomal system. The UPS regulates and maintains protein levels by abolishing mutant, misfolded, or damaged proteins (Glickman and Ciechanover, 2002). There are two pathways for the UPS; Ub dependent or Ub independent. In the Ub dependent pathway, proteins' lysines are covalently conjugated to a Ub molecule or a chain of Ub molecules (Glickman and Ciechanover, 2002). The chain of Ub is then recognized by the proteasome. Once recognized, the protein is passed through the proteasome and proteolysed by trypsin like, chymotrypsin like, and postglutamyl activities into small proteolytic fragments (Glickman and Ciechanover, 2002; Lee et al., 2013). In comparison with the Ub independent pathway, substrate proteins are able to proceed directly to the proteasome for degradation (Glickman and Ciechanover, 2002; Lee et al., 2013). As stated above, tau can be processed through both UPS pathways (Lee et al., 2013). More specifically, full length monomeric tau is degraded through the UPS while truncated and insoluble forms of tau go through the autophagy—lysosomal system (Lee et al., 2013; Dolan and Johnson, 2010).

Under normal conditions, tau binds to microtubules and assists with their formation and stabilization. In addition, tau also plays an important role in axonal transport and microtubule stabilization, induction of neurite outgrowth, maintenance of nucleolar organization, induction of insulin resistance, and maintenance of neuronal polarity (Fig. 8.5). Under pathological conditions, tau dissociates from axonal microtubules and missorts to pre and postsynaptic terminals. It is reported that pathogenic tau binds to synaptic vesicles via its N terminal domain and interferes with presynaptic functions, including synaptic vesicle mobility and release rate, lowering neurotransmission in fly and rat neurons (Zhou et al., 2017). Converging evidence suggests that hyperphosphorylation, misfolding, and fibrillization of tau ("tau pathology") impair synaptic plasticity and cause degeneration (Wang and Mandelkow, 2016), with a large agreement toward a toxic gain of function. However, constitutive deletion of tau does not lead to lethality or neurodegeneration (Wang and Mandelkow, 2016), presumably because of compensatory mechanisms (Harada et al., 1994). Furthermore, tau is obviously needed for normal brain function, because tau deletion has been associated with brain iron accumulation (Lei et al., 2012) and deficits in synaptic plasticity and cognition (Kimura et al., 2014; Ahmed et al., 2015).

Tau contains 85 putative phosphorylation sites, including 45 serine, 35 threonine, and 5 tyrosine residues, which comprise 53%, 41%, and 6% of

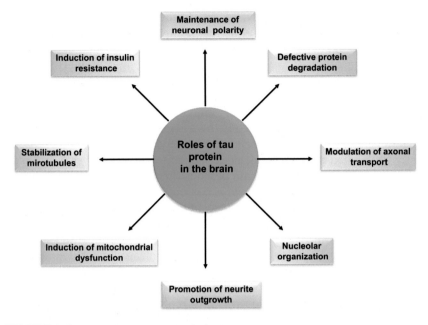

FIGURE 8.5   Roles of tau protein in the brain.

the phosphorylatable residues on tau, respectively (Hanger et al., 2009). Hyperphosphorylation of tau is catalyzed by a number of protein kinases including cyclin dependent kinase-5, glycogen synthase kinase-3, CaM kinase II, casein kinase II, stress activated kinase, c-Jun N terminal kinase (SAPK/JNK), kinase p38, and Fyn kinase (Gong and Iqbal, 2008). It is not yet known which of the many tau phosphorylation sites that have been identified are essential for the pathogenesis of CTE and which sites may become phosphorylated only after the formation of tau pathology in other tauopathies. Phosphorylation of tau decreases normally with age and coincides with the development of phosphatases (Murray et al., 2014). However, in tauopathies, the aberrant phosphorylation of tau leads to abnormal accumulations of p-tau in the brain (Stoothoff and Johnson, 2005). Dephosphorylation of tau is crucial for the normal functional status of the tau protein. Collective evidence suggests that the biological function of the microtubule associated tau protein (Weingarten et al., 1975) is regulated by several kinases and phosphatases (Gail and Judith, 1999). An imbalance in activity between kinases and phosphatases results in the abnormal phosphorylation of 38 or more serine and/or threonine amino acids on tau in another tauopathy called AD (Tanaka et al., 1998; Iqbal et al., 2005). There are two protein phosphatases (PPs): PP2A and PP2B (calcineurin) (Tanaka et al., 1998). PP2B is a calcium/calmodulin-activated serine/threonine phosphatase, regulated by *RCAN1* (previously also known as Adapt78, DSCR1, or calcipressin1). *RCAN1* overexpression leads to inhibition of PP2B and increased tau phosphorylation (Ermak et al., 2002). PP2A appears to be a major phosphatase regulating tau phosphorylation in the brain (Kins et al., 2001), but downregulation of PP2A alone, in animal brains, does not produce paired helical filaments (Kins et al., 2001). In addition, tau undergoes acetylation within the lysine rich microtubule binding region (Cohen et al., 2011). While the full complement of enzymes controlling tau acetylation has not been well characterized, in vitro and cell based experiments have indicated that CREB-binding protein or the highly homologous p300 acetylates tau with high affinity in the lysine rich microtubule-binding region (Cohen et al., 2011). Acetylation at residues K280/K281 is critical for normal and pathological tau functions. Site specific tau acetylation not only alters the tau posttranslational profile but also impairs tau mediated microtubule stability and accelerates tau aggregation. Furthermore, acetylation of full length tau makes it more susceptible to seed dependent tau aggregation supporting the view that tau acetylation plays an important role in in the pathophysiology of tauopathies (Cohen et al., 2011) (Fig. 8.6). Collective evidence suggests that tau is mainly an

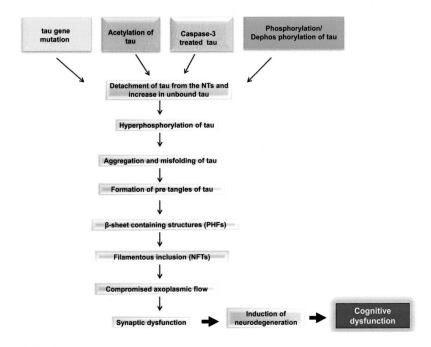

FIGURE 8.6 Hypothetical mechanism associated with formation of neurofibrillary tangles in tauopathies.
PHFs, Paired helical filaments; *NFTs*, neurofibrillary tangles.

axonal protein. However, in tauopathies, it is also present at dendritic spines where they may play a toxic role. This toxic role may be the consequence of tau modifications like phosphorylation, truncation, or acetylation. The knowledge of the role of acetylated tau in tauopathies has increased in recent years. For example, Tracy et al. (2016) have described a possible mechanism explaining the role of acetylated tau (at lysines 274 and 281). Based on detailed investigations, it is suggested that aberrant acetylation at K274 and K281 in tau may be a contributing factor in memory loss related to tauopathies, including AD. It is also reported that dementia in AD is linked with elevated levels of acetylated K274 and acetylated K281, which correlate negatively with those of KIBRA, a synaptic protein, which is not only involved in synaptic function, cell polarity, vesicular transport, and neuronal plasticity (Schneider, et al., 2010) but also plays a critical in AMPAR trafficking. Mimicking acetylation of these lysines in transgenic mice impairs synaptic plasticity and memory retention, likely due to deficient activity dependent actin polymerization and AMPAR trafficking (Tracy et al., 2016). Elevating KIBRA in neurons expressing acetyl mimicking tau was sufficient to reestablish actin polymerization and AMPAR insertion during plasticity (Tracy et al., 2016). It is also shown that acetylated tau (at lysines 274 and 281) destabilizes the cytoskeleton in the axon initial segment (Sohn et al., 2016).

In other tauopathies, tau protein also undergoes proteolytic cleavage by several proteolytic enzymes. Caspase-3 cleaves tau at aspartate (D) residue 421 (Rissman et al., 2004). Calpain-1 and caspase-6 hydrolyze tau at N terminal of tau (Park and Ferreira, 2005; Horowitz et al., 2004), respectively. The tau fragments, which are produced by above proteases, have been detected in affected regions of human tauopathy brain (Rissman et al., 2004; Ferreira and Bigio, 2011). Tau fragments, which are generated by caspase-3, show an increased tendency and propensity to aggregate and act as a seeding nidus for the aggregation and fibrillization of full length tau species (Binder et al., 2005). In contrast, breakdown of tau by calpain may partially inhibit tau aggregation (Ferreira and Bigio, 2011). The temporal and homeostatic relationship between tau cleavage and phosphorylation is unclear, with data showing that phosphorylation of different tau residues precedes (Rametti et al., 2004), follows (Rissman et al., 2004), and inhibits (Guillozet-Bongaarts et al., 2006) the proteolytic cleavage of tau by caspase-3. However, substantial studies support the view that caspase-3-mediated breakdown of tau species results in generation of tau fragments, which are particularly prone to phosphorylation in both primary neuronal cells (Garwood et al., 2011) and human tauopathy brain (Rissman et al., 2004). In addition, phosphorylated and caspase-3-generated tau species readily form aggregates in cells (Cho and Johnson, 2004). Converging evidence therefore support the view that phosphorylation and caspase mediated cleavage of tau are important events during the development of the characteristic tau aggregates that accumulate in AD and other tauopathies.

Phosphorylation of tau changes its shape and regulates its biological activity. The molecular mechanisms by which accumulation, hyperphosphorylation, and aggregation of p-tau contribute to the pathogenesis of CTE and other tauopathies (Goedert et al., 2000; Hutton, 2000; Spillantini et al., 2000). These diseases share a common histopathological hallmark known as NFTs that consist of an accumulation of fibrillar tau deposits initially produced from p-tau protein aggregation (Ballatore et al., 2007). In addition, tauopathies are also characterized by the abnormal expression of BDNF, a key modulator of neuronal survival, synaptic plasticity, and memory consolidation (Gezen-Ak et al., 2013). The severity of these pathological hallmarks correlates with the degree of cognitive impairment in patients. However, how tau pathology specifically modifies BDNF signaling and affects neuronal function during early prodromal stages of tauopathy remain unclear (Mazzaro et al., 2016).

On the basis of mathematical modeling experiments, it is proposed that the bulk accumulation of p-tau aggregates in cell bodies may depress neuronal energy metabolism through molecular crowding leading to long term alterations in neuronal physiology (Fig. 8.7) (Vazquez, 2013). Hyperphosphorylation of tau makes this protein resistant to calcium activated proteases, calpains, and the Ub—proteasome pathway. As stated above, hyperphosphorylation of tau produces neurotoxic effects not only by inducing mitochondrial dysfunction, increasing oxidative stress, and promoting collapse of the microtubule based cytoskeleton, but also by promoting neuronal apoptosis and inducing neuritic dystrophy (Fig. 8.7) (Arnaud et al., 2006; Oddo et al, 2008). These processes contribute to brain swelling, axonal injury and hypoxia, disruption of BBB function, and induction of neuroinflammation leading to cognitive impairment. In tauopathies, hyperphosphorylation of tau disengages tau from microtubules, with consequent misfolding and deposition into inclusions that not only affect neurons but also to some extent glial cells. Under pathological conditions (tauopathies), normal tau becomes hyperphosphorylated, causing it to fall off the microtubules and be relocated to the somatodendritic compartment (Stoothoff and Johnson, 2005). Here, it is subjected to further phosphorylation and conformational change, which leads to the formation of paired helical and straight filaments of abnormal tau. These filamentous or fibrillar forms of tau aggregate into mature NFT (Kuret et al., 2005; Farías et al., 2011). Tau oligomers also have ability to enter and exit cells, propagating from disease-affected regions to unaffected areas. While the mechanism by which the spreading of misfolded tau occurs has yet to be

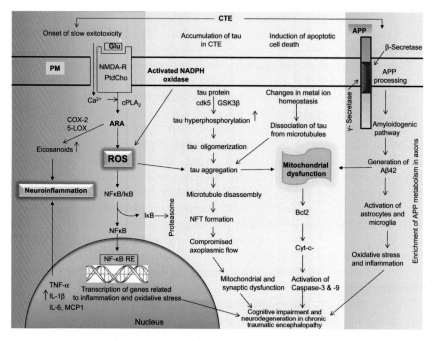

FIGURE 8.7   Hypothetical diagram showing signal transduction processes associated with neurodegeneration in chronic traumatic encephalopathy.

Glu, Glutamate; *NMDA-R*, NMDA receptor; *PtdCho*, phosphatidylcholine; *cPLA₂*, cytosolic phospholipase A₂; *lyso-PtdCho*, lyso-phosphatidylcholine; *COX-2*, cyclooxygenase-2; *5-LOX*, 5-lipoxygenase; *ARA*, arachidonic acid; *ROS*, reactive oxygen species; *NF-κB*, nuclear factor κB; *NF-κB-RE*, nuclear factor κB-response element; *I-κB*, inhibitory subunit of NF-κB; *TNF-α*, tumor necrosis factor-α; *IL-1β*, interleukin-1β; *IL-6*, interleukin-6; *MCP-1*, monocyte chemoattractant protein-1; *Cdk5*, cyclin dependent kinase 5; *Bcl-2*, B-cell lymphoma 2; *cyto-c*, cytochrome; *APP*, amyloid precursor protein.

elucidated, there are a few different models which have been proposed, including cell membrane stress and pore formation, endocytosis and exocytosis, and nontraditional secretion of protein not enclosed by a membrane (Gerson and Kayed, 2013; Gerson et al., 2016). It is proposed that tau oligomers potentiate neuronal damage, leading to neurodegeneration not only in neurotraumatic but also in neurodegenerative diseases (Hawkins et al., 2013; Gerson et al, 2016; Sengupta et al., 2015). Additionally, injections of these tau oligomers produce accelerated onset of cognitive deficits into brains of Htau mice supporting the view that tau oligomers may be responsible for seeding the spread of pathology post TBI. Tau oligomers have been implicated in synaptic loss as shown in studies of wild type human tau transgenic mice (Clavaguera et al., 2009, 2013). When the oligomer lengthens, it adapts a β-sheet structure and transforms into a detergent insoluble aggregate with granular appearance under atomic force microscopy. As these granular tau oligomers fuse together, they form tau fibrils, which ultimately form NFTs (Takashima, 2013). These steps support the view that tau oligomers contribute to neuronal dysfunction prior to NFT formation (Maeda et al., 2006). In tauopathies, neurodegeneration is a complex, progressive, and multifactorial process (Fig. 8.7). It is initiated by alterations in signal transduction processes due to the accumulation and aggregation of hyper p-tau protein leading not only to impairment in axoplasmic flow, but also in slow progression of retrograde degeneration and loss of connectivity in affected neurons. Studies on the correlation between cognitive impairment and histopathological changes have indicated that the number of NFTs, and not the plaques, correlates best with the presence and or the degree of dementia in not only in AD (Arriagada et al., 1992), but also in a number of tauopathies such as progressive supranuclear palsy (PSP), Pick's disease, frontotemporal dementia, cortico basal degeneration, and variants of PD and Lewy body dementia (LBD) (Fig. 8.8). The crossing of human APP transgenic mice with human tau transgenic mice lead to marked increase in aggregation of tau with concomitant dendritic spine loss and acceleration in cognitive impairment (Chabrier et al., 2014). On the basis of extensive investigation, it is proposed that the crosstalk between Aβ and tau not only contributes to

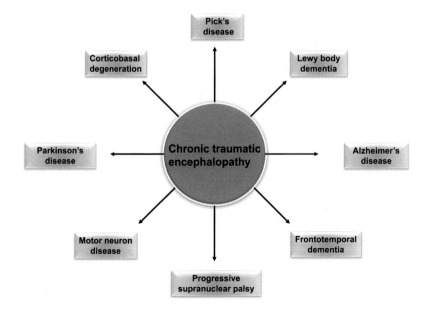

FIGURE 8.8 Neurological disorders mediated by chronic traumatic encephalopathy.

induction and enhancement of tau phosphorylation, but also to the Aβ-mediated proteasomal impairment of tau degradation and dysregulation of axonal transport with possible bidirectional effects, leading to increase in Aβ as well as tau (Blurton-Jones and Laferla, 2006). Accumulation of Aβ and phosphorylation of tau has been reported to downregulate the density and function of synapses leading to abnormalities in signal transduction processes in neuronal network within the brain (Iqbal et al., 2009).

Clinically, CTE is characterized by behavioral changes, executive dysfunction, memory deficits, cytoskeletal disruption, and cognitive impairments that begin insidiously and most often progress slowly over decades (Fig. 8.9) (McKee et al., 2009). The majority of CTE cases (>85%) also show abnormal accumulations of phosphorylated 43 kDa TAR DNA binding protein (TDP-43) that are partially colocalized with p-tau protein (McKee et al., 2013). Wild type TDP43 regulates the transcription of thousands of genes (Hebron et al., 2013). Repeated mTBI causes an upregulation of Ca^{2+}-permeable AMPA receptors, which in turn lead to carboxy terminal-cleaved TDP43 fragments (Yamashita et al., 2012). These fragments translocate to the cytosol, mediated in part by the process of ubiquitination.[19] These fragments accumulate and form intracellular aggregates that are found in several neurodegenerative diseases including: AD, PD, amyotrophic lateral sclerosis, and CTE (Bandyopadhyay et al., 2013). The role of TDP-43 in neuronal degeneration in CTE is not understood. However, several mechanisms have been proposed. One mechanism by which TDP43

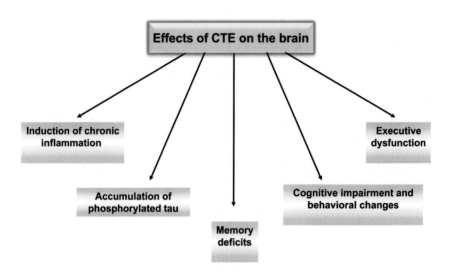

FIGURE 8.9   Effects of chronic traumatic encephalopathy on neuronal metabolism.

mediates its neurotoxicity involves the aggregation of TDP43. These TDP43 aggregates produce misfolding of Cu/Zn superoxide dismutase (SOD1), which predisposes surrounding neuronal cells to free radical damage (Bandyopadhyay et al., 2013). The clinical symptoms of TDP43 pathology include cognitive and motor impairment (Yamashita et al., 2012). Another mechanism of TDP43 neurotoxicity involves abnormal phosphorylation of TDP-43, which has been reported to disrupt important signaling pathways, leading to neuronal dysfunction (Forman et al., 2007). Furthermore, TDP-43 has been reported to suppress tau expression by promoting its mRNA instability through the UG repeats of its 3'-untranslated region (Gu et al., 2017) supporting the view that TDP-43 suppresses tau expression by promoting the instability of its mRNA. Downregulation of TDP-43 may be involved not only in the tau neuropathology of AD but also in other related neurodegenerative disorders such as CTE (Gu et al., 2017). In addition, β-amyloid precursor protein processing, apolipoprotein E, presenilin, and neprilysin genes along with axonal injury and neuroinflammation may also contribute to the pathogenesis of CTE. Although definitive diagnosis of CTE requires neuropathological examination, a major current research goal is the identification of biomarkers for disease diagnosis and prognosis. Collective evidence suggests that RMBT can trigger self propagating cycles of neuronal injury involving axonal injury, tau hyperphosphorylation, misfolding and aggregation, cytoskeletal breakdown, and disrupted axonal transport leading to synaptic loss in CTE. In contrast, during acute TBI, the brain undergoes shear deformation producing acute injury to axons, small blood vessels, and astrocytes (Johnson et al., 2012a; McKee et al., 2009). Although research on the long term effects of severe TBI is advancing quickly, the incidence and prevalence of posttraumatic neurodegeneration and CTE are unknown. Critical knowledge gaps include elucidation of molecular and pathogenic mechanisms, identification of genetic risk factors, and clarification of relevant variables—including age at exposure to trauma, history of prior and subsequent head trauma, substance use, gender, stress, and comorbidities—all of which may contribute to risk profiles and the development of posttraumatic neurodegeneration and CTE (McKee et al., 2009, 2013).

NEUROCHEMICAL CHANGES IN CHRONIC TRAUMATIC ENCEPHALOPATHY

The molecular mechanisms associated with the pathogenesis of CTE remain unknown. However, it is becoming increasingly evident that

DAI, accumulation of p-tau, onset of slow neuronal excitotoxicity, dys-regulation of ion homeostasis, and activation of microglial cells, astrocy-tosis, neuroinflammation, microvascular injury, and microhemorrhages are closely associated with the pathogenesis of CTE. These processes not only produce increase in proinflammatory cytokines but also cause neuroglial energy crisis contributing to slow neurodegeneration in CTE (Fig. 8.10) (McKee et al., 2013; Ling et al., 2012, 2015). Depending on the severity and extent of DAI, these changes can manifest acutely as immediate loss of consciousness or confusion along with cognitive dysfunction. As stated above, hyperphosphorylation of tau in axons produces neurotoxic effects not only by disengaging it from microtu-bules, inducing mitochondrial dysfunction, increasing oxidative stress,

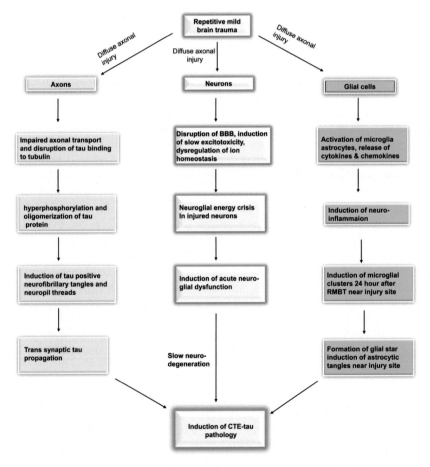

FIGURE 8.10   Neurochemical changes associated with the pathogenesis of CTE.

and promoting collapse of the microtubule based cytoskeleton, but also by promoting neuronal apoptosis and inducing neuritic dystrophy (Fig. 8.10) (Arnaud et al., 2006; Oddo et al, 2008; Ling et al., 2015). Several recent studies have indicated that tau can be physiologically released to the extracellular fluid both in vivo and in cultured cells, and such release is probably regulated by neuronal activity (Yamada et al., 2014). Although roles of intracellular tau are becoming increasingly evident, the physiological function of extracellular tau remains elusive. In vitro and in vivo studies have shown that exogenous tau aggregates can be internalized by neurons and act as seeds to induce the aggregation of other tau proteins (Frost et al., 2009; Clavaguera et al., 2009). Based on these findings, it is proposed that the release and uptake of tau underlies the spreading of tau pathology (Mohamed et al., 2013). However, how and what tau species are released by donor neurons and then taken up by recipient neurons is not clear.

Studies on whole RNA sequencing analysis of postmortem brain tissue from CTE patients have indicated that the genes related to the MAP kinase and calcium signaling pathways are significantly downregulated in CTE (Seo et al., 2017). Alterations in the expression of PPs in these networks further support the view that the tauopathy observed in CTE involves common pathological mechanisms similar to AD (Seo et al., 2017; Turner et al., 2016). Using cell lines and animal models, it is reported that reduction in PPP3CA/PP2B phosphatase activity is directly associated with increases in phosphorylation of tau proteins. These findings provide important insights into PP dependent neurodegeneration in CTE (Seo et al., 2017).

RISK FACTORS FOR CHRONIC TRAUMATIC ENCEPHALOPATHY

Professional athletes and soldiers are at greatest risk for development of CTE (Peskind et al., 2013). In addition, individuals with one or two copies of the apolipoprotein ε4 allele have poorer outcome following head trauma and are at increased risk for developing CTE following TBI (Spillantini et al., 2011). Athletes exposed to subconcussive and concussive injury, as well as soldiers exposed to even a single blast, can develop behavioral and psychiatric problems within a single year following injury (Bailes et al., 2013). An area in need of further investigation is how acute neurotrauma relates to and/or causes chronic neurodegenerative diseases in susceptible individuals.

BIOCHEMICAL MARKERS FOR CHRONIC TRAUMATIC ENCEPHALOPATHY

Earlier studies on biomarkers of CTE have indicated that levels of neuronal biomarkers (tau and neurofilament protein) or glial injury (GFAP and S-100β) as well as CSF/serum albumin ratio, hemoglobin, and bilirubin content in CSF are not affected by brain damage in CTE (Blennow et al., 2011). However, Shahim et al. (2017) have reported that serum axonal protein neurofilament light (NFL) levels are increased in boxers 7–10 days after bout as compared to the levels after 3 months rest as well as compared with controls ($P = 0.0007$ and $P < 0.0001$, respectively). Levels of NFL are decreased following 3 months of rest but were still higher than in controls ($P < 0.0001$). It is also reported that boxers, who received many (>15) hits to the head or were groggy after bout, had higher concentrations of serum NFL as compared to those who received fewer hits to the head ($P = 0.0023$). Serum NFLs are increased over time in hockey players and the levels returned to normal at return to play (Shahim et al., 2017).

NEUROLOGICAL DISORDERS ASSOCIATED WITH CHRONIC TRAUMATIC ENCEPHALOPATHY

CTE is associated with the development of several neurodegenerative disorders such as LBD, AD, FTLD, and motor neuron disease (MND) (Fig. 8.8) (McKee et al., 2013; Hazrati et al., 2013). According to Stein et al. (2014), among 71 combined cases of pathologically confirmed CTE, 17% were linked with LBD, 11% were associated with MND, 12% with AD, and 6% with FTLD. In another study of 313 AD patients, 27% were linked with LBD, 2.6% were associated with FTLD, and none had MND. Furthermore, the average age at death of subjects with CTE is younger than those with AD, supporting the view that these comorbidities are not simply age related. Indeed, the frequent presence of comorbid pathologies in CTE suggests that either repetitive trauma or the accumulation of tau pathology in CTE provokes the deposition of other abnormal proteins (Aβ peptide, α-synuclein, TDP-43) contributing to neurodegenerative process (McKee et al., 2013; Hazrati et al., 2013). Pathological processes linking CTE with above neurodegenerative diseases are not clearly understood. However, it is becoming increasingly evident that there is significant overlap between CTE and other tauopathies, like AD. Knowing that similarities exist between CTE and AD makes it less daunting; a lot of information is available on pathogenesis and diagnostic methods of AD (Farooqui, 2017). This information can be used for devising diagnostic methods for CTE. However, it is vital to differentiate CTE from other neurodegenerative diseases so they can be properly diagnosed and treated. The recent consensus statement goes a long way. A team of neuropathologists was established to differentiate between digitized slides from 25 cases of tauopathy including CTE, AD, Parkinson dementia complex of Guam, PSP, corticobasal degeneration, primary age related tauopathy, and argyrophilic grain disease by the National Institute of Health (NIH).

Molecular mechanisms that link CTE with other neurodegenerative tauopathies are not fully understood. However, CTE mediated neurochemical changes in axolemma permeability, massive calcium influx, activation of calcium dependent enzymes (phospholipases A_2, nitric oxide synthases, endonucleases, nitric oxide synthases, PPs, and various protein kinases, matrix metalloproteinases and calpains), and changes in levels of lipid mediators promote the misfolding, truncation, phosphorylation and aggregation of many proteins, including tau and TDP-43 and the breakdown of the microtubules and neurofilaments. These processes not only alter neural membrane homeostasis but also disrupt axonal transport. It is also likely that RMBTs and accumulation of misfolded p-tau aggregates may either interfere with normal clearance mechanisms of accumulated proteins or induce a decrease in availability of neurotrophins allowing induction and spreading of neurodegeneration and induction of synaptic dysfunction in the brains of CTE patients (Frost et al., 2009; Hall and Patuto, 2012). Another possibility is that the tau protein itself serves as the toxic agent, which may promote transcellular propagation and neurodegeneration (Frost et al., 2009; Hall and Patuto, 2012). Among above calcium dependent enzymes, continued calpain hyperactivation in CTE may contribute to neuropathological changes. Calpain mediated proteolysis regulates the activity of key tau kinases (cdk5) which may not only increase tau phosphorylation but also promote tau mediated neurodegeneration in vivo (Noble et al., 2013). Effect of calpain inhibitors in animal models of CTE is not known. Availability of this information can open many avenues for the treatment of CTE in human patients of CTE.

EFFECTS OF CONCUSSIONS AND CHRONIC TRAUMATIC ENCEPHALOPATHY ON COGNITIVE FUNCTION

Concussion and CTE are known to produce both short and long term deficits in cognitive function including attention, learning and memory, and higher order executive functions. Post injury cognitive deficits following concussion and CTE can be attributed to damage in certain vulnerable brain regions including the medial temporal regions, dorsolateral prefrontal cortex as well as subcortical WM tracts (McAllister, 2011). The risk of cognitive impairment increases with the number of insults suffered. One study has demonstrated a fivefold increase in mild cognitive disorders and a threefold prevalence of significant memory problems in players who suffered three or more concussions (Guskiewicz et al., 2005). While the case for repetitive insults producing chronic neurodegeneration and cognitive impairment is solid, it is becoming increasingly evident that a single moderate to severe head trauma is sufficient to cause chronic neurodegeneration and the development of a neurodegenerative disorder such as AD in some individuals (Plassman et al., 2000; Fleminger et al., 2003; Johnson et al., 2012b). A direct physical impact to the brain or shear forces (due to rapid angular acceleration/deceleration) from the primary injury produces mechanical damage not only to neuronal and glial cells but also to vasculature and axons. The damage from the primary injury following concussion or CTE is immediate and irreversible. The primary injury is followed by secondary injury, which involves both systemic complications and neural cell injury, which develops over the course of hours to several weeks following concussion and mTBI. Systemic impairments including edema, increase in intracranial pressure and hemorrhage. These processes contribute to decrease in CBF and impaired metabolism through the involvement of glutamate mediated excitotoxicity, increase in calcium influx, free radical generation, mitochondrial dysfunction, onset of neuroinflammatory events, and pro apoptotic gene activation (Fig. 8.11).

Among above processes, impaired calcium homeostasis following mTBI affects signaling pathways involving calcium dependent enzymes (phospholipases A_2, calpains, and nitric oxide synthases) and protein kinases (CaMKII and MAPK), which play important roles in phosphorylating downstream effectors involved in the induction of long term potentiation (LTP) and long term depression (LTD), two of the major molecular mechanisms underlying learning and memory (Walker and Tesco, 2013).

Synapses are the principal sites for chemical communication between neurons and are essential for performing the dynamic functions of the brain. The flow of neural information between neurons is ignited from presynaptic terminals by the release of a small chemical ingredient called neurotransmitter. As stated above, in normal brain, native tau plays an important role in synaptic function due to its regulation of microtubule stability and thus axonal transport. In mild and severe TBI, AD, and related tauopathies, synapses are exposed to disease phosphorylated and acetylated tau, which may cause the loss of synaptic contacts resulting in initiation of disease process. In these pathological conditions, development of tau containing neurofibrillary pathology

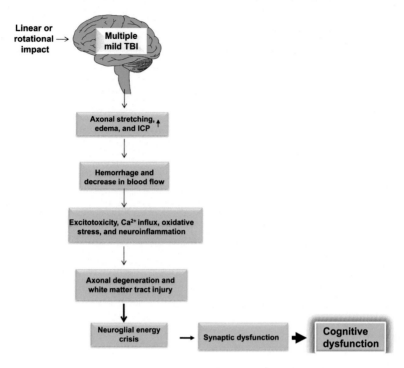

FIGURE 8.11   Effects of multiple mild TBI on cognitive impairment.

correlates well not only with synaptic loss but also with cognitive impairment (Wakade et al., 2010; Farooqui, 2017; Bae and Kim, 2017). Moreover, several transgenic models of tauopathy expressing various forms of tau protein exhibit structural synaptic deficits. The pathological tau proteins cause the dysregulation of synaptic proteome and lead to the functional abnormalities of synaptic transmission. Given the large number of proteins needed for synaptic function, the proliferation of defective proteins and the subsequent loss of protein homeostasis may be a leading cause of synaptic dysfunction. The localization of tau within synapses in both healthy and CTE brains indicates that tau may play a role in normal synaptic function, which may be disrupted in CTE. Accumulation of *cis* p-tau may impact synaptic activity in several ways (Du et al., 2010; Christoffel et al., 2011; Bhat et al., 2015; Cai and Tammineni, 2017). Several studies have indicated that *cis* p-tau interacts directly with postsynaptic signaling complexes, regulating glutamatergic receptor content in dendritic spines leading to disruption of synaptic mitochondrial function. Early trials of *cis* p-tau-targeted immunotherapy reduce tau pathology and synapse loss, indicating that the toxic effects of *cis* p-tau may be reversible within a certain time frame. Thus, understanding the role of *cis* p-tau in both normal and degenerating synapses is crucial for the development of therapeutic strategies designed to ameliorate synapse loss and prevent CTE pathogenesis (Cai and Tammineni, 2017). These processes result in neurodegeneration not only through necrotic (rapid, uncontrolled) and apoptotic (delayed) cell death (Stoica and Faden, 2010) but also through necroptosis (Christofferson and Yuan, 2010) and autophagy (Decuypere et al., 2012). Collectively, these studies suggest that modified tau protein plays a key role in the synaptic impairment of human tauopathies.

Advancements in imaging techniques have allowed the detection of extensive WM tract damage in concussions and CTE (Miller et al., 2016). Originally, it was reported that the majority of axonal separation took place due to tearing and shearing of the axons during the primary injury. However, it is becoming increasingly evident that concussion and CTE mediated axonal degeneration is produced by secondary injury through the involvement of NMDA receptor mediated excitotoxicity, calcium influx, free radical generation, mitochondrial dysfunction, and apoptosis (Kraus et al., 2007). All these processes contribute to the deficit in cognitive dysfunction. Concussion and CTE are known to induce abnormalities in neurotransmitter systems (e.g., cholinergic, monoaminergic, and catecholamine), which play important roles in cognition (McAllister, 2011). Similarly, impaired calcium homeostasis following injury also affects signaling pathways including those of the protein kinases CaMKII and MAPK, which play important roles in phosphorylating downstream effectors involved in the induction of LTP and LTD, two of the major molecular mechanisms underlying learning and memory.

CONCLUSION

Public awareness of the pathological consequences of concussion and CTE has increased considerably because of contact sports such as American football, wrestling, rugby, hockey, lacrosse, soccer, and skiing as well as military veterans, who have exposed themselves to an explosive blast during their deployment in in Iraq and Afghanistan. Annually, more than 1.5 million Americans sustain concussion or mTBIs with no loss of consciousness and without hospitalization; an equal number sustain injuries sufficient to impair consciousness but insufficiently severe to necessitate long term hospitalization. Neurochemical changes in concussion are mediated by the induction of oxidative stress, cytoskeletal and axonal alterations, impairments in neurotransmission resulting in decrease in neuroplasticity, memory loss, and behavioral changes and vulnerability to delayed cell death. In most players, symptoms and consequences of concussion are resolved in 7–10 days. However, in some players, even one concussion after a period of latency (15–20 years) result in dementia. In contrast, CTE is a progressive neurodegenerative tauopathy associated with RMBT. Neurochemical changes in CTE are accompanied with the accumulation of p-tau, induction of mitochondrial dysfunction, increasing oxidative stress, collapse of the microtubule based cytoskeleton, and induction of neuronal apoptosis. The regulation of tau binding to Microtubules (MTs) depends on phosphorylation of serine/threonine predominantly in the proline rich region and also by lysine acetylation directly within the MT binding repeat region. These two posttranslational tau modifications act in concert to decrease tau–MT binding affinity. While tau hyperphosphorylation has been extensively characterized in association with NFT pathology in AD. Although tau hyperphosphorylation is widely considered to be the major trigger of tau malfunction, tau undergoes several posttranslational modifications at lysine residues including acetylation, methylation, ubiquitylation, SUMOylation, and glycation. These processes contribute to brain swelling, axonal injury and hypoxia, disruption of BBB, and increases in inflammatory responses leading to cognitive impairment. The exact relationship between concussion and CTE is not clear. However, it is possible that repetitive axonal injury initiates a series of metabolic, ionic, and cytoskeletal disturbances that trigger a pathological cascade leading to CTE in susceptible individuals.

References

Ahmed, T., Blum, D., Burnouf, S., Demeyer, D., Buée-Scherrer, V., et al., 2015. Rescue of impaired late phase long term depression in a tau transgenic mouse model. Neurobiol. Aging 36, 730–739.

Albayram, O., Herbert, M.K., Kondo, A., Tsai, C.Y., Baxley, S., et al., 2016. Function and regulation of tau conformations in the development and treatment of traumatic brain injury and neurodegeneration. Cell Biosci. 6, 59.

Amos, T., Stein, D.J., Ipser, J.C., 2014. Pharmacological interventions for preventing posttraumatic stress disorder (PTSD). Cochrane Database Syst Rev. 7, CD006239.

Arnaud, L., Robakis, N.K., Figueiredo-Pereira, M.E., 2006. It may take inflammation, phosphorylation and ubiquitination to 'tangle' in Alzheimer's disease. Neurodegener. Dis. 3, 313–319.

Arriagada, P.V., Growdon, J.H., Hedley-Whyte, E.T., Hyman, B.T., 1992. Neurofibrillary tangles but not senile plaques parallel duration and severity of Alzheimer's disease. Neurology 42, 631–639.

Bae, J.R., Kim, S.H., 2017. Synapses in neurodegenerative diseases. BMB Rep. 50, 237–246.

Bailes, J.E., Petraglia, A.L., Omalu, B.I., Nauman, E., Talavage, T., 2013. Role of subconcussion in repetitive mild traumatic brain injury. J. Neurosurg. 119, 1235–1245.

Ballatore, C., Lee, V.M., Trojanowski, J.Q., 2007. Tau-mediated neurodegeneration in Alzheimer's disease and related disorders. Nat. Rev. Neurosci. 8, 663–672.

Bandyopadhyay, U., Cotney, J., Nagy, M., Oh, S., Leng, J., et al., 2013. RNA-Seq profiling of spinal cord motor neurons from a presymptomatic SOD1 ALS mouse. PLoS ONE 8, e53575.

Barkhoudarian, G., Hovda, D.A., Giza, C.C., 2011. The molecular pathophysiology of concussive brain injury. Clin. Sports Med. 30, 33–48.

Barr, W.B., McCrea, M., 2001. Sensitivity and specificity of standardized neurocognitive testing immediately following sports concussion. J. Int. Neuropsychol. Soc. 7, 693–702.

Baugh, C.M., Stamm, J.M., Riley, D.O., Gavett, B.E., Shenton, M.E., et al., 2012. Chronic traumatic encephalopathy: neurodegeneration following repetitive concussive and subconcussive brain trauma. Brain Imaging Behav. 6, 244–254.

Baugh, C.M., Kiernan, P.T., Kroshus, E., Daneshvar, D.H., Montenigro, P.H., et al., 2015. Frequency of head-impact-related outcomes by position in NCAA division I collegiate football players. J. Neurotrauma 32, 314–326.

Bazarian, J.J., McClung, J., Shah, M.N., Cheng, Y.T., Flesher, W., et al., 2005. Mild traumatic brain injury in the United States, 1998–2000. Brain Inj. 19, 85–91.

Bazarian, J.J., Blyth, B., Mookerjee, S., He, H., McDermott, M.P., 2010. Sex differences in outcome after mild traumatic brain injury. J. Neurotrauma 27, 527–539.

Bazarian, J.J., Zhu, T., Blyth, B., Borrino, A., Zhong, J., 2012. Subject-specific changes in brain white matter on diffusion tensor imaging after sportsrelated concussion. Magn. Reson. Imaging 30, 171–180.

Bennett, R.E., Brody, D.L., 2014. Acute reduction of microglia does not alter axonal injury in a mouse model of repetitive concussive traumatic brain injury. J. Neurotrauma 31, 1647–1663.

Bhat, A.H., Dar, K.B., Anees, S., Zargar, M.A., Masood, A., Sofi, M.A., et al., 2015. Oxidative stress, mitochondrial dysfunction and neurodegenerative diseases: a mechanistic insight. Biomed. Pharmacother. 74, 101–110.

Binder, L.I., Guillozet-Bongaarts, A.L., Garcia-Sierra, F., Berry, R.W., 2005. Tau, tangles, and Alzheimer's disease. Biochim. Biophys. Acta 1739, 216–223.

Blennow, K., Jonsson, M., Andreasen, N., Rosengren, L., Wallin, A., et al., 2011. No neurochemical evidence of brain injury after blast overpressure by repeated explosions or firing heavy weapons. Acta Neurol. Scand. 123, 245–251.

Blurton-Jones, M., Laferla, F.M., 2006. Pathways by which Abeta facilitates tau pathology. Curr. Alzheimer Res. 3, 437–448.

Bremner, J.D., Randall, P., Scott, T.M., Capelli, S., Delaney, R., et al., 1995. Deficits in short term memory in adult survivors of childhood abuse. Psychiatry Res. 59, 97–107.

Brenner, L.A., 2011. Neuropsychological and neuroimaging findings in traumatic brain injury and posttraumatic stress disorder. Dialogues Clin. Neurosci. 13, 311–323.

Brod, S.A., 2000. Unregulated inflammation shortens human functional longevity. Inflamm. Res. 49, 561–570.

Broglio, S.P., Eckner, J.T., Paulson, H.L., Kutcher, J.S., 2012. Cognitive decline and aging: the role of concussive and subconcussive impacts. Exerc. Sport Sci. Rev. 40, 138–144.

Cai, Q., Tammineni, P., 2017. Mitochondrial aspects of synaptic dysfunction in Alzheimer's disease. J. Alzheimers Dis. 57, 1087–1103.

Cantu, R.C., 1998. Second impact syndrome. Clin. Sports Med. 17, 37–44.

Cassidy, J.D., Carroll, L.J., Peloso, P.M., et al., 2004. Incidence, risk factors and prevention of mild traumatic brain injury: results of the WHO Collaborating Centre Task Force on Mild Traumatic Brain Injury. J. Rehabil. Med. 43 (Suppl), 28–60.

Centers for Disease Control and Prevention (CDC), 2006. Sports related injuries among high school athletes in the United States. MMWR Morb. Mortal Wkly Rep. 55, 1037–1040.

Chabrier, M.A., Cheng, D., Castello, N.A., Green, K.N., LaFerla, F.M., 2014. Synergistic effects of amyloid-beta and wild type human tau on dendritic spine loss in a floxed double transgenic model of Alzheimer's disease. Neurobiol. Dis. 64, 107–117.

Charney, D.S., Deutch, A.Y., Krystal, J.H., Southwick, S.M., Davis, M., 1993. Psychobiologic mechanisms of posttraumatic stress disorder. Arch. Gen. Psychiatry 50, 295–305.

Cho, J.H., Johnson, G.V., 2004. Glycogen synthase kinase 3 beta induces caspase-cleaved tau aggregation in situ. J. Biol. Chem. 279, 54716–54723.

Christoffel, D.J., Golden, S.A., Russo, S.J., 2011. Structural and synaptic plasticity in stress related disorders. Rev. Neurosci. 22, 535–549.

Christofferson, D.E., Yuan, J., 2010. Necroptosis as an alternative form of programmed cell death. Curr. Opin. Cell Biol. 22, 263–268.

Chun, K.A., Manley, G.T., Stiver, S.I., Aiken, A.H., Phan, N., et al., 2010. Interobserver variability in the assessment of CT imaging features of traumatic brain injury. J. Neurotrauma 27, 325–330.

Churchill, N.W., Hutchison, M.G., Richards, D., Leung, G., Graham, S.J., et al., 2017. Neuroimaging of sport concussion: persistent alterations in brain structure and function at medical clearance. Sci. Rep. 7, 8297.

Clark, A.J., Auguste, K.I., Sun, P.P., 2011. Cervical spinal stenosis and sports related cervical cord neurapraxia. Neurosurg. Focus 31, E7.

Clark, A.L., Bangen, K.J., Sorg, S.F., Schiehser, D.M., Evangelista, N.D., et al., 2016. Dynamic association between perfusion and white matter integrity across time since injury in veterans with history of TBI. Neuroimage Clin. 14, 308–315.

Clavaguera, F., Bolmont, T., Crowther, R.A., Abramowski, D., Frank, S., et al., 2009. Transmission and spreading of tauopathy in transgenic mouse brain. Nat. Cell Biol. 11, 909–913.

Clavaguera, F., Akatsu, H., Fraser, G., Crowther, R.A., Frank, S., et al., 2013. Brain homogenates from human tauopathies induce tau inclusions in mouse brain. Proc. Natl. Acad. Sci. U.S.A. 110, 9535–9540.

Cohen, T.J., Guo, J.L., Hurtado, D.E., Kwong, L.K., Mills, I.P., et al., 2011. The acetylation of tau inhibits its function and promotes pathological tau aggregation. Nat. Commun. 2, 252.

Combs, H.L., Berry, D.T., Pape, T., Babcock-Parziale, J., Smith, B., et al., 2015. The effects of mild traumatic brain injury, posttraumatic stress disorder, and combined mild traumatic brain injury/posttraumatic stress disorder on returning veterans. J. Neurotrauma 32, 956–966.

Cornelius, C., Crupi, R., Calabrese, V., Graziano, A., Milone, P., Pennisi, G., et al., 2013. Traumatic brain injury: oxidative stress and neuroprotection. Antioxid. Redox Signal. 19, 836–853.

Crisco, J.J., Fiore, R., Beckwith, J.G., Chu, J.J., Brolinson, P.G., et al., 2010. Frequency and location of head impact exposures in individual collegiate football players. J. Athl. Train. 45, 549–559.

Croall, I.D., Cowie, C.J., He, J., Peel, A., Wood, J., et al., 2014. White matter correlates of cognitive dysfunction after mild traumatic brain injury. Neurology 83, 494–501.

Cubon, V.A., Putukian, M., Boyer, C., Dettwiler, A., 2011. A diffusion tensor imaging study on the white matter skeleton in individuals with sports related concussion. J. Neurotrauma (28), 189–201.

Decuypere, J.-P., Parys, J.B., Bultynck, G., 2012. Regulation of the autophagic Bcl-2/Beclin 1 interaction. Cells 1, 284–312.

Defense and Veterans Brain Injury Center, 2016. Department of Defense Numbers for TBI—Worldwide Totals. <http://dvbic.dcoe.mil/files/tbi-numbers/DoD-TBI-Worldwide-Totals_2016_Q1_May-16-2016_v1.0_2016-06-24_1>.

Del Bigio, M.R., Johnson, G.E., 1989. Clinical presentation of spinal cord concussion. Spine 14, 37–40.

Delouche, A., Attyé, A., Heck, O., Grand, S., Kastler, A., et al., 2016. Diffusion MRI: pitfalls, literature review and future directions of research in mild traumatic brain injury. Eur. J. Radiol. 85, 25–30.

Di Battista, A.P., Buonora, J.E., Rhind, S.G., Hutchison, M.G., Baker, A.J., et al., 2015. Blood biomarkers in moderate to-severe traumatic brain injury: potential utility of a multi-marker approach in characterizing outcome. Front Neurol. 6, 110.

Doherty, C.P., O'Keefe, E., Wallace, E., Loftus, T., Keaney, J., et al., 2016. Blood–brain barrier dysfunction as a hallmark pathology in chronic traumatic encephalopathy. J. Neuropathol. Exp. Neurol. 75, 656–662.

Dolan, P.J., Johnson, G.V., 2010. A caspase-cleaved form of tau is preferentially degraded through the autophagy pathway. J. Biol. Chem. 285, 21978–21987.

Dong, H., Goico, B., Martin, M., Csernansky, C.A., Bertchume, A., et al., 2004. Modulation of hippocampal cell proliferation, memory, and amyloid plaque deposition in APPsw (Tg2576) mutant mice by isolation stress. Neuroscience 127, 601–609.

Du, H., Guo, L., Yan, S., Sosunov, A.A., McKhann, G.M., Yan, S.S., 2010. Early deficits in synaptic mitochondria in an Alzheimer's disease mouse model. Proc. Natl. Acad. Sci. U.S.A. 107, 18670–18675.

Eierud, C., Craddock, R.C., Fletcher, S., Aulakh, M., King-Casas, B., et al., 2014. Neuroimaging after mild traumatic brain injury: review and meta-analysis. NeuroImage 4, 283–294.

Ermak, G., Harris, C.D., Davies, K.J.A., 2002. The DSCR1 (Adapt78) isoform 1 protein calcipressin 1 inhibits calcineurin and protects against acute calcium mediated stress damage, including transient oxidative stress. FASEB J. 16, 814–824.

Erol, A., 2008. An integrated and unifying hypothesis for the metabolic basis of sporadic Alzheimer's disease. J. Alzheimers Dis. 13, 241–253.

Farías, G., Cornejo, A., Jiménez, J., Guzmán, L., Maccioni, R.B., 2011. Mechanisms of tau self aggregation and neurotoxicity. Curr. Alzheimer Res. 8, 608–614.

Farooqui, A.A., 2010. Neurochemical Aspects of Neurotraumatic and Neurodegenerative Diseases. Springer Science + Business Media. L.L.C, New York.

Farooqui, A.A., 2014. Inflammation and Oxidative Stress in Neurological Disorders. Springer International Publishing, Switzerland.

Farooqui, A.A., 2017. Neurochemical Aspects of Alzheimer Disease. Academic Press, Cambridge, MA.

Ferreira, A., Bigio, E.H., 2011. Calpain mediated tau cleavage: a mechanism leading to neurodegeneration shared by multiple tauopathies. Mol. Med. 17, 676–685.

Fleminger, S., Oliver, D.L., Lovestone, S., Rabe-Hesketh, S., Giora, A., 2003. Head injury as a risk factor for Alzheimer's disease: the evidence 10 years on a partial replication. J. Neurol. Neurosurg. Psychiatry 74, 857–862.

Forman, M.S., Trojanowski, J.Q., Lee, V.M.Y., 2007. TDP-43: a novel neurodegenerative proteinopathy. Curr. Opin. Neurobiol. 17, 548–555.

Fortier, C.B., Amick, M.M., Grande, L., McGlynn, S., Kenna, A., et al., 2014. The Boston Assessment of Traumatic Brain Injury-Lifetime (BAT-L) semistructured interview: evidence of research utility and validity. J. Head Trauma Rehabil. 29, 89–98.

Faul, M., Coronado, V., 2015. Epidemiology of traumatic brain injury. Handb. Clin. Neurol. 127, 3–13.

Fife, T.D., Giza, C., 2013. Posttraumatic vertigo and dizziness. Semin. Neurol. 33, 238–243.

Fischer, I., Haas, C., Raghupathi, R., Jin, Y., 2016. Spinal cord concussion: studying the potential risks of repetitive injury. Neural Regen. Res. 11, 58–60.

Frost, B., Jacks, R.L., Diamond, M.I., 2009. Propagation of tau misfolding from the outside to the inside of a cell. J. Biol. Chem. 284, 12845–12852.

Gail, V.W.J., Judith, A.H., 1999. Tau protein in normal and Alzheimer's disease brain: an update. J. Alzheimers Dis. 1, 329–351.

Garwood, C.J., Pooler, A.M., Atherton, J., Hanger, D.P., Noble, W., 2011. Astrocytes are important mediators of Abeta-induced neurotoxicity and tau phosphorylation in primary culture. Cell Death Dis. 2, e167.

Gavett, B.E., Stern, R.A., McKee, A.C., 2011. Chronic traumatic encephalopathy: a potential late effect of sport related concussive and subconcussive head trauma. Clin. Sports Med. 30, 179–188.

Gerson, J.E., Kayed, R., 2013. Formation and propagation of tau oligomeric seeds. Front. Neurol. 4, 93.

Gerson, J., Castillo-Carranza, D.L., Sengupta, U., Bodani, R., Prough, D.S., et al., 2016. Tau oligomers derived from traumatic brain injury cause cognitive impairment and accelerate onset of pathology in Htau mice. J. Neurotrauma 33, 2034–2043.

Gezen-Ak, D., Dursun, E., Hanaðasý, H., Bilgiç, B., Lohman, E., et al., 2013. BDNF, TNFα, HSP90, CFH, and IL-10 serum levels in patients with early or late onset Alzheimer's disease or mild cognitive impairment. J. Alzheimers Dis. 37, 185–195.

Giza, C.C., Hovda, D.A., 2014. The new neurometabolic cascade of concussion. Neurosurgery 75 (Suppl 4), S24–S33.

Giza, C.G., Kutcher, J.S., 2014. An introduction to sports concussions. Continuum (Minneap. Minn.) 20, 1545–1551.

Giza, C.C., Kutcher, J.S., Ashwal, S., Barth, J., Getchius, T.S., et al., 2013. Summary of evidence based guideline update: evaluation and management of concussion in sports. Neurology 80, 2250–2257.

Glickman, M.H., Ciechanover, A., 2002. The ubiquitin–proteasome proteolytic pathway: destruction for the sake of construction. Physiol. Rev. 82, 373–428.

Goedert, M., Ghetti, B., Spillantini, M.G., 2000. Tau gene mutations in frontotemporal dementia and parkinsonism linked to chromosome 17 (FTDP-17). Their relevance for understanding the neurogenerative process. Ann. N.Y. Acad. Sci. 920, 74–83.

Gong, C.X., Iqbal, K., 2008. Hyperphosphorylation of microtubule associated protein tau: a promising therapeutic target for Alzheimer disease. Curr. Med. Chem. 15, 2321–2328.

Greve, M.W., Zink, B.J., 2009. Pathophysiology of traumatic brain injury. Mt. Sinai J. Med. 76, 97–104.

Gu, J., Wu, F., Xu, W., Shi, J., Hu, W., et al., 2017. TDP-43 suppresses tau expression via promoting its mRNA instability. Nucleic Acids Res. 45, 6177–6193.

Guillozet-Bongaarts, A.L., Cahill, M.E., Cryns, V.L., Reynolds, M.R., Berry, R.W., et al., 2006. Pseudophosphorylation of tau at serine 422 inhibits caspase cleavage: in vitro evidence and implications for tangle formation in vivo. J. Neurochem. 97, 1005–1014.

Guskiewicz, K.M., McCrea, M., Marshall, S.W., Cantu, R.C., Randolph, C., et al., 2003. Cumulative effects associated with recurrent concussion in collegiate football players: the NCAA Concussion Study. JAMA 290, 2549–2555.

Guskiewicz, K.M., Marshall, S.W., Bailes, J., McCrea, M., Cantu, R.C., et al., 2005. Association between recurrent concussion and late life cognitive impairment in retired professional football players. Neurosurgery 57, 719–726.

Haber, Y.O., Chandler, H.K., Serrador, J.M., 2016. Symptoms associated with vestibular impairment in veterans with posttraumatic stress disorder. PLoS ONE 11, e0168803.

Hall, G., Patuto, B., 2012. Is tau ready for admission to the prion club? Prion 6, 223–233.

Hanger, D.P., Anderton, B.H., Noble, W., 2009. Tau phosphorylation: the therapeutic challenge for neurodegenerative disease. Trends Mol. Med. 15, 112–119.

Harada, A., Oguchi, K., Okabe, S., Kuno, J., Terada, S., et al., 1994. Altered microtubule organization in small calibre axons of mice lacking tau protein. Nature 369, 488–491.

Hawkins, B.E., Krishnamurthy, S., Castillo-Carranza, D.L., Sengupta, U., Prough, D.S., et al., 2013. Rapid accumulation of endogenous tau oligomers in a rat model of traumatic brain injury: possible link between traumatic brain injury and sporadic tauopathies. J. Biol. Chem. 288, 17042–17050.

Hazrati, L.N., Tartaglia, M.C., Diamandis, P., Davis, K.D., Green, R.E., et al., 2013. Absence of chronic traumatic encephalopathy in retired football players with multiple concussions and neurological symptomatology. Front. Hum. Neurosci. 6, 222.

Hebron, M.L., Lonskaya, I., Sharpe, K., Weerasinghe, P.P., Algarzae, N.K., et al., 2013. Parkin ubiquitinates Tar-DNA binding protein-43 (TDP-43) and promotes its cytosolic accumulation via interaction with histone deacetylase 6 (HDAC6). J. Biol. Chem. 288, 4103–4115.

Hoge, C.W., McGurk, D., Thomas, J.L., Cox, A.L., Engel, C.C., et al., 2008. Mild traumatic brain injury in U.S. soldiers returning from Iraq. N. Engl. J. Med. 358, 453–463.

Holly, E.N., DeBold, J.F., Miczek, K.A., 2015. Increased mesocorticolimbic dopamine during acute and repeated social defeat stress: modulation by corticotropin releasing factor receptors in the ventral tegmental area. Psychopharmacology (Berl.) 232, 4469–4479.

Holm, L., Cassidy, J.D., Carroll, L.J., et al., 2005. Summary of the WHO collaborating centre for neurotrauma task force on mild traumatic brain injury. J. Rehabil. Med. 37, 137–141.

Hootman, J.M., Dick, R., Agel, J., 2007. Epidemiology of collegiate injuries for 15 sports: summary and recommendations for injury prevention initiatives. J. Athl. Train. 42, 311–319.

Horowitz, P.M., Patterson, K.R., Guillozet-Bongaarts, A.L., Reynolds, M.R., Carroll, C.A., Weintraub, S.T., et al., 2004. Early N-terminal changes and caspase-6 cleavage of tau in Alzheimer's disease. J. Neurosci. 24, 7895–9902.

Hovda, D., Le, H., Lifshitz, J., Berry, J., Badie, H., Yoshino, A., et al., 1994. Long term changes in metabolic rates for glucose following mild, moderate and severe concussive head injuries in adult rats. J. Neurosci. 20, 845.

Hovda, D.A., 1996. Metabolic dysfunction. In: Narayan, R.K., Wilberger, J.E., Povlishock, J.T. (Eds.), Neurotrauma. McGraw-Hill, New York, pp. 1459–1478.

Hutton, M., 2000. Molecular genetics of chromosome 17 tauopathies. Ann. N.Y. Acad. Sci. 920, 63–73.

Iqbal, K., Del, C., Alonso, A., Chen, S., Chohan, M.O., et al., 2005. Tau pathology in Alzheimer disease and other tauopathies. Biochim. Biophys. Acta 1739, 198–210.

Iqbal, K., Liu, F., Gong, C.X., Alonso, A.C., Grundke-Iqbal, I., 2009. Mechanisms of tau induced neurodegeneration. Acta Neuropathol. 118, 53–69.

Ito, H., Kanno, I., Fukuda, H., 2005. Human cerebral circulation: positron emission tomography studies. Ann. Nucl. Med. 19, 65–74.

Jin, K., Peel, A.L., Mao, X.O., Xie, L., Cottrell, B.A., et al., 2004. Increased hippocampal neurogenesis in Alzheimer's disease. Proc. Natl. Acad. Sci. U.S.A 101, 343–347.

Jin, Y., Bouyer, J., Haas, C., Fischer, I., 2015. Evaluation of the anatomical and functional consequences of repetitive mild cervical contusion using a model of spinal concussion. Exp. Neurol. 271, 175–188.

Johnson, V.E., Stewart, W., Smith, D.H., 2012a. Axonal pathology in traumatic brain injury. Exp. Neurol. 6, 35–43.

Johnson, V.E., Stewart, W., Smith, D.H., 2012b. Widespread tau and amyloid-beta pathology many years after a single traumatic brain injury in humans. Brain Pathol. 22, 142–149.

Johnson, V.E., Stewart, W., Weber, M.T., Cullen, D.K., Siman, R., et al., 2016. SNTF Immunostaining reveals previously undetected axonal pathology in traumatic brain injury. Acta Neuropathol. 131, 115–135.

Kawata, K., Liu, C.Y., Merkel, S.F., Ramirez, S.H., Tierney, R.T., et al., 2016. Blood biomarkers for brain injury: what are we measuring? Neurosci. Biobehav. Rev. 68, 460–473.

Kimura, T., Whitcomb, D.J., Jo, J., Regan, P., Piers, T., et al., 2014. Microtubule associated protein tau is essential for long term depression in the hippocampus. Philos. Trans. R. Soc. Lond. B: Biol. Sci. 369, 20130144.

King, P.R., Donnelly, K.T., Donnelly, J.P., Dunnam, M., Warner, G., et al., 2012. Psychometric study of the neurobehavioral symptom inventory. J. Rehabil. Res. Dev. 49, 879–888.

Kins, S., Crameri, A., Evans, D.R., Hemmings, B.A., Nitsch, R.M., et al., 2001. Reduced protein phosphatase 2A activity induces hyperphosphorylation and altered compartmentalization of tau in transgenic mice. J. Biol. Chem. 276, 38193–38200.

Kraus, M.F., Susmaras, T., Caughlin, B.P., Walker, C.J., Sweeney, J.A., et al., 2007. White matter integrity and cognition in chronic traumatic brain injury: a diffusion tensor imaging study. Brain 130, 2508–2519.

Kraus, N., Thompson, E.C., Krizman, J., Cook, K., White-Schwoch, T., et al., 2016. Auditory biological marker of concussion in children. Sci. Rep. 6, 39009.

Kulbe, J.R., Geddes, J.W., 2016. Current status of fluid biomarkers in mild traumatic brain injury. Exp. Neurol. 275 (Pt. 3), 334–352.

Kuret, J., Congdon, E.E., Li, G., Yin, H., Yu, X., Zhong, Q., 2005. Evaluating triggers and enhancers of tau fibrillization. Microsc. Res. Technol. 67, 141–155.

Laker, S.R., 2011. Epidemiology of concussion and mild traumatic brain injury. PM&R 3, S354–S358.

Lam, J.M., Hsiang, J.N., Poon, W.S., 1997. Monitoring of autoregulation using Doppler flowmetry in patients with head injury. J. Neurosurg. 86, 438–445.

Langlois, J.A., Rutland-Brown, W., Wald, M.M., 2006. The epidemiology and impact of traumatic brain injury: a brief overview. J Head Trauma Rehabil. 21, 375–378.

Lee, M.J., Lee, J.H., Rubinsztein, D.C., 2013. Tau degradation: the ubiquitinproteasome system versus the autophagy–lysosome system. Prog. Neurobiol. 105, 49–59.

Lehman, E.J., 2013. Epidemiology of neurodegeneration in American style professional football players. Alzheimers Res. Ther. 5, 34.

Lei, P., Ayton, S., Finkelstein, D.I., Spoerri, L., Ciccotosto, G.D., Wright, D.K., et al., 2012. Tau deficiency induces parkinsonism with dementia by impairing APP-mediated iron export. Nat. Med. 18, 291–295.

Li, H.H., Lee, S.M., Cai, Y., Sutton, R.L., Hovda, D.A., 2004. Differential gene expression in hippocampus following experimental brain trauma reveals distinct features of moderate and severe injuries. J. Neurotrauma 21, 1141–1153.

Li, B., Yamamori, H., Tatebayashi, Y., Shafit-Zargado, B., et al., 2008. Failure of neuronal maturation in Alzheimer disease dentate gyrus. J. Neuropathol. Exp. Neurol. 67, 78–84.

Lim, J., Lu, K.P., 2005. Pinning down phosphorylated tau and tauopathies. Biochim. Biophys. Acta 1739, 311–322.

Ling, J.M., Pena, A., Yeo, R.A., Merideth, F.L., Klimaj, S., et al., 2012. Biomarkers of increased diffusion anisotropy in semi acute mild traumatic brain injury: a longitudinal perspective. Brain 135, 1281–1292.

Ling, H., Hardy, J., Zetterberg, H., 2015. Neurological consequences of traumatic brain injuries in sports. Mol Cell Neurosci. 66, 114–122.

Lippa, S.M., Pastorek, N.J., Benge, J.F., Thornton, G.M., 2010. Postconcussive symptoms after blast and nonblast-related mild traumatic brain injuries in Afghanistan and Iraq war veterans. J. Int. Neuropyschol. Soc. 16, 856–866.

Liu, S.W., Huang, L.C., Chung, W.F., Chang, H.K., Wu, J.C., et al., 2017. Increased risk of stroke in patients of concussion: a nationwide cohort study. Int. J. Environ. Res. Public Health 14. pii: E230.

Longhi, L., Saatman, K.E., Fujimoto, S., Raghupathi, R., Meaney, D.F., et al., 2005. Temporal window of vulnerability to repetitive experimental concussive brain injury. Neurosurgery 56, 364–374.

Lu, D., Mahmood, A., Goussev, A., Schallert, T., Qu, C., et al., 2004. Atorvastatin reduction of intravascular thrombosis, increase in cerebral microvascular patency and integrity, and enhancement of spatial learning in rats subjected to traumatic brain injury. J. Neurosurg. 101, 813–821.

MacFarlane, M.P., Glenn, T.C., 2015. Neurochemical cascade of concussion. Brain Inj. 29, 139–153.

Maeda, S., Sahara, N., Saito, Y., Murayama, S., Ikai, A., et al., 2006. Increased levels of granular tau oligomers: an early sign of brain aging and Alzheimer's disease. Neurosci. Res. 54, 197–201.

Mazzaro, N., Barini, E., Spillantini, M.G., Goedert, M., Medini, P., et al., 2016. Tau-driven neuronal and neurotrophic dysfunction in a mouse model of early tauopathy. J. Neurosci. 36, 2086–2100.

McAllister, T.W., 2011. Neurobiological consequences of traumatic brain injury. Dialogues Clin. Neurosci. 13, 287–300.

McCrea, M., Guskiewicz, K.M., Marshall, S.W., et al., 2003. Acute effects and recovery time following concussion in collegiate football players: the NCAA concussion study. JAMA 290, 2556–2563.

McCrea, M., Barr, W.B., Guskiewicz, K., et al., 2005. Standard regression based methods for measuring recovery after sport-related concussion. J. Int. Neuropsychol. Soc. 11, 58–69.

McCrory, P., 2001. Does second impact syndrome exist? J. Clin. Sport Med. 11, 144–149.

McCrory, P., Meeuwisse, W., Johnston, K., Dvorak, J., Aubry, M., Molloy, M., et al., 2009. Consensus statement on Concussion in Sport: 3rd International Conference on Concussion in Sport held in Zurich, November 2008. Clin. J. Sport Med.: Off. J. Can. Acad. Sport Med. 19, 185–200.

McCrory, P., Meeuwisse, W., Aubry, M., Cantu, B., Dvořák, J., Echemendia, R., et al., 2013. Consensus statement on Concussion in Sport: The 4th International Conference on Concussion in Sport held in Zurich, November 2012. Br. J. Sports Med. 47, 250–258.

McKee, A.C., Cantu, R.C., Nowinski, C.J., Hedley-Whyte, E.T., Gavett, B.E., et al., 2009. Chronic traumatic encephalopathy in athletes: progressive tauopathy after repetitive head injury. J. Neuropathol. Exp. Neurol. 68, 709–735.

McKee, A.C., Stern, R.A., Nowinski, C.J., Stein, T.D., Alvarez, V.E., et al., 2013. The spectrum of disease in chronic traumatic encephalopathy. Brain 136, 43–64.

McKee, A.C., Daneshvar, D.H., Alvarez, V.E., Stein, T.D., 2014. The neuropathology of sport. Acta Neuropathol. 127, 29–51.

McKee, A.C., Cairns, N.J., Dickson, D.W., Folkerth, R.D., Dirk Keene, C., et al., 2015. The first NINDS/NIBIB consensus meeting to define neuropathological criteria for the diagnosis of chronic traumatic encephalopathy. Acta Neuropathol. 131, 75–86.

Meaney, D.F., Smith, D.H., Shreiber, D.I., Bain, A.C., Miller, R.T., et al., 1995. Biomechanical analysis of experimental diffuse axonal injury. J. Neurotrauma 12, 689–694.

Miller, D.R., Hayes, J.P., Lafleche, G., Salat, D.H., Verfaellie, M., 2016. White matter abnormalities are associated with chronic postconcussion symptoms in blast related mild traumatic brain injury. Hum. Brain Mapp. 37, 220–229.

Mohamed, N.V., Herrou, T., Plouffe, V., Piperno, N., Leclerc, N., 2013. Spreading of tau pathology in Alzheimer's disease by cell-to-cell transmission. Eur J Neurosci. 37, 1939–1948.

Montenigro, P.H., Alosco, M.L., Martin, B.M., Daneshvar, D.H., Mez, J., et al., 2016. Cumulative head impact exposure predicts later life depression, apathy, executive dysfunction, and cognitive impairment in former high school and college football players. J. Neurotrauma 34, 328–340.

Moore, A.H., Osteen, C.L., Chatziioannou, A.F., Hovda, D.A., Cherry, S.R., 2000. Quantitative assessment of longitudinal metabolic changes in vivo after traumatic brain injury in the adult rat using FDG-microPET. J. Cereb. Blood Flow Metab. 20, 1492–1501.

Morrison, F.G., Ressler, K.J., 2014. From the neurobiology of extinction to improved clinical treatments. Depress. Anxiety 31, 279–290.

Murray, M.E., Kouri, N., Lin, W.-L., Jack, C.R., Dickson, D.W., et al., 2014. Clinicopathologic assessment and imaging of tauopathies in neurodegenerative dementias. Alzheimers Res. Ther. 6, 1–13.

Nashner, L.M., Peters, J.F., 1990. Dynamic posturography in the diagnosis and management of dizziness and balance disorders. Neurol. Clin. 8, 331–349.

Niogi, S.N., Mukherjee, P., 2010. Diffusion tensor imaging of mild traumatic brain injury. J. Head Trauma Rehabil. 25, 241–255.

Noble, J.M., Hesdorffer, D.C., 2013. Sport related concussions: a review of epidemiology, challenges in diagnosis, and potential risk factors. Neuropsychol. Rev. 23, 273–284.

Noble, W., Hanger, D.P., Miller, C.C.J., Lovestone, S., 2013. The importance of tau phosphorylation for neurodegenerative diseases. Front. Neurol. 4, 88–98.

Oddo, S., Caccamo, A., Tseng, B., Cheng, D., Vasilevko, V., et al., 2008. Blocking Abeta42 accumulation delays the onset and progression of tau pathology via the C terminus of heat shock protein70-interacting protein: a mechanistic link between Abeta and tau pathology. J. Neurosci. 28, 12163–12175.

Olivier, B., 2015. Serotonin: a never ending story. Eur. J. Pharmacol. 753, 2–18.

Ommaya, A.K., Grubb Jr., R.L., Naumann, R.A., 1971. Coup and contre-coup injury: observations on the mechanics of visible brain injuries in the rhesus monkey. J. Neurosurg. 35, 503–516.

Omalu, B.I., DeKosky, S.T., Minster, R.L., 2005. Chronic traumatic encephalopathy in a National Football League player. Neurosurgery 57, 128–134.

Omalu, B.I., Fitzsimmons, R.P., Hammers, J., Bailes, J., 2010. Chronic traumatic encephalopathy in a professional American wrestler. J. Forensic Nurs. 6, 130–136.

Ouchterlony, D., Masanic, C., Michalak, A., Topolovec-Vranic, J., Rutka, J.A., 2016. Treating benign paroxysmal positional vertigo in the patient with traumatic brain injury: effectiveness of the canalith repositioning procedure. J. Neurosci. Nurs. 48, 90–99.

Papa, L., 2016. Potential blood based biomarkers for concussion. Sports Med. Arthrosc. 24, 108–115.

Park, S.Y., Ferreira, A., 2005. The generation of a 17 kDa neurotoxic fragment: an alternative mechanism by which tau mediates beta-amyloid-induced neurodegeneration. J. Neurosci. 25, 5365–5375.

Pellman, E.J., Powell, J.W., Viano, D.C., Casson, I.R., Tucker, A.M., et al., 2004. Concussion in professional football: epidemiological features of game injuries and review of the literature—part 3. Neurosurgery 54, 81–96.

Peskind, E.R., Brody, D., Cernak, I., McKee, A., Ruff, R.L., 2013. Military and sports-related mild traumatic brain injury: clinical presentation, management, and long term consequences. J. Clin. Psychiatry (74), 180–188.

Plassman, B.L., Havlik, R.J., Steffens, D.C., Helms, M.J., Newman, T.N., et al., 2000. Documented head injury in early adulthood and risk of Alzheimer's disease and other dementias. Neurology 55, 1158–1166.

Povlishock, J.T., 1992. Traumatically induced axonal injury: pathogenesis and pathobiological implications. Brain Pathol. 2, 1–12.

Povlishock, J.T., Katz, D.I., 2005. Update of neuropathology and neurological recovery after traumatic brain injury. J. Head Trauma Rehabil. 20, 76–94.

Prins, M.L., Alexander, D., Giza, C.C., Hovda, D.A., 2013. Repeated mild traumatic brain injury: mechanisms of cerebral vulnerability. J. Neurotrauma 30, 1557–9042.

Qaseem, A., Snow, V., Cross Jr., J., Forciea, M.A., Hopkins Jr., R., et al., 2008. Current pharmacologic treatment of dementia: a clinical practice guideline from the American College of Physicians and the American Academy of Family Physicians. Ann. Intern. Med. 148, 370–378.

Rametti, A., Esclaire, F., Yardin, C., Terro, F., 2004. Linking alterations in tau phosphorylation and cleavage during neuronal apoptosis. J. Biol. Chem. 279, 54518–54528.

Riemann, B.L., Guskiewicz, K.M., 2000. Effects of mild head injury on postural stability as measured through clinical balance testing. J. Athl. Train. 35, 19–25.

Riggio, S., Wong, M., 2009. Neurobehavioral sequelae of traumatic brain injury. Mt. Sinai J. Med. 76, 163–172.

Rissman, R.A., Poon, W.W., Blurton-Jones, M., Oddo, S., Torp, R., Vitek, M.P., et al., 2004. Caspase cleavage of tau is an early event in Alzheimer disease tangle pathology. J. Clin. Invest. 114, 121–130.

Ritchie, K., Lovestone, S., 2002. The dementias. Lancet 360, 1759–1766.

Roher, A.E., Debbins, J.P., Malek-Ahmadi, M., Chen, K., Pipe, J.G., et al., 2012. Cerebral blood flow in Alzheimer's disease. Vasc. Health Risk Manage. 8, 599–611.

Romeo, R.D., 2016. The impact of stress on the structure of the adolescent brain: implications for adolescent mental health. Brain Res. 1654, 185–191.

Ruff, R.L., Blake, K., 2016. Pathophysiological links between traumatic brain injury and posttraumatic headaches. F1000Res 5. pii: F1000 Faculty Rev-2116.

Rutherford, G.W., Corrigan, J.D., 2009. Long term consequences of traumatic brain injury. J. Head Trauma Rehabil. 24 (6), 421–423.

Salim, A., Hadjizacharea, P., Brown, C., Inaba, K., Teixeira, P.G., et al., 2008. Significance of troponin elevation after severe traumatic brain injury. J. Trauma 64, 46–57.

Schneider, A., Huentelman, M.J., Kremerskothen, J., Duning, K., Spoelgen, R., et al., 2010. KIBRA: a new gateway to learning and memory? Front. Aging Neurosci. 2, 4.

Sengupta, U., Guerrero-Muñoz, M.J., Castillo-Carranza, D.L., Lasagna-Reeves, C.A., Gerson, J.E., et al., 2015. Pathological interface between oligomeric alpha-synuclein and tau in synucleinopathies. Biol. Psychiatry 78, 672–683.

Seo, J.S., Lee, S., Shin, J.Y., Hwang, Y.J., Cho, H., et al., 2017. Transcriptome analyses of chronic traumatic encephalopathy show alterations in protein phosphatase expression associated with tauopathy. Exp. Mol. Med. 49, e333.

Shahim, P., Zetterberg, H., Tegner, Y., Blennow, K., 2017. Serum neurofilament light as a biomarker for mild traumatic brain injury in contact sports. Neurology 88, 1788–1794.

Shaw, N.A., 2002. The neurophysiology of concussion. Prog. Neurobiol. 67, 281–344.

Silverberg, N.D., Iverson, G.L., 2011. Etiology of the postconcussion syndrome: physiogenesis and psychogenesis revisited. NeuroRehabilitation 29, 317–329.

Siman, R., Giovannone, N., Hanten, G., Wilde, E.A., McCauley, S.R., et al., 2013. Evidence that the blood biomarker SNTF predicts brain imaging changes and persistent cognitive dysfunction in mild TBI patients. Front. Neurol. 4, 190.

Slobounov, S.M., Walter, A., Breiter, H.C., Zhu, D.C., Bai, X., et al., 2017. The effect of repetitive subconcussive collisions on brain integrity in collegiate football players over a single football season: a multi modal neuroimaging study. Neuroimage Clin. 14, 708–718.

Sohn, P.D., Tracy, T.E., Son, H.I., Zhou, Y., Leite, R.E., et al., 2016. Acetylated tau destabilizes the cytoskeleton in the axon initial segment and is mislocalized to the somatodendritic compartment. Mol. Neurodegener. 11, 47.

Sonnen, J.A., Larson, E.B., Haneuse, S., Woltjer, R., Li, G., et al., 2009. Neuropathology in the adult changes in thought study: a review. J. Alzheimers Dis. 18, 703–711.

Spillantini, M.G., Van Swieten, J.C., Goedert, M., 2000. Tau gene mutations in frontotemporal dementia and parkinsonism linked to chromosome 17 (FTDP-17). Neurogenetics 2, 193–205.

Spillantini, M.G., Lovino, M., Vuono, R., 2011. Release of growth factors by neuronal precursor cells as a treatment for diseases with tau pathology. Arch. Ital. Biol. 149, 215–223.

Stein, T.D., Alvarez, V.E., McKee, A.C., 2014. Chronic traumatic encephalopathy: a spectrum of neuropathological changes following repetitive brain trauma in athletes and military personnel. Alzheimers Res. Ther. 6, 4.

Stein, T.D., Montenigro, P.H., Alvarez, V.E., Xia, W., Crary, J.F., et al., 2015. Beta-amyloid deposition in chronic traumatic encephalopathy. Acta Neuropathol. 130, 21–34.

Stoica, B.A., Faden, A.I., 2010. Cell death mechanisms and modulation in traumatic brain injury. Neurotherapeutics 7, 3–12.

Stoothoff, W.H., Johnson, G.V.W., 2005. Tau phosphorylation: physiological and pathological consequences. Biochim. Biophys. Acta 1739, 280–297.

Takashima, A., 2013. Tauopathies and tau oligomers. J. Alzheimers Dis. 37, 565–568.

Tanaka, T., Zhong, J., Iqbal, K., Trenkner, E., Grundke-Iqbal, I., 1998. The regulation of phosphorylation of tau in SY5Y neuroblastoma cells: the role of protein phosphatases. FEBS Lett. 426, 248–254.

Tavazzi, B., Vagnozzi, R., Signoretti, S., et al., 2007. Temporal window of metabolic brain vulnerability to concussions: oxidative and nitrosative stresses—part II. Neurosurgery 61, 390–395.

Teasdale, G., Maas, A., Lecky, F., Manley, G., Stocchetti, N., et al., 2014. The Glasgow Coma Scale at 40 years: standing the test of time. Lancet Neurol. 13, 844–854.

Tempel, Z.J., Bost, J.W., Norwig, J.A., Maroon, J.C., 2015. Significance of T2 hyperintensity on magnetic resonance imaging after cervical cord injury and return to play in professional athletes. Neurosurgery 77, 23–31.

Thomas, S., Prins, M.L., Samii, M., Hovda, D.A., 2000. Cerebral metabolic response to traumatic brain injury sustained early in development: a 2-deoxy-D-glucose autoradiographic study. J. Neurotrauma 17, 649–665.

Torg, J.S., Corcoran, T.A., Thibault, L.E., Pavlov, H., Sennett, B.J., et al., 1997. Cervical cord neurapraxia: classification, pathomechanics, morbidity, and management guidelines. J. Neurosurg. 87, 843–850.

Tracy, T.E., Sohn, P.D., Minami, S.S., Wang, C., Min, S.W., et al., 2016. Acetylated tau obstructs KIBRA-mediated signaling in synaptic plasticity and promotes tauopathy-related memory loss. Neuron 90, 245–260.

Turner, R.C., Lucke-Wold, B.P., Robson, M.J., Lee, J.M., Bailes, J.E., 2016. Alzheimer's disease and chronic traumatic encephalopathy: distinct but possibly overlapping disease entities. Brain Inj. 30, 1279–1292.

Vazquez, A., 2013. Metabolic states following accumulation of intracellular aggregates: implications for neurodegenerative diseases. PLoS ONE 8, e63822.

Wakade, C., Sukumari-Ramesh, S., Laird, M.D., Dhandapani, K.M., Vender, J.R., 2010. Delayed reduction in hippocampal postsynaptic density protein-95 expression temporally correlates with cognitive dysfunction following controlled cortical impact in mice. J. Neurosurg. 113, 1195–1201.

Walker, K.R., Tesco, G., 2013. Molecular mechanisms of cognitive dysfunction following traumatic brain injury. Front. Aging Neurosci. 5, 29.

Wang, Y., Mandelkow, E., 2016. Tau in physiology and pathology. Nat. Rev. Neurosci. 17, 5–21.

Weingarten, M.D., Lockwood, A.H., Hwo, S.Y., Kirschner, M.W., 1975. A protein factor essential for microtubule assembly. Proc. Natl. Acad. Sci. U.S.A. 72, 1858–1862.

Werner, C., Engelhard, K., 2007. Pathophysiology of traumatic brain injury. Br. J. Anaesth. 99, 4–9.

Xu, W.L., Qiu, C.X., Wahlin, A., Winblad, B., Fratiglioni, L., 2004. Diabetes mellitus and risk of dementia in the Kungsholmen project: a 6-year follow up study. Neurology 63, 1181–1186.

Yokobori, S., Hosein, K., Burks, S., Sharma, I., Gajavelli, S., 2013. Biomarkers for the clinical differential diagnosis in traumatic brain injury—a systematic review. CNS Neurosci. Ther. 19, 556—565.

Yamada, K., Holth, J.K., Liao, F., Stewart, F.R., Mahan, T.E., et al., 2014. Neuronal activity regulates extracellular tau in vivo. J. Exp. Med. 211, 387—393.

Yamashita, T., Hideyama, T., Hachiga, K., Teramoto, S., Takano, J., Iwata, N., et al., 2012. A role for calpain dependent cleavage of TDP-43 in amytrophic lateral sclerosis pathology. Nat. Commun. 3, 1307—1321.

Yoshino, A., Hovda, D.A., Kawamata, T., Katayama, Y., Becker, D.P., 1991. Dynamic changes in local cerebral glucose utilization following cerebral concussion in rats: evidence of a hyper and subsequent hypometabolic state. Brain Res. 561, 106—119.

Yurgil, K.A., Barkauskas, D.A., Vasterling, J.J., Nievergelt, C.M., Larson, G.E., et al., 2014. Association between traumatic brain injury and risk of posttraumatic stress disorder in active duty marines. JAMA Psychiatry 71, 149—157.

Zhang, Y., Bhavnani, B.R., 2006. Glutamate induced apoptosis in neuronal cells is mediated via caspase dependent and independent mechanisms involving calpain and caspase-3 proteases as well as apoptosis inducing factor (AIF) and this process is inhibited by equine estrogens. BMC Neurosci. 7, 49.

Zhang, K., Johnson, B., Pennell, D., Ray, W., Sebastianelli, W., et al., 2010. Are functional deficits in concussed individuals consistent with white matter structural alterations: combined FMRI & DTI study. Exp. Brain Res. 204, 57—70.

Zhou, L., McInnes, J., Wierda, K., Holt, M., Herrmann, A.G., et al., 2017. Tau association with synaptic vesicles causes presynaptic dysfunction. Nat Commun. 8, 15295.

Zwimpfer, T.J., Bernstein, M., 1990. Spinal cord concussion. J. Neurosurg. 72, 894—900.

Potential Neuroprotective Strategies for Concussion and Chronic Traumatic Encephalopathy

INTRODUCTION

Public awareness of concussion has grown in recent years among young college students (age ≤ 18 years). The incidence of concussions among minors has increased 57% between 2008 and 2009 (Center for Disease Control and Prevention, 2011), and among high school athletes, the incidences have increased by 4.2-fold over an 11-year consecutive period beginning in 1998 (Lincoln et al., 2011). Annually, over 300,000 people suffer sports-related concussions in the United States and those between the ages of 15−24 years are most commonly affected (Harmon et al., 2013a,b). Conservative estimates of the combined direct and indirect annual costs for the treatment of concussion are approximately $12 billion (Finkelstein et al., 2006). Symptoms of concussion are imperative in making decisions regarding diagnosis, treatment, and prevention of concussion. This is particularly problematic for young people because of the potential cumulative or long-term deleterious effects of concussion (Zemper, 2003). The Centre for Disease Control recently declared that sport concussions are reaching "epidemic levels" and deserve further research (Bazarian et al, 2006). Under normal daily mechanical loading conditions, axons can easily stretch to at least twice their resting length and relax back unharmed to their prestretch straight geometry (Tang-Schomer et al., 2010). However, following concussion, rapid stretching of axons results in physically breaking of the axonal cytoskeleton, a process, which is observed not only in preclinical traumatic brain injury (TBI) models, but also in human TBI (Smith et al., 1999;

381

Tang-Schomer et al., 2012). Because microtubules (MTs) essentially serve as the anatomical tracks for protein transport, proteins pile up at points of individual microtubule disconnection, resulting in varicose swellings distributed periodically along the injured axon (Johnson et al., 2013; Tang-Schomer et al., 2012) as well as partial transport interruption (Tang-Schomer et al., 2012) rather than complete transport failure in an entire region of the axon. During this event, some protein transport continues through areas of swelling along remaining intact MTs, but may be derailed farther along the axon because of MT disruption there (Smith, 2016).

As stated in Chapter 8, Molecular Aspects of Concussion and Chronic Traumatic Encephalopathy, concussion is a complex neurological syndrome caused by traumatic biomechanical acceleration and deceleration forces initiated by either a direct blow to the head, face or neck or via excessive force elsewhere on the body transmitted to the head (McCrory et al., 2009). During concussion rotational acceleration, diffuse shear and strain forces produce variable degrees of injury not only to axons, neuronal membranes, glia, but also to vascular structures, leading to transitory ionic functional disturbances with clinical manifestations. Collective evidence suggests that concussion-mediated brain injury not only involves bioenergetic challenges, oxidative stress, and neuroinflammation, but also abnormalities in signal transduction processes due to axonal injury leading to impairments in neurotransmission, decrease in neuroplasticity, memory loss, and behavioral changes along with alterations in blood−brain barrier (BBB) permeability and increase in leukocyte infiltration into the brain (Barkhoudarian et al., 2011; Giza and Hovda, 2014). At the molecular level, concussion cascade begins with the release of excitatory neurotransmitters, which result in cellular membrane disruption and ionic imbalances. Increasing amounts of adenosine triphosphate (ATP) are required in an attempt to correct these ionic imbalances, and an increase in glucose metabolism is observed within the first 24 hours after concussion (MacFarlane and Glenn, 2015). This increased glucose metabolism, combined with an initial decrease in cerebral blood flow (CBF), results in a mismatch between the energy required and that available to brain structures. The increase in glucose metabolism is followed by a period of reduced glucose uptake and metabolism, which may last for as long as 1 month (Giza and Hovda, 2001). It is also suggested that the loss of function of axonal sodium channels throughout the brain network may also underlie common neurocognitive symptoms of concussion, such as loss of consciousness, decreased processing speed, and memory dysfunction. With too much sodium entering the axon, the capacity to generate action potentials (the rapid exchange of ions across the neural membrane) is lost or dysfunctional, interrupting or slowing signaling in the axon and throughout the neural network of the brain (Johnson et al., 2013). To correct concussion-mediated neurochemical changes and restore metabolic homeostasis, neural cells are forced to function at an increased capacity, resulting in a tremendous need for ATP, and these demands for ATP can be met through glycolytic pathways. Although neurons in this hypermetabolic state quickly produce ATP, this process is inefficient and results not only in excessive production of lactate and the generation of oxygen radicals, which can damage key cellular components, such as DNA and neural membrane phospholipids. Furthermore, excessive Ca^{2+} influx reduces the polarization of mitochondrial membranes, resulting in mitochondrial dysfunction, which leads to induction of oxidative stress, as well as impairment in lactate metabolism (Giza and Hovda, 2001; Barkhoudarian et al., 2011).

CBF is an important factor, which is altered by the concussion (Len and Neary, 2011; Wang et al., 2016). In humans, CBF may be assessed noninvasively using arterial spin labeling (ASL). This procedure is a form of magnetic resonance imaging (MRI) which uses radio-frequency pulses to magnetically "tag" inflowing arterial blood, producing an endogenous tracer which can be used to quantify tissue perfusion. Using ASL, it is reported that CBF is reduced following concussion and mTBI (Grossman et al., 2013; Meier et al., 2015), although in some cases perfusion may be initially unaltered or even elevated at early injury (Churchill et al., 2017). Very little is known about the relationship between CBF and physical and mental functioning of the brain. However, it is reported that decrease in CBF may lead to neuroglial energy crisis, disruption of intracortical circuits resulting in mild cognitive impairment (MCI). Moreover, CBF is also linked with neuronal metabolism at the microvascular level and observed changes following concussion observed can be due to a relative uncoupling of neuronal activity with the astrocytic and vascular components of the neurovascular unit (Venkat et al., 2016). Thus patients with concussion 1 month after injury exhibit regional hypoperfusion compared to controls, but more severe symptoms such as dizziness is accompanied with higher regional CBF (Lin et al., 2016) in frontal and occipital lobes. Similarly, a study of persistent postconcussive symptoms in children reported elevated CBF in symptomatic individuals but decreased CBF in asymptomatic individuals, relative to controls (Barlow et al., 2016). These studies support the view that there may be reliable cerebral perfusion correlates of postconcussion symptoms following mild TBI throughout the concussion recovery timeline. Although the molecular mechanisms associated with the pathogenesis of concussion has yet to be fully elucidated, it is becoming increasingly clear that not only cerebrovascular alterations play a significant role in the evolution of injury sequelae, but posttraumatic brain repair processes are also associated with concussion (Tan et al., 2014;

Pop and Badaut, 2011). Collective evidence suggests that in the acute phase of concussion, metabolic changes among neural cells are not only supported by alterations in neuronal depolarization, ion transport, glycolysis, mitochondrial function, and excitatory neurotransmitter release, but also by reductions in global and regional CBF. These changes are linked to cognitive, vestibular, and oculomotor dysfunction of various brain systems or domains (Giza and Hovda, 2001; McCrory et al., 2013a). The short-term symptoms of concussions depend on the severity of the injury. Symptoms often include headache, cognitive impairment (i.e., diminished reaction times or "feeling foggy"), sensitivity to light and sound, irritability, sleep disturbances, and loss of consciousness. Symptoms typically resolve within 7–10 days for adults (McCrory et al., 2013b), but the presence of abnormal neurometabolic function may persist for up to 4 weeks after injury (Shrey et al., 2011). Postconcussion treatment and recovery is primarily limited to cognitive and physical rest until symptoms resolve. For athletes, returning to play after a concussion involves a gradual increase in the intensity of physical activity once cognitive and balance symptoms have resolved fully (Harmon et al., 2013a,b). Concussion is known to adversely affect a person's cognitive, emotional, and social functioning, and create lasting personal, familial, and societal implications. In approximately 10%–15% of individuals who have sustained concussion, persistent symptoms can impact an individual's ability to return to daily functioning (Carroll et al., 2004). As stated in Chapter 8, Molecular Aspects of Concussion and Chronic Traumatic Encephalopathy, physical symptoms of concussion include headache, nausea, fatigue, and dizziness, cognitive symptoms include memory, attention, and executive function impairments, and mental health concerns are associated with depression, anxiety, and posttraumatic stress disorders. These symptoms can negatively impact individual's ability to recover from concussion (Cancelliere et al., 2014). Many studies have indicated that 22%–36% of patients report three or more of such posttraumatic symptoms at 6 months postmild TBI (Hou et al., 2012) with about 23% not being recovered by 1 year postinjury (Cassidy et al., 2014).

Studies on animal models of concussion have indicated that cascade of concussion occurs over a period of hours rather than minutes and thus explains why some signs and symptoms of concussion may be delayed. Although the temporal course of these metabolic processes has been well documented in animal studies, the magnitude and duration of these pathophysiological alterations in humans remain poorly understood. Neuroimaging studies indicate that concussion produces functional changes without obvious structural damage to the brain (Chen et al., 2007; Zhang et al., 2010). As stated earlier, signs and symptoms of concussion are nonspecific, but may include sudden confusion, lack of balance or coordination, vision abnormalities, and memory impairment. The recent position statement of the National Athletic Trainers' Association (NATA) recommends the use of symptom checklists, neuropsychological testing, and postural stability assessment (Guskiewicz et al., 2003; Yengo-Kahn et al., 2016). Baseline testing on these measures is important for athletes participating in contact sports with a high concussion risk; however, if resources allow, then all athletes should receive baseline assessment. Follow-up testing should be conducted to aid in the decision process for return to play. Using all the available information may be the best approach to safely returning an athlete to play after a concussion. These tools can also be used to monitor recovery (Scorza et al., 2012; Yengo-Kahn et al., 2016). Thus recognizing the symptoms of concussion is imperative in making decisions regarding diagnosis, and prevention of concussion.

MANAGEMENT OF CONCUSSION

Cognitive and physical rest are the cornerstones of initial management of concussion. There are no specific treatments for concussion; therefore focus is on managing symptoms of concussion. Current management of concussion consists of early education, rest until symptom free, with gradual return to school, physical activity protocol, and finally to play. Although this management strategy is effective for most concussion patients, it is not an appropriate strategy for concussion patients with persistent postconcussion symptoms. Prolonged rest and periods of restricted activity may promote at risk for secondary issues and contribute to the chronicity of postconcussion symptoms. Active rehabilitation protocol for concussion patients who are slow to recover from concussion is needed. It is hypothesized that an active rehabilitation intervention can reduce persistent postconcussion symptoms, improve function, and facilitate return to activity (Reed et al., 2015). Because concussion recovery is variable, rigid classification systems have mostly been abandoned in favor of an individualized approach. The complexity of concussion requires clinicians to use a variety of tools for information, but the current tendency is to base the return-to-play decision on the athlete's self-reporting of symptoms and ability to perform sport-specific tasks without a recurrence of concussion symptoms (Scorza et al., 2012; Schneider et al., 2013). Relying solely on this information can be dangerous because it creates an incomplete picture of the injury. Programs aimed to limit repeated concussion, particularly before recovery from an initial concussion, like return-to-play and return-to-work are all based on the provision of an accurate knowledge of the history of concussion symptoms by the patient to a doctor or another person such as a coach or an athletic trainer. Recognizing and understanding the symptoms of concussion such as headaches, dizziness, sensitivity to light and sound, difficulty focusing or concentrating, sleep disturbance, and fatigue is paramount for accurate patient management and for the prevention of future events (Cao et al., 2014). Because some athletes, in particular children, may not have the vocabulary to express subtle aspects of their symptoms, it is important that physicians and coaches ask specifically about fixed or transient neurological deficits such as monocular blurred vision or transient weakness or numbness that can point to focal injury to central and peripheral nervous system structures. Not recognizing symptoms of concussion may result in inappropriately early return to play in sports and potentially may have negative and serious consequences. Concerns over the short- and long-term effects of concussion among professional athletes have brought these subjects to the global scale. Recent media attention has focused on the short-term memory loss, headache, and migraine suffered 10−20 years following concussion in sports such as football and hockey (Meehan and Bachur, 2009). Pharmacologic interventions and biofeedback have been used to address headache, and psychotherapy to address emotional and behavioral adjustment (Andrasik, 2010). Neurofeedback, although still considered experimental, has been used to "normalize" brain wave patterns, in the hopes of reducing symptoms, although rigorously controlled research has not yet clearly demonstrated its efficacy (Thatcher, 2009; Thornton and Carmody, 2009). Vestibular therapy has been reported to give promising results for postconcussive symptoms of dizziness and balance problems (Herdman, 2000; Alsalaheen et al., 2010). Although patients with concussion are advised to restrict physical and cognitive activity until all symptoms resolve. However, recent research suggests that prolonged rest beyond the first couple of days after a concussion may hinder rather than aid recovery (Leddy et al., 2016a,b). Humans do not respond well to removal from their social and physical environments, and sustained rest adversely affects the physiology of concussion and can lead to physical deconditioning and reactive depression (Leddy et al., 2016a). A test called Buffalo Concussion Treadmill Test has been designed to systematically evaluate exercise tolerance in persons with prolonged symptoms after concussion. Buffalo Concussion Treadmill Test is the only functional test known to safely and reliably reveal exercise intolerance in humans with postconcussion syndrome (PCS). New research suggests that absolute rest beyond the first few days after concussion may be detrimental to concussion recovery (Leddy et al., 2016b). However, further research is required to determine the appropriate mode, duration, intensity, and frequency of exercise during the acute recovery phase of a concussion prior to making specific exercise recommendations. For patients with PCS, subsymptom threshold exercise improves activity tolerance and is an appropriate treatment option for this patient population (Imhoff et al., 2016).

OMEGA-3 FATTY ACIDS AND CONCUSSION

It is known that omega-3 fatty acids (docosahexaenoic acid and eicosapentaenoic acid) occur abundantly in the brain and play a crucial role in essential neuronal functions, such as axonal guidance, synapse and dendrite formation, and neurotransmission (Farooqui, 2009). As stated in Chapter 8, Molecular Aspects of Concussion and Chronic Traumatic Encephalopathy, omega-3 fatty acids can be used as potential therapeutic agent for the treatment of TBI (Lewis et al., 2013). Lewis has also suggested that omega-3 fatty acids can also be used for the treatment of concussion (Lewis, 2016). Following experimental TBI, omega-3 fatty acids exert potent neuroprotective effects through multifaceted actions, e.g., amelioration of oxidative stress, mitigation of endoplasmic reticulum stress, modulation of microglial activation, and improvement of white matter integrity (Farooqui, 2009; Barrett et al., 2014). At the molecular level, omega-3 fatty acids produce their beneficial effects on neurotraumatic diseases by generating omega-3 fatty acid-derived lipid mediators called docosanoids (resolvins, neuroprotectins, and maresins) (Bazan et al., 2011; Serhan, 2005; Farooqui, 2009, 2011). These mediators produce antioxidant, antiinflammatory, and antiapoptotic effects and protect neuronal cells from neurodegeneration in neurotraumatic and neurodegenerative diseases (Farooqui, 2010, 2011). Studies with aged rodents have consistently shown that omega-3 fatty acids supplementation improves neurogenesis and synaptogenesis, executive functions and learning abilities, while omega-3 PUFA deficiency is associated with memory deficits and impaired hippocampal plasticity (Denis et al., 2013; Luchtman and Song, 2013; Maruszak et al., 2014). Furthermore, omega-3 fatty acids can also normalize levels of brain-derived neurotrophic factor (BDNF), synapsin I, and cyclic AMP-response element binding protein and restore learning and memory disability (Wu et al., 2003, 2004, 2005; Farooqui, 2009). The use of omega-3 fatty acids to treat TBI has not hitherto been translated to the clinic, although there are sporadic case studies using omega-3 fatty acids acutely after human TBI (Lewis and Bailes, 2011; Lewis et al., 2013; Roberts et al., 2008). A large portion of the preclinical studies on omega-3 fatty acids have indicated that pre-TBI treatment with omega-3 fatty acids produces beneficial effects in TBI (Wu et al., 2004; Pu et al., 2013). However, these observations have provided limited information on the use of omega-3 fatty acids in human TBI. While some studies delivered invaluable mechanistic insights of post-TBI omega-3 fatty acids treatment (Shin and Dixon, 2011) concerns still remain over the short delivery time window or the lack of long-term functional evaluation. To facilitate future investigations on omega-3 fatty acids in concussion and TBI patients, information should be obtained on clinical feasibility of omega-3 fatty acids using optimal doses, manageable delivery routes, and time window. In addition, other anecdotal, alternative/ complementary treatments such as Epsom salts footbaths (for magnesium intake) and craniosacral therapy have also been used to manage symptoms of concussion (Greenman and McPartland, 1995).

REHABILITATION AND CONCUSSION

It is well known that brain has life-long capacity to induce experience-dependent plasticity, which allows brain to adapt to new environments or to changes in the environment, and to changes in internal brain states such as occurs following concussion or brain damage. Physical therapists manage (treat) concussion patients by teaching and training them for balance to correct balance dysfunctions, gaze stabilization activities, vestibular habituation activities, and canalith repositioning (Alsalaheen et al., 2010, 2013). Following concussion, oculomotor control is compromised through axonal injury or blunt trauma to the visual control systems (Brosseau-Lachaine et al., 2008; Heitger et al., 2008). Physical therapists treat patients with concussion by addressing impairments in oculomotor control such as convergence (Thiagarajan and Ciuffreda, 2013), smooth pursuits (Kongsted et al., 2007), saccades (Heitger et al., 2009), and ocular fixation (Ciuffreda et al., 2007).

CHRONIC TRAUMATIC ENCEPHALOPATHY

As stated in Chapter 8, Molecular Aspects of Concussion and Chronic Traumatic Encephalopathy, chronic traumatic encephalopathy (CTE) is a progressive tauopathy, which is caused by repeated concussive or subconcussive blows to the head. CTE commonly occurs in athletes. CTE takes years to decades to develop, often providing a significant latent period between when the neurotrauma occurs and when symptoms develop. Originally described in boxers, CTE has been reported to occur in a variety of contact sports, including American football, professional wrestling, professional hockey, soccer, as well as other activities associated with mild repetitive head trauma (Gavett et al., 2011). Neuropathological changes in CTE include cerebral atrophy, cavum septum pellucidum with fenestrations, shrinkage of the mammillary bodies, dense tau immunoreactive inclusions (neurofibrillary tangles (NFTs), glial tangles, and neuropil neurites), and diffuse axonal injury (DAI). As stated in Chapter 8, Molecular Aspects of Concussion and Chronic Traumatic Encephalopathy, pathologically, DAI consists of a spectrum of abnormalities from primary mechanical breaking of the axonal cytoskeleton, to transport interruption, swelling and proteolysis, through secondary physiological changes. Depending on the severity and extent of trauma, these alterations can manifest acutely as immediate loss of consciousness or confusion and persist as coma and/or cognitive dysfunction. In addition, recent evidence suggests that TBI may induce long-term neurodegenerative processes, such as insidiously progressive axonal pathology. Indeed, axonal degeneration has been found to continue even years after injury in humans, and appears to play a role in the development of Alzheimer's disease (AD)-like pathological changes. In addition, in some patients with CTE also show TDP-43 proteinopathy as well as low-grade diffuse white matter rarefaction, microglial activation, and presence of reactive astrocytes (Gavett et al., 2011). White matter is primarily composed of myelin and myelinated axons. Structural and functional completeness of myelin is critical for the reliable and efficient transmission of information. Changes in white matter tracts may contribute to the development of demyelinating diseases. Activation of microglial cells and presence of reactive astrocytes lead to neuroinflammation, a process which occurs in the brain after repeated TBI prior to, or independently, from the formation of NFTs (Yoshiyama et al., 2007; Jaworski et al., 2011). Therefore it is likely that tau oligomers, which are formed prior to NFTs, may contribute to the neuroinflammation (Patterson et al., 2011). This inflammatory response may induce a self-perpetuating cycle, whereby tau oligomers increase neuroinflammation, causing more damage to the neurons, which in turn may increase the rate of tau oligomer formation. Furthermore, neuroinflammation directly influences the rate of disease progression and the extent of neuronal loss (Golde, 2009), supporting the view that disrupting neuroinflammation can provide a novel neuroprotective intervention for tauopathies. CTE is characterized by the accumulation and deposition of hyperphosphorylated tau (p-tau) protein as NFT beginning perivascularly and at the depths of the cortical sulci. Later stage p-tau pathology becomes more widespread, particularly dense in the medial temporal lobes, also present in the white matter, and leads to prominent neuronal loss and gliosis. These neuropathological changes in CTE patients may be responsible for disordered memory and executive functioning, behavioral, and personality disturbances (apathy, depression, irritability, impulsiveness, aggression, and suicidality) that usually begin 8−10 years after experiencing repetitive mild TBI (McKee et al., 2009). Early behavioral symptoms of CTE usually do not appear until the mid-1930s, and cognitive impairment does not begin until the early 1960s (Baugh et al., 2014). At the present time, there are no formal clinical or pathological diagnostic criteria for CTE (Gavett et al., 2011). Postmortem microscopic diagnosis of CTE is almost exclusively limited to the use of antibodies directed against p-tau protein, with p-tau immunoreactivity observed in a perivascular pattern and at the depths of the sulci in addition to p-tau immune-positive glial and neuronal profiles in subpial regions and astrocytic p-tau positive plaques (Omalu, 2014). Two conformations of phosphorylated tau (*cis* p-tau and *trans* p-tau) are present in the brain. These conformation forms can be distinguished on the basis of their polyclonal and monoclonal antibodies (Ab). The *trans* p-tau is physiologic. It promotes MT assembly and neuronal survival, whereas the *cis* is early pathogenic and its presence leads to tauopathy in AD, TBI, and CTE (Lu et al., 2016; Albayram et al., 2016). Peptidyl-prolyl isomerase (Pin1) is a unique peptidyl-prolyl *cis*−*trans* isomerase, which catalyzes prolyl isomerization and plays a critical role in regulating a subset of phosphoproteins by specifically catalyzing conformational change on the phosphorylated Ser/Thr-Pro motifs (Lu and Zhou, 2007; Lee et al., 2011). Pin1 is colocalized with phosphorylated tau in brain tissue from AD and other tauopathies. In line with its diverse physiological role, Pin1 not only prevents the accumulation of the pathogenic *cis* p-tau into nonpathogenic *trans* p-tau, but also plays an important protective role in the brain against AD by maintaining tau and amyloid precursor protein in their proper forms. Histological studies have indicated that the appearance of robust *cis* p-tau in the early stages of human MCI, AD, and CTE brains, as well as after sport- and military-related TBI. Notably, the presence of *cis* p-tau has been reported to occur within hours after closed head injury and long before other known pathogenic p-tau conformations including oligomers, prefibrillary tangles, and NFTs. Importantly, *cis* p-tau monoclonal antibody treatment not only eliminates *cis* p-tau induction and tau pathology, but also restores many neuropathological and functional outcomes in TBI mouse models. Thus *cis* p-tau is an early driver of tau pathology in TBI and CTE and detection of *cis* p-tau in human bodily fluids can potentially provide new diagnostic and prognostic tools. This information can be used to develop treatment for AD, TBI, and CTE (Albayram et al., 2016). It should also be noted that AD is also characterized by a relatively uniform distribution of tau containing NFTs in layers containing large projection neurons, such as layers III and V (Gavett et al., 2011). In contrast, CTE is exemplified by an irregular distribution of tau in more superficial cortical layers such as II and III. Similarly, the progressive topographic involvement of regions of the brain as seen in CTE differs from what is seen in other neurodegenerative diseases like AD. Most cases of CTE do not show beta-amyloid deposition and the presence of positive neuritic plaques. Most CTE patients show the evidence of axonal injury, which ranges from multifocal axonal varicosities in earlier stage pathology to axonal loss in later stage pathology. Stage I and II CTE can present macroscopically with mild enlargement of the lateral ventricles or third ventricle and/or mild septal abnormalities. In contrast, neuritic amyloid plaques are seen in AD supporting the view that neuritic amyloid plaques are not characteristic features of CTE, and are less frequently seen in CTE (Gavett et al., 2011). More recently, it is reported that tau has been shown to propagate from cell to cell potentially acting as a signaling molecule that contributes to disease progression. In addition, in CTE tau translocate itself to dendrites leading to synaptic dysfunction. This translocation of tau may subsequently contribute to neurodegeneration. Collective evidence suggests that clinically CTE is a chronic composite syndrome, which is accompanied by alterations in mood, neuropsychiatric disturbances, and cognitive impairment (McKee et al., 2009; Omalu et al., 2010, 2011; Stern et al., 2013; Turner et al., 2012). Behavioral abnormalities such as irritability, judgment issues, increased risk-taking, and depression are characteristic and prominent early in the course of CTE. As stated in Chapter 8, Molecular Aspects of Concussion and Chronic Traumatic Encephalopathy, additional symptoms of CTE are difficulty in sleeping, poor concentration, or memory impairment (McKee et al., 2009; Omalu et al., 2010, 2011; Stern et al., 2013; Turner et al., 2012). Definitive and confirmatory diagnosis of CTE is still based on direct tissue histochemical and immunohistochemical analyses, which reveal topographically multifocal or diffuse cortical and subcortical hyperphosphorylated tauopathy, which is accompanied by isomorphic fibrillary astrogliosis and microglial activation. Cherry et al. (2017) have recently reported that levels of CCL11 (eotaxin-1), a chemokine, which contributes to age-associated cognitive decline, are markedly increased in the brain and cerebrospinal fluid (CSF) in CTE compared to AD. Due to the limited sample size, this study has been most likely too underpowered to observe an effect of CSF CCL11 on CTE severity. Thus these preliminary data suggest that CCL11 may be a novel biomarker to aid in the detection of CTE neuropathology and to discriminate CTE from AD.

RISK FACTORS FOR CHRONIC TRAUMATIC ENCEPHALOPATHY

It well known that repetitive concussive or subconcussive blows to the head may increase the risk for CTE (McKee et al., 2009; Daneshvar et al., 2011; Gavett et al., 2011). This pathological condition is found not only in athletes who participate in contact sports (American football, boxing, hockey, soccer, and professional wrestling), but also other groups at risk for repetitive head trauma and CTE are military veterans, epileptics, and victims of domestic abuse (McKee et al., 2009). It has been reported that approximately 17% of professional retired boxers will exhibit CTE (Omalu et al., 2010). Although each group listed earlier has a unifying factor of head trauma, they differ in particular aspects that may influence the severity or chronicity of their injury (Fig. 9.1). Crisco et al. (2010) have reported that that the average number of impacts received by an individual football player during a single season varies from 380 to 420. These impacts vary in severity based on their position. Offensive linemen, defensive linemen, and line backers receive the most frequent impacts, while quarterbacks and running backs received the greatest magnitude of head impacts (Crisco et al., 2011).

Lifestyle, pollution, stress are other important risk factors, which can prone and promote the pathogenesis of TBI, CTE, and AD after trauma. The common denominators of these factors are oxidative stress and inflammatory response. Chronic low-grade oxidative stress and systemic inflammation during physiological aging and immune-senescence are intertwined in the pathogenesis of premature aging (Farooqui, 2014). The latter has been associated with frailty, morbidity, and mortality in elderly subjects. However, it is unknown to what extent oxidative stress and neuroinflammation is controlled by epigenetic events in early life. Today, human diet is believed to have a major influence on both the development and prevention of age-related diseases (Farooqui, 2014). Long-term

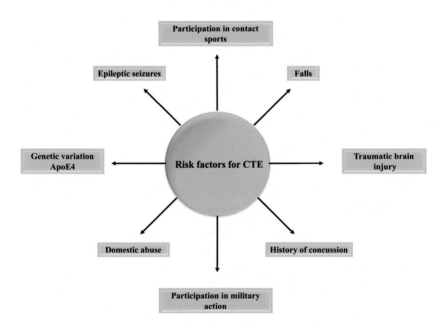

FIGURE 9.1   Risk factors for chronic traumatic encephalopathy (CTE).

consumption of western diet, lack exercise, sleep deprivation, high intake of alcohol (alcohol abuse), use of recreational and performance enhancing drugs can lead to personality changes and neuropsychiatric difficulties (Almeida et al., 2014; Zahr et al., 2011; Hartgens and Kuipers, 2004; Sheidow et al., 2012; Farooqui, 2014). Long-term consumption of western diet along with physical inactivity, genetic and environmental factors is associated with a higher risk for developing chronic visceral diseases (obesity, cardiovascular diseases, diabetes, and metabolic syndrome) as well as neurotraumatic (stroke) and neurodegenerative diseases (AD and Parkinson's disease (PD)) (Farooqui, 2014). This is due to the enrichment of high levels of omega-6 fatty acids (arachidonic acid (ARA)), low fiber, and high salt contents in western diet. ARA is metabolized to proinflammatory prostaglandins (PGs), leukotrienes (LTs), and thromboxanes (TXs). In addition, consumption of western diet increases the levels of proinflammatory cytokines (TNF-α, IL-1β, and IL-6). These mediators contribute to oxidative stress and neuroinflammatory responses (Farooqui, 2010, 2011, 2014). Based on this information, it can be proposed that long-term consumption of western diet, lack exercise, sleep deprivation, high consumption of alcohol (alcohol abuse), use of recreational and performance enhancing drugs can prone one to worst consequences of TBI, CTE, and AD. Thus, consequences of TBI among people consuming western diet may be bad than people consuming Mediterranean diet. Components of Mediterranean diet (whole grain, fruits and vegetables (polyphenols), olive oil, fish, and garlic components) increase energy and neuroplasticity (Farooqui, 2012; Gomez-Pinilla and Tyagi, 2013). Population-based studies have demonstrated that diets rich in polyphenols promote better performance in several cognitive abilities in a dose-dependent manner (Nurk et al., 2009) and lower the risk of cognitive decline (Devore et al., 2012; Rabassa et al., 2015) in older persons and patients with neurotraumatic and neurodegenerative diseases. Converging evidence supports the view that a healthy diet may promote healthy brain aging and preserve cognitive function, especially in aging adults and patients with neurotraumatic and neurodegenerative diseases.

POTENTIAL TREATMENT STRATEGIES FOR TAUOPATHIES

Interest in the treatment of CTE has increased considerably due to its association with neurodegenerative diseases such as AD, PD, dementia, and Lewy body dementia (LBD). Many strategies have been suggested to treat tauopathies. Some of these strategies include kinase inhibitors, immunotherapy, tau aggregation inhibitors, and microtubule-stabilizing compounds. However, none these strategies have been effective in stopping CTE-mediated tau pathology nor do they address tau degradation pathways. Thus there are no approved treatments for diseases with only tau inclusions such as CTE, progressive supranuclear palsy (PSP), Pick's disease, frontotemporal dementia (FTD), corticobasal degeneration (CBD), and LBD (Karakaya et al., 2012), whereas the currently approved drugs for AD and PD temporarily relieve symptoms without altering disease progression (Anand et al., 2014).

INDOLETHYLBENZAMIDE FOR TAUOPATHIES

The synthesis of Novel indolethylbenzamides (Fig. 9.2) for the treatment of tauopathies has been described but no information is available on the effects of these drugs in animal models or CTE patients (Rosse, 2012). It will be important to test the efficacy of these drugs to block tau pathology in CTE.

EPOTHILONE FOR TAUOPATHIES

It is well known that MTs are essential for a wide range of dynamic cellular processes in the brain. MTs not only control neuronal migration, differentiation, and formation of synaptic connections during development, but also play essential roles in the mature nervous system by

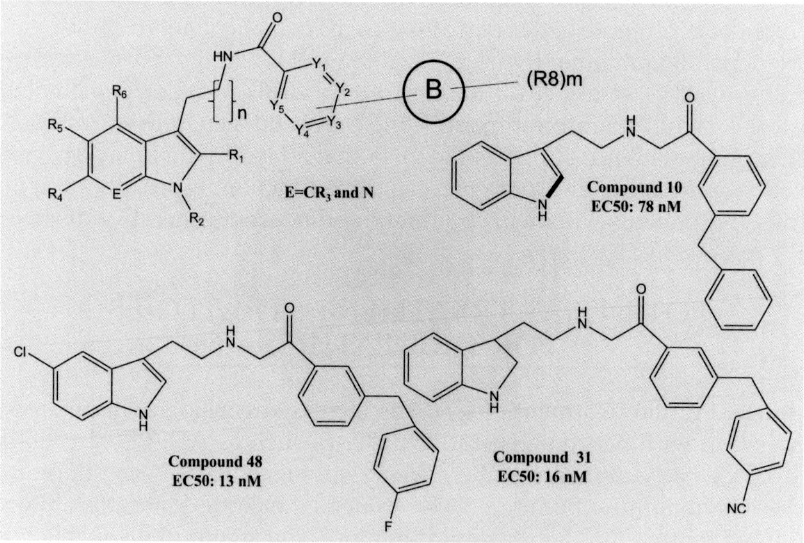

FIGURE 9.2   Chemical structures for indolethylbenzamides.

providing architectural support and serving as major tracks for antero-grade and retrograde transport of organelles and other cargos. Indeed, nerve injury causes disorganization of MTs (Hur et al., 2012). Perturbation of MT dynamics is a common feature in a number of neurodevelopmental (Kapitein and Hoogenraad, 2015) and neurodegenerative diseases (Eira et al., 2016). Epothilone D (EpoD) (Fig. 9.3), a MT-stabilizing agent, which has ability to cross BBB, can be used to treat tau pathology in PS19 tau Tg mice (Brunden et al., 2010; Zhang et al., 2012). EpoD not only has ability to attenuate axonal deficits, but also promote the suppression of cognitive impairments in PS19 mice suggesting that this compound may have potential to treat tauopathies and AD. PS19 mice have been treated with weekly doses of 0.3 or 1 mg/kg of EpoD from 9 to 12 months of age (Zhang et al., 2011). At both doses the EpoD has no effect on axonal dystrophy in Tg mice.

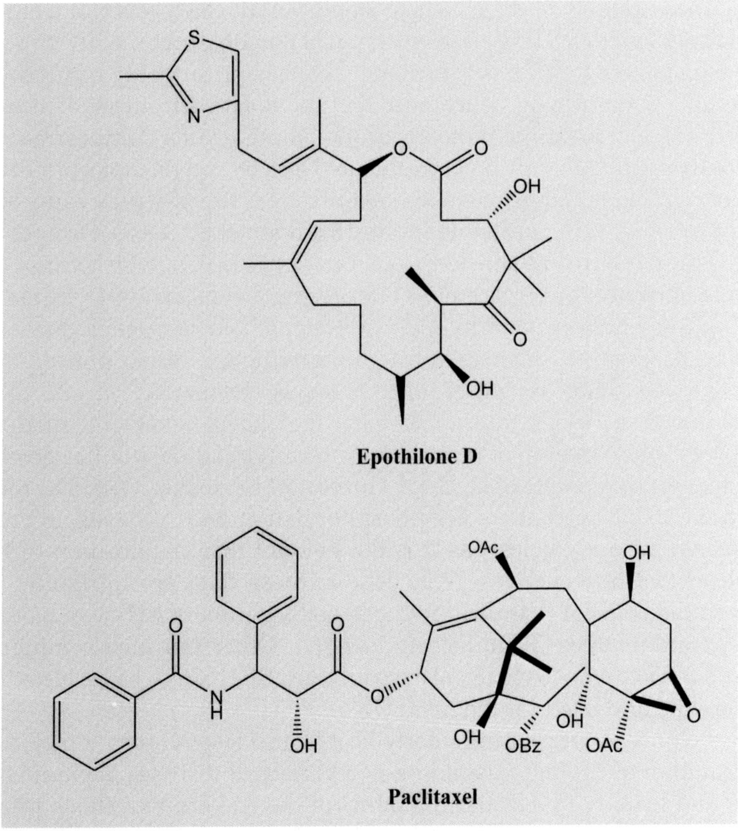

Epothilone D

Paclitaxel

FIGURE 9.3   Chemical structures for paclitaxel and epothilone D.

However, it normalizes the impaired fast axonal transport. Moreover, the treatment of 12-month-old PS19 mice with higher doses of EpoD results in an improvement of both working and spatial memory performance indicating the greatest change. Furthermore, immunohistochemical staining of phospho-tau and misfolded tau indicates the extent of tau pathology in the brains of the aged PS19 mice is reduced by EpoD. Moreover, the EpoD-treated PS19 mice also display a lower amount of insoluble tau within the brain as determined by ELISA quantification. Importantly, EpoD treatment results in diminution of the hippocampal neuron and synapse loss that is normally observed in the aged PS19 mice as they accumulate increasing amounts of tau pathology (Yoshiyama et al., 2007). Notably, no adverse effects of EpoD have been observed in the interventional study with aged PS19 mice, which is highly significant for AD and related tauopathies supporting the view that EpoD or a related MT-stabilizing intervention therapy will require chronic administration of the drug for months to years.

Paclitaxel (Fig. 9.3), drug, which stabilizes MT also work in a similar way (Brunden et al., 2009). However, paclitaxel does not readily cross the BBB, the observed paclitaxel-mediated changes presumably result due to the uptake at peripheral neuromuscular junctions with subsequent retrograde transport to spinal motor neurons. These results demonstrate that tau loss of function can be compensated for by small molecule drugs, and that MT-stabilizing agents that readily cross the BBB may cause similar improvements in tauopathy brains (Brunden et al., 2009). Octapeptide NAP (Asn-Ala-Pro-Val-Ser-Ile-Pro-Gln or NAPVSIPQ), which crosses the BBB also promotes MT assembly (Gozes and Divinski, 2004). Intranasal NAP administration for 3 months to 9-month old transgenic mice that develop Aβ and tau deposits results in a reduction of tau phosphorylation as well as a lowering of Aβ levels (Matsuoka et al., 2007). Furthermore, in older transgenic mice that have developed moderate pathology, NAP treatment reduces tau phosphorylation, but has no effect on Aβ levels (Matsuoka et al., 2008; Gozes and Divinski, 2004). The mechanism whereby NAP alters tau phosphorylation and Aβ levels in young transgenic mice is unclear, as it is not evident that stabilization of MTs will lead to these changes. Nonetheless, these data are intriguing and support the concept that drug-induced stabilization of MTs can be beneficial in tauopathies (Brunden et al., 2009). Other tau kinase inhibitors (SRN-003-556, AR-A014418, alsterpaullone, SB216763) have also been synthesized and used for the treatment of AD (Fig. 9.4).

Heat shock proteins (particularly Hsp70 and Hsp90) play a major role in regulation of protein misfolding in a variety of diseases, including tau levels and toxicity in AD and inhibitors of the 90-kDa heat shock protein (Hsp90) have been used to treat tauopathies (Dickey et al., 2007). Hsp90 acts as a molecular chaperone, which interacts with other proteins to

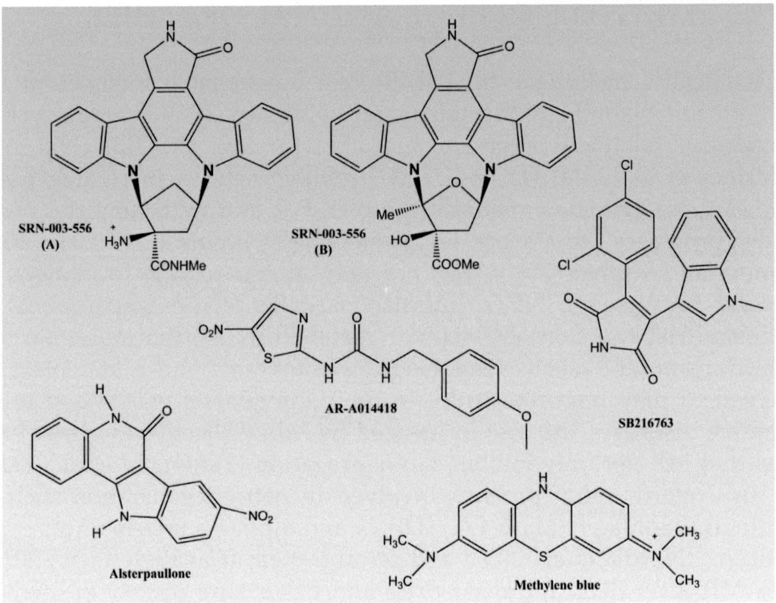

FIGURE 9.4   Chemical structure for tau kinase inhibitors.

form a complex that assists in the refolding of denatured proteins in an ATP-dependent process (Dickey et al., 2007; Brunden et al., 2009). The ATPase activity of Hsp90 is inhibited with molecules such as geldana-mycin. According to these authors (Dickey et al., 2007), the composition of the refolding complexes changes in such a way that stabilization of proteins by Hsp90 can be targeted for degradation by the proteasome (Dickey et al., 2007; Zhang and Burrows, 2004). Hsp90 inhibitors have been extensively used for the treatment of cancer. It is reported that many oncogenic proteins are not only stabilized by Hsp90, but interactions between proteins and Hsp90 inhibitors reduce the levels of tau phosphorylation at proline-directed kinase sites Ser202/Thr205 and Ser396/Ser404 in cells overexpressing mutated human tau (Dickey et al., 2006). Furthermore, Hsp90 inhibitors decrease the levels of modified tau in cells. Thus treating transgenic mice, which express human tau with BBB-permeable Hsp90 inhibitor (EC102) for 7 days, or PU24FCl for a month results in reduction in the amount of hyperphosphorylated tau in the brain (Dickey et al., 2007; Luo et al., 2007). Although Hsp90 inhibitors reduce the levels of phosphorylated and misfolded monomeric tau through the ubiquitin-proteasome system, it is unlikely that this pathway can affect larger tau oligomers and fibrils. Thus more studies are required on this important topic.

METHYLENE BLUE AND TAUOPATHIES

Chemically, methylene blue (MB) is a bioavailable member of the phenothiazine family with high water solubility. It is a redox-cycling compound, relatively nontoxic and able to pass the BBB (Fig. 9.4) (Schirmer et al., 2011; Oz et al., 2009), which acts by increasing heme synthesis, cytochrome c oxidase (complex IV), and mitochondrial respiration, processes, which are impaired in AD brains (Oz et al., 2009; Atamna and Kumar, 2010). MB not only attenuates the formations of amyloid plaques and NFTs, but also partially repairs impairments in mitochondrial function and cellular metabolism. Furthermore, various neurotransmitter systems (cholinergic, serotonergic and glutamatergic), believed to play important roles in the pathogenesis of AD and other cognitive disorders, are also influenced by MB. Collective evidence suggests that MB not only inhibits tau aggregation (Taniguchi et al., 2005), but also retards other proteins involved in neurodegeneration such as huntingtin (Sontag et al., 2012), TDP-43 and alpha-synuclein (Arai et al., 2010), Aβ (Necula et al., 2007) and prion protein (Cavaliere et al., 2013). Thus MB is an FDA-approved drug and has a long history of medical use, mainly as an antiseptic and antimalaria compound. In this Phase II clinical trial, a daily dose of 3×60 mg Rember (a derivative of the oxidized form of MB) over 1 year appeared to show a slow-down of cognitive decline in mild and moderate AD patients. In AD, MB also produces beneficial effects by targeting microtubule affinity-regulating kinase (MARK4) (Sun et al., 2016). MB partially rescues the synaptic toxicity in Drosophila larva overexpressing PAR1 (MARK analog). In 293T culture, MB decreases MARK4-mediated tau phosphorylation in a dose-dependent manner. Further studies revealed a twofold mechanism by MB including downregulation of MARK4 protein level through ubiquitin-proteasome pathway and inhibition of MARK4 kinase activity in vitro (Sun et al., 2016).

CR8 FOR CHRONIC TRAUMATIC ENCEPHALOPATHY

CR8, a potent second-generation cyclin-dependent kinase (CDK) inhibitor (Fig. 9.5), reduces cell cycle activation and cortical, hippocampal, and thalamic neuronal loss, and inhibits cortical microglial and astrocyte activation. It has been used in the lateral fluid percussion (LFP) injury model of TBI. It enables DNA synthesis in neurons, microglia/macrophages, and astrocytes to occur after 7 and 14 days post TBI (Taupin, 2007). In LFP injury, CR8 downregulates the expression of cell cycle markers such as CDK1, n-myc phosphorylation (Kabadi et al.,

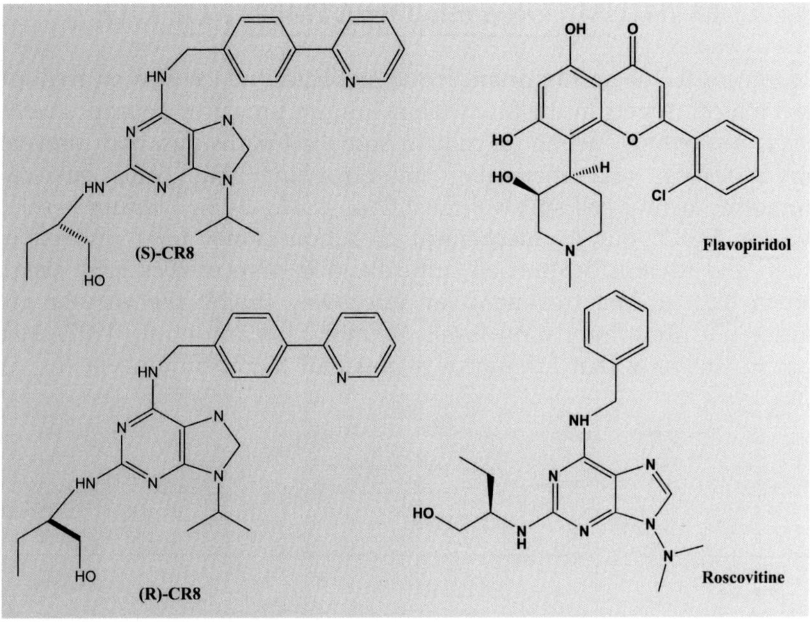

FIGURE 9.5   Chemical structures for (S)-CR8, (R)-CR8, flavopiridol, and roscovitine.

2012a), and other cell cycle proteins (Kabadi et al., 2012b; Wu et al., 2012a,b). CR8 not only provides neuroprotection, but also improves memory retention and reduces LFP-induced impairment in fear-based contextual and emotional memory function in the passive avoidance task (Kabadi and Faden, 2014; Kabadi et al., 2014). Furthermore, CR8 also preserves neurons in the hippocampus and surrounding areas, resulting in cognitive improvements. Signs of depression, which are normally present in LFP injured rats are greatly reduced after treatment with CR8. At the cellular level, CR8 decreases microglia and astrocyte activation, thereby preventing further damage to the CNS. Collective evidence suggests that CR8 treatment not only attenuates sensorimotor and cognitive deficits, alleviates depressive-like symptoms, but also decreases lesion volume. Cell cycle activation occurs in both neurons as well as glial cells (Byrnes and Faden, 2007; Stoica et al., 2009). Administration of another cell cycle inhibitor (CR3) after TBI also result in significant increase in neuronal survival and reduction in both microglial and astroglial activation (Hilton et al., 2008; Kabadi et al., 2014). These studies support the view that cell cycle activation may contribute to the progression of neurodegeneration and chronic neuroinflammation following TBI in animal models (Kabadi and Faden, 2014; Kabadi et al., 2014). Based on this information, it can be suggested that CR3 and CR8 can be used for the treatment of CTE in animal models.

LITHIUM FOR THE TREATMENT OF CTE

Lithium (Li) is an important mood stabilizer, which acts on multiple biochemical targets in the brain. Thus lithium produces neuroprotective effects not only by acting on cellular signaling pathways, both preventing apoptosis and increasing neurotrophins (Fig. 9.6), but also promoting neural cell survival (Dell'Osso et al., 2016). Lithium is selective for GSK3, but its mechanism of action is not fully understood (Klein and Melton, 1996). Cell culture and in vivo studies have clearly shown that lithium treatment can effectively inhibit the enzyme and reduce tau phosphorylation levels (Munoz-Montano et al., 1997), supporting the view that lithium as a potential therapeutic agent for AD

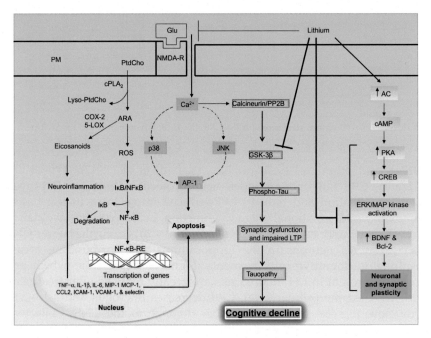

FIGURE 9.6   Effect of lithium on cognitive decline. Hypothetical diagram showing the site of action lithium. *AC*, adenylyl cyclase; *AP-1*, activator protein-1; *ARA*, arachidonic acid; *BDNF*, brain-derived neurotrophic factor; *cAMP*, cyclic AMP; *COX-2*, cyclooxygenase-2; *cPLA$_2$*, cytosolic phospholipase A$_2$; *CREB*, cyclic AMP-response element binding protein; *ERK1*, extracellular signal-regulated kinase-1; *Glu*, glutamate; *GSK*, glycogen synthase kinase-3 beta; *I-κB*, inhibitory subunit of NF-κB; *IL-1β*, interleukin-1β; *IL-6*, interleukin-6; *JNK*, c-Jun NH(2)-terminal kinase; *5-LOX*, 5-lipoxygenase; *lyso-PtdCho*, lysophosphatidylcholine; *MAP*, mitogen-activated protein kinase (p38); *MCP-1*, monocyte chemoattractant protein-1; *NF-κB*, nuclear factor-κB; *NF-κB-RE*, nuclear factor-κB-response element; *NMDA-R*, NMDA receptor; *PKA*, protein kinase A; proto-oncogene bcl-2; *PtdCho*, phosphatidylcholine; *ROS*, reactive oxygen species; *TNF-α*, tumor necrosis factor-α.

and other tauopathies (Alvarez et al., 2002; Caccamo et al., 2007). Furthermore, lithium produces positive effects on neurogenesis, brain remodeling, angiogenesis, and mesenchymal stem cells functioning. Lithium also inhibits and neuroinflammation by blocking the glycogen synthase kinase-3 (Dell'Osso et al., 2016).

It is also well known that lithium produces neuroprotective effects in preclinical studies on TBI (Leeds et al., 2014). Lithium pretreatment not only attenuates interleukin-1β expression, brain edema, hippocampal neurodegeneration, and loss of hemispheric tissues, but also improves memory and spatial learning leading to alleviation of depressive behaviors in mouse models of mild TBI (Shapira et al., 2007; Zhu et al., 2010). Postinjury injections with therapeutic doses of lithium also reduce lesion volume and attenuate TBI-induced neuroinflammation by inhibiting microglia activation and cyclooxygenase-2 induction, while BBB integrity is maintained through the inhibition of matrix metallopeptidase-9 expression. Furthermore, in mild TBI, lithium treatment also suppresses hyperlocomotor activity, anxiety-like behaviors, and impairments in motor coordination (Yu et al., 2012). In addition, lithium administration also increases GSK-3β phosphorylation with subsequent β-catenin accumulation, and reduce neuronal loss in the hippocampal CA3 region, as well as decrease in hippocampal-dependent deficits in learning and memory (Leeds et al., 2014; Dash et al., 2011; Yu et al., 2012). Because the pathogenesis of CTE is linked neuropsychiatric disorders (bipolar disorders, depression, manic episodes), it is proposed that lithium may produce beneficial effects in CTE.

HYPERBARIC OXYGEN THERAPY FOR TAUOPATHIES

Hyperbaric oxygen therapy (HBOT) is a neurotherapeutic method, which promotes brain repair by providing oxygen-enriched air to patients in a closed chamber pressurized above one atmosphere absolute (1 ATA). The combination of hyperoxia and hyperbaric pressure results in significant improvements in tissue oxygenation as well as mitochondrial metabolism with antiapoptotic and antiinflammatory effects (Chen et al., 2010; Huang and Obenaus, 2011; Lin et al., 2012). Hyperbaric oxygen has been shown to produce neuroprotective effects against ischemic and hemorrhagic brain injury and CTE (Qin et al., 2007; Stoller, 2011). It is demonstrated that HBOT treatment performed 2 days postinjury not only produces significant reduction in overall neurological deficit scores, but also causes a decrease in neuronal apoptosis in brain tissues. It is proposed that 12 hours post TBI is an effective window for HBOT administration (Wang et al., 2010; Hu et al., 2016). Another randomized clinical trial on the effect of HBOT in on military service member suffering from persistent postconcussion symptoms (PCS) has indicated that supplemental administration of breathing with 100% oxygen at 1.5 ATA or air at 1.2 ATA for 60 min improves symptoms and quality of life compared with local care management of those without HBOT chamber intervention. However, no differences are observed between HBOT and sham group receiving air at 1.2 ATA supporting the view that the observed improvements were not due to the oxygen but may reflect nonspecific improvements related to placebo effects (Reis et al., 2015). The molecular mechanism associated with the effect of HBOT is not fully understood. However, it is suggested that HBOT reduces apoptosis, upregulates growth factors, promotes antioxidant levels, and inhibits inflammatory cytokines in animal models, and hence, it is likely that HBOT can be advantageous in treating at least the secondary phase of TBI, CTE, and PTSD. In addition, it is also reported that HBOT exposure produces a putative prophylactic or preconditioning benefit in animal models of TBI and CTE, and the optimal time frame for treatment is yet to be determined (Eve et al., 2016). Discussions continue regarding the effectiveness of HBOT, but recent publications regarding the cognitive benefits of HBOT leave the medical community with an opportunity to pursue and conduct further research into its therapeutic benefits for the growing population of TBI and CTE patients. It must be noted that HBOT administration has several side effects. At high pressures (>3 ATA), prolonged oxygen exposure can cause convulsions, though whether this is detrimental is under debate since the seizures abate on removal of oxygen at the high pressure. Animal studies suggest that the seizures may result from increased nitric oxide synthesis (Elayan et al., 2000; Uusijarvi et al., 2015). Fortunately, these observations are at 3 ATA than those being used in the study; hence, with limited exposure times (60–90 minutes at a time), this should reduce the likelihood of convulsions as a side effect.

Collective evidence suggests that HBOT can produce some potential side effects such as acute cerebral toxicity and more reactive oxygen species with long-term use, and therefore, studies on determining optimal exposure duration to HBOT for maximal benefit is very important (Eve et al., 2016).

TAU ANTIBODIES FOR THE TREATMENT OF CHRONIC TRAUMATIC ENCEPHALOPATHY

Considerable progress has been made on immunotherapy of AD in animal models. Thus NFTs can be labeled in situ with antibodies against a variety of neuronal proteins, including vimentin, actin, ubiquitin, MAP2, and β-amyloid in animal models of AD. In crude preparations, paired helical filaments (PHFs) can be detected with antibodies against MAP2, neurofilament, ubiquitin, and tau (Wilcock and Colton, 2008; Santa-Maria et al., 2012). In animal models, treatment with a phospho-tau peptide (containing the phosphorylated PHF-1 epitopes Ser396, Ser404) injected prior to the onset of pathology produces retardation of tau aggregates in the Tg P301L mouse tau model (Asuni et al., 2007). Phosphorylation at these specific epitopes increases the fibrillogenic character of tau and enhances PHFs formation (Fath et al., 2002). However, almost all studies have failed to give beneficial effects in AD patients.

Targeting oligomeric tau species through immunotherapy may be superior to targeting NFTs across the spectrum of neurodegenerative tauopathies and, therefore, this approach can be used for disease-modifying intervention in AD as well as CTE (Lasagna-Reeves et al., 2011a,b; Castillo-Carranza et al., 2013a,b). Injections of native tau increase the risk of developing autoimmunity and/or other related complications. To protect against negative side effects of autoimmunity, a novel anti-tau oligomer-specific mouse monoclonal antibody (anti-TOMA) has been developed (Castillo-Carranza et al., 2014; Schroeder et al., 2017). This antibody recognizes tau oligomers specifically and does not recognize monomeric functional tau or mature metastable NFTs. This antibody has been used to study tau oligomers in a mouse model of tauopathy, JNPL3. JNPL3 is expressed in the mutant human tau protein (P301L), which is responsible for FTD (Lewis et al., 2000). TOMAs have ideal characteristics for immunotherapy. TOMAs are not only unique for their specificity for tau oligomers, but also have high affinity, and ability to sequester tau oligomer toxicity in vitro. Furthermore, other IgG antibodies have been shown to enter the brain in P301L mice, supporting the ability of TOMA to cross the BBB if administered intravenously (Asuni et al., 2007). Treatment of male homozygous P301L mice with TOMA indicates that TOMA has ability to modulate the pathological effects of tau oligomers in vivo. TOMA dose used in above-mentioned studies was 5- to 10-fold lower than those previously used to nonselectively target tau aggregates by passive immunotherapy (Boutajangout et al., 2010, 2011; Chai et al., 2011). This may contribute to increased safety of antibodies while maintaining efficacy because oligomeric tau represents a small percentage of total tau in the brain. Moreover, these experiments have provided evidence that intravenous delivery of IgG antibodies can be detected within the P301L mouse brain, suggesting that the BBB may be impaired in this mouse model (Asuni et al., 2007). Large double-blind trials on TOMA have not been performed in AD patients. So, nothing is known about the ability of TOMA for crossing BBB as well as affinity and specificity of TOMA in normal human subjects and AD patients.

Another antibody is called tauC3 antibody (Fig. 9.7). This antibody shows a very high binding specificity for the target caspase-cleaved tau protein when tested against the recombinant tauC3 protein versus the full-length protein in both western blotting and in surface plasmon resonance (SPR) experiments (Nicholls et al., 2017). Anti-tauC3 antibody significantly block the seeding properties of AD lysate as determined by the tauFRET2 seeding biosensor assay. Depletion of p-tau species also results in the inhibition of tau seeding in tau-transgenic mouse lines rTg4510 (Takeda et al., 2015) suggesting that tauC3 may be one of several species responsible for tau aggregation and seeding activity, or, at the very least, closely associated with the seed competent forms of tau. Since, there are several cleavage sites upstream of the caspase cleavage site at D421, which may determine a larger portion of the tau species present in the high molecular weight fraction, especially in later stage AD patients. None of above antibodies have been tested in animal models or CTE patients. However, antibodies have been developed to distinguish between *cis* p-tau and *trans* p-tau (Kondo et al., 2015; Lu et al., 2016). Based on the discovery of *cis* p-tau, it is proposed that this form is not only a precursor of tau-induced pathological changes, but an early

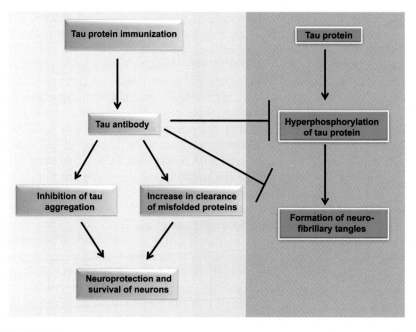

FIGURE 9.7   Production of tau antibodies. Tau antibody blocks the hyperphosphorylation of tau protein.

driver of neurodegeneration that directly links mild TBI to CTE and possibly to AD. Within hours of mild TBI in mice or neuronal stress in vitro, neurons prominently produce *cis* p-tau, which causes and spreads *cis* p-tau pathologic changes, termed cistauosis, a condition, which eventually leads to widespread tau-mediated neurodegeneration and brain atrophy. Cistauosis is effectively blocked by the *cis* p-tau antibody, which targets intracellular *cis* p-tau for proteasome-mediated degradation and prevents extracellular *cis* p-tau from spreading to other neurons (Kondo et al., 2015; Lu et al., 2016). Treating mild TBI mice with *cis* p-tau antibody not only blocks early cistauosis but also prevents development and spreading of tau-mediated neurodegeneration and brain atrophy and restores brain histopathologic features and functional outcomes. Thus cistauosis is a common early disease mechanism for AD, mild TBI, and CTE, and *cis* p-tau and its antibody may be useful for early diagnosis, treatment, and prevention of these devastating diseases (Kondo et al., 2015; Lu et al., 2016).

From above information, it is clear that most current therapies to treat CTE have failed and there is no treatment for concussion and CTE. The easiest way to reduce the incidence of CTE is to decrease the number of concussions (McKee et al., 2009). In athletes, this can be achieved by limiting exposure to neurotrauma, e.g., by penalizing intentional hits to the head (as is happening in football and hockey) and adhering to strict "return to play" guidelines. Proper care and management of mild TBI in general and particularly in sports will also reduce CTE. No reliable or specific measures of neurological dysfunction after concussion currently exist, and most recommendations are centered on the resolution of acute symptoms such as headache, confusion, and sensitivity to light (Cantu, 2003). Persistent decreases in P300 amplitudes in response to an auditory stimulus have been reported in asymptomatic patients at least 5 weeks after a concussion. This observation casts doubt on the validity of the absence of symptoms as a guidepost (Gosselin et al., 2006; Mayers, 2008). Neuropsychological tests have been used to provide estimates of the appropriate time for athletes to return to practice and play. In concussed athletes, positron emission tomography (PET), diffusion tensor imaging, and MRI can be used to detect abnormalities in gait abnormalities. These tests can also be used to study the effects of transcranial magnetic stimulation and balance testing in concussed athletes or nonathletes with TBI (Gosselin et al., 2006; De Beaumont et al., 2007). Information from these tests can be used to determine time for complete recovery and safe return to play (Mayers, 2008). In addition, animal model studies have indicated that early return to play or overactivity within a week of concussion results in the inhibition of functional recovery (Kozlowski et al., 1996).

BENEFICIAL EFFECTS OF EXERCISE ON CONCUSSION AND CHRONIC TRAUMATIC ENCEPHALOPATHY

It is well known that neurons have ability to change and reorganize continuously to meet the dynamic demands of the internal and external environment. This process is called as neuroplasticity. This process depends on neural membrane depolarization, stimulus-mediated synaptic activity, and subsequent changes in dendritic morphology. Neural plasticity is a central hallmark of learning and memory. It is modulated by exercise (Cotman et al., 2007; Farooqui, 2014; Phillips, 2017). Clinical studies have indicated that moderate exercise restores cerebrovascular function and autonomic balance following concussion (Baker et al., 2012; Leddy et al., 2016a,b). In addition, exercise produces neuroprotective effects on the brain by inducing the expression of brain-derived neurotropic factors (BDNFs) (Seifert et al., 2010; Farooqui, 2014). This leads to increase in neuroplasticity (Hotting and Roder, 2013; Farooqui, 2014). These processes not only promote structural integrity of the brain, but also preserve the cognition function (Tseng et al., 2013; Farooqui, 2014). It has been postulated that the introduction of exercise during rehabilitation may have a positive impact on the chronic symptoms following concussion (Baker et al., 2012; Archer, 2012). Thus Gagnon et al. (2009, 2016) have reported that children and adolescents who participated in light aerobic exercise show improved postconcussion outcomes compared to those who did not. Their patients exercised at 50%−60% of their predicted max heart rate (220-age). Studies on the effect of exercise on concussion are also supported by other investigators (Reed et al., 2015) in young athletes as well as in college athletes (Reed et al., 2015; Maerlender et al., 2015).

The neuroprotective benefits of exercise have been demonstrated in patients as well as in animal models of stroke, AD, and other neurodegenerative diseases such as PD, CBD, and PSP (Farooqui, 2014; Steffen et al., 2007, 2014). It is also suggested that exercise decreases $A\beta$ accumulation and development NFTs (Dao et al., 2014). Steffen et al. have reported a case of improved motor function and an attenuated rate of brain volume loss in a patient with CBD and PSP after 2.5 and 10 years of exercise (Steffen et al., 2007, 2014; Leem et al., 2009). Based on these observations, it can be proposed that regular exercise can produce beneficial effects in patients with CTE.

CONCLUSION

Concussion is a clinical syndrome of biomechanically induced alteration of brain dysfunction, typically affecting memory and orientation, which may involve chronic pain, headaches, vestibular dysfunction, depression, and sometime loss of consciousness. Millions of concussions occur annually, many of them related to sports. Biologically, a complex sequence of neurochemical processes occurs following repetitive concussions. These processes include initial ionic flux, glutamate release, and axonal damage to longer term neurodegeneration, which may result not only in persistent neurocognitive changes (De Beaumont et al., 2012), but also in increased risk of CTE, posttraumatic stress, dementia, depression, and neurodegenerative diseases (AD and PD) (Jordan, 2013; Lucke-Wold et al., 2014). However, there is a paucity of prospective or longitudinal studies examining repetitive concussions and long-term neurodegeneration. At present it is not possible to establish a causal relationship among repetitive concussions, CTE, and neurodegenerative diseases.

Neuropathologically, both AD and CTE are characterized by abnormal accumulations of hyperphosphorylated tau proteins. However, recent neuropathological studies have indicated that CTE shows a unique pattern of tau pathology in neurons and astrocytes, and accumulation of other misfolded proteins such as TDP-43. Currently, no reliable biomarkers of late-onset neurodegenerative diseases following TBI are available, and a definitive diagnosis can be made only via postmortem neuropathological examination. Development in neuroimaging techniques such as tau and amyloid PET imaging might not only enable early diagnosis of CTE, but also contribute to the interventions for prevention of late-onset neurodegenerative diseases following TBI (Chen et al., 2004). Further studies are necessary to elucidate the mechanisms of neurodegeneration in the living brain of patients with TBI.

References

Albayram, O., Herbert, M.K., Kondo, A., Tsai, C.Y., Baxley, S., et al., 2016. Function and regulation of tau conformations in the development and treatment of traumatic brain injury and neurodegeneration. Cell Biosci. 6, 59.

Almeida, O.P., Hankey, G.J., Yeap, B.B., Golledge, J., Flicker, L., 2014. Alcohol consumption and cognitive impairment in older men: a Mendelian randomization study. Neurology 82, 1038–1044.

Alsalaheen, B.A., Mucha, A., Morris, L.O., et al., 2010. Vestibular rehabilitation for dizziness and balance disorders after concussion. J. Neurol. Phys. Ther. 34, 87–93.

Alsalaheen, B.A., Whitney, S.L., Mucha, A., Morris, L.O., Furman, J.M., Sparto, P.J., 2013. Exercise prescription patterns in patients treated with vestibular rehabilitation after concussion. Physiother. Res. Int. 18, 100–108.

Alvarez, G., Munoz-Montano, J.R., Satrustegui, J., Avila, J., Bogonez, E., Diaz-Nido, J., 2002. Regulation of tau phosphorylation and protection against beta-amyloid-induced neurodegeneration by lithium. Possible implications for Alzheimer's disease. Bipolar Disord. 4, 153–165.

Anand, R., Gill, K.D., Mahdi, A.A., 2014. Therapeutics of Alzheimer's disease: past, present and future. Neuropharmacology 76 (Pt A), 27–50.

Andrasik, F., 2010. Biofeedback in headache: an overview of approaches and evidence. [Review]. Cleve. Clin. J. Med. 77 (Suppl. 3), S72—S76.

Arai, T., Hasegawa, M., Nonoka, T., Kametani, F., Yamashita, M., et al., 2010. Phosphorylated and cleaved TDP-43 in ALS, FTLD and other neurodegenerative disorders and in cellular models of TDP-43 proteinopathy. Neuropathology 30, 170—181.

Archer, T., 2012. Influence of physical exercise on traumatic brain injury deficits: scaffolding effect. Neurotox. Res. 21, 418—434.

Asuni, A.A., Boutajangout, A., Quartermain, D., Sigurdsson, E.M., 2007. Immunotherapy targeting pathological tau conformers in a tangle mouse model reduces brain pathology with associated functional improvements. J. Neurosci. 27, 9115—9129.

Atamna, H., Kumar, R., 2010. Protective role of methylene blue in Alzheimer's disease via mitochondria and cytochrome c oxidase. J. Alzheimers Dis. 20 (Suppl. 2), S439—S452.

Baker, J.G., Freitas, M.S., Leddy, J.J., Kozlowski, K.F., Willer, B.S., 2012. Return to full functioning after graded exercise assessment and progressive exercise treatment of postconcussion syndrome. Rehabil. Res. Pract. 2012, 705309.

Barkhoudarian, G., Hovda, D.A., Giza, C.C., 2011. The molecular pathophysiology of concussive brain injury. Clin. Sports Med. 30, 33—48.

Barlow, K.M., Marcil, L.D., Dewey, D., Carlson, H.L., MacMaster, F.P., et al., 2016. Cerebral perfusion changes in post-concussion syndrome: a prospective controlled cohort study. J. Neurotrauma 34, 996—1004.

Barrett, E.C., McBurney, M.I., Ciappio, E.D., 2014. ω-3 fatty acid supplementation as a potential therapeutic aid for the recovery from mild traumatic brain injury/concussion. Adv. Nutr. 5, 268—277.

Baugh, C.M., Robbins, C.A., Stern, R.A., McKee, A.C., 2014. Current understanding of chronic traumatic encephalopathy. Curr. Treat. Options Neurol. 16, 306.

Bazan, N.G., Molina, M.F., Gordon, W.C., 2011. Docosahexaenoic acid signalolipidomics in nutrition: significance in aging, neuroinflammation, macular degeneration, Alzheimer's, and other neurodegenerative diseases. Annu. Rev. Nutr. 31, 321—351.

Bazarian, J.J., Veazie, P., Mookerjee, S., Lerner, E.B., 2006. Accuracy of mild traumatic brain injury case ascertainment using ICD-9 codes. Acad. Emerg. Med. 13, 31—38.

Boutajangout, A., Quartermain, D., Sigurdsson, E.M., 2010. Immunotherapy targeting pathological tau prevents cognitive decline in a new tangle mouse model. J. Neurosci. 30, 16559—16566.

Boutajangout, A., Ingadottir, J., Davies, P., Sigurdsson, E.M., 2011. Passive immunization targeting pathological phospho-tau protein in a mouse model reduces functional decline and clears tau aggregates from the brain. J. Neurochem. 118, 658—667.

Brosseau-Lachaine, O., Gagnon, I., Forget, R., Faubert, J., 2008. Mild traumatic brain injury induces prolonged visual processing deficits in children. Brain Inj. 22, 657—668.

Brunden, K.R., Trojanowski, J.Q., Lee, V.M., 2009. Advances in tau-focused drug discovery for Alzheimer's disease and related tauopathies. Nat. Rev. Drug Discov. 8, 783—793.

Brunden, K.R., Zhang, B., Carroll, J., Yao, Y., Potuzak, J.S., et al., 2010. Epothilone D improves microtubule density, axonal integrity and cognition in a transgenic mouse model of tauopathy. J. Neurosci. 30, 13861—13866.

Byrnes, K.R., Faden, A.I., 2007. Role of cell cycle proteins in CNS injury. Neurochem. Res. 32, 1799—1807.

Caccamo, A., Oddo, S., Tran, L.X., LaFerla, F.M., 2007. Lithium reduces tau phosphorylation but not A beta or working memory deficits in a transgenic model with both plaques and tangles. Am. J. Pathol. 170, 1669—1675.

Cantu, R.C., 2003. Recurrent athletic head injury: risks and when to retire. Clin. Sports Med. 22, 593—603.

Cao, Z.J., Chen, Y., Wang, S.M., 2014. Health belief model based evaluation of school health education programme for injury prevention among high school students in the community context. BMC Public Health 14, 26.

Cancelliere, C., Hincapie, C.A., Keightley, M., Godbolt, A.K., Cote, P., et al., 2014. Systematic review of prognosis and return to play after sport concussion: results of the international collaboration on mild traumatic brain injury prognosis. Arch. Phys. Med. Rehabil. 95 (3S), S210–S229.

Carroll, L.J., Cassidy, J.D., Peloso, P.M., Borg, J., von Holst, H., et al., 2004. Prognosis for mild traumatic brain injury: results of the WHO Collaborating Centre Task Force on Mild Traumatic Brain Injury. J. Rehabil. Med. (43 Suppl.), 84–105.

Cassidy, J.D., Boyle, E., Carroll, L.J., 2014. Population-based, inception cohort study of the incidence, course, and prognosis of mild traumatic brain injury after motor vehicle collisions. Arch. Phys. Med. Rehabil. 95 (3 Suppl.), S278–S285.

Castillo-Carranza, D.L., Lasagna-Reeves, C.A., Kayed, R., 2013a. Tau aggregates as immunotherapeutic targets. Front. Biosci. (Schol. Ed.) 5, 426–438.

Castillo-Carranza, D.L., Guerrero-Muñoz, M.J., Kayed, R., 2013b. Immunotherapy for the treatment of Alzheimer's disease: amyloid-β or tau, which is the right target? Immunotargets Ther. 3, 19–28.

Castillo-Carranza, D.L., Sengupta, U., Guerrero-Muñoz, M.J., Lasagna-Reeves, C.A., Gerson, J.E., et al., 2014. Passive immunization with Tau oligomer monoclonal antibody reverses tauopathy phenotypes without affecting hyperphosphorylated neurofibrillary tangles. J. Neurosci. 34, 4260–4272.

Cavaliere, P., Torrent, J., Prigent, S., Granata, V., Pauwels, K., et al., 2013. Binding of methylene blue to a surface cleft inhibits the oligomerization and fibrillization of prion protein. Biochim. Biophys. Acta 1832, 20–28.

Centers for Disease Control and Prevention, 2011. Nonfatal traumatic brain injuries related to sports and recreation activities among persons aged ≤19 years–United States, 2001–2009. MMWR Morb. Mortal. Wkly. Rep. 60, 1337–1342.

Chai, X., Wu, S., Murray, T.K., Kinley, R., Cella, C.V., et al., 2011. Passive immunization with anti-Tau antibodies in two transgenic models: reduction of Tau pathology and delay of disease progression. J. Biol. Chem. 2011 (286), 34457–34467.

Chen, J.-K., Johnston, K.M., Frey, S., Petrides, M., Worsley, K., et al., 2004. Functional abnormalities in symptomatic concussed athletes: an fMRI study. Neuroimage 22, 68–82.

Chen, J.K., Johnston, K.M., Collie, A., McCrory, P., Ptito, A., 2007. A validation of the post concussion symptom scale in the assessment of complex concussion using cognitive testing and functional MRI. J. Neurol. Neurosurg. Psychiatry 78, 1231–1238.

Chen, Z., Ni, P., Lin, Y., Xiao, H., Chen, J., Qian, G., et al., 2010. Visual pathway lesion and its development during hyperbaric oxygen treatment: a bold- fMRI and DTI study. J. Magn. Reson. Imaging 31, 1054–1060.

Cherry, J.D., Stein, T.D., Tripodis, Y., Alvarez, V.E., Huber, B.R., et al., 2017. CCL11 is increased in the CNS in chronic traumatic encephalopathy but not in Alzheimer's disease. PLoS One 12, e0185541.

Churchill, N.W., Hutchison, M.G., Richards, D., Leung, G., Graham, S.J., et al., 2017. The first week after concussion: blood flow, brain function and white matter microstructure. Neuroimage Clin. 14, 480–489.

Ciuffreda, K.J., Kapoor, N., Rutner, D., Suchoff, I.B., Han, M.E., et al., 2007. Occurrence of oculomotor dysfunctions in acquired brain injury: a retrospective analysis. Optometry 78, 155–161.

Cotman, C.W., Berchtold, N.C., Christie, L.A., 2007. Exercise builds brain health: key roles of growth factor cascades and inflammation. Trends Neurosci. 30, 464–472.

Crisco, J.J., Fiore, R., Beckwith, J.G., Chu, J.J., Brolinson, P.G., et al., 2010. Frequency and location of head impact exposures in individual collegiate football players. J. Athl. Train. 45, 549–559.

Crisco, J.J., Wilcox, B.J., Beckwith, J.G., et al., 2011. Head impact exposure in collegiate football players. J. Biomech. 44, 2673–2678.

Daneshvar, D.H., Baugh, C.M., Nowinski, C.J., McKee, A.C., Stern, R.A., Cantu, R.C., 2011. Helmets and mouth guards: the role of personal equipment in preventing sport-related concussions. Clin. Sports Med. 30, 145–163.

Dao, A.T., Zagaar, M.A., Salim, S., Eriksen, J.L., Alkadhi, K.A., 2014. Regular exercise prevents non-cognitive disturbances in a rat model of Alzheimer's disease. Int. J. Neuropsychopharmacol. 17, 593–602.

Dash, P.K., Johnson, D., Clark, J., et al., 2011. Involvement of the glycogen synthase kinase-3 signaling pathway in TBI pathology and neurocognitive outcome. PLoS One 6, e24648.

De Beaumont, L., Brisson, B., Lassonde, M., Jolicoeur, P., 2007. Long-term electrophysiological changes in athletes with a history of multiple concussions. Brain Inj. 21, 631–644.

De Beaumont, L., Henry, L.C., Gosselin, N., 2012. Long-term functional alterations in sports concussion. Neurosurg. Focus 33, 1–7.

Dell'Osso, L., Del Grande, C., Gesi, C., Carmassi, C., Musetti, L., 2016. A new look at an old drug: neuroprotective effects and therapeutic potentials of lithium salts. Neuropsychiatr. Dis. Treat. 12, 1687–1703.

Denis, I., Potier, B., Vancassel, S., Heberden, C., Lavialle, M., 2013. Omega-3 fatty acids and brain resistance to ageing and stress: body of evidence and possible mechanisms. Ageing Res. Rev. 12, 579–594.

Devore, E.E., Kang, J.H., Breteler, M.M., Grodstein, F., 2012. Dietary intakes of berries and flavonoids in relation to cognitive decline. Ann. Neurol. 72, 135–143.

Dickey, C.A., Dunmore, J., Lu, B., Wang, J.W., Lee, W.C., et al., 2006. HSP induction mediates selective clearance of tau phosphorylated at proline-directed Ser/Thr sites but not KXGS (MARK) sites. FASEB J. 20, 753–755.

Dickey, C.A., Kamal, A., Lundgren, K., Klosak, N., Bailey, R.M., Dunmore, J., et al., 2007. The high-affinity HSP90-CHIP complex recognizes and selectively degrades phosphorylated tau client proteins. J. Clin. Invest. 117, 648–658.

Eira, J., Silva, C.S., Sousa, M.M., Liz, M.A., 2016. The cytoskeleton as a novel therapeutic target for old neurodegenerative disorders. Prog. Neurobiol. 141, 61–82.

Elayan, I.M., Axley, M.J., Prasad, P.V., Ahlers, S.T., Auker, C.R., 2000. Effect of hyperbaric oxygen treatment on nitric oxide and oxygen free radicals in rat brain. J. Neurophysiol. 83, 2022–2029.

Eve, D.J., Steele, M.R., Sanberg, P.R., Borlongan, C.V., 2016. Hyperbaric oxygen therapy as a potential treatment for post-traumatic stress disorder associated with traumatic brain injury. Neuropsychiatr. Dis. Treat. 12, 2689–2705.

Farooqui, A.A., 2009. Beneficial Effects of Fish Oil on Human Brain. Springer, New York, NY.

Farooqui, A.A., 2010. Neurochemical Aspects of Neurotraumatic and Neurodegenerative Diseases. Springer, New York, NY.

Farooqui, A.A., 2011. Lipid Mediators and Their Metabolism in the Brain. Springer International Publishing, Switzerland.

Farooqui, A.A., 2012. Phytochemicals, Signal Transduction, and Neurological Disorders. Springer International Publishing, Switzerland.

Farooqui, A.A., 2014. Inflammation and Oxidative Stress in Neurological Disorders. Springer International Publishing, Switzerland.

Fath, T., Eidenmuller, J., Brandt, R., 2002. Tau-mediated cytotoxicity in a pseudohyperphosphorylation model of Alzheimer's disease. J. Neurosci. 22, 9733–9741.

Finkelstein, E.A., Corso, P.S., Miller, T.R., 2006. The Incidence and Economic Burden of Injuries in the United States. Oxford University Press, New York, NY.

Gagnon, I., Grilli, L., Friedman, D., Iverson, G.L., 2016. A pilot study of active rehabilitation for adolescents who are slow to recover from sport-related concussion. Scand. J. Med. Sci. Sports 26, 299–306.

Gagnon, I., Galli, C., Friedman, D., Grilli, L., Iverson, G.L., 2009. Active rehabilitation for children who are slow to recover following sport-related concussion. Brain Inj. 23, 956–964.

Gavett, B.E., Stern, R.A., McKee, A.C., 2011. Chronic traumatic encephalopathy: a potential late effect of sport-related concussive and subconcussive head trauma. Clin. Sports Med. 30, 179–188.

Giza, C.C., Hovda, D.A., 2001. The neurometabolic cascade of concussion. J. Athl. Train. 36, 228–235.

Giza, C.C., Hovda, D.A., 2014. The new neurometabolic cascade of concussion. Neurosurgery 75 (Suppl. 4), S24–S33.

Golde, T.E., 2009. The therapeutic importance of understanding mechanisms of neuronal cell death in neurodegenerative disease. Mol. Neurodegener. 4, 8.

Gomez-Pinilla, F., Tyagi, E., 2013. Diet and cognition: interplay between cell metabolism and neuronal plasticity. Curr. Opin. Clin. Nutr. Metab. Care 16, 726–733.

Gosselin, N., Theriault, M., Leclerc, S., Montplaisir, J., Lassonde, M., et al., 2006. Neurophysiological anomalies in symptomatic and asymptomatic concussed athletes. Neurosurgery 58, 1151–1161.

Gozes, I., Divinski, I., 2004. The femtomolar-acting NAP interacts with microtubules: novel aspects of astrocyte protection. J. Alzheimer Dis. 6, S37–S41.

Greenman, P.E., McPartland, J.M., 1995. Cranial findings and iatrogenesis from craniosacral manipulation in patients with traumatic brain syndrome. J. Am. Osteopath. Assoc. 95, 182–188; 191–192.

Grossman, E., Jensen, J., Babb, J., Chen, Q., Tabesh, A., et al., 2013. Cognitive impairment in mild traumatic brain injury: a longitudinal diffusional kurtosis and perfusion imaging study. Am. J. Neuroradiol. 34, 951–957.

Guskiewicz, K.M., McCrea, M., Marshall, S.W., Cantu, R.C., Randolph, C., et al., 2003. Cumulative effects associated with recurrent concussion in collegiate football players: the NCAA Concussion Study. JAMA 290, 2549–2555.

Harmon, K.G., Drezner, J.A., Gammons, M., Guskiewicz, K.M., Halstead, M., et al., 2013a. American Medical Society of Sports Medicine position statement: concussion in sport. Br. J. Sports Med. 47, 15–26.

Harmon, K.G., Drezner, J.A., Gammons, M., Guskiewicz, K., Halstead, M., Herring, S.A., et al., 2013b. American Medical Society for Sports Medicine position statement: concussion in sport. Clin J. Sport Med. 47, 15–26.

Hartgens, F., Kuipers, H., 2004. Effects of androgenic-anabolic steroids in athletes. Sports Med. (Auckland, NZ) 34, 513–554.

Heitger, M.H., Jones, R.D., Anderson, T.J., 2008. A new approach to predicting postconcussion syndrome after mild traumatic brain injury based upon eye movement function. Conf. Proc. IEEE Eng. Med. Biol. Soc. 2008, 3570–3573.

Heitger, M.H., Jones, R.D., Macleod, A.D., Snell, D.L., Frampton, C.M., Anderson, T.J., 2009. Impaired eye movements in post-concussion syndrome indicate suboptimal brain function beyond the influence of depression, malingering or intellectual ability. Brain. 132, 2850–2870.

Herdman, S., 2000. Vestibular Rehabilitation, third ed F.A. Davis Company, Philadelphia, PA.

Hilton, G.D., Stoica, B.A., Byrnes, K.R., Faden, A.I., 2008. Roscovitine reduces neuronal loss, glial activation, and neurologic deficits after brain trauma. J. Cereb. Blood Flow Metab. 11, 1845–1859.

Hotting, K., Roder, B., 2013. Beneficial effects of physical exercise on neuroplasticity and cognition. Neurosci. Biobehav. Rev. 9 (Pt B), 2243–2257.

Hou, R., Moss-Morris, R., Peveler, R., Mogg, K., Bradley, B.P., et al., 2012. When a minor head injury results in enduring symptoms: a prospective investigation of risk factors for postconcussional syndrome after mild traumatic brain injury. J. Neurol. Neurosurg. Psychiatry 83, 217–223.

Hu, Q., Manaenko, A., Xu, T., Guo, Z., Tang, J., et al., 2016. Hyperbaric oxygen therapy for traumatic brain injury: bench-to-bedside. Med. Gas Res. 6, 102–110.

Huang, L., Obenaus, A., 2011. Hyperbaric oxygen therapy for traumatic brain injury. Med. Gas Res. 1, 21.

Hur, E.-M., Saijilafu, Zhou, F.-Q., 2012. Growing the growth cone: remodeling the cytoskeleton to promote axon regeneration. Trends Neurosci. 35, 164–174.

Imhoff, S., Fait, P., Carrier-Toutant, F., Boulard, G., 2016. Efficiency of an active rehabilitation intervention in a slow-to-recover paediatric population following mild traumatic brain injury: a pilot study. J. Sports Med. (Hindawi Publ. Corp.) 2016, 5127374.

Jaworski, T., Lechat, B., Demedts, D., Gielis, L., Devijver, H., et al., 2011. Dendritic degeneration, neurovascular defects, and inflammation precede neuronal loss in a mouse model for tau-mediated neurodegeneration. Am. J. Pathol. 179, 2001–2015.

Johnson, V.E., Stewart, W., Smith, D.H., 2013. Axonal pathology in traumatic brain injury. Exp. Neurol. 246, 35–43.

Jordan, B.D., 2013. The clinical spectrum of sport-related traumatic brain injury. Nat. Rev. Neurol. 9, 222–3010.

Kabadi, S.V., Faden, A.I., 2014. Selective CDK inhibitors: promising candidates for future clinical traumatic brain injury trials. Neural Regen. Res. 9, 1578–1580.

Kabadi, S.V., Stoica, B.A., Loane, D.J., Byrnes, K.R., Hanscom, M., et al., 2012a. Cyclin D1 gene ablation confers neuroprotection in traumatic brain injury. J. Neurotrauma 29, 813–827.

Kabadi, S.V., Stoica, B.A., Hanscom, M., Loane, D.J., Kharebava, G., et al., 2012b. CR8, a selective and potent CDK inhibitor, provides neuroprotection in experimental traumatic brain injury. Neurotherapeutics 9, 405–421.

Kabadi, S.V., Stoica, B.A., Loane, D.J., Luo, T., Faden, A.I., 2014. CR8, a novel inhibitor of CDK, limits microglial activation, astrocytosis, neuronal loss, and neurologic dysfunction after experimental traumatic brain injury. J. Cereb. Blood Flow Metab. 34, 502–513.

Kapitein, L.C., Hoogenraad, C.C., 2015. Building the neuronal microtubule cytoskeleton. Neuron 87, 492–506.

Karakaya, T., Fusser, F., Prvulovic, D., Hampel, H., 2012. Treatment options for tauopathies. Curr. Treat. Options Neurol. 14, 126–136.

Klein, P.S., Melton, D.A., 1996. A molecular mechanism for the effect of lithium on development. Proc. Natl. Acad. Sci. USA 93, 8455–8459.

Kondo, A., Shahpasand, K., Mannix, R., Qiu, J., Moncaster, J., et al., 2015. Antibody against early driver of neurodegeneration cis P-tau blocks brain injury and tauopathy. Nature 523, 431–436.

Kongsted, A., Jorgensen, L.V., Bendix, T., Korsholm, L., Leboeuf-Yde, C., 2007. Are smooth pursuit eye movements altered in chronic whiplash-associated disorders? A cross-sectional study. Clin. Rehabil. 2, 1038–1049.

Kozlowski, D.A., James, D.C., Schallert, T., 1996. Use-dependent exaggeration of neuronal injury after unilateral sensorimotor cortex lesions. J. Neurosci. 16, 4776–4786.

Lasagna-Reeves, C.A., Castillo-Carranza, D.L., Sengupta, U., Clos, A.L., Jackson, G.R., et al., 2011a. Tau oligomers impair memory and induce synaptic and mitochondrial dysfunction in wild-type mice. Mol. Neurodegener. 6, 39.

Lasagna-Reeves, C.A., Castillo-Carranza, D.L., Jackson, G.R., Kayed, R., 2011b. Tau oligomers as potential targets for immunotherapy for Alzheimer's disease and tauopathies. Curr. Alzheimer Res. 8, 659–665.

Leddy, J., Hinds, A., Sirica, D., Willer, B., 2016a. The role of controlled exercise in concussion management. PM R. 8 (3 Suppl.), S91–S100.

Leddy, J.J., Baker, J.G., Willer, B., 2016b. Active rehabilitation of concussion and post-concussion syndrome. Phys. Med. Rehabil. Clin. North Am. 27, 437–454.

Lee, T.H., Pastorino, L., Lu, K.P., 2011. Peptidyl-prolyl cis-trans isomerase Pin1 in ageing, cancer and Alzheimer disease. Expert Rev. Mol. Med. 13, e21.

Leeds, P.R., Yu, F., Wang, Z., Chiu, C.T., Zhang, Y., et al., 2014. A new avenue for lithium: intervention in traumatic brain injury. ACS Chem. Neurosci. 5, 422–433.

Leem, Y.H., Lim, H.J., Shim, S.B., Cho, J.Y., Kim, B.S., et al., 2009. Repression of tau hyperphosphorylation by chronic endurance exercise in aged transgenic mouse model of tauopathies. J. Neurosci. Res. 87, 2561–2570.

Len, T., Neary, J., 2011. Cerebrovascular pathophysiology following mild traumatic brain injury. Clin. Physiol. Funct. Imaging 31, 85–93.

Lewis, J., McGowan, E., Rockwood, J., Melrose, H., Nacharaju, P., et al., 2000. Neurofibrillary tangles, amyotrophy and progressive motor disturbance in mice expressing mutant (P301L) tau protein. Nat. Genet. 25, 402–405.

Lewis, M., Ghassemi, P., Hibbeln, J., 2013. Therapeutic use of omega-3 fatty acids in severe head trauma. Am. J. Emerg. Med. 31, 273.e5–e8.

Lewis, M.D., 2016. Concussions, traumatic brain injury, and the innovative use of omega-3s. J. Am. Coll. Nutr. 35, 469–475.

Lewis, M.D., Bailes, J., 2011. Neuroprotection for the warrior: dietary supplementation with omega-3 fatty acids. Mil. Med. 176, 1120–1127.

Lin, C.-M., Tseng, Y.-C., Hsu, H.-L., Chen, C.-J., Chen, D.Y.-T., et al., 2016. Arterial spin labeling perfusion study in the patients with subacute mild traumatic brain injury. PLoS One 11, e149109.

Lin, K.-C., Niu, K.-C., Tsai, K.-J., Kuo, J.-R., Wang, L.-C., et al., 2012. Attenuating inflammation but stimulating both angiogenesis and neurogenesis using hyperbaric oxygen in rats with traumatic brain injury. J. Trauma Acute Care Surg. 72, 650–659.

Lincoln, A.E., Caswell, S.V., Almquist, J.L., Dunn, R.E., Norris, J.B., et al., 2011. Trends in concussion incidence in high school sports: a prospective 11-year study. Am. J. Sports Med. 39, 958–963.

Lu, K.P., Zhou, X.Z., 2007. The prolyl isomerase PIN1: a pivotal new twist in phosphorylation signalling and disease. Nat. Rev. Mol. Cell Biol. 8, 904–916.

Lu, K.P., Kondo, A., Albayram, O., Herbert, M.K., Liu, H., et al., 2016. Potential of the antibody against cis-phosphorylated tau in the early diagnosis, treatment, and prevention of Alzheimer disease and brain injury. JAMA Neurol. 73, 1356–1362.

Luchtman, D.W., Song, C., 2013. Cognitive enhancement by omega-3 fatty acids from child-hood to old age: findings from animal and clinical studies. Neuropharmacology 64, 550–565.

Lucke-Wold, B.P., Turner, R.C., Logsdon, A.F., Bailes, J.E., Huber, J.D., et al., 2014. Linking traumatic brain injury to chronic traumatic encephalopathy: identification of potential mechanisms leading to neurofibrillary tangle development. J. Neurotrauma 31, 1129–1138.

Luo, W.J., Dou, F., Rodina, A., Chip, S., Kim, J., et al., 2007. Roles of heat-shock protein 90 in maintaining and facilitating the neurodegenerative phenotype in tauopathies. Proc. Natl. Acad. Sci. USA 104, 9511–9516.

MacFarlane, M.P., Glenn, T.C., 2015. Neurochemical cascade of concussion. Brain Inj. 29, 139–153.

Maerlender, A., Rieman, W., Lichtenstein, J., Condiracci, C., 2015. Programmed physical exertion in recovery from sports-related concussion: a randomized pilot study. Dev. Neuropsychol. 40, 273–278.

Maruszak, A., Pilarski, A., Murphy, T., Branch, N., Thuret, S., 2014. Hippocampal neurogenesis in Alzheimer's disease: is there a role for dietary modulation? J. Alzheimers Dis. 38, 11–38.

Matsuoka, Y., Gray, A.J., Hirata-Fukae, C., Minami, S.S., Waterhouse, E.G., et al., 2007. Intranasal NAP administration reduces accumulation of amyloid peptide and tau hyperphosphorylation in a transgenic mouse model of Alzheimer's disease at early pathological stage. J. Mol. Neurosci. 31, 165–170.

Matsuoka, Y., Jouroukhin, Y., Gray, A.J., Ma, L., Hirata-Fukae, C., et al., 2008. A neuronal microtubule-interacting agent, NAPVSIPQ, reduces tau pathology and enhances cognitive function in a mouse model of Alzheimer's disease. J. Pharmacol. Exp. Ther. 325, 146–153.

Mayers, L., 2008. Return-to-play criteria after athletic concussion: a need for revision. Arch Neurol. 65, 1158–1161.

McCrory, P., Meeuwisse, W., Johnston, K., Dvorak, J., Aubry, M., Molloy, M., et al., 2009. Consensus statement on Concussion in Sport 3rd International Conference on Concussion in Sport held in Zurich, November 2008. Clin. J. Sport Med. 19, 185–200.

McCrory, P., Meeuwisse, W., Aubry, M., Cantu, B., Dvorak, J., Echemendia, R., et al., 2013a. Consensus statement on Concussion in Sport–the 4th International Conference on Concussion in Sport held in Zurich, November 2012. J. Sci. Med. Sport 16, 178–189.

McCrory, P., Meeuwisse, W.H., Aubry, M., Cantu, B., Dvorák, J., et al., 2013b. Consensus statement on concussion in sport: the 4th International Conference on Concussion in Sport held in Zurich. Br. J. Sports Med. 47, 250–258.

McKee, A.C., Cantu, R.C., Nowinski, C.J., Hedley-Whyte, E.T., Gavett, B.E., et al., 2009. Chronic traumatic encephalopathy in athletes: progressive tauopathy after repetitive head injury. J. Neuropathol. Exp. Neurol. 68, 709–735.

Meehan 3rd, W.P., Bachur, R.G., 2009. Sport-related concussion. Pediatrics 123, 114.

Meier, T., Bellgowan, P., Singh, R., Kuplicki, R., Polanski, D., et al., 2015. Recovery of cerebral blood flow following sports-related concussion. JAMA Neurol. 72, 530–538.

Munoz-Montano, J.R., Moreno, F.J., Avila, J., Diaz-Nido, J., 1997. Lithium inhibits Alzheimer's disease-like tau protein phosphorylation in neurons. FEBS Lett. 411, 183–188.

Necula, M., Breydo, L., Milton, S., Kayed, R., van der Veer, W.E., et al., 2007. Methylene blue inhibits amyloid Abeta oligomerization by promoting fibrillization. Biochemistry 46, 8850–8860.

Nicholls, S.B., DeVos, S.L., Commins, C., Nobuhara, C., Bennett, R.E., et al., 2017. Characterization of TauC3 antibody and demonstration of its potential to block tau propagation. PLoS One 12, e0177914.

Nurk, E., Refsum, H., Drevon, C.A., et al., 2009. Intake of flavonoid-rich wine, tea, and chocolate by elderly men and women is associated with better cognitive test performance. J. Nutr. 139, 120–127.

Omalu, B., 2014. Chronic traumatic encephalopathy. Prog. Neurol. Surg. 28, 38–49.

Omalu, B., Bailes, J., Hamilton, R.L., Kamboh, M.I., Hammers, J., et al., 2011. Emerging histomorphologic phenotypes of chronic traumatic encephalopathy in American athletes. Neurosurgery 69, 173–183.

Omalu, B.I., Bailes, J., Hammers, J.L., Fitzsimmons, R.P., 2010. Chronic traumatic encephalopathy, suicides and parasuicides in professional American athletes: the role of the forensic pathologist. Am. J. Forens. Med. Pathol. 31, 130–132.

Oz, M., Lorke, D.E., Petroianu, G.A., 2009. Methylene blue and Alzheimer's disease. Biochem. Pharmacol. 78, 927–932.

Patterson, K.R., Remmers, C., Fu, Y., Brooker, S., Kanaan, N.M., et al., 2011. Characterization of prefibrillar Tau oligomers in vitro and in Alzheimer disease. J. Biol. Chem. 286, 23063–23076.

Phillips, C., 2017. Physical activity modulates common neuroplasticity substrates in major depressive and bipolar disorder. Neural Plast. 2017, 37.

Pop, V., Badaut, J., 2011. A neurovascular perspective for long-term changes after brain trauma. Transl. Stroke Res. 2, 533–545.

Pu, H., Guo, Y., Zhang, W., Huang, L., Wang, G., et al., 2013. Omega-3 polyunsaturated fatty acid supplementation improves neurologic recovery and attenuates white matter injury after experimental traumatic brain injury. J. Cereb. Blood Flow Metab. 33, 1474–1484.

Qin, Z., Song, S., Xi, G., Silbergleit, R., Keep, R.F., et al., 2007. Preconditioning with hyperbaric oxygen attenuates brain edema after experimental intracerebral hemorrhage. Neurosurg. Focus. 22, E13.

Rabassa, M., Cherubini, A., Zamora-Ros, R., et al., 2015. Low levels of a urinary biomarker of dietary polyphenol are associated with substantial cognitive decline over a 3-year period in older adults: the Invecchiare in Chianti Study. J. Am. Geriatr. Soc. 63, 938−946.

Reed, N., Greenspoon, D., Iverson, G.L., et al., 2015. Management of persistent postconcussion symptoms in youth: a randomised control trial protocol. BMJ Open 5, e008468.

Reis, C., Wang, Y., Akyol, O., Ho, W.M., Ii, R.A., et al., 2015. What's new in traumatic brain injury: update on tracking, monitoring and treatment. Int. J. Mol. Sci. 16, 11903−11965.

Roberts, L., Bailes, J., Dedhia, H., Zikos, A., Singh, A., et al., 2008. Surviving a mine explosion. J. Am. Coll. Surg. 207, 276−283.

Rosse, G., 2012. Novel indolethylbenzamides for the treatment of tauopathies: patent highlight. ACS Med. Chem. Lett. 3, 877−878.

Santa-Maria, I., Varghese, M., Ksiezak-Reding, H., Dzhun, A., Wang, J., et al., 2012. Paired helical filaments from Alzheimer Disease brain induce intracellular accumulation of tau protein in aggresomes. J Biol Chem. 287, 20522−20533.

Schirmer, R.H., Adler, H., Pickhardt, M., Mandelkow, E., 2011. Lest we forget you--methylene blue.... Neurobiol. Aging 32, 2325.e7−16.

Schneider, K.J., Iverson, G.L., Emery, C.A., McCrory, P., Herring, S.A., et al., 2013. The effects of rest and treatment following sport-related concussion: a systematic review of the literature. Br. J. Sports Med. 47, 304−307.

Schroeder, S., Joly-Amado, A., Soliman, A., Sengupta, U., Kayed, R., et al., 2017. Oligomeric tau-targeted immunotherapy in Tg4510 mice. Alzheimers Res. Ther. 9, 46.

Scorza, K.A., Raleigh, M.F., O'Connor, F.G., 2012. Current concepts in concussion: evaluation and management. Am. Fam. Physician 85, 123−132.

Seifert, T., Brassard, P., Wissenberg, M., Rasmussen, P., Nordby, P., et al., 2010. Endurance training enhances BDNF release from the human brain. Am. J. Physiol. Regul. Integr. Comp. Physiol. 298, R372−R377.

Serhan, C.N., 2005. Novel eicosanoid and docosanoid mediators: resolvins, docosatrienes, and neuroprotectins. Curr. Opin. Clin. Nutr. Metab. Care 8, 115−121.

Shapira, M., Licht, A., Milman, A., Pick, C.G., Shohami, E., et al., 2007. Role of glycogen synthase kinase-3beta in early depressive behavior induced by mild traumatic brain injury. Mol. Cell. Neurosci. 34, 571−577.

Sheidow, A.J., McCart, M., Zajac, K., Davis, M., 2012. Prevalence and impact of substance use among emerging adults with serious mental health conditions. Psychiatr. Rehabil. J. 35, 235−243.

Shin, S.S., Dixon, C.E., 2011. Oral fish oil restores striatal dopamine release after traumatic brain injury. Neurosci. Lett. 496, 168−171.

Shrey, D.W., Griesbach, G.S., Giza, C.C., 2011. The pathophysiology of concussions in youth. Phys. Med. Rehabil. Clin. North Am. 22, 577−602.

Smith, D.H., 2016. Neuromechanics and pathophysiology of diffuse axonal injury in concussion. Bridge (Wash DC) 46, 79−84.

Smith, D.H., Wolf, J.A., Lusardi, T.A., Lee, V.M., Meaney, D.F., 1999. High tolerance and delayed elastic response of cultured axons to dynamic stretch injury. J. Neurosci. 19, 4263−4269.

Sontag, E.M., Lotz, G.P., Agrawal, N., Tran, A., Aron, R., et al., 2012. Methylene blue modulates huntingtin aggregation intermediates and is protective in Huntington's disease models. J. Neurosci. 32, 11109−11119.

Steffen, T.M., Boeve, B.F., Mollinger-Riemann, L.A., Petersen, C.M., 2007. Long-term loco-motor training for gait and balance in a patient with mixed progressive supranuclear palsy and corticobasal degeneration. Phys. Ther. 87, 1078—1087.

Steffen, T.M., Boeve, B.F., Petersen, C.M., Dvorak, L., Kantarci, K., 2014. Long-term exercise training for an individual with mixed corticobasal degeneration and pro-gressive supranuclear palsy features: 10-year case report follow-up. Phys. Ther. 94, 289—296.

Stern, R.A., Daneshvar, D.H., Baugh, C.M., Seichepine, D.R., Montenigro, P.H., et al., 2013. Clinical presentation of chronic traumatic encephalopathy. Neurology 81, 1122—1129.

Stoica, B.A., Byrnes, K.R., Faden, A.I., 2009. Cell cycle activation and CNS injury. Neurotox. Res. 16, 221—237.

Stoller, K.P., 2011. Hyperbaric oxygen therapy (1.5 ATA) in treating sports related TBI/CTE: two case reports. Med. Gas Res. 1, 17.

Sun, W., Lee, S., Huang, X., Liu, S., Inayathullah, M., et al., 2016. Attenuation of synaptic toxicity and MARK4/PAR1-mediated Tau phosphorylation by methylene blue for Alzheimer's disease treatment. Sci. Rep. 6, 34784.

Takeda, S., Wegmann, S., Cho, H., DeVos, S.L., Commins, C., et al., 2015. Neuronal uptake and propagation of a rare phosphorylated high-molecular-weight tau derived from Alzheimer's disease brain. Nat. Commun. 6, 8490.

Tan, C.O., Meehan, W.P., Iverson, G.L., Taylor, J.A., 2014. Cerebrovascular regulation, exercise, and mild traumatic brain injury. Neurology 83, 1665—1672.

Tang-Schomer, M.D., Patel, A.R., Baas, P.W., Smith, D.H., 2010. Mechanical breaking of microtubules in axons during dynamic stretch injury underlies delayed elasticity, micro-tubule disassembly, and axon degeneration. FASEB J. 24, 1401—1410.

Tang-Schomer, M.D., Johnson, V.E., Baas, P.W., Stewart, W., Smith, D.H., 2012. Partial interruption of axonal transport due to microtubule breakage accounts for the for-mation of periodic varicosities after traumatic axonal injury. Exp. Neurol. 233, 364—372.

Taniguchi, S., Suzuki, N., Masuda, M., Hisanaga, S., Iwatsubo, T., et al., 2005. Inhibition of heparin-induced tau filament formation by phenothiazines, polyphenols, and porphyr-ins. J. Biol. Chem. 280, 7614—7623.

Taupin, P., 2007. BrdU immunohistochemistry for studying adult neurogenesis: para-digms, pitfalls, limitations, and validation. Brain Res. Rev. 53, 198—214.

Thatcher, R.W., 2009. EEG evaluation of traumatic brain injury and EEG biofeedback treat-ment. In: Budzynski, T.H., Budzynski, H.K., Evans, J.R., Abarbanel, A. (Eds.), Introduction to Quantitative EEG and Neurofeedback: Advanced Theory and Applications, second ed. Elsevier, Inc, Burlington, MA, pp. 269—294.

Thiagarajan, P., Ciuffreda, K.J., 2013. Effect of oculomotor rehabilitation on vergence responsivity in mild traumatic brain injury. J. Rehabil. Res. Dev. 50, 1223—1240.

Thornton, K.E., Carmody, D.P., 2009. Traumatic brain injury rehabilitation: QEEG biofeed-back treatment protocols. Appl. Psychophysiol. Biofeedback 34, 59—68.

Tseng, B.Y., Uh, J., Rossetti, H.C., Cullum, C.M., Diaz-Arrastia, R.F., et al., 2013. Masters athletes exhibit larger regional brain volume and better cognitive performance than sedentary older adults. J. Magn. Reson. Imaging 38, 1169—1176.

Turner, R.C., Lucke-Wold, B.P., Robson, M.J., Omalu, B.I., Petraglia, A.L., et al., 2012. Repetitive traumatic brain injury and development of chronic traumatic encephalopa-thy: a potential role for biomarkers in diagnosis, prognosis, and treatment? Front. Neurol. 3, 186.

Uusijarvi, J., Eriksson, K., Larsson, A.C., Nihlén, C., Schiffer, T., et al., 2015. Effects of hyperbaric oxygen on nitric oxide generation in humans. Nitric Oxide 44, 88—97.

Venkat, P., Chopp, M., Chen, J., 2016. New insights into coupling and uncoupling of cere-bral blood flow and metabolism in the brain. Croat. Med. J. 57, 223—228.

Wang, G.-H., Zhang, X.-G., Jiang, Z.-L., Li, X., Peng, L.-L., et al., 2010. Neuroprotective effects of hyperbaric oxygen treatment on traumatic brain injury in the rat. J. Neurotrauma 27, 1733–1743.

Wang, Y., Nelson, L.D., LaRoche, A.A., Pfaller, A.Y., Nencka, A.S., et al., 2016. Cerebral blood flow alterations in acute sport-related concussion. J. Neurotrauma 33, 1227–1236.

Wilcock, D.M., Colton, C.A., 2008. Anti-amyloid-beta immunotherapy in Alzheimer's disease: relevance of transgenic mouse studies to clinical trials. J. Alzheimers Dis. 15, 555–569.

Wu, A., Molteni, R., Ying, Z., Gomez-Pinilla, F., 2003. A saturated-fat diet aggravates the outcome of traumatic brain injury on hippocampal plasticity and cognitive function by reducing brain-derived neurotrophic factor. Neuroscience 119, 365–375.

Wu, A., Ying, Z., Gomez-Pinilla, F., 2004. Dietary omega-3 fatty acids normalize BDNF levels, reduce oxidative damage, and counteract learning disability after traumatic brain injury in rats. J. Neurotrauma 21, 1457–1467.

Wu, A., Ying, Z., Gomez-Pinilla, F., 2005. Omega-3 fatty acids supplementation restores homeostatic mechanisms disrupted by traumatic brain injury. J. Neurotrauma 22, 1212.

Wu, J., Kharebava, G., Piao, C., Stoica, B.A., Dinizo, M., et al., 2012a. Inhibition of E2F1/CDK1 pathway attenuates neuronal apoptosis in vitro and confers neuroprotection after spinal cord injury in vivo. PLoS One 7, e42129.

Wu, J., Pajoohesh-Ganji, A., Stoica, B.A., Dinizo, M., Guanciale, K., et al., 2012b. Delayed expression of cell cycle proteins contributes to astroglial scar formation and chronic inflammation after rat spinal cord contusion. J. Neuroinflammation 9, 169.

Yengo-Kahn, A.M., Hale, A.T., Zalneraitis, B.H., Zuckerman, S.L., Sills, A.K., et al., 2016. The Sport Concussion Assessment Tool: a systematic review. Neurosurg Focus. 40, E6.

Yoshiyama, Y., Higuchi, M., Zhang, B., Huang, S.M., Iwata, N., et al., 2007. Synapse loss and microglial activation precede tangles in a P301S tauopathy mouse model. Neuron 53, 337–351.

Yu, F., Wang, Z., Tchantchou, F., Chiu, C.T., Zhang, Y., et al., 2012. Lithium ameliorates neurodegeneration, suppresses neuroinflammation, and improves behavioral performance in a mouse model of traumatic brain injury. J. Neurotrauma 29, 362–374.

Zahr, N.M., Kaufman, K.L., Harper, C.G., 2011. Clinical and pathological features of alcohol-related brain damage. Nat. Rev. Neurol. 7, 284–294.

Zemper, E.D., 2003. Two-year prospective study of relative risk of a second cerebral concussion. Am. J. Phys. Med. Rehabil. 82, 653–659.

Zhang, H., Burrows, F., 2004. Targeting multiple signal transduction pathways through inhibition of Hsp90. J. Mol. Med. 82, 488–499.

Zhang, B., Carroll, J., Trojanowski, J.Q., Yao, Y., Iba, M., et al., 2011. The microtubule-stabilizing agent, epothilone D, reduces axonal dysfunction, neurotoxicity, cognitive deficits and Alzheimer-like pathology in an interventional study with aged tau transgenic mice. J. Neurosci. 32, 3601–3611.

Zhang, B., Carroll, J., Trojanowski, J.Q., Yao, Y., Iba, M., et al., 2012. The microtubule-stabilizing agent, epothilone D, reduces axonal dysfunction, neurotoxicity, cognitive deficits and Alzheimer-like pathology in an interventional study with aged tau transgenic mice. J. Neurosci. 32, 3601–3611.

Zhang, K., Johnson, B., Pennell, D., Ray, W., Sebastianelli, W., et al., 2010. Are functional deficits in concussed individuals consistent with white matter structural alterations: combined FMRI & DTI study. Exp. Brain Res. 204, 57–70.

Zhu, Z.F., Wang, Q.G., Han, B.J., William, C.P., 2010. Neuroprotective effect and cognitive outcome of chronic lithium on traumatic brain injury in mice. Brain Res. Bull. 83, 272–277.

10

Summary, Perspective, and Direction for Future Research on Neurotraumatic Diseases

INTRODUCTION

Stroke, spinal cord injury (SCI), and traumatic brain injury (TBI)—mediated brain injuries are a major public health burden, with 7 million people being victims of stroke in the United States. Approximately 17,000 new SCI cases occur each year, and 3.17–5.3 million people suffer from TBI (Faul et al., 2010; Roger et al., 2012; Jullienne and Badaut, 2013). Every year, 795,000 people visit the intensive care unit and are diagnosed with a stroke, representing an average of one victim of stroke every 40 seconds (Roger et al., 2012). Among them, majority (87%) are ischemic strokes and 13% are brain hemorrhages. According to WHO, 500,000 people suffer an SCI each year. People with spinal cord injuries are two to five times more likely to die prematurely, with worse survival rates in low- and middle-income countries. Up to 90% of SCI cases are due to traumatic causes such as road traffic crashes, falls, and violence. An estimated 3.8 million people in the United States sustain a TBI every year, resulting in 60 billion dollars in annual healthcare costs (Langlois et al., 2006; Faul et al., 2010; Faul and Coronado, 2015). A higher number of people (approximately 1.7 million) are admitted to the emergency room for a TBI in the United States. TBI afflicts people of all ages and genders and represents the major cause of disability and death in developed countries, accounting for 30.5% of all injury-related deaths in the United States (Faul et al., 2010). In ischemic stroke, the lesion is a result of an occlusion of a cerebral blood vessel (cerebral artery in most cases) by a clot (thrombus). In most cases, TBI results from a physical blow to the head during traumatic events such as falls, motor vehicle collisions, or contact sports—related injuries (Rutland-Brown et al., 2006; Fu et al., 2016; Jordan, 2013). This type of brain injury can also be inflicted by exposure to explosive blasts (Cernak, Noble-Haeusslein 2010). As stated in Chapter 6, Neurochemical Aspects of Traumatic Brain Injury, TBIs are classified as mild, moderate, or severe, based on clinical observations and history such as duration of loss of consciousness and posttraumatic amnesia. Approximately 80% of TBIs are classified as "mild" head injuries (Harmon et al., 2013; Faul and Coronado, 2015; Malec et al., 2007). However, diagnosis is primarily by exclusion of injuries requiring specific intervention (Carroll et al., 2004). Furthermore, inconsistent clinical definitions between governing organizations present challenges in comparing incidence rates of mild traumatic brain injury (mTBI); (Summers et al., 2009; Faul and Coronado, 2015). This difficulty in diagnosis can be a serious concern due to acute effects such as second impact syndrome (Jordan, 2013) or through chronic effects arising from repetitive mTBI (Stern et al., 2011). In Western countries, Federal and State governments, along with many sports governing bodies, are introducing and implementing rule and policy changes to protect athletes and to standardize medical care. There is an inherent risk in many contact sports (American football, wrestling, rugby, hockey, lacrosse, and soccer) for repetitive TBI that athletes subject themselves to. It may be up to coaches and physicians to protect athletes of their well-being. It is important to understand that athletes are a unique demographic of patients who have many behavioral *heterogeneities* that may be different from the "violent crime, rape, war" patients. Long-term effects of repeated mTBI include chronic motor and neuropsychological deficits (de Beaumont et al., 2007; de Beaumont et al., 2009). It is reported that among 400 collegiate football players, with two or more previous mTBIs, independently predicted long-term deficits of executive function, processing speed, and self-reported symptom severity (Collins et al., 1999). The nature, burden, and duration of the clinical postconcussive symptoms may be more important than the presence or duration of amnesia alone (McCrory et al., 2000). A telephone-based survey study performed by the University of Michigan Institute of Social Research, in association with the National Football League of 1063 retired NFL players, found a 19-fold increase in rate of age and memory-related diseases (Alzheimer's disease and Parkinson's disease) in the 35- to 49-year-old age group and a 5-fold increase in ages older than 50 years when compared to national control groups.

SIMILARITIES AND DIFFERENCES IN ACUTE AND CHRONIC BRAIN DISEASES

Stroke, SCI and severe TBI are considered acute brain disorders, which are accompanied by neurodegeneration that occurs at the injury site or the location of clot in the blood vessel anywhere in the brain. Despite the difference in the origin of the pathology, stroke, SCI, and severe TBI share several similarities regarding their pathophysiology (Farooqui, 2010). Thus, stroke, SCI, and severe TBI are accompanied by overstimulation of glutamate receptor, a massive influx of Ca^{2+}, prolonged decrease in ATP, stimulation of Ca^{2+}-dependent enzyme, induction of mitochondrial dysfunction, increase in oxidative and nitrosative stress, hyperexcitability, and onset of acute neuroinflammation due to the activation of microglia and astrocytes around injury site (Fig. 10.1) (Farooqui, 2010). In addition, stroke, SCI, and severe TBI are also accompanied by induction of apoptotic cell death. These processes result in neurodegeneration and irreversible loss of neurologic function, not only through the breakdown of cellular and subcellular integrity, but also through alterations in redox and free-radical generation (Farooqui, 2010). Severe single-incident of severe TBI, with or without skull fracture, can lead to permanent brain damage, with incomplete recovery and residual sensory, motor, and cognitive deficits leading to increased risk of late onset Alzheimer's disease (AD) (Sivanandam and Thakur, 2012). In contrast, repetitive mTBI results in chronic neurodegeneration as observed in chronic traumatic encephalopathy (CTE), a pathological condition that has a significant τ pathology including phosphorylated τ in neurofibrillary tangles, neurites, and glial deposits (Omalu et al., 2005; McKee et al., 2013). Some cases of CTE also demonstrate diffused $A\beta$ plaques and pathological accumulations of phosphorylated forms of the DNA-binding protein TDP-43 (McKee et al., 2013). Preclinical studies have indicated that sustained microglial activation after repetitive mTBI may play an important role in the chronic neurodegeneration, which may contribute to the loss of neurological function (Farooqui, 2010; Byrnes et al., 2012).

It is well known that microglia play important roles in the brain, including synaptic pruning, CNS repair, and mediating the immune response against peripheral infection (Farooqui, 2017). Microglial cells may also contribute to the removal of cellular debris by phagocytosis and promote the release of neurotrophic factors, which may not only prevent neuronal injury but also restore tissue integrity in the injured brain. Brain contains two types of microglial phenotypes. M1-like microglia are proinflammatory, whereas M2-like microglia are immunosuppressive phenotypes. M1-like microglia promote neurotoxicity via

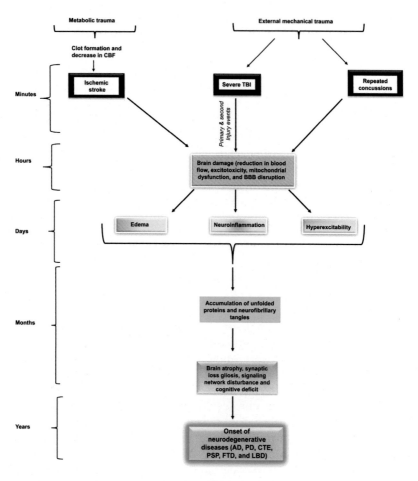

FIGURE 10.1 Neurochemical processes, which are common in stroke, severe TBI, and neurodegenerative diseases. PSP, Progressive supranuclear palsy; FTD, frontotemporal dementia; LBD, Lewy body dementia.

the release of several proinflammatory mediators, such as nitric oxide (NO), interleukin (IL)-1β, and tumor necrosis factor alpha (TNF-α) (Block et al., 2001). Conversely, M2-like microglia produce neuroprotective, neurosupportive, and immunosupportive effects via several mechanisms. For example, neuroprotective roles of M2-like microglia include glutamate uptake (Byrnes et al., 2009), removal of dead cell debris and abnormally accumulated proteins (Diaz-Aparicio et al., 2016), and production of neurotrophic factors such as insulin-like growth factor-1 (Thored et al., 2009), glial cell-derived neurotrophic factor (Lu et al., 2005), and brain-derived neurotrophic factor (Batchelor et al., 1999). Thus, following stroke or severe TBI, microglial cells produce neurotoxic effects in the brain (Loane and Byrnes, 2010; Farooqui, 2010) by releasing inflammatory factors such as proinflammatory eicosanoids, cytokines and chemokines, (TNF-α, IL-6, IL-1β, interferon-γ, and several chemokines) (Boche et al., 2013), reactive oxygen and nitrogen species, and NO as well as antiinflammatory cytokines, and growth factors (TGF-β, CD206, and Arg1) (Farooqui, 2014). Following repetitive mTBI, microglial cells undergo chronic activation producing low levels of above-mentioned mediators, which may cause chronic neurodegeneration. Thus, high levels of reactive oxygen species (ROS), eicosanoids, proinflammatory cytokines, and chemokines promote acute brain injury (stroke and severe TBI), whereas low levels of above metabolites are associated with chronic neurodegenerative disorders such as AD, Parkinson's disease (PD), Huntington's disease (HD), amyotrophic lateral sclerosis (ALS), and CTE (Eikelenboom et al., 2002; Byrnes and Faden, 2007; Farooqui, 2010; Farooqui, 2011).

MOLECULAR MECHANISM OF NEURODEGENERATION IN STROKE, SCI, AND TBI

As stated above, stroke, SCI, and TBI are accompanied by upregulation of interplay among excitotoxicity, oxidative stress, and neuroinflammation resulting in rapid neurodegeneration (in a matter of minutes, hours to days) because of a sudden lack of oxygen, rapid decrease in ATP, disturbance in transmembrane potential, and sudden collapse of ion gradients at very early stage (Fig. 10.1) (Farooqui, 2010). In contrast, in neurodegenerative diseases, oxygen, nutrients, and low levels of ATP continue to be available to neurons and glial cell leading to maintenance of cellular homeostasis to a limited extent. The interplay among excitotoxicity, oxidative stress, and neuroinflammation occurs at a slow rate, leading to a neurodegenerative process that occurs gradually in a specific brain region of the brain and takes many years to develop (Farooqui, 2010). For example, in AD, due to downregulation excitotoxicity, oxidative stress, and neuroinflammation, neurons die in the nucleus basalis, hippocampal region, and entorhinal cortex after 65 years of age. In PD, neurodegeneration occurs in the substantia nigra after midlife. Degeneration of striatal medium spiny neurons is involved in the pathogenesis of HD, and ALS is characterized by damage to motor neurons in the brain and spinal cord at relatively younger age compared to AD and PD (Farooqui, 2010). It is not clear when a neurodegenerative disease actually starts and how long it takes for neuropathological changes to appear. Onset of neurodegeneration in a specific population of neurons in a specific region provides the basis for the selective vulnerability. The underlying mechanisms for selective vulnerability are probably related to specific properties of neurons, including size, axonal length, connections, metabolism, and gene mutations (Farooqui, 2010). This neurodegeneration contributes to tragic neurological and behavioral disabilities ranging from memory loss to paralysis. For example, in AD neurodegeneration in nucleus basalis, hippocampal, and entorhinal cortical regions is responsible for the memory disturbances. Furthermore, neurochemical changes in AD not only involve abnormalities in immune system but also the accumulation of misfolded protein (Aβ and its oligomer) promoting chronic mild oxidative stress and neuroinflammation, which lingers for years, causing continued insult to the brain tissue and ultimately reaching the threshold of detection many years after the onset of the neurodegenerative diseases (Farooqui et al., 2007; Farooqui, 2014). These processes also initiate vicious cycles of aberrant neuronal activity and compensatory alterations in neurotransmitter receptor signaling, leading to loss of synapse, disintegration of neural networks, and, ultimately, failure of neurological functions. In contrast, stroke-mediated injury affects multiple different neuronal population and phenotypes. For example, an infarct might involve the thalamus, hippocampus, and striate visual cortex, affecting three or more very different neuronal populations including neurons, oligodendrocytes, astrocytes, and endothelial cells (Savitz et al., 2003, 2004). The size and position of the affected region depends on which vessel is occluded. Brain is particularly vulnerable to oxidative damage not only due to high oxygen consumption and the presence of polyunsaturated fatty acids in neural membrane phospholipids but also because of high amounts of redox-active transition metals and relatively low activities of antioxidant enzymes (Farooqui, 2010). Despite above differences, induction of oxidative stress, onset of neuroinflammation, changes in levels of lipid mediators, and neuronal cell death by apoptosis are common processes associated with stroke, TBI, and AD.

LINK BETWEEN STROKE AND ALZHEIMER'S DISEASE

It is well known that stroke shares common mechanisms such as disturbed cellular calcium and energy homeostasis and accumulation of toxic metabolites (ROS, NO, cytokines, and chemokines) with AD. Thus, a link between stroke and AD is not only constituted by the upregulation of amyloid precursor protein (APP), a larger Type I transmembrane spanning glycoprotein, which not only plays a pivotal role in the pathogenesis of AD but is also associated with neurochemical changes in regulation of calcium homeostasis in stroke, repetitive mTBI, and severe TBI (Fig. 10.2) (Kocki et al., 2015; Hefter et al., 2016). The full-length APP has cell adhesion and receptor-like properties. Full-length APP consists of four main domains: the extracellular domains E1 (Dahms et al., 2010) and E2; a transmembrane sequence (Dahms et al., 2012); and the APP intracellular domain (AICD) (Radzimanowski et al., 2008; Coburger et al., 2014). APP is cleaved by a large number of proteases, which are grouped into α-, β-, and γ-secretases, depending on the cleavage site. AICD not only regulates its own production via induction of APP and β-secretase (BACE1) gene expression but also modulates levels of Aβ peptide by upregulating neprilysin (NEP) gene expression (Fig. 10.3). In a pathological situation like AD this cycle seems to be disturbed resulting in enhanced Aβ production along with reduced NEP levels leading to the severe accumulation of Aβ in brain tissue. The occurrence of proteases, which cleaves APP outside the cell membrane, has also been reported (Baranger et al., 2016). In addition to precursor for beta-amyloid (Aβ), APP also plays important roles in ion transport,

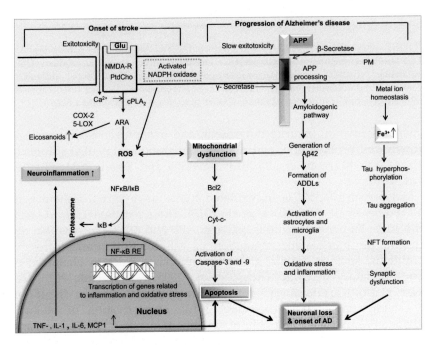

FIGURE 10.2 Molecular mechanisms that are common between stroke and AD. Glu, Glutamate; PtdCho, phosphatidylcholine; cPLA$_2$, cytosolic phospholipase A$_2$; COX-2, cyclooxygenase-2; 5-LOX, 5-lipoxygenase; ARA, arachidonic acid; NF-κB-RE, nuclear factor-κB-response element; I-κB, inhibitory subunit of NF-κB; MCP-1, monocyte chemoattractant protein-1; Bcl-2, B-cell lymphoma 2; cyto-c, cytochrome.

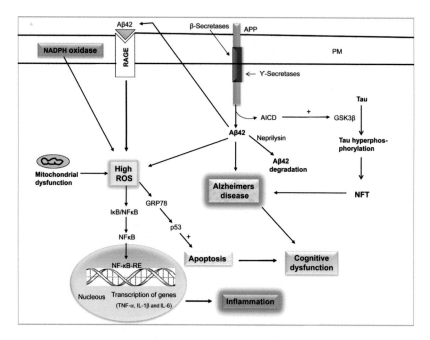

FIGURE 10.3   Effects of APP-derived products (Aβ and AICD) on the pathogenesis od AD. PM, Plasma membrane; RAGE, receptor for advanced glycation end products; GSH, glutathione; NF-κB-RE, nuclear factor-κB-response element; I-κB, inhibitory subunit of NF-κB; NTF, neurofibrillary tangle; GRP78, a major endoplasmic reticulum (ER) chaperone protein; p53, a tumor suppressor protein; GSK3β, glycogen synthase kinase 3 beta.

synapse formation, neurite outgrowth, and synaptogenesis, as well as growth, cell proliferation, and neuronal migration (Fig. 10.4) (Muresan et al., 2009; Muresan et al., 2013; Dawkins and Small, 2014; Hughes et al., 2014).

Metabolism of APP is upregulated following hypoxia, ischemia, or TBI (Pottier et al., 2012; Kocki et al., 2015). These reactions coincide well with some known interactions between APP and other proteins that are relevant for homeostatic regulation of cell integrity under stressful conditions, such as certain glutamate receptors, calcium channels, or gene regulatory networks (Russo et al., 2005; Kocki et al., 2015). Aβ exerts neurotoxic effects via a variety of mechanisms, such as disruption of calcium homeostasis (Berridge, 2010), overactivation of mGluR5 (Zhang et al., 2015), impairment of synaptic transmission, plasticity, and network function (Palop and Mucke, 2010), mitochondrial dysfunction (Chen and Zhong, 2013), and apoptosis (Umeda et al., 2011). Remarkably, it is also able to translocate into the nucleus and influence apoptosis-related gene transcription (Barucker et al., 2014; Multhaup et al., 2015). The accumulation of Aβ is a critical component of AD

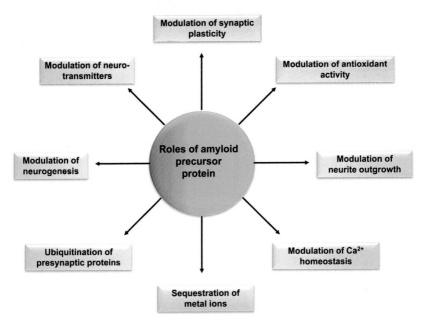

FIGURE 10.4   Role of APP in the brain.

pathogenesis (Farooqui, 2017). Furthermore, hypoxia modulates the expression and activity of Aβ-metabolizing enzymes, resulting in increased Aβ peptides, including the deleterious Aβ(1-42) (Guglielmotto et al., 2009; Pluta et al., 2013). Abnormal Aβ and the change of synaptic plasticity appear simultaneously during the early stage of AD. However, the association between synaptic plasticity and Aβ is complicated. Synaptic activity regulates Aβ levels in AD, which are primarily associated with the regulation of APP endocytosis and cleavage (Farooqui, 2017). The complex interrelations between stroke and AD are also supported by immune exhaustion, induction of mitochondrial dysfunction, disruption of blood–brain barrier (BBB), and activation of microglia and astrocytes. Onset of atherosclerosis, cardiovascular disease, stroke, and AD are made worse by the inflammatory cascade released during immune exhaustion (Brod, 2000). Furthermore, the risk for immune exhaustion is magnified in both stroke and AD with comorbidities such as diabetes, obesity, insulin resistance, and hypertension (Purkayastha and Cai, 2013; Pinti et al., 2014). Additionally, neurochemical changes in the onset of stroke and progression of AD produce damage to pericytes, astrocytes, and endothelial cells (Kelleher and Soiza, 2013) and PKC activity, which regulates tight junction proteins. In both pathological conditions, the integrity of tight junction complexes is compromised (Kook et al., 2013). In addition, biomarkers for onset of stroke and progression of AD (cyclooxygenase-2 and IL-6) interact with PKC through Toll-like receptors (Mesquita et al., 2014; Yang et al., 2014; Mesquita et al., 2014). This pathway is associated not only with decrease in BBB disruption but also with prevention of immune exhaustion. Nowadays, several investigators proposed that the ischemic episodes, which eventually lead to neurodegeneration especially in hippocampus, also accompanied by the accumulation of Aβ, tau protein pathology, and irreversible dementia of Alzheimer type (Pluta et al., 2013). The most persuasive evidence supporting this hypothesis comes from investigations on stroke patients and from experimental ischemic brain studies that mimic Alzheimer type dementia (Ikonomovic et al., 2017). It is reported that brain ischemia dysregulates expression of APP and amyloid-processing enzyme genes, which ultimately compromise brain functions, leading over time to the complex alterations that characterize advanced sporadic AD. The identification of the genes involved in AD induced by ischemia may enable to further define the events leading to sporadic AD-related abnormalities. Collectively, these studies suggest that upregulation of APP, disturbed cellular calcium and energy homeostasis, mitochondrial dysfunction, accumulation of toxic metabolites (ROS, NO, cytokines, and chemokines), disruption of BBB, activation of microglia and astrocytes, and immune exhaustion are common processes associated with the pathogenesis of stroke and AD.

LINK BETWEEN TBI AND ALZHEIMER'S DISEASE

It is reported that about 55.5% of TBI patients may show deteriorated condition, from acute post-TBI cognitive deficits to then meeting diagnostic criteria for AD supporting the view that TBI may be a risk factor for late onset AD (Bogoslovsky et al., 2017). The molecular mechanisms contributing to the link between TBI and AD are still elusive. However, both conditions are accompanied by a decrease in blood flow, cerebral hypoperfusion, ischemia, hypoxia, hemorrhage, BBB disruption edema, alterations in APP metabolism, hyperphosphorylation of tau, disturbed cellular calcium and energy homeostasis, mitochondrial dysfunction, accumulation of toxic metabolites (ROS, NO, cytokines, and chemokines), disruption of BBB, and activation of microglia and astrocytes resulting in neurological dysfunction across a host of physiological and psychological domains. These neurochemical changes are common to the neuropathology of TBI and AD. Studies on the progression of AD in the aftermath of TBI as potential risk factor for developing AD are in progress. The pathology of TBI is complex and dependent on injury severity, age-at-injury, and length of time between injury and neuro-pathological evaluation. In addition, the mechanisms involved in pathology and recovery after TBI and onset and progression of AD may likely involve not only genetic/epigenetic factors but also peripheral factors (age, vascular health, hemorheological abnormalities). Thus, with advanced age and vascular dysfunction, TBI can trigger self-propagating cycles of neuronal injury, pathological protein aggregation, and synaptic loss promoting the onset of AD (Ikonomovic et al., 2017). It is also reported that a single moderate to severe TBI increases the risk of developing late-onset AD, whereas repeat mTBI increases the risk of developing CTE and PD (Washington et al., 2016). Human postmortem studies on both single TBI and repeat mTBI have indicated that the accumulation of Aβ, hyperphosphorylated tau, TDP-43, and Lewy body pathology indicating that the onset of neuropathology of TBI, which is best described as a "polypathology" (Washington et al., 2016). Preclinical studies confirm that multiple proteins associated with the development of neurodegenerative disease accumulate in the brain after TBI. The chronic sequelae of both single TBI and repeat mTBI share common neuropathological features and clinical symptoms of classically defined neurodegenerative disorders (Washington et al., 2016). Clinically, TBI, CTE, and AD are characterized by progressive deficits in cognition (memory, executive dysfunction), behavior (explosivity, aggression), mood (depression, suicidality), and motor function (Parkinsonism), which correlate with the anatomic distribution of brain pathology.

TBI is also a risk factor for dementia (Veitch et al., 2013; Mortimer et al., 1991; Wang et al., 2012), suggesting that in certain vulnerable individuals, TBI may contribute to progressive cognitive decline. The majority of TBI-exposed older adults, however, do not develop dementia (Barnes et al., 2014; Wang et al., 2012). Risk factors for post-TBI cognitive decline remain to be elucidated (Gardner and Yaffes, 2015).

FUTURE STUDIES ON THE TREATMENT OF NEUROTRAUMATIC AND NEURODEGENERATIVE DISEASES

The United States is in the midst of a national crisis. The number of patients with neurotraumatic and neurodegenerative diseases is increasing at a constant rate. As baby boomer generation grows older, enormous impact of neurotraumatic and neurodegenerative diseases will be felt by the American society (Hodes, 2006; Trojanowski, 2008; Trojanowski et al., 2010). In 2005, number of patients with neurotraumatic and neurodegenerative diseases in the world was about

25–30 million, with more than 3 million new cases occurring each year. It is estimated that the number of people affected will double every 20 years, to 80–100 million by 2050; if a cure of neurotraumatic and neurodegenerative diseases is not discovered, our health support system (Medicare and Medicaid) will go bankrupt seriously affecting US economy. Thus, developing strategies for the treatment of neurotraumatic and neurodegenerative diseases and the use of substances that protect and promote a healthy nervous system is extremely important (Hodes, 2006; Trojanowski, 2008). To solve this problem, the National Institute on Aging/National Institutes of Health (NIA/NIH) should establish an extensive national network of neurotraumatic and neurodegenerative research facilities at academic institutions including AD, PD, HD, and ALS Centers, consortium to establish a registry for neurotraumatic and neurodegenerative diseases, neurotraumatic and neurodegenerative disease drug discovery programs, national neurotraumatic and neurodegenerative disease coordinating center, and neurotraumatic and neurodegenerative neuroimaging initiative. These programs may not only contribute to future challenges on neurotraumatic and neurodegenerative diseases but also provide beneficial information on risk factors, biomarker, molecular mechanisms, and treatment of these pathological conditions (Hodes, 2006; Trojanowski, 2008; Trojanowski et al., 2010).

DIRECTION OF FUTURE RESEARCH ON NEUROTRAUMATIC AND NEURODEGENERATIVE DISEASES

Neurotraumatic and neurodegenerative diseases are major public health problems worldwide. The devastating impact of these diseases may not only lead to economic loss worldwide but also cause loss of human potential across the globe, especially in low- and middle-income countries. Although some progress has been made on risk factors, biomarkers, neurochemical alterations, and treatment of stroke, SCI, TBI, AD, and PD in animal models, this information is still in the infancy (Farooqui, 2010), and more studies are required on risk factors, biomarkers, molecular mechanisms, and treatment of these pathological conditions in human patients. Treatment options are lacking for the early neuropathological and neurobehavioral deficits associated with stroke, SCI, TBI, AD, and PD in human subjects. Upregulation of interplay among excitotoxicity, oxidative stress, and neuroinflammation appears to be major mediators of stroke and TBI-mediated neurodegeneration. These processes are being intensively studied in animal models and human translational studies, with the hopes of not only understanding the mechanisms of stroke, SCI, TBI, AD, and PD and developing therapeutic strategies but also improving the outcomes of the millions of people impacted by stroke, SCI, and TBIs each year.

Very little is known about risk factors, biomarkers, molecular mechanisms, and treatment of CTE in patients (Turner et al., 2015; Turner et al., 2016). Thus, studies are needed not only on molecular mechanisms of CTE but also on the treatment and characterization of specific biomarkers, and better animal model of CTE. The first step in creating a preclinical model of CTE is to choose a model that can be used to generate a combination of biochemical and behavioral changes posttrauma consistent with the CTE-like phenotype. Specifically, tauopathy or a precursor of tauopathy (tau hyperphosphorylation), must be present. An ideal animal model of CTE should be able to reproduce all neurochemical and behavioral characteristics of CTE. Behavioral changes must be induced by repetitive mild brain trauma. These changes should persist or worsen at chronic time points postinjury. In animal models of CTE much of the tau accumulation occurs in dilated axons via an Aβ-independent but cjun N-terminal kinase—dependent mechanism. This should be confirmed in human patients with CTE. Levels of lipid mediators, cytokines, and chemokines should be determined in animal models and human patients of CTE using proteomics and lipidomics. In addition, many questions related to CTE development and onset still remain unanswered (Turner et al., 2016). These include the role of impact severity, the time interval between impacts, the age at which impacts occur, and the total number of impacts sustained. Other important variables such as the location of impacts, character of impacts, and effect of environment/lifestyle and genetics also warrant further study. Although, some investigators have developed animal models that show some symptoms of CTE but not all. Thus, it is clear that more studies are required to understand the development of neuropathological and neurobehavioral features in animal models consistent with human CTE. Specifically, acute and chronic injury studies are needed that characterize the development of human tau-based pathology in animal models. Does repetitive TBI cause dendritic spine loss? If so, which regions are vulnerable and what are the temporal dynamics? Does spine loss correlate with behavioral impairments? Finally, does genetic vulnerability play a role in the susceptibility to injury and response to concussive TBI? Large-scale multicenter and double-blind studies involving thousands of thousands of CTE patients are needed to obtain this important information.

Several studies have indicated that TBI is a risk factor for the development of AD, PD, CTE, and other dementias (Bazarian et al., 2009; Fleminger et al., 2003; Guskiewicz et al., 2005; Plassman et al., 2000; Reitz et al., 2011). Plassman and colleagues have reported that both moderate and severe head injuries sustained during early adulthood contribute to increased risk of AD, PD, and other dementia, whereas the relationship between mild head injury and AD is inconclusive (Plassman et al., 2000). A meta-analysis of 75 published studies has indicated that dementia of the AD type is associated with moderate and severe TBI but not with mTBI unless there is a loss of consciousness (Bazarian et al., 2009). Availability of this information may not only facilitate better diagnosis and planning of clinical trials (shorter or longer) but also promote the evaluation of many therapeutic agents with shorter or longer half-lives. The discovery and introduction of inexpensive drugs and innovative interventions, including mobile technologies and e-health applications, which are focused on policy management improvement, are essential for the treatment of neurotraumatic and neurodegenerative diseases.

In addition, mammalian brain has ability to undergo experience-mediated adaptations. This property is reflected in the ability of neural cells to continuously modify the neural circuitry not only to the feelings and behavior but also to interact effectively with their environment and to cope better with neural injuries and neurodegenerative diseases through the stimulation of neural plasticity. Four core factors have been reported to modulate neural plasticity. They include reduced schedules of brain activity, noisy processing, weakened neuromodulatory control, and negative learning. The locus of this plasticity occurs at the level of synapses, the specialized junctions where one neuron receives chemical signals from another (Fleming and England, 2010). Synaptic connections become stronger or weaker in response to specific patterns of activity. This activity modulates changes not only in the release of neurotransmitters at presynaptic neurons but also in the receptors localized on postsynaptic neurons. It is proposed that accumulation of abnormal aggregated proteins in neurotraumatic and neurodegenerative diseases may impair the integrity or function of presynaptic terminals and postsynaptic specializations through interplay among excitotoxicity, neuroinflammation, and oxidative stress (Farooqui and Horrocks, 2007; Palop and Mucke, 2010).

CONCLUSION

Neurotraumatic and neurodegenerative diseases are multifactorial diseases. Because the number of patients with neurotraumatic and neurodegenerative diseases is increasing with a significant rate, the discovery and use of inexpensive drugs and innovative interventions to prevent and lower the risk of these pathological conditions is a crucial matter. Although, some information is available on risk factors (dietary habits, genetics and heredity, age, lifestyle, and exposure to neurotoxins) and treatment for neurotraumatic and neurodegenerative diseases is available in animal models, information on optimal preventive strategies as well as drugs for the treatment of these conditions in humans is still in infancy. The hypothesis that upregulation of interplay among excitotoxicity, oxidative stress, and neuroinflammation may result in rapid neurodegeneration (in a matter of minutes, hours to days) in neurotraumatic disease seems to be plausible. In contrast, in neurodegenerative diseases, the interplay among excitotoxicity, oxidative stress, and neuroinflammation occurs at a slow rate, leading to a neurodegenerative process, which is accompanied by the accumulation of unfolded proteins occurs gradually in a specific brain region of the brain and takes many years to develop. This hypothesis can be the basis of the therapeutic potential of cocktail of antioxidants and antiinflammatory agents that prevent protein misfolding and aggregation. The principal routes of intracellular protein metabolism are the ubiquitin proteasome system and the autophagy–lysosome pathway. These routes collaborate to degrade wasted proteins, and their interplay is involved in coping with the neurological diseases, in which neurochemical pathways (NF-κB and Nrf2) may play a collective role by assisting the protein targeting to the proteasome or autophagy. Although, the molecular mechanisms of different pathologies with regard to the neurodegenerative disease development remain unknown but alterations in gene expression, protein–protein interactions, neuroplasticity, and synaptic dysfunction are closely associated with neurodegenerative process in neurotraumatic and neurodegenerative diseases. Drugs that block oxidative stress, neuroinflammation, and misfolding and facilitate the removal of misfolded protein from neurons may prevent or delay the pathogenesis of above chronic diseases.

References

Barnes, D.E., Kaup, A., Kirby, K.A., Byers, A.L., Diaz-Arrastia, R., et al., 2014. Traumatic brain injury and risk of dementia in older veterans. Neurology 83, 312–319.

Baranger, K., Marchalant, Y., Bonnet, A.E., Crouzin, N., Carrete, A., et al., 2016. MT5-MMP is a new pro-amyloidogenic proteinase that promotes amyloid pathology and cognitive decline in a transgenic mouse model of Alzheimer's disease. Cell. Mol. Life Sci. 73, 217–236.

Barucker, C., Harmeier, A., Weiske, J., Fauler, B., Albring, K.F., et al., 2014. Nuclear translocation uncovers the amyloid peptide Aβ42 as a regulator of gene transcription. J. Biol. Chem. 289, 20182–20191.

Batchelor, P.E., Liberatore, G.T., Wong, J.Y., Porritt, M.J., Frerichs, F., et al., 1999. Activated macrophages and microglia induce dopaminergic sprouting in the injured striatum and express brain-derived neurotrophic factor and glial cell line-derived neurotrophic factor. J. Neurosci. 19, 1708–1716.

Bazarian, J.J., Cernak, I., Noble-Haeusslein, L., Potolicchio, S., Temkin, N., 2009. Longterm neurologic outcomes after traumatic brain injury. J. Head Trauma Rehabil. 24, 439–451.

Berridge, M.J., 2010. Calcium hypothesis of Alzheimer's disease. Pflugers Arch. 459, 441–449.

Block, F., Schmidt, W., Nolden-Koch, M., Schwarz, M., 2001. Rolipram reduces excitotoxic neuronal damage. NeuroReport 12, 1507–1511.

Boche, D., Perry, V.H., Nicoll, J.A., 2013. Review: activation patterns of microglia and their identification in the human brain. Neuropathol. Appl. Neurobiol. 39, 3–18.

Bogoslovsky, T., Wilson, D., Chen, Y., Hanlon, D., Gill, J., et al., 2017. Increases of plasma levels of glial fibrillary acidic protein, tau, and amyloid β up to 90 days after traumatic brain injury. J. Neurotrauma. 34, 66–73.

Brod, S.A., 2000. Unregulated inflammation shortens human functional longevity. Inflamm. Res. 49, 561–570.

Byrnes, K., Faden, A., 2007. Role of cell cycle proteins in CNS injury. Neurochem. Res. 32, 1799–1807.

Byrnes, K.R., Loane, D.J., Faden, A.I., 2009. Metabotropic glutamate receptors as targets for multipotential treatment of neurological disorders. Neurotherapeutics. 6, 94–107.

Byrnes, K.R., Loane, D.J., Stoica, B.A., Zhang, J., Faden, A.I., 2012. Delayed mGluR5 activation limits neuroinflammation and neurodegeneration after traumatic brain injury. J. Neuroinflamm. 9, 43.

Carroll, L., Cassidy, J.D., Peloso, P., Borg, J., Von Holst, H., Holm, L., et al., 2004. Prognosis for mild traumatic brain injury: results of the WHO collaborating Centre task force on mild traumatic brain injury. J. Rehabil. Med. 36, 84–105.

Cernak, I., Noble-Haeusslein, L.J., 2010. Traumatic brain injury: an overview of pathobiology with emphasis on military populations. J. Cereb. Blood Flow Metab. 30, 255–266.

Chen, Z., Zhong, C., 2013. Decoding Alzheimer's disease from perturbed cerebral glucose metabolism: implications for diagnostic and therapeutic strategies. Prog. Neurobiol. 108, 21–43.

Coburger, I., Hoefgen, S., Than, M.E., 2014. The structural biology of the amyloid precursor protein APP—a complex puzzle reveals its multi-domain architecture. Biol. Chem. 395, 485–498.

Collins, M.W., Grindel, S.H., Lovell, M.R., et al., 1999. Relationship between concussion and neuropsychological performance in college football players. J. Am. Med. Assoc. 282, 964–970.

Dahms, S.O., Hoefgen, S., Roeser, D., Schlott, B., Gührs, K.-H., et al., 2010. Structure and biochemical analysis of the heparin-induced E1 dimer of the amyloid precursor protein. Proc. Natl. Acad. Sci. U S A 107, 5381–5386.

Dahms, S.O., Könnig, I., Roeser, D., Gührs, K.-H., Mayer, M.C., et al., 2012. Metal binding dictates conformation and function of the amyloid precursor protein (APP) E2 domain. J. Mol. Biol. 416, 438–452.

Dawkins, E., Small, D.H., 2014. Insights into the physiological function of the β-amyloid precursor protein: beyond Alzheimer's disease. J. Neurochem. 129, 756–769.

de Beaumont, L., Lassonde, M., Leclerc, S., Théoret, H., 2007. Long-term and cumulative effects of sports concussion on motor cortex inhibition. Neurosurgery 61, 329–336.

de Beaumont, L., Thoret, H., Mongeon, D., et al., 2009. Brain function decline in healthy retired athletes who sustained their last sports concussion in early adulthood. Brain 132 (part 3), 695–708.

Diaz-Aparicio, I., Beccari, S., Abiega, O., Sierra, A., 2016. Clearing the corpses: regulatory mechanisms, novel tools, and therapeutic potential of harnessing microglial phagocytosis in the diseased brain. Neural. Regen. Res. 11, 1533–1539.

Eikelenboom, P., Bate, C., van Gool, W.A., Hoozemans, J.J.M., Rozemuller, J.M., et al., 2002. Neuroinflammation in Alzheimer's disease and prion disease. Glia 40, 232–239.

Farooqui, A.A., 2010. Neurochemical Aspects of Neurotraumatic and Neurodegenerative Diseases. Springer, New York.

Farooqui, A.A., 2011. Lipid Mediators and Their Metabolism in the Brain. Springer, New York.

Farooqui, A.A., 2014. Inflammation and Oxidative Stress in Neurological Disorders. Springer, New York.

Farooqui, A.A., 2017. Neurochemical Aspects if Alzheimer's Disease. Academic Press, San Diego, CA.

Farooqui, A.A., Horrocks, L.A., 2007. Glycerophospholipids in Brain. Springer, New York.

Farooqui, A.A., Horrocks, L.A., Farooqui, T., 2007. Modulation of inflammation in brain: a matter of fat. J. Neurochem. 101, 577–599.

Faul, M., Xu, L., Wald, M.M., Coronado, V., Dellinger, A.M., 2010. Traumatic brain injury in the United States: national estimates of prevalence and incidence, 2002-2006. Inj. Prev. 16, A268.

Faul, M., Coronado, V., 2015. Epidemiology of traumatic brain injury. Handb. Clin. Neurol. 127, 3–13.

Fleming, J.J., England, P.M., 2010. AMPA receptors and synaptic plasticity: a chemist's perspective. Nat. Chem. Biol. 6, 89–97.

Fleminger, S., Oliver, D., Lovestone, S., Rabe-Hesketh, S., Giora, A., 2003. Head injury as a risk factor for Alzheimer's disease: the evidence 10 years on: a partial replication. J. Neurol. Neurosurg. Psychiatry 74, 857–862.

Fu, T.S., Jing, R., McFaull, S.R., Cusimano, M.D., 2016. Health & economic burden of traumatic brain injury in the emergency department. Can. J. Neurol. Sci. 43, 238–247.

Gardner, R.C., Yaffe, K., 2015. Epidemiology of mild traumatic brain injury and neurodegenerative disease. Mol. Cell. Neurosci. 66 (Pt B), 75–80.

Guglielmotto, M., Aragno, M., Autelli, R., Giliberto, L., Novo, E., et al., 2009. The upregulation of BACE1 mediated by hypoxia and ischemic injury: role of oxidative stress and HIF1alpha. J. Neurochem. 108, 1045–1056.

Guskiewicz, K.M., Marshall, S.W., Bailes, J., McCrea, M., Cantu, R.C., et al., 2005. Association between recurrent concussion and late-life cognitive impairment in retired professional football players. Neurosurgery 57, 719–726.

Harmon, K.G., Drezner, J.A., Gammons, M., Guskiewicz, K.M., Halstead, M., et al., 2013. American Medical Society for Sports Medicine position statement: concussion in sport. Br. J. Sports Med. 47, 15–26.

Hefter, D., Kaiser, M., Weyer, S.W., Papageorgiou, I.E., Both, M., et al., 2016. Amyloid precursor protein protects neuronal network function after hypoxia via control of voltage-gated calcium channels. J. Neurosci. 36, 8356–8371.

Hodes, R.J., 2006. Public funding for Alzheimer's disease research in United States. Nat. Med. 12, 770–773.

Hughes, T.M., Lopez, O.L., Evans, R.W., Kamboh, M.I., Williamson, J.D., Klunk, W.E., et al., 2014. Markers of cholesterol transport are associated with amyloid deposition in the brain. Neurobiol. Aging 35, 802–807.

Ikonomovic, M.D., Mi, Z., Abrahamson, E.E., 2017. Disordered APP metabolism and neurovasculature in trauma and aging: Combined risks for chronic neurodegenerative disorders. Ageing Res. Rev. 34, 51–63.

Jordan, B.D., 2013. The clinical spectrum of sport-related traumatic brain injury. Nat. Rev. Neurol. 9, 222–230.

Jullienne, A., Badaut, J., 2013. Molecular contributions to neurovascular unit dysfunctions after brain injuries: lessons for target-specific drug development. Future Neurol. 8, 677–689.

Kelleher, R.J., Soiza, R.L., 2013. Evidence of endothelial dysfunction in the development of Alzheimer's disease: is Alzheimer's a vascular disorder? Am. J. Cardiovasc. Dis. 3, 197–226.

Kocki, J., Ułamek-Kozioł, M., Bogucka-Kocka, A., Januszewski, S., Jabłoński, M., et al., 2015. Dysregulation of amyloid-β protein precursor, β-secretase, presenilin 1 and 2 genes in the rat selectively vulnerable CA1 subfield of hippocampus following transient global brain ischemia. J. Alzheimer's Dis. 47, 1047–1056.

Kook, S.Y., Seok Hong, H., Moon, M., Mook-Jung, I., 2013. Disruption of blood-brain barrier in Alzheimer disease pathogenesis. Tissue Barriers 1, e23993.

Langlois, J.A., Rutland-Brown, W., Wald, M.M., 2006. The epidemiology and impact of traumatic brain injury: a brief overview. J. Head Trauma. Rehabil. 21, 375–378.

Loane, D.J., Byrnes, K.R., 2010. Role of microglia in neurotrauma. Neurotherapeutics 7, 366–377.

Lu, Y.Z., Lin, C.H., Cheng, F.C., Hsueh, C.M., 2005. Molecular mechanisms responsible for microglia-derived protection of Sprague-Dawley rat brain cells during in vitro ischemia. Neurosci. Lett. 373, 159–164.

Malec, J.F., Brown, A.W., Leibson, C.L., Flaada, J.T., Mandrekar, J.N., et al., 2007. The Mayo classification system for traumatic brain injury severity. J. Neurotrauma. 24, 1417–1424.

McCrory, P.R., Ariens, M., Berkovic, S.F., 2000. The nature and duration of acute concussive symptoms in Australian football. Clin. J. Sport. Med. 10, 235–238.

McKee, A.C., Stern, R.A., Nowinski, C.J., Stein, T.D., Alvarez, V.E., et al., 2013. The spectrum of disease in chronic traumatic encephalopathy. Brain 136, 43–64.

Mesquita, R.F., Paul, M.A., Valmaseda, A., Francois, A., Jabr, R., et al., 2014. Protein kinase Cepsilon-calcineurin cosignaling downstream of toll-like receptor 4 downregulates fibrosis and induces wound healing gene expression in cardiac myofibroblasts. Mol. Cell. Biol. 34, 574–594.

Mortimer, J.A., van Duijn, C.M., Chandra, V., Fratiglioni, L., Graves, A.B., et al., 1991. Head trauma as a risk factor for Alzheimer's disease: a collaborative re-analysis of case-control studies. EURODEM Risk Factors Research Group. Int. J. Epidemiol 20 (Suppl 2), S28–S35.

Multhaup, G., Huber, O., Buée, L., Galas, M.C., 2015. Amyloid precursor protein (APP) metabolites APP intracellular fragment (AICD), Aβ42 and tau in nuclear roles. J. Biol. Chem. 290, 23515–23522.

Muresan, V., Varvel, N.H., Lamb, B.T., Muresan, Z., 2009. The cleavage products of amyloid-β precursor protein are sorted to distinct carrier vesicles that are independently transported within neurites. J. Neurosci. 29, 3565–3578.

Muresan, V., Villegas, C., Ladescu Muresan, Z., 2013. Functional interaction between amyloid-beta precursor protein and peripherin neurofilaments: a shared pathway leading to Alzheimer's disease and amyotrophic lateral sclerosis. Neurodegener. Dis. 13, 122–125.

Omalu, B.I., DeKosky, S.T., Minster, R.L., Kamboh, M.I., Hamilton, R.L., et al., 2005. Chronic traumatic encephalopathy in a National Football League player. Neurosurgery 57, 128–134.

Palop, J.J., Mucke, L., 2010. Amyloid-β induced neuronal dysfunction in Alzheimer's disease: from synapses toward neural networks. Nat. Neurosci. 13, 812–818.

Pinti, M., Cevenini, E., Nasi, M., De Biasi, S., Salvioli, S., et al., 2014. Circulating mitochondrial DNA increases with age and is a familiar trait: Implications for "inflammaging". Eur. J. Immunol 44, 1552–1562.

Plassman, B.L., Havlik, R.J., Steffens, D.C., Helms, M.J., Newman, T.N., et al., 2000. Documented head injury in early adulthood and risk of Alzheimer's disease and other dementias. Neurology 55, 1158–1166.

Pluta, R., Jabłoński, M., Ułamek-Kozioł, M., Kocki, J., Brzozowska, J., et al., 2013. Sporadic Alzheimer's disease begins as episodes of brain ischemia and is chemically dysregulated Alzheimer's disease genes. Mol. Neurobiol. 48, 500–515.

Pottier, C., Wallon, D., Lecrux, A.R., Maltete, D., Bombois, S., et al., 2012. Amyloid-β protein precursor gene expression in Alzheimer's disease and other conditions. J. Alzheimers. Dis. 28, 561–566.

Purkayastha, S., Cai, D., 2013. Neuroinflammatory basis of metabolic syndrome. Mol. Metab. 2, 356–363.

Radzimanowski, J., Simon, B., Sattler, M., Beyreuther, K., Sinning, I., et al., 2008. Structure of the intracellular domain of the amyloid precursor protein in complex with Fe65-PTB2. EMBO Rep. 9, 1134–1140.

Reitz, C., Brayne, C., Mayeux, R., 2011. Epidemiology of Alzheimer disease. Nat. Rev. Neurol. 7, 137–152.

Roger, V.L., Go, A.S., Lloyd-Jones, D.M., et al., 2012. Heart disease and stroke statistics—2012 update: a report from the American Heart Association. Circulation 125, e2–e220.

Russo, C., Venezia, V., Repetto, E., Nizzari, M., Violani, E., et al., 2005. The amyloid precursor protein and its network of interacting proteins: physiological and pathological implications. Brain Res. Rev. 2005 (48), 257–264.

Rutland-Brown, W., Langlois, J.A., Thomas, K.E., Xi, Y.L., et al., 2006. Incidence of traumatic brain injury in the United States, 2003. J. Head Trauma. Rehabil. 21, 544.

Savitz, S.I., Malhotra, S., Gupta, G., Rosenbaum, D.M., 2003. Cell transplants offer promise for stroke recovery. J. Cardiovasc. Nurs. 18, 57–61.

Savitz, S.I., Dinsmore, J.H., Wechsler, L.R., Rosenbaum, D.M., Caplan, L.R., 2004. Cell therapy for stroke. NeuroRx 1, 406–414.

Sivanandam, T.M., Thakur, M.K., 2012. Traumatic brain injury: a risk factor for Alzheimer's disease. Neurosci. Biobehav. Rev. 36, 1376–1381.

Stern, R.A., Riley, D.O., Daneshvar, D.H., Nowinski, C.J., Cantu, R.C., et al., 2011. Long-term consequences of repetitive brain trauma: chronic traumatic encephalopathy. PM&R 3, S460–S467.

Summers, C.R., Ivins, B., Schwab, K.A., 2009. Traumatic brain injury in the United States: an epidemiologic overview. Mt. Sinai J. Med. J. Transl. Pers. Med. 76, 105–110.

Thored, P., Heldmann, U., Gomes-Leal, W., Gisler, R., Darsalia, V., et al., 2009. Long-term accumulation of microglia with proneurogenic phenotype concomitant with persistent neurogenesis in adult subventricular zone after stroke. Glia 57, 835–849.

Trojanowski, J.Q., 2008. PENN neurodegenerative disease research-in the spirit of Benjamin Franklin. Neurosignals 16, 5–10.

Trojanowski, J.Q., Arnold, S.E., Karlawish, J.H., Brunden, K., Cary, M., et al., 2010. Design of comprehensive Alzheimer disease centers to address unmet national needs. Alzheimer's Dement. 6, 150–155.

Turner, R.C., Lucke-Wold, B.P., Logsdon, A.F., Robson, M.J., Lee, J.M., et al., 2015. Modeling chronic traumatic encephalopathy: the way forward for future discovery. Front. Neurol. 6, 223.

Turner, R.C., Lucke-Wold, B.P., Robson, M.J., Lee, J.M., Bailes, J.E., 2016. Alzheimer's disease and chronic traumatic encephalopathy: distinct but possibly overlapping disease entities. Brain Inj. 30, 1279–1292.

Umeda, T., Tomiyama, T., Sakama, N., Tanaka, S., Lambert, M.P., et al., 2011. Intraneuronal amyloid ß oligomers cause cell death via endoplasmic reticulum stress, endosomal/lysosomal leakage and mitochondrial dysfunction in vivo. J. Neurosci. Res. 89, 1031–1042.

Veitch, D.P., Friedl, K.E., Weiner, M.W., 2013. Military risk factors for cognitive decline, dementia and Alzheimer's disease. Curr. Alzheimer Res. 10, 907–930.

Wang, H.K., Lin, S.H., Sung, P.S., Wu, M.H., Hung, K.W., Wang, L.C., et al., 2012. Population based study on patients with traumatic brain injury suggests increased risk of dementia. J. Neurol. Neurosurg. Psychiatry 83, 1080–1085.

Washington, P.M., Villapol, S., Burns, M.P., 2016. Polypathology and dementia after brain trauma: does brain injury trigger distinct neurodegenerative diseases, or should they be classified together as traumatic encephalopathy? Exp. Neurol. 275 (Pt 3), 381–388.

Yang, X.S., Liu, M.Y., Zhang, H.M., Xue, B.Z., Shi, H., et al., 2014. Protein kinase C-delta mediates sepsis-induced activation of complement 5a and urokinase-type plasminogen activator signaling in macrophages. Inflamm. Res. 63, 581–589.

Zhang, H., Wu, L., Pchitskaya, E., Zakharova, O., Saito, T., et al., 2015. Neuronal store-operated calcium entry and mushroom spine loss in amyloid precursor protein knock-in mouse model of Alzheimer's disease. J. Neurosci. 2015 (35), 13275–13286.

Index

Note: Page numbers followed by "*f*" and "*t*" refer to figures and tables, respectively.

Mesenchymal stem cells. *See* Mesenchymal stromal cells (MSCs)
Mesenchymal stromal cells (MSCs), 125–128, 314–315
Messenger RNA (mRNA), 113–116, 313
Metabolic syndrome, 392–393
Metalloproteases, 42–45
3-Methyl-1-phenyl-2-pyrazolin-5-one. *See* Edaravone
1-Methyl-4-phenyl-1,2,3,6-tetrahydropyridine, 24–25
Methyl-CpG-binding-domain (MBD), 48–49
Methylene blue (MB), 398
and tauopathies, 398
Methylprednisolone (MP), 204f, 205–209
harmful effects, 208f
hypothetical diagram showing beneficial effects, 207f
Methylprednisolone sodium succinate (MPSS), 203–205, 207–209
Mevastatin, 299f
MHC. *See* Major histocompatibility complex (MHC)
Microarray studies, 181–182
Microglia(l), 47–48, 184–185, 421–423
activation, 303–304
cells, 421–423
OX-42 expression, 213–214
Micronutrient density, 29
MicroRNAs (miRNAs), 8–10, 120–121, 181–182, 313
brain-specific, 120–121
and traumatic brain injury, 313–314
Microstructural injury, 335–339
Microtubule affinity-regulating kinase (MARK4), 398
Microtubule-associated protein 2 (MAP2), 13–14, 349
Microtubules (MTs), 381–382, 394–396
dynamics, 394–396
Middle cerebral artery occlusion (MCAO), 10–12, 48–49, 105
Mild cognitive impairment (MCI), 383–384
Mild hyperhomocysteinemia, 5–7
Mild traumatic brain injuries (mTBIs), 335–339
symptoms, 287–288
Mild traumatic injuries, 335–339
Minocycline, 198–199, 213–214, 213f, 300f
and stroke therapy, 116–117, 117f
and traumatic brain injury, 302–304

MIP-1α. *See* Macrophage inflammatory proteins-1α (MIP-1α)
miR-155 inhibition, 120–121
miRNAs. *See* MicroRNAs (miRNAs)
Miserable minority, 239–241
Mitochondria(l), 47–48
depolarization, 47–48
dysfunction, 42–45, 382–383
matrix, 47–48
membrane potential, 47–48
Mitochondrial DNA (mtDNA), 62–63
Mitochondrial nitric oxide synthases (mtNOS), 165–166
Mitogen-activated protein kinases (MAPKs), 42–45, 213–214, 259, 302–303, 363, 366
MK 801 drug, 100–102
MKP-1. *See* MAPK phosphatase-1 (MKP-1)
MMPs. *See* Matrix metalloproteinases (MMPs)
Mn-SOD. *See* Manganese-superoxide dismutase (Mn-SOD)
MNCs. *See* Mononuclear cells (MNCs)
MND. *See* Motor neuron disease (MND)
Moderate TBI, 245–247
diagnosis, 239–241
Modifiable risk factors, 5–7
Molecular
chaperone, 396–397
mechanism, 316–317, 361–363, 365, 383–384
Monoaminergic, 368
Monoclonal Abs, 351–352
Monocyte chemoattractant protein-1 (MCP-1), 66–68, 174–176, 342
Mononuclear cells (MNCs), 125–128
Monosialoganglioside (GM1), 205
ganglioside, 105–106, 204f, 209
Mood dysfunction, 352–353
Motor neuron disease (MND), 364–365
Mouse double minute 2 (MDM2), 125–128
MP. *See* Methylprednisolone (MP)
MPSS. *See* Methylprednisolone sodium succinate (MPSS)
MPT. *See* Membrane permeability transition (MPT)
MRI. *See* Magnetic resonance imaging (MRI)
mRNA. *See* Messenger RNA (mRNA)
MSCs. *See* Mesenchymal stromal cells (MSCs)
mTBIs. *See* Mild traumatic brain injuries (mTBIs)